Master Techniques
in General Surgery

COLON AND RECTAL SURGERY: ABDOMINAL OPERATIONS

Master Techniques in General Surgery

Also available in this series:

Master Techniques in Breast Surgery

December 2010
Kirby I. Bland, MD
V. Suzanne Klimberg, MD

Master Techniques in Colon and Rectal Surgery: Anorectal Operations

November 2011
Steven D. Wexner, MD
James W. Fleshman, MD

Coming Soon

Master Techniques in Hernia Surgery

September 2012
Daniel Jones, MD

Master Techniques in Stomach Surgery

September 2012
Michael S. Nussbaum, MD
Jeffrey H. Peters, MD

Master Techniques in Hepatobiliary and Pancreatic Surgery

December 2012
Keith Lillemoe, MD
William Jarnagin, MD

Master Techniques in Esophageal Surgery

March 2013
James Luketich

Master Techniques in General Surgery

COLON AND RECTAL SURGERY: ABDOMINAL OPERATIONS

Edited by

Steven D. Wexner, MD, FACS, FRCS, FRCS(Ed)
Chairman, Department of Colorectal Surgery
Chief Academic Officer and Emeritus Chief of Staff
Cleveland Clinic Florida
Weston, Florida

Professor and Associate Dean for Academic Affairs
Florida Atlantic University
Boca Raton, Florida

Professor and Assistant Dean for Clinical Education
Florida International University College of Medicine
Miami, Florida

Professor of Surgery, Ohio State University
Columbus, Ohio

Affiliate Professor
Department of Surgery, Division of General Surgery
University of South Florida College of Medicine
Tampa, Florida

Affiliate Professor of Surgery
University of Miami, Miller School of Medicine
Miami, Florida

James W. Fleshman, MD
Professor of Surgery at Washington University in
   St. Louis
Chief of Colon and Rectal Surgery
Chief of Surgery
Barnes Jewish West County Hospital
St. Louis, Missouri

Series Editor

Josef E. Fischer, MD
William V. McDermott Professor of Surgery
Harvard Medical School
Chairman of Surgery, Emeritus
Beth Israel Deaconess Hospital
Boston, Massachusetts

Chairman of Surgery
Christian R. Holmes Professor of Surgery Emeritus
University of Cincinnati College of Medicine
Cincinnati, Ohio

Illustrations by: BodyScientific International, LLC.

 Wolters Kluwer | Lippincott Williams & Wilkins
Health
Philadelphia • Baltimore • New York • London
Buenos Aires • Hong Kong • Sydney • Tokyo

Acquisitions Editor: Brian Brown
Product Manager: Brendan Huffman
Production Manager: Bridgett Dougherty
Senior Manufacturing Manager: Benjamin Rivera
Marketing Manager: Lisa Lawrence
Design Coordinator: Doug Smock
Production Service: Aptara, Inc.

© 2012 by LIPPINCOTT WILLIAMS & WILKINS, a WOLTERS KLUWER business
Two Commerce Square
2001 Market Street
Philadelphia, PA 19103 USA
LWW.com

Printed in China

Library of Congress Cataloging-in-Publication Data

Colon and rectal surgery : abdominal operations / edited by Steven D. Wexner, James W. Fleshman, Josef E. Fischer.
      p. ; cm. – (Master techniques in general surgery)
   Includes bibliographical references and index.
   ISBN 978-1-60547-643-8 (hardback : alk. paper)
   I. Wexner, Steven D. II. Fleshman, James. III. Fischer, Josef E., 1937- IV. Series: Master techniques in general surgery.
   [DNLM: 1. Colon–surgery. 2. Rectum–surgery. 3. Abdomen–surgery. 4. Digestive System Surgical Procedures–methods. WI 650]
   617.5'547–dc23

                                   2011039286

Since books are tools by which teaching occurs, I dedicate this book to my loving sons, Wesley and Trevor who certainly taught me at least as many things as I have taught them. This book is also dedicated to that very special person who taught me the true meaning of life.

Steven D. Wexner

Herand Abcarian, MD, FACS
Chairman, Division of Colon and Rectal Surgery
John H. Stroger Hospital of Cook County
Professor of Surgery
University of Illinois at Chicago
Chicago, Illinois

Christine M. Bartus, MD, FACS, FACRS
Associate Professor of Surgery
University of Connecticut
Farmington, Connecticut

Badma Bashankaev, MD
Staff Surgeon, Department of Colorectal Surgery
National Research Center of Surgery of Russian Academy of
    Medical Sciences
Moscow, Russia

David E. Beck, MD
Chairman, Department of Colon and Rectal Surgery
Ochsner Clinic Foundation
New Orleans, Louisiana

Edward Borrazzo, MD
Attending Surgeon
Department of Surgery
Fletcher Allen Health Care
Associate Professor of Surgery
University of Vermont College of Medicine
Burlington, Vermont

Marylise Boutrose, MD, FRCS
Colorectal Fellow
Colorectal Surgery
Cleveland Clinic Florida
Weston, Florida

Susan M. Cera, MD, FACS, FASCRS
Physicians Regional Medical Group
Colorectal Surgeon, Division of Colorectal Surgery
Chief, Robotic Surgery
Chief of Endoscopy
Chief of Pharmacy and Therapeutics
Director, Anorectal Physiology Lab
Physicians Regional Medical Center
Naples, Florida
Clinical Professor
Department of Colorectal Surgery
Cleveland Clinic
Weston, Florida

Christopher L.H. Chan, BSc (Hons), PhD, FRCS (Gen Surg)
Senior Lecturer/Honorary Consultant Colorectal Surgeon
Academic Surgical Unit, Barts and The London NHS Trust
Institute Cellular & Molecular Science
Queen Mary's School of Medicine and Dentistry
University of London
Edinburgh, United Kingdom

Hester Yui Shan Cheung, FRACS
Department of Surgery
Pamela Youde Nethersole Eastern Hospital
Chai Wan, Hong Kong
China

Chi Chiu Chung, FRCSEd
Department of Surgery
Pamela Youde Nethersole Eastern Hospital
Chai Wan, Hong Kong
China

Robert R. Cima, MD, MA
Mayo Clinic, Rochester
Department of Surgery
Division of Colon and Rectal Surgery
Mayo Clinic
Consultant, Division of Colon and Rectal Surgery
Associate Professor of Surgery
Mayo Clinic College of Medicine
Rochester, Minnesota

Jeffrey L. Cohen, MD, FACS, FACRS
President of Connecticut Surgical Group
Clinical Professor of Surgery
University of Connecticut
Farmington, Connecticut

Conor P. Delaney, MD, PhD
Jeffrey L. Ponsky, MD, Professor of Surgical Education
Chief, Division of Colorectal Surgery
Director, Institute of Colorectal Surgery
Director, Institute of Surgical Innovation
University Hospitals Case Medical Center
Cleveland, Ohio

Ashwin deSouza, MD, MRCSEd, DNB, FCPS, MNAMS
Fellow, Laparoscopic and Minimally Invasive Colon and
    Rectal Surgery
University of Illinois Medical Center
Chicago, Illinois

David W. Dietz, MD
Vice-Chairman
Department of Colorectal Surgery
Digestive Disease Institute
Cleveland Clinic
Cleveland, Ohio

Eric J. Dozois, MD
Program Director, Colon and Rectal Surgery
Professor of Surgery
Mayo Clinic
Rochester, MN

David B. Earle, MD, FACS
Director of Minimally Invasive Surgery
Baystate Medical Center
Assistant Professor of Surgery
Tufts University School of Medicine
Springfield, Massachusetts

Jonathan Edward Efron, MD
Associate Professor of Surgery
Chief of Ravitch Service
The Mark M. Ravitch, M.D. Endowed Professorship in
    Gastrointestinal Surgery
The Johns Hopkins Hospital
Baltimore, MD

C. Neal Ellis, MD, FACS, FASCRS, FACG
Professor of Surgery
Temple University
System Director, Division of Colon and Rectal Surgery
West Penn Allegheny Health System
Pittsburgh, PA

**Victor W. Fazio, AO, MB, MS, MD (Hon), FRACS, FRACS (Hon),
FACS, FRCS, FRCS (Ed), FRCSI**
Rupert B. Turnbull Jr, MD, Chair
Chairman Digestive Diseases Institute
Cleveland Clinic Foundation
Cleveland, Ohio

Alessandro Fichera, MD, FACS, FASCRS
Associate Professor
Program Director, Colon and Rectal Surgery Training
    Program
Department of Surgery
University of Chicago Medical Center
Chicago, Illinois

James W. Fleshman, MD
Professor of Surgery at Washington University in St. Louis
Chief of Colon and Rectal Surgery
Chief of Surgery
Barnes Jewish West County Hospital
St. Louis, Missouri

Morris E. Franklin Jr, MD, FACS
Texas Endosurgery Institute
San Antonio, Texas

Jared C. Frattini, MD
Assistant Professor of Surgery
Department of Colon and Rectal Surgery
University of South Florida
Tampa, Florida

Joseph L. Frenkel, MD
Division of Colorectal Surgery
Lankenau Medical Center and Institute for Medical
    Research
Wynnewood, Pennsylvania

Makram Gedeon, MD
General Surgeon
Bristol Hospital
Bristol, CT

Hak Su Goh, BSc (Hons), MBBS (Lond), FRCS, FAMS
Consultant Surgeon
Goh Hak Su Colon and Rectal Center
Singapore

Sarah W. Grahn, MD
Clinical Instructor
Department of Surgery, Division of Colon and Rectal
    Surgery
University of California
San Francisco, California

Abdullah Al Haddad, MD
Assistant Professor of Clinical Surgery
University of Miami, Miller School of Medicine
Miami, Florida

Jason F. Hall, MD
Staff Surgeon
Department of Colon and Rectal Surgery
Lahey Clinic
Burlington, Massachusetts
Assistant Professor of Surgery
Department of Surgery
Tufts University School of Medicine
Boston, Massachusetts

Terry C. Hicks, MD
Vice Chair
Department of Colon Rectal Surgery
Ochsner Clinic Foundation
New Orleans, Louisiana

Farah A. Husain, MD
Clinical Instructor at Emory University in Atlanta
Minimally-Invasive Surgery and Endosurgery
Emory University
Atlanta, GA

Neil Hyman, MD
Chief, Division of General Surgery
Fletcher Allen Health Care
Samuel B. and Michelle D. Labow Professor of Surgery
University of Vermont College of Medicine
Burlington, Vermont

Myles R. Joyce, MB, Bch, BAO, MD, MMedSci, FRSCI
Colorectal Surgeon
Digestive Disease Institute
Cleveland Clinic Foundation
Cleveland, Ohio

Hasan T. Kirat, MD
Department of Colorectal Surgery
Cleveland Clinic Foundation
Cleveland, Ohio

Ira J. Kodner, MD, FACS
Solon & Bettie Gershman Professor, Surgery
Division of General Surgery
Section of Colon and Rectal Surgery
Director, Center for Colorectal and Pelvic Floor Disorders
    (COPE)
Washington University School of Medicine
St. Louis, MO

Dean C-S Koh, MBBS, FRCSE, FRCSG, FAMS
Consultant Surgeon
Division of Colorectal Surgery
University Surgical Cluster
National University Hospital
Singapore

Jorge A. Lagares-Garcia, MD, FACS, FASCRS
Program Director, Colorectal Surgery Residency Program
Clinical Assistant Professor of Surgery
Warren Alpert Brown University School of Medicine
Clinical Instructor of Surgery
Boston University
R.I. Colorectal Clinic, LLC
Pawtucket, Rhode Island

Ron G. Landmann, MD
Assistant Professor of Surgery
Mayo School of Graduate Medical Education
Senior Associate Consultant, Colon & Rectal Surgery
Mayo Clinic
Jacksonville, Florida

Sang W. Lee, MD
Associate Professor of Clinical Surgery
Division of Colorectal Surgery
New York Presbyterian Hospital
Weill-Cornell Medical College
New York, New York

Michael Ka Wah Li, FRCS (Eng), FRCSEd
Department of Surgery
Pamela Youde Nethersole Eastern Hospital
Chai Wan, Hong Kong
China

Edward Lin, DO, FACS
Associate Professor of Surgery
Director, Emory Endosurgery Unit
Emory University School of Medicine
Atlanta, GA

Martin Luchtefeld, MD
Ferguson Clinic-Michigan Medical PC
Spectrum Health
Grand Rapids, Michigan

Helen M. Macrae, MD
Associate Professor
Mount Sinai Hospital
Department of Surgery
University of Toronto
Toronto, Ontario
Canada

Robert D. Madoff, MD, FACS
Professor of Surgery
Chief, Division of Colon and Rectal Surgery
University of Minnesota
Minneapolis, Minnesota

Peter W. Marcello, MD, FACS, FASCRS
Vice Chairman, Department of Colon & Rectal Surgery
Lahey Clinic
Burlington, Massachusetts

Jorge E. Marcet, MD, FACS, FACRS
Professor of Surgery
Department of Colon and Rectal Surgery
University of South Florida
Tampa, Florida

Floriano Marchetti, MD
Associate Professor of Clinical Surgery
Division of Colon and Rectal Surgery
Director, Colon and Rectal Surgery Residency Program
DeWitt Daughtry Family Department of Surgery
Miller School of Medicine–University of Miami
Miami, Florida

Slawomir Marecik, MD
Clinical Assistant Professor of Surgery
University of Illinois Medical School at Chicago
Chicago, Illinois
Attending Surgeon
Section Head, Robotic Colon and Rectal Surgery
Advocate Lutheran General Hospital
Park Ridge, Illinois

David A. Margolin, MD, FACS, FASCRS
Director of Colon and Rectal Research
Department of Colon and Rectal Surgery
Ochsner Clinical Foundation
New Orleans, Louisiana

John H. Marks, MD
Medical Director, Lankenau Hospital Colorectal Center
Chief of Colorectal Surgery, Main Line Health Systems
Director of Minimally Invasive Colorectal Surgery and
    Rectal Cancer Management Fellowship
Lankenau Medical Center
Professor, Lankenau Institute of Medical Research
Marks Colorectal Surgical Associates
Lankenau Medical Center and Institute for Medical
    Research
Wynnewood, Pennsylvania

Brent D. Matthews, MD
Chief, Section of Minimally Invasive Surgery
Professor of Surgery
Washington University School of Medicine
Barnes-Jewish Hospital
St. Louis, Missouri

Timothy Mayfield, MD
Department of Surgery
SurgixTM Minimally Invasive Surgery Institute
Shawnee Mission Medical Center
Shawnee Mission, Kansas

Genevieve B. Melton-Meaux, MD, MA
Assistant Professor of Surgery
Division of Colon and Rectal Surgery
University of Minnesota
Minneapolis, Minnesota

Fabrizio Michelassi, MD
Lewis Atterbury Stimson Professor and Chairman
Department of Surgery
Weill Cornell Medical College
Surgeon-in-Chief
New York Presbyterian Hospital—Weill Cornell Medical
    Center
New York, New York

John Migaly, MD
Assistant Professor of Surgery
Section of Colon and Rectal Surgery
Division of General Surgery
Duke University Medical Center
Durham, North Carolina

Jeffrey W. Milsom, MD
Jerome J. DeCosse, MD, Professor of Surgery
Division of Colon & Rectal Surgery
New York Presbyterian Hospital
Weill-Cornell Medical College
New York, New York

Neil Mortensen, MD
Department of Colorectal Surgery
Oxford Radcliffe Hospitals
Oxford, United Kingdom

Roberta L. Muldoon, MD, FACS
Assistant Professor of Surgery
Department of Surgery
Vanderbilt University
Nashville, Tennessee

Matthew G. Mutch, MD
Associate Professor of Surgery
Department of Surgery, Section of Colon and Rectal Surgery
Washington University School of Medicine
St. Louis, Missouri

Martin I. Newman, MD, FACS
Associate Program Director
Director of Education
Department of Plastic Surgery
Cleveland Clinic Florida
Weston, Florida

R. John Nicholls, MD, FRCS
Professor of Colorectal Surgery
Imperial College of London
Department of Biosurgery and Surgical Technology
St. Mary's Campus
London, United Kingdom

Juan J. Nogueras, MD, FACS, FASCRS
Affiliate Professor of Clinical Biomedical Sciences
Charles Schmidt College of Medicine
Florida Atlantic University
Clinical Professor of Surgery
Herbert Wertheim College of Medicine
Florida International University
Chief of Staff
Cleveland Clinic Florida
Weston, Florida

Philip B. Paty, MD
Vice Chair, Department of Surgery
Member, Colorectal Service
Memorial Sloane-Kettering Cancer Center
New York, New York

William J. Peche, MD
Assistant Professor of Colon and Rectal Surgery
University of Utah
Department of Surgery
Salt Lake City, Utah

Joseph B. Petelin, MD, FACS
Clinical Associate Professor
Department of Surgery
University of Kansas School of Medicine
Kansas City, Kansas
Director, SurgixTM Minimally Invasive Surgery Institute
    and Fellowship
Shawnee Mission, Kansas

Guillermo Portillo, MD
Texas Endosurgery Institute
San Antonio, Texas

Leela M. Prasad, MD, MS (Surg), FRCS(E), FRCS(C), FACS, FASCRS
Turi Josefson Professor
Chief, Division of Colon & Rectal Surgery/Minimally
    Invasive and Robotic Colon & Rectal Surgery
Vice Chairman & Professor of Clinical Surgery
Department of Surgery
University of Illinois Medical School at Chicago
Chicago, Illinois
Director, Center for Robotic Surgery
Vice Chairman, Department of Surgery
Advocate Lutheran General Hospital
Park Ridge, Illinois

Sonia L. Ramamoorthy, MD
Assistant Professor of Surgery, Colon and Rectal Surgery
Division of Surgical Oncology
UC San Diego Medical Center
The John and Rebecca Moores' Cancer Center
La Jolla, California

Arthur L. Rawlings, MD, MDiv
Clinical Fellow, Minimally Invasive Surgery
Washington University School of Medicine
Barnes-Jewish Hospital
St. Louis, Missouri

Thomas E. Read, MD, FACS, FASCRS
Professor of Surgery
Tufts University School of Medicine
Staff Surgeon, Department of Colon and Rectal Surgery
Program Director, Colon & Rectal Surgery Residency
Lahey Clinic Medical Center
Burlington, Massachusetts

Feza H. Remzi, MD
Chairman
Department of Colorectal Surgery
Cleveland Clinic Foundation
Cleveland, Ohio

David Rivadeneira, MD, FACS, FASCRS
Chief, Department of Colon and Rectal Surgery
Director, Colon and Rectal Program
St. Catherine of Siena Medical Center
Smithtown, New York

Patricia L. Roberts, MD
Chair
Department of Colon and Rectal Surgery
Lahey Clinic
Burlington, Massachusetts
Professor of Surgery
Department of Surgery
Tufts University School of Medicine
Boston, Massachusetts

Howard M. Ross, MD, FACS, FASCRS
Chief, Colon and Rectal Surgery
Director, Center for Crohn's and Colitis Management
Riverview Medical Center
Red Bank, New Jersey
Clinical Associate Professor
University of Medicine and Dentistry of New Jersey
Newark, New Jersey

David A. Rothenberger, MD
Deputy Chairman and Professor
Department of Surgery
University of Minnesota
Minneapolis, Minnesota

Karla Russek, MD
Texas Endosurgery Institute
San Antonio, Texas

Laurence R. Sands, MD, FACS, FASCRS
Associate Professor of Clinical Surgery
Chief, Division of Colon and Rectal Surgery
University of Miami Miller School of Medicine
Miami, Florida

Deborah R. Schnipper, MD
Chief Resident, General Surgery
Integrated Residency Program
University of Connecticut
Farmington, Connecticut

Christina J. Seo, MD
Colorectal Surgeon
Barash-White, MD, PA
Bergen County, NJ

Joy C. Singh, MD
Department of Colorectal Surgery
Oxford Radcliffe Hospitals
Oxford, United Kingdom

Bradford Sklow, MD
Associate Professor of Colon and Rectal Surgery
University of Utah
Department of Surgery
Salt Lake City, Utah

Toyooki Sonoda, MD
Section of Colon and Rectal Surgery
Weill Medical College of Cornell University
New York Presbyterian Hospital
New York, New York

Michael J. Stamos, MD, FACS, FASCRS
Professor and the John E. Connolly Chair, Surgery
University of California, Irvine
School of Medicine
Orange, CA

Scott R. Steele, MD, FACS
Chief, Colon and Rectal Surgery
Madigan Army Medical Center
Tacoma, Washington

Sharon L. Stein, MD
Assistant Professor of Surgery
Division of Colorectal Surgery
University Hospitals Case Medical Center
Cleveland, Ohio

Paul R. Sturrock, MD
Assistant Professor of Surgery
Department of Surgery, Division of Colon and Rectal
    Surgery
University of Massachusetts Medical School
Worcester, Massachusetts

Paris P. Tekkis, MD, FRCS
Reader in Surgery and Consultant Colorectal Surgeon
Imperial College of London
The Royal Marsden Hospital, London
London, United Kingdom

William Timmerman, MD
Colon and Rectal Specialists, Ltd
Associate Clinical Professor of Surgery
Medical College of Virginia, Virginia Commonwealth
    University
Richmond, Virginia

Petr Tsarkov, MD, PhD
Head of Department of Colorectal and Pelvic Floor Surgery
National Research Center for Surgery of Russian Academy
    of Medical Sciences
Moscow, Russia

Madhulika G. Varma, MD
Associate Professor of Surgery
Chief, Section of Colorectal Surgery
Department of Surgery
University of California
San Francisco, California

Anthony M. Vernava, MD, FACS, FASCRS
Chief of Colorectal Surgery
Physicians Regional Health Care System
Naples, Florida

Dirk Weimann, MD
Chirurg, Viseralchirurg, EBSQ Coloproctology
Ludwig burg, Germany

Martin R. Weiser, MD
Associate Member, Colorectal Service
Department of Surgery
Memorial Sloane-Kettering Cancer Center
New York, New York

Eric G. Weiss, MD, FACS, FASCRS, FACG
Vice Chairman of Colorectal Surgery
Cleveland Clinic Florida
Weston, Florida

Richard Whelan, MD, FACS, FASCRS
Chief of Division, Colorectal Surgery and Surgical Oncology
Professor of Clinical Surgery, Columbia University

Charles B. Whitlow, MD
Residency Program Director
Ochsner Clinic Foundation
New Orleans, Louisiana

Norman S. Williams, MS, FRCS
Professor of Surgery
Academic Surgical Unit, Barts and The London NHS Trust
Institute Cellular & Molecular Science
Queen Mary's School of Medicine and Dentistry
University of London
Edinburgh, United Kingdom

Paul E. Wise, MD, FACS, FASCRS
Assistant Professor of Surgery
Director, Vanderbilt Hereditary Colorectal Cancer Registry
Department of General Surgery, Division of General Surgery
Vanderbilt University Medical Center
Nashville, Tennessee

W. Douglas Wong, MD
Chief, Colorectal Service
Department of Surgery
Memorial Sloane-Kettering Cancer Center
New York, New York

Tonia M. Young-Fadok, MD, MS, FACS, FASCRS
Chair, Division of Colon and Rectal Surgery
Mayo Clinic
Professor of Surgery
Mayo Clinic Foundation
Phoenix, Arizona

We live in a high technology world where the "miracles" of modern surgery make headline news around the globe. It is no longer surprising to hear of yet another start-up medical technology company that promises a new surgical device that will save countless lives, improve outcomes, and significantly decrease pain and suffering. People find themselves mesmerized by watching "key hole surgery" broadcast in high definition to their home television and find it surprisingly elegant and bloodless compared to their prior mental picture of surgeons at work. So it is perhaps understandable that many patients today go online to find surgeons and institutions offering the newest approaches and latest technology. It seems as though the modern surgeon armed with high tech devices and digitalized equipment should be invincible. Indeed, it is easy for surgeons to be inappropriately swept up by the siren song of technical innovation.

In this kind of world, one might question the utility of yet another surgical textbook, especially one devoted to operative technique. Fortunately, editors Steven Wexner and James Fleshman have created a unique publication that is a far cry from the traditional textbook of the past. The list of contributing authors includes seasoned master surgeons schooled in traditional techniques and highly innovative researchers and entrepreneurs who are exploring new frontiers of surgical technology. Over the course of their busy clinical careers, the editors themselves have successfully bridged both perspectives. Their unique experiences are apparent in this new, tightly edited and highly practical textbook that emphasizes tried and true open techniques and new, less invasive techniques.

Drs. Wexner and Fleshman understand that surgical outcomes are dependent on many factors including clinical acumen and mature judgment to guide individualized decision-making. But they also know that surgeons must master basic operative skills and develop a full reservoir of different techniques that can be used to fit the demands of the case at hand. As importantly, they know that no matter how revolutionary or exciting, technology has its limits. Innovation is providing new tools but it is the surgeon's skill in deciding what tools to use and the way in which they are used that determines the surgical outcome. Operative technique remains critical to minimize patient morbidity, cure cancer and other life-threatening conditions, and preserve function and quality of life. All colon and rectal surgeons will find this book to be a valuable adjunct to their practice. The artist's color drawings are superb and anatomically correct. The text is easy to read, very focused, and useful for busy surgeons. I congratulate the editors for bringing this book to us.

David A. Rothenberger, MD
August 1, 2011

The Mastery of Colorectal Surgery textbook is a two volume compendium that demonstrates virtually all of the currently employed techniques for abdominal and anorectal surgery. All of the chapters have been written by internationally acclaimed experts, each of whom was given literary license to allow the book to be more creative and less rigorously formatted. Although some techniques are self-explanatory and the authors therefore concentrated their verbiage upon results and controversies surrounding a particular technique, other procedures are described in a more algorithmic manner. Specifically, some techniques require a much more heavily weighted description of preoperative and/or postoperative parameters rather than intraoperative variables. The matching of illustrations and videos has also been tailored to suit the needs of each chapter. Because of the quantity of material, the book is divided into two volumes: one that includes the abdominal and one that includes anorectal procedures. While many textbooks vie for the attention of surgeons in training and surgeons in practice, the Mastery series, edited by Dr. Josef Fischer, has established itself as the resource for expert management of each theme. Therefore, this book was deliberately crafted to augment rather than to replace several other excellent recently published textbooks. It is our hope that these volumes be used in that context so that the reader can learn the fundamentals and basics using many other excellent source materials and then rely upon the Mastery of Colorectal Surgery books for more clarity in terms of review of very specific procedures. In that same manner, these books perform a ready preoperative resource before embarking upon individual procedures.

We wish to thank Josef Fischer with having entrusted us with this latest of his literary offspring. The project took a considerable amount of time and effort and we certainly thank him for his patience. In addition, we thank our respective staff in Weston and in Saint Louis, especially Liz Nordike, Heather Dean, Dr. Fabio Potenti, and Debbie Holton for their extensive efforts as well as Nicole Dernoski at Wolters Kluwer. We wish to express our sincerest and deepest gratitude to each and every contributor for their time, attention, expertise, and commitment to the project. Without our individual chapter authors, this work would not exist. We know that each of them has many significant competing obligations for their limited time and thank them for having participated to such an important degree in this project. Last, our appreciation goes to our families for their love and support as it is always time away from them that allows us to produce these type of books. In particular, appreciation goes to Linda Fleshman and to Wesley and Trevor Wexner.

PART III: LOW ANTERIOR RESECTION

PART IV: TOTAL COLECTOMY WITH ILEORECTAL ANASTOMOSIS

PART V: TOTAL PROCTOCOLECTOMY WITH ILEOSTOMY

PART VI: RESTORATIVE PROCTOCOLECTOMY

PART VII: ABDOMINOPERINEAL RESECTION

PART VIII: PELVIC EXENTERATION

PART IX: SURGERY FOR POSTERIOR COMPARTMENT DYSFUNCTION

PART X: COLOSTOMY

PART XI: ILEOSTOMY

PART XII: STOMAL COMPLICATIONS

PART XIII: HARTMANN'S REVERSAL

PART XIV: ABDOMINAL OPERATIONS FOR RECTAL PROLAPSE

PART XV: VENTRAL HERNIA REPAIR

PART XVI: SMALL BOWEL STRICTUREPLASTY

1 Open Medial to Lateral

David W. Dietz

Introduction and Historical Perspective

With the wide acceptance of laparoscopic surgery for colon cancer, most patients with right colon pathology, both benign and malignant, are being treated by the "minimally invasive" approach. Within our department, the number of open right colectomies has dropped precipitously over the past 10 years. However, due to our department's reputation as a national referral center for complex colorectal problems, approximately 50% of right colectomies are still performed using an open technique. The principle indications in these cases are locally advanced colon cancer and recurrent inflammatory bowel disease.

In most centers, open right colectomy is most commonly performed using a "lateral-to-medial" approach where the tumor is manipulated prior to ligation of the venous drainage. In the 1950s, however, seminal work by Barnes (1) and Turnbull (2) led to the development of a "no touch" isolation approach to segmental colectomies in patients with cancer. The principles of the "no touch" technique were based on the observations by several investigators that cancer cells were actively shed into the bloodstream during tumor manipulation. This concept was first introduced by Tyzzer (3) in 1913 who found that the vigorous manipulation of implanted chest wall tumors in mice resulted in the development of extensive liver metastases. In 1954, Cole et al. (4) reported the finding of shed cancer cells in the portal venous blood of a perfused resected cancer-bearing segment of human colon. One year later, Fisher and Turnbull (5) reported cancer cells in the portal venous blood of 8 of 25 resected colectomy specimens.

In 1952, Barnes (1) described a technique for right colectomy whereby the vascular pedicles and adjacent lymphatic channels were ligated prior to mobilization of the colon and manipulation of the tumor. The procedure began with division of the mid-transverse colon. Beginning with the middle colic vessels, the mesenteric dissection proceeded toward the terminal ileum, dividing and ligating the right branch of the middle colic artery and vein, right colic vessels, and ileocolic pedicle. The terminal ileum was then divided. Only at this point, with the vascular and lymphatic drainage of the right colon controlled, was the tumor manipulated to allow division of the lateral attachments of the right colon and completion of the operation. Barnes noted that this technique was proposed in order to "prevent forcing, by such manipulation, malignant cells into the areas beyond the site of surgery via the blood and lymph channels." The

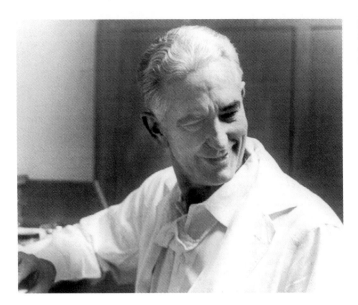

Figure 1.1   Rupert B. Turnbull, M.D. Chairman of the Department of Colorectal Surgery at the Cleveland Clinic 1961–1978.

author also stated that a literature search, as well as personal visits to some of the largest surgical clinics of the time, led him to believe that these principles were being ignored by surgeons of the day and most right colectomies were being performed in nononcologic fashion; similar to the lateral-to-medial approach taught to most residents and fellows today! Barnes concluded that "the procedure now seems so reasonable and based on such good surgical principles that I cannot believe it to be a new departure, but merely the dusting off of a very old (albeit long forgotten) technique."

In 1953, Turnbull (2) (Fig. 1.1), who was then the chairman of the Department of Colon and Rectal Surgery at the Cleveland Clinic, devised a similar operation that followed these basic oncologic principles. Termed the "no-touch isolation technique," it involved a unique medial-to-lateral approach to vascular ligation prior to tumor manipulation. His initial report on the results of the technique, presented to the American Surgical Association in 1967, was hailed by discussants as "the most important advance in the surgical treatment in carcinoma of the colon in the (preceding) thirty years" (2). Turnbull compared 664 patients operated upon using his "no touch" technique with 232 patients undergoing "conventional" colectomy and found a marked improvement in 5-year survival rates (50.8% vs. 34.8%). This overall survival rate of 50% was unheard of at the time, as the usual rate for colon cancer was between 25% and 35%. Further examination of the data revealed that the greatest advantage for the "no touch" technique was in patients with stage C (lymph node positive) tumors (58% vs. 28%).

Subsequent studies, however, have failed to firmly demonstrate this advantage for Turnbull's "no touch" technique. Despite this, a "no touch" segmental colectomy is still performed by many of the colorectal surgeons in our department.

 INDICATIONS/CONTRAINDICATIONS

In addition to its theoretical merits related to lymphovascular dissemination of malignant cells in any colon cancer, a medial-to-lateral approach right colectomy is also advantageous in patients with locally advanced carcinoma of the cecum or ascending colon. Elevation of the right colon mesentery off of the retroperitoneum with ligation of the ileocolic pedicle early in the procedure allows the surgeon to better define the retroperitoneal structures prior to attacking areas of transmural tumor invasion that may be involving the ureter, kidney, duodenum, or major vascular structures.

Contraindications to the medial-to-lateral approach are conditions wherein the right colon mesentery is not easily separated from the retroperitoneum. These include the finding of significant malignant adenopathy involving the ileocolic pedicle and the extremely thickened and fibrotic mesentery seen in some patients with Crohn's disease.

PREOPERATIVE PLANNING

The most important aspect of preoperative planning related to performing a medial-to-lateral right colectomy is the realization that the procedure may be required. As stated in the preceding text, a common indication is a locally advanced colon cancer that is invading retroperitoneal structures. This finding is best appreciated on CT scan of the abdomen and pelvis, a study that should be obtained in all patients with colon cancer as part of the preoperative staging workup. If invasion of the vena cava, aorta, or iliac vessels is suggested, then a subsequent magnetic resonance angiogram should be obtained for precise definition and operative planning. Involvement of a vascular surgeon to assist in en bloc tumor resection and vascular reconstruction is suggested.

Ureteric stents should be considered in all cases of retroperitoneal tumor invasion as well as in cases of large, bulky tumors that do not appear to be directly invasive. A urologist should also be involved if ureter resection and reconstruction is anticipated.

Mechanical bowel preparation is not routinely performed in our institution for patients undergoing right colectomy. A recent Cochrane review found no beneficial effect in terms of reduced rates of wound infection or anastomotic leak in patients undergoing segmental colectomy (6).

 SURGERY

The patient is placed on the operating table in the supine position. After insertion of a Foley catheter, the skin of the abdomen is prepped and draped. After intravenous administration of a broad-spectrum antibiotic, the peritoneal cavity is entered via a midline incision and a self-retaining retractor is placed. The abdomen is explored to determine the presence and extent of any metastatic disease and to also rule out unexpected pathology. An assessment of tumor resectability is made with special attention paid to the duodenum, pancreas, great vessels, and right kidney and ureter. This is mostly achieved by visual inspection, as the tumor should not be manipulated prior to vascular ligation. The small bowel is first retracted to the patient's right side in order to expose the base of its mesentery (Fig. 1.2A). The peritoneum overlying the base of the small bowel mesentery is then incised just above its border with the fourth portion of the duodenum and this incision is extended caudally for approximately 6 cm (Fig. 1.2B). Careful dissection is then undertaken in a plane posterior to the superior mesenteric vessels to separate the mesentery from the retroperitoneum. This dissection proceeds in a medial-to-lateral direction until the surgeon can insert the second and third fingers of his nondominant hand behind the superior mesenteric vessels and the fingertips come to lie on either side of the ileocolic vascular pedicle (Fig. 1.2C). The small bowel and its mesentery are then reflected back to the patient's left to set up vascular division (Fig. 1.2D). Mesenteric windows are then opened on either side of the ileocolic pedicle near its origin using the fingertips of the surgeon's nondominant hand as a guide (Fig. 1.2E). After clearing lymphatic tissue from the vessel origins, clamps are applied and the vessels are divided and ligated with #1 chromic ties (Fig. 1.2F). Through this window in the mesentery, the plane between the ascending mesocolon, and the retroperitoneal structures is developed in a cephalad direction. The surgeon will encounter the most medial aspect of Gerota's fascia and the anterior surface of the duodenum and pancreatic head during this portion of the operation. As dissection proceeds above the duodenum, a plane between the first portion of the duodenum and the transverse mesocolon will be entered. It is at this point that the right branch of the middle colic artery and vein are mobilized to their origin (Fig. 1.2G). The right branch of the middle colic artery and vein are then divided between clamps at their origin and are ligated with #1 chromic ties. The remaining mesentery adjacent to the mid-transverse colon, which includes the marginal artery, is then divided. Pulsatile arterial bleeding should be confirmed from the distal end of the divided marginal artery prior to ligation (Fig. 1.2H). This indicates adequate blood supply on the colon side for creation of the ileocolic anastomosis. Likewise the remaining mesentery adjacent to the terminal ileum containing the two marginal ileal vessels is also divided (Fig. 1.2I).

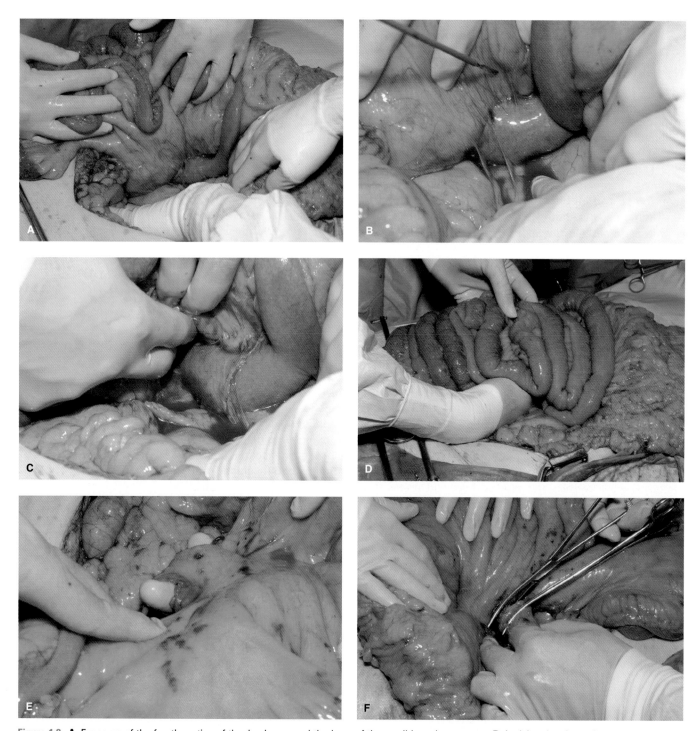

Figure 1.2. **A.** Exposure of the fourth portion of the duodenum and the base of the small bowel mesentery. **B.** Incising the visceral peritoneum of the small bowel mesentery near its base. **C.** Developing the avascular plane between the small bowel mesentery and retroperitoneum. **D.** Reflecting the small bowel back toward the patient's right side. Surgeon's hand is under the mesentery and its vessels. **E.** The ileocolic vessels are isolated near their origin from the superior mesenteric artery and vein. **F.** High division and ligation of the ileocolic vessels. (*continued*)

With the lymphovascular drainage of the right colon now interrupted, the tumor may be manipulated without fear of disseminating malignant cells. Attention is turned to the omentum and its attachments to the transverse colon. Beginning at the anticipated site of division in the mid-transverse colon, the omentum is separated from the transverse colon itself and the transverse mesocolon by developing the avascular plane (Fig. 1.2J). This dissection proceeds from the mid-transverse colon toward the hepatic

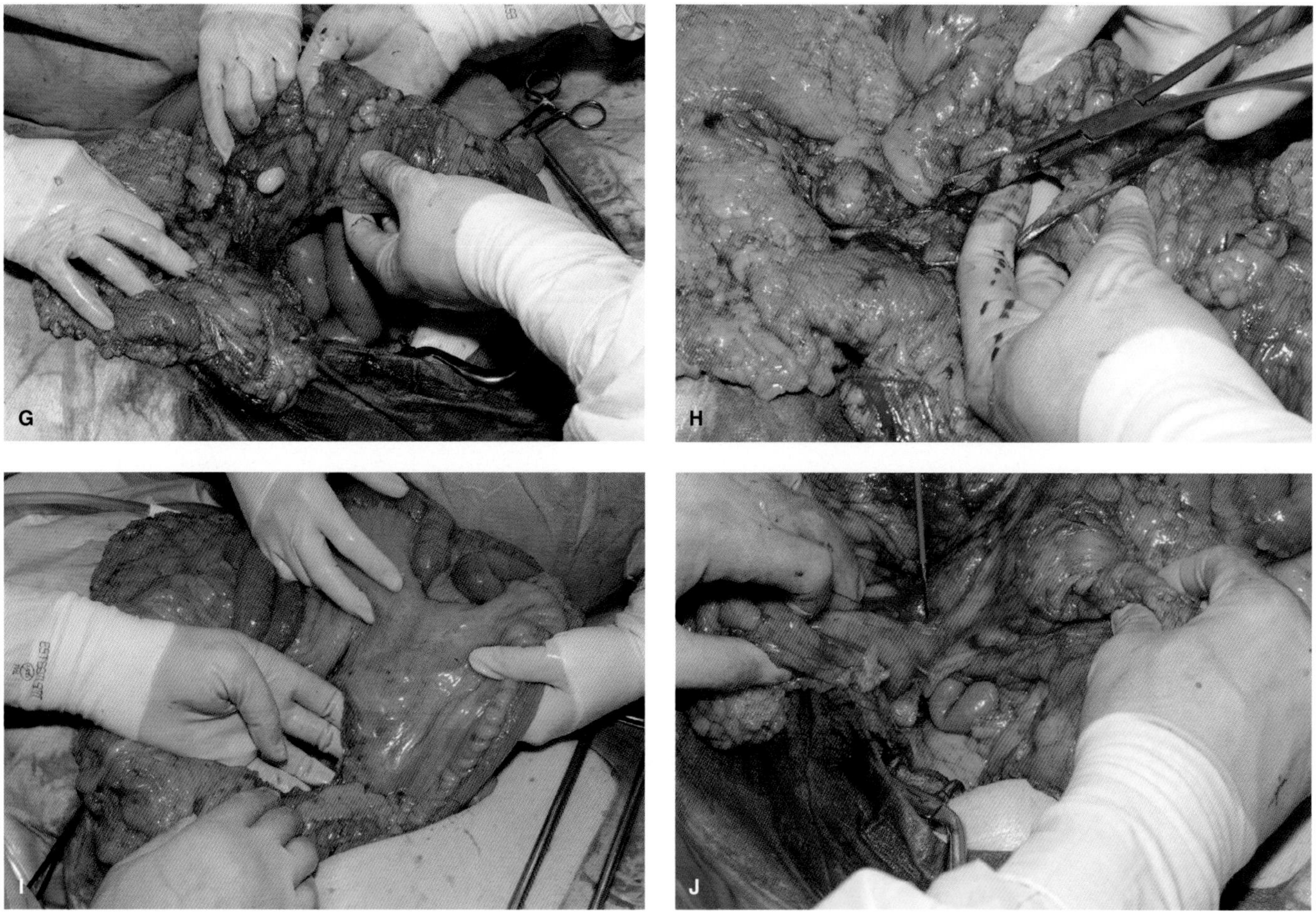

Figure 1.2. (*Continued*) **G.** Right branch of the middle colic artery and vein isolated. **H.** Pulsatile bleeding from the marginal vessel adjacent to the transverse colon. **I.** Marginal vessels along the terminal ileum. **J.** Separating the omentum from the transverse colon and mesocolon. (*continued*)

flexure. A "crossing" vein between the omentum and the proximal transverse mesocolon is often encountered at this point in the operation. After this vein has been divided and ligated the omentum should be completely free from the proximal half of the transverse colon and its mesocolon and the lesser sac fully exposed. The lateral attachments of the right colon are carefully mobilized and the hepatic flexure attachments divided, taking care to identify the right ureter during the course of this dissection. Precise dissection at the junction of the pericolic fat and lateral areolar tissue, rather than in the middle of the areolar tissue plane itself, will minimize risk of injury to the ureter (Fig. 1.2K). The mid-transverse colon (Fig. 1.2L) and the terminal ileum (Fig. 1.2M) are then divided between clamps and the right colectomy specimen is removed from the operative field and sent to pathology.

Ileocolic anastomosis is performed according to the surgeon's preference. In cases where either the wall of colon or ileum is abnormal, a hand-sewn anastomosis is most reliable. My routine is to use interrupted vertical mattress sutures of 3-0 Vicryl to construct the posterior (mesenteric) wall and interrupted seromuscular sutures of the same for the anterior (anti-mesenteric) wall. In cases where a stapled anastomosis is favored, I prefer an end to side ileocolic anastomosis using a circular stapler introduced through the open end of the colon (Fig. 1.2N). The spike of the stapler should be brought through the antimesenteric wall of the colon approximately 6 cm proximal to the end of the colonic stump. The anvil is placed in the end of the ileum and the bowel wall is "purse-stringed" around the post with a 0 Prolene suture. The open end of the colonic stump is then closed with a linear stapler. The mesentery of the ileum and transverse colon are

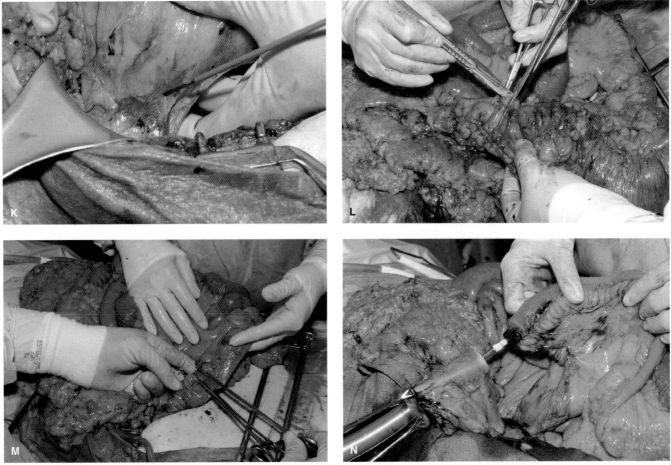

Figure 1.2. (*Continued*) **K.** Dividing the lateral attachments of the right colon. Line of dissection is at the junction of the areolar tissue and the pericolic fat. **L.** Dividing the mid-transverse colon. **M.** Dividing the terminal ileum. **N.** Creating the end-to-side ileocolic anastomosis using the circular stapler introduced through the end of the colon.

reapproximated with a running absorbable suture and the omentum is laid over the anastomosis. Incorporating the tip of the omentum into the tie at the end of the mesentery closure suture line will ensure that it stays in place over the anastomosis.

→ POSTOPERATIVE MANAGEMENT

Postoperative management of the patient should follow an accelerated care pathway. Nasogastric tubes are not used routinely. The patient is allowed a clear liquid diet on the first postoperative day and is ambulated in the hallway with the assistance of the nursing staff. Intravenous narcotic pain medication is replaced by an oral analgesic once the patient is reliably tolerating oral intake. Empiric antibiotics are discontinued within the first 24 hours after surgery and the Foley catheter is removed by the second postoperative day. The patient is advanced to a soft diet on the return of bowel function and is subsequently discharged from the hospital. The average length of stay after open medial-to-lateral right colectomy is 5 days at our institution.

↘ COMPLICATIONS

Complications following open medial-to-lateral right colectomy include prolonged ileus, wound infection, intra-abdominal abscess, urinary tract infection, hemorrhage, deep venous thrombosis, and anastomotic leak. The incidence of wound infection following open right colectomy ranges from 10% to 15% while the risk of intra-abdominal abscess is approximately 3%. Ileocolic anastomotic leak occurs in less than 2% of patients. Intra-abdominal bleeding that requires blood transfusion occurs in 5% of cases. Postoperative mortality (death within 30 days of surgery) is extremely rare and is typically related to cardiovascular or thromboembolic events in high-risk patients.

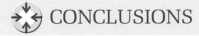 ## RESULTS

Despite the theoretical merits of the no touch technique for the resection of colon cancer, modern studies have not found a clear survival advantage when compared to more common methods of segmental colectomy. One randomized prospective trial has been conducted to examine this question. Wiggers et al. randomized 236 patients with curable colorectal cancer to undergo colectomy either by conventional resection or the no touch isolation technique (7). After appropriate exclusions and a minimum of 5 years of follow-up there were 117 patients remaining to be analyzed in the no touch group and 119 in the conventional group. There were no differences in postoperative morbidity or mortality. Analysis of tumor recurrence, disease-free survival, and overall survival found no statistically significant differences between the two groups. However, in all analyses of oncologic endpoints the no touch group had better outcomes. Liver metastases occurred in fewer patients in the no touch group (14 vs. 22, $p = 0.14$) and tended to occur at a later point in time (22.4 vs. 12.6 months). Disease-related death occurred in 24.7% of patients in the no touch group as compared to 31.1% in the conventional resection group. Subgroup analysis revealed that patients with the highest risk tumors gained particular benefit from the no touch technique. In patients whose tumors demonstrated angiolymphatic invasion, disease-related death occurred in 52% of patients in the conventional group versus 31% in the "no touch" group. The authors concluded that, although no statistically significant differences were found between the two techniques, the "no touch" approach should be used for all tumors in areas of the colon where it is easily applicable, as even small improvements in prognosis are valuable in patients with colorectal cancer.

CONCLUSIONS

Both colorectal and general surgeons should be familiar with a medial-to-lateral approach to right colectomy. This technique has theoretical advantages related to dissemination of cancer cells into the venous drainage and early studies demonstrated a survival advantage for patients undergoing a "no touch" segmental colectomy. A more recent randomized controlled trial found a trend toward fewer liver metastases and cancer-related deaths in the "no touch" group, but it did not reach statistical significance. Medial-to-lateral right colectomy is also useful in cases of tumor fixation to retroperitoneal structures and in patients with severe inflammatory bowel disease involving the terminal ileum and right colon.

References

1. Barnes J. Physiologic resection of the right colon. *Surg Gynecol Obstet* 1952;94(6):722–726.
2. Turnbull RB, Kyle K, Watson FR, Spratt J. Cancer of the colon: the influence of the no-touch isolation technic on survival rates. *Ann Surg* 1967;166:420–425.
3. Tyzzer EE. Factors in the production and growth of tumor metastases. *J Med Res* 1913;28:309.
4. Cole WH, Packard D, Southwick HW. Carcinoma of the colon with special reference to prevention of recurrence. *JAMA* 1954;155:1549.
5. Fisher ER, Turnbull RB. The cytologic demonstration and significance of tumor cells in the mesenteric venous blood in patients with colorectal carcinoma. *Surg Gynecol Obstet* 1955; 100:102.
6. Guenaga KK, Matos D, Wille-Jorgensen P. Mechanical bowel preparation for elective colorectal surgery. *Cochrane Database Syst Rev* 2009;(1):CD001544.
7. Wiggers T, Jeekel J, Arends JW, et al. No-touch isolation technique in colon cancer: a controlled prospect trial. *Br J Surg* 1988; 75(5):409–415.

2 Open Lateral to Medial

Farah Husain, Ira Kodner, and Edward Lin

In this section, the open surgical technique with a lateral to medial approach will be outlined.

Location continues to be the major determinant of the type and extent of colon resection, influencing the degree of resection based on the arterial, venous, and lymphatic drainage of the affected colon segment. Furthermore, there is increasing reliance, by medical societies and health care payers, on the adequacy of lymph node resection. Therefore, the number of lymph nodes examined histologically serves as a benchmark of satisfactory oncologic therapy.

 ## SURGICAL ANATOMY

Colon

Topography
Oncologic colon resection and lymph node harvest are based on the vascular supply of their subsegments. The colon and rectum are derived from the embryologic midgut and hindgut, with the blood supplies following the superior mesenteric artery and inferior mesenteric arteries, respectively. Derivatives of the midgut include the cecum and the right half to two-thirds of the transverse colon. While the derivatives of the hindgut are the left one-third to one-half of the transverse colon, the descending colon, sigmoid colon, rectum, and the superior portion of the anal canal.

Cecum
The cecum is located in the right iliac fossa and is approximately 10 cm long, with the widest transverse diameter of all the colon segments averaging 7.5 cm. It is completely enveloped with visceral peritoneum and is typically mobile. The gonadal vessels and the right ureter typically course posterior to the medial border of the cecum.

The terminal ileum empties from a medial-to-lateral direction into the cecum through a thickened invagination called the ileocecal valve. The valve prevents retrograde flow from the colon into the small bowel, but in approximately 25–30% of individuals, the ileocecal valve is incompetent. The incompetent valve is most evident during colonoscopies when colonic air readily passes into the small intestines, resulting in marked abdominal distention and patient discomfort. Patients with distal colonic obstructions and functional ileocecal valves typically have colonic dilatation on radiography that mimic a closed-loop obstruction. While the cecum is quite distensible, a diameter greater than 12 cm can result in ischemic necrosis and perforation.

Ascending Colon

From the cecum, the ascending colon is the 12–20 cm segment that runs upward toward the liver on the right side. With the exception of its posterior surface that is fixed to the retroperitoneum, the ascending colon is covered laterally and anteriorly by visceral peritoneum. The psoas muscle, second portion of the duodenum, the right ureter, and the inferior pole of the right kidney all have important anatomic relationships to the posterior aspect of the ascending colon.

Laterally, the ascending colon is attached to the parietal peritoneum via an embryonic fusion plane between the visceral and parietal peritoneum. This subtle anatomic landmark is relatively avascular and serves as the classic landmark for surgical mobilization of the ascending colon away from its retroperitoneal attachments.

The hepatic flexure of the ascending colon rests under the right liver and turns medially and anteriorly into the transverse colon. The hepatic flexure can often be identified during colonoscopy by a purplish impression on the superior aspect of the colon wall when the scope reaches the right side.

Transverse Colon

The transverse colon is suspended between the hepatic flexure and the splenic flexure on its mesentery and spans 40–50 cm, sharing important anatomic relationships with the stomach, tail of pancreas, spleen, and left kidney. It is completely invested with peritoneum and has a long mesentery known as the transverse mesocolon and may reach into the pelvis. Anatomically, the transverse colon is attached to the greater curvature of the stomach by the gastrocolic ligament or omentum. The greater omentum is attached by a thin relatively avascular membrane to the antimesenteric surface of the transverse colon. Locally advanced tumors of the transverse colon may involve the stomach, pancreas and duodenum posteriorly, as well as the spleen and omentum.

Blood Supply

Arteries

The right colon and up to two-thirds of the proximal transverse colon are derived from the midgut, a region supplied by the superior mesenteric artery. The distal transverse colon and left colon are derived from the hindgut, supplied by the inferior mesenteric artery. All the terminal vessels that vascularize a limited area of bowel wall are supplied by these arteries. Collateralization is excellent along marginal arteries at the mesenteric border, serving as an important source of a segment's blood supply when a major vessel is occluded. The presence of these marginal arteries also allows the sacrifice of major vessels, facilitating the colon's mobilization for anastomosis. The lymphatics and innervation of the colon follow the vascular supply.

The superior mesenteric artery (SMA) supplies the entire small bowel with 12–18 jejunal and ileal branches to the left and 3 major colonic branches to the right. The ileocolic vessel is the most constant of these branches and supplies the terminal ileum, appendix, and cecum. The right colic artery is the most variable blood supply of the colon, and may be absent in up to 20% of patients. When present, the right colic artery can originate from the SMA, as a branch of the ileocolic artery or middle colic artery. The right colic artery communicates with the middle colic artery through the marginal arteries.

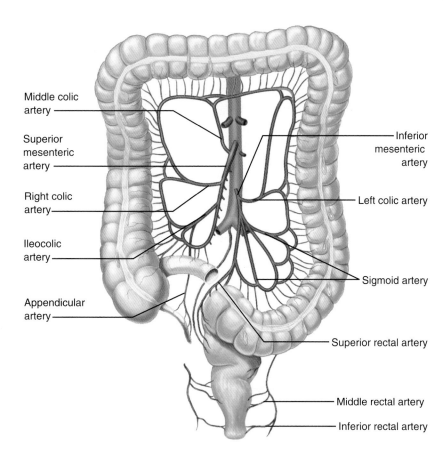

Figure 2.1   Arterial supply to the colon and rectum.

The middle colic artery is a major blood supply to the colon and is an important surgical landmark when planning a colon resection because it is a demarcation point for the clinical definition of a right or left hemicolectomy (Fig. 2.1). This artery arises proximally as the SMA enters the small bowel mesentery at the inferior border of the pancreas. The middle colic artery then ascends into the transverse mesocolon, and typically divides into the right and left colon blood supplies through the marginal artery. The middle colic may also be absent in some patients and the presence of an accessory middle colic artery may be found in 10% of patients.

Veins

The colon's venous anatomy parallels the arterial supply of the corresponding midgut- or hindgut-derived segments. Drainage of the midgut-derived right colon is achieved by the superior mesenteric venous system, which includes the ileocolic, right colic, and middle colic veins. This configuration forms the superior mesenteric vein and joins the splenic vein to empty into the portal venous system.

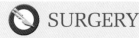 SURGERY

Surgical resection continues to be the primary therapeutic method for malignant tumors of the colon. The value of screening colonoscopy and possibly CT colonography cannot be overestimated in the detection of early or premalignant disease. However, endoscopically unresectable polyps require resection, and the vascular supply and lymphatic drainage to the mesenteric segment define the limits of resection.

Most patients undergoing elective colon resection for tumor have had cancer staging to determine distant metastasis or synchronous colonic lesions. Currently, this includes biochemical evaluations, positive emission tomography CT scan, possibly MRI, and additional colonoscopic evaluations. Aside from the cecum and rectum, the accuracy of exact tumor location cannot always be ascertained by colonoscopy. Surgical strategy can be anticipated if precise tumor localization can be marked preoperatively by double contrast colonography when feasible or endoscopic ink tattooing or clip marking. Intraoperative colonoscopy to localize the tumor is time consuming and may unnecessarily induce bowel distention.

Bowel preparation for right colectomy is not necessary. Resection of obstructing tumors with primary anastomosis is acceptable.

The major surgical procedures for the right colon include right hemicolectomy and extended right hemicolectomy. Three main considerations in re-establishing intestinal continuity that may alter the rate of anastomotic complications include lack of demonstrable pulsatile arterial blood flow, tension at the anastomosis, and perianastomotic hematoma or contamination. Other issues that may increase anastomotic complications include: sepsis, circulatory shock, carcinoma at the anastomosis, and preoperatiel radiation.

Most surgical resections for tumors should include the intermediate lymph nodes. The Intergroup 0089 trial for adjuvant chemotherapy in Stages II and III colon cancer treatment showed that the best survival is evident when greater than 20 negative lymph nodes are evaluated for Stage II cancer, and greater than 40 lymph nodes evaluated for Stage III cancer. For the present, the National Cancer Institute Guidelines 2000 recommend a minimum of 12 lymph nodes in the resected specimen for adequate tumor staging, which also serves as a benchmark for adequate oncologic resection.

STANDARD RESECTIONS FOR RIGHT-SIDED COLON TUMORS (FIG. 2.2)

Tumor location	Resection
Cecum/appendix	Right hemicolectomy
Ascending colon	Right hemicolectomy
Hepatic flexure	Extended right hemicolectomy
Transverse colon	Extended right hemicolectomy

Right Hemicolectomy

The patient is generally placed in supine position, with the surgeon standing on the patient's left side. Tumors located in the appendix, cecum, or ascending colon require a right hemicolectomy, the anatomic boundaries of which span the cecum to the proximal half of the transverse colon.

An extended right hemicolectomy includes the transverse colon to the splenic flexure. This procedure includes the left branch of the middle colic artery. The procedure is appropriate for tumors at the hepatic flexure and in the transverse colon. Many surgeons avoid isolated transverse colon resections because a hepatic flexure to splenic flexure anastomosis is a potentially problematic one.

Abdominal incisions used to perform a right hemicolectomy may vary, with choices including a midline, paramedian, transverse supraumbilical, or even a Pfannenstiel incision. The peritoneal cavity is inspected for gross metastasis. The small bowel should be evaluated from the ligament of Treitz to the ileocecal valve and the liver is closely examined. A solitary hepatic metastasis may be resected at the same time, but with appropriate presurgical evaluations, this occurrence is generally anticipated rather than unexpected. The uterus and ovaries should be identified and examined. The mass should be identified and the surrounding tissue assessed for extension beyond the colon; as in most cases, an en bloc resection is planned. If a complete resection is not possible, the primary tumor is often resected to avoid the complications of obstruction and hemorrhage.

Figure 2.2

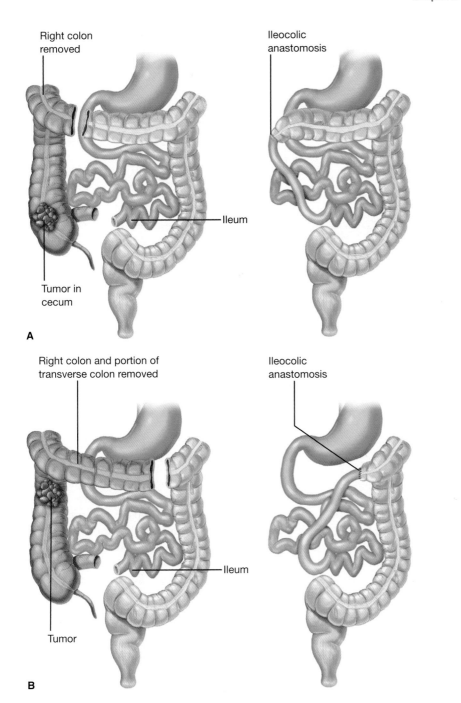

Right colon
removed

Ileocolic
anastomosis

Ileum

Tumor in
cecum

A

Right colon and portion of
transverse colon removed

Ileocolic
anastomosis

Ileum

Tumor

B

The planned resection for right hemicolectomy includes the final 6–10 cm of the ileum and the proximal transverse colon. Tumors of the cecum, to include appendiceal masses, should include 10–15 cm of the ileum.

Mobilization of the right colon can begin from the cecum toward the hepatic flexure. In this case, the peritoneal attachments to the cecum are incised with electrocautery. The colon is retracted anteriorly and medially so that electrocautery can be used to further release the lateral peritoneal attachments along the right gutter. Blunt dissection with a sponge can be used to divide any remaining thin attachments to the retroperitoneum. This maneuver will aid in insuring the gonadal vessels and ureter remains posterior to the specimen. Awareness of the course of the ureter and gonadal vessels is important. The right ureter should be readily visible as it courses from the posterior aspect of the duodenum toward the bifurcation of the iliac vessels.

The colon is freed distally from lateral attachments, which can be accomplished by placing the left index finger behind the peritoneal attachments while using electrocautery

Figure 2.3

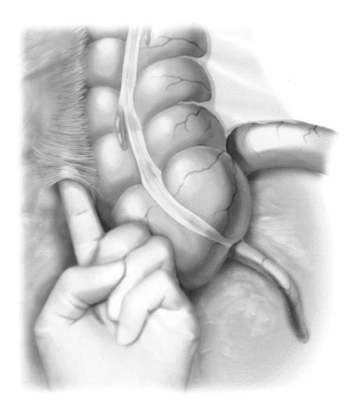

above the finger (Fig. 2.3). Mobilization of the right colon is completed when the hepatic flexure is freed superiorly from the liver and posteriorly from the duodenum. The duodenum and head of the pancreas can be visualized when the hepatic flexure dissection is completed. The renocolic ligament that anchors the hepatic flexure may be thick and either be ligated with 2-0 silk or divided with ultrasonic shears or electrothermal bipolar device (LigaSure, Covidien, Boulder, CO). The gastrocolic ligament can be divided just below the gastroepiploic arcade of the stomach using the same energy sources. The omentum attached to the resected colon can also be taken with the specimen. Three areas require caution during cephalad mobilization of the right colon: (1) excessive mobilization deep to the mesentery and entering Gerota's fascia, (2) avulsion of a collateral venous branch between the inferior pancreaticoduodenal and middle colic veins, and (3) injury to the second and third portion of the duodenum.

The ileocolic, right colic, and right branch of the middle colic vessels require ligation at their origins for adequate oncologic procedures. To identify the ileocolic pedicle, the right colon is retracted caudally away from the midline; the ileocolic pedicle becomes visible as a pulsatile ridge. The mesenteric window at the vascular base is opened on either side of the pedicle before dividing the pedicle. Once divided, the ileocolic pedicle is lifted anteriorly like a handle, and blunt dissection along the avascular retroperitoneal plane is achieved by lifting the mesentery and simultaneously sweeping the retroperitoneum posteriorly. The mesentery and cecum should be free from posterior attachments.

The remainder of the mesentery can be divided from the ileocolic pedicle down to the right branch of the middle colic artery. The right colic vessel commonly branches from the ileocolic artery, and therefore, may not need to be individually ligated. The ultimate landmark of the cephalad dissection is to identify the duodenum and remain anterior to the duodenum as well as to protect the ureter and duodenum. The right branch of the middle colic or the root of the middle colic can be suture ligated at this junction, or if safe, a bipolar cutting and sealing device can be used. Care should be taken to not injure the main middle colic artery. Although for tumors located in the transverse colon, the middle colic vessel should be ligated before the bifurcation at the inferior border of the pancreas. It is probably best to avoid direct manipulation of the tumor during the dissection, but this technique is more a surgeon preference than a data supported fact.

The transverse colon can be divided with linear cutting staplers, usually with a blue cartridge. Similarly the appropriate site of the ileum is divided with the same stapler. Intestinal continuity can be restored by hand-sewn (one- or two-layer) or stapled technique with equivalent functional results, but the stapled technique does save some time.

The stapled anastomosis begins by aligning the two ends of the bowel along the end of the antimesenteric borders. The general spillage of bowel content is minimal during this procedure and therefore, it is unnecessary to place bowel clamps proximal and distal to the anastomosis. The antimesenteric corner of the staple line is excised on both bowel ends, and the forks of the blue-cartridge linear cutting stapler instrument are inserted into the ileum and colon. After firing the instrument the internal staple line is checked for bleeding, and the resultant ileocolostomy edges are aligned using Allis clamps or anchored with stay sutures. The opening of the ileocolostomy can be closed either with a linear stapler or with another application of the linear cutting stapler. It is also acceptable to close the common opening using interrupted 3-0 silk sutures or running 3-0 vicryl sutures followed by Lembert sutures. The merits of closing the mesenteric defect are unknown, but a running suture should suffice if closure is desired (Fig. 2.4).

For extended right hemicolectomy, we prefer to bring the ileum directly to the proximal descending colon and not to the splenic flexure to avoid the risk of involving the watershed area.

The fascial incision is closed with heavy absorbable sutures such as running 1-0 polydioxanone suture.

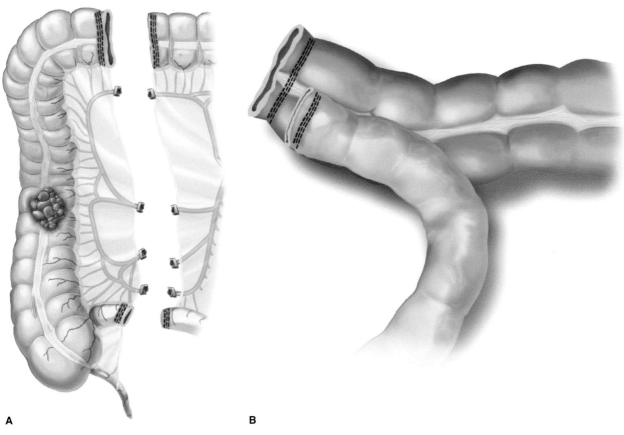

A   **B**

Figure 2.4

Suggested Readings

Beck DE, Wolff BG, Fleshman JW, Pemberton JH, Wexner SD, eds. *The ASCRS Textbook on Colon and Rectal Surgery.* New York: Springer, 2006.

Delaney CP, Neary P, Heriot AG, Senagore AJ, eds. *Operative Techniques in Laparoscopic Colorectal Surgery.* New York: Springer, 2006.

Garcia-Ruiz A, Milsom JW, Ludwig KA, Marchesa P. Right colonic arterial anatomy. Implications for laparoscopic surgery. *Dis Colon Rectum* 1996;39:906–911.

Goldenberg EA, Khaitan L, Huang IP, Smith CD, Lin E. Surgeon-initiated screening colonoscopy program based on SAGES and ASCRS recommendations in a general surgery practice. *Surg Endosc* 2006;20(6):964–966.

Goldstein NS. Lymph node recoveries from 2427 pT3 colorectal resection specimens spanning 45 years: recommendations for a minimum number of recovered lymph nodes based on predictive probabilities. *Am J Surg Pathol* 2002;26:179–189.

Gordon PH, Nivatvongs S, eds. *Principles and Practice of Surgery for the Colon, Rectum, and Anus.* 2nd Ed. St. Louis, MO: Quality Medical Publishing, 1999.

Kahokehr A, Sammour T, Zargar-Shoshtari K, Srinivasa S, Hill AG. Recovery after open and laparoscopic right hemicolectomy: a comparison. *J Surg Res* 2010;162(1):11–16.

Kaisser AM, Nunoo-Mensah JW, Beart RW. Tumors of the colon. In: Zinner MJ, Ashley SW, eds. *Maingot's Abdominal Operations.* 11th ed. New York: McGraw-Hill, 2007:625–659.

Koopmann MC, Heise CP. Laparoscopic and minimally invasive resection of malignant colorectal disease. *Surg Clin North Am* 2008;88:1047–1072.

Le Voyer TE, Sigurdson ER, Hanlon AL, et al. Colon cancer survival is associated with increasing number of lymph nodes analyzed: a secondary survey of intergroup trial INT-0089. *J Clin Oncol* 2003;21:2912–2919.

Marcello PW, Roberts PL, Rusin LC, Holubkov R, Schoetz DJ. Vascular pedicle ligation technique during laparoscopic colectomy. A prospective randomized trial. *Surg Endosc* 2006;20:263–269.

Milsom JW, Böhm B, Nakajima K, Tonohira Y, eds. *Laparoscopic Colorectal Surgery.* New York: Springer, 2006.

Nelson H, Petrelli N, Carlin A, et al. Guidelines 2000 for colon and rectal cancer surgery. *J Natl Cancer Inst* 2001;93:583–596.

Pappas TN, Pryor AD, Harnisch MC, eds. Atlas of Laparoscopic Surgery. 3rd ed. New York: Springer, 2008.

Scott-Conner CEH, Henselmann C. *Chassin's Operative Strategy in Colon and Rectal Surgery.* New York: Springer, 2006.

The Clinical Outcomes of Surgical Therapy Study Group. A comparison of laparoscopically assisted and open colectomy for colon cancer. *N Engl J Med* 2004;350:2050–2059.

3 Laparoscopic Medial to Lateral

Toyooki Sonoda

 INDICATIONS AND CONTRAINDICATIONS

The laparoscopic dissection of the right colon is generally thought to be more straightforward than the transverse colon, left colon, or the rectum. There are two general approaches, one where the colon is mobilized from its lateral attachment first (the lateral approach), and one where the vascular pedicles are initially ligated, followed by colonic mobilization (the medial approach). Both accomplish the same dissection, but advantages to the medial-to-lateral approach include the following:

- Early ligation of the vascular pedicles in cancer may theoretically prevent the liberation of tumor cells into the mesenteric circulation during mobilization (the Turnbull "no-touch" technique)
- Preservation of the lateral colonic ligament until the end of the mobilization keeps the right colon fixed in place, limiting the need to manipulate a floppy colon

Indications

The most common indications for a laparoscopic right colectomy include malignant neoplasm, benign polyp not amenable to colonoscopic removal, and Crohn's disease. Uncommon yet possible indications are right-sided diverticulitis, chronic volvulus, hemorrhage, and ischemia.

Contraindications

There are both absolute and relative contraindications to the laparoscopic approach to colectomy. Absolute contraindications include:

- Hemodynamic instability
- Known history of extensive adhesions from prior surgery

The relative contraindications to laparoscopy depend on each clinical circumstance, and the skills and comfort levels of the surgeon, including

- Large tumor size (>8 cm)
- Tumor invading other structures
- Bowel dilation from obstruction or ileus
- Emergency surgery
- History of prior surgery

A patient may have had many operations in the past, but the amount of adhesions may not prohibit a subsequent laparoscopic colectomy. For example, even patients who have undergone one or two open ileocolic resections for Crohn's disease may still be candidates for laparoscopic ileocolectomy. When extensive adhesions are present and a conversion to open surgery is necessary, it is important that the decision to convert is made early in the operation. Omental adhesions to the abdominal wall, even if extensive, can be favorable for the laparoscopic approach; significant intraloop adhesions are usually not as easily managed.

 PREOPERATIVE PLANNING

The patient should be prepared for surgery as usual, with attention paid to preoperative comorbidities. Neoplasms should be evaluated with preoperative computed tomographic scan, complete colonoscopy whenever possible, and magnetic resonance imaging or positron emission tomographic scan when appropriate. Patients with Crohn's disease should undergo colonoscopy and complete imaging of the small intestine using a computed tomographic or magnetic resonance enterography.

Whenever a lesion is present, especially one that may not be visible on the serosal surface, an endoscopic tattoo should be placed using India ink. This maneuver allows for laparoscopic identification of the tumor-bearing segment, and helps eliminate the possibilities of removing an incorrect segment of intestine or resecting a tumor with inadequate lateral margins. The tattoo should be placed in a uniform manner, in multiple quadrants to assure that the tattoo is visible on the serosal surface and not hidden by the mesentery. The author favors a tattoo in three quadrants, distal to the tumor. Placing a tattoo both proximally and distally may lead to confusion if only one area is visible.

The use of mechanical bowel preparation prior to surgery is controversial. Several randomized prospective trials do not show advantages to bowel preparation in terms of anastomotic leaks and wound infections. However, with the laparoscopic approach, the ability to palpate the bowel is limited. If the location of a tumor or polyp cannot be ascertained during laparoscopic surgery, an intraoperative colonoscopy should be performed rather than a blind resection. This, of course, would be difficult in the setting of an unprepared colon. The use of CO_2 colonoscopy limits bowel distension during surgery, and this can be performed without any proximal bowel occlusion due to the rapid absorption of intraluminal CO_2. If air colonoscopy is used, however, the terminal ileum should be occluded with a bowel grasper to avoid small bowel distension.

 SURGERY

Patients undergoing laparoscopic bowel resection should receive appropriate intravenous antibiotics within one hour of skin incision. For a lengthy operation, the antibiotics must be redosed intraoperatively based on their pharmacokinetics. Prophylaxis against deep vein thrombosis should be preoperatively given.

Positioning

A gel pad is placed on the operating table to avoid patient slippage during extreme tilt. Although a laparoscopic right colectomy can be performed in the supine position, the author prefers to use the modified lithotomy position, with both the arms tucked at the sides. The hip flexion must be kept to a minimum, or the thighs will obstruct the laparoscopic instruments during upper abdominal dissection. The advantages of this positioning are as follows:

- In a difficult right colectomy, the surgeon or assistant can stand between the legs and help with retraction through an additional port
- When a lesion (or tattoo) is difficult to identify, an intraoperative colonoscopy can be performed
- In cases of ileal Crohn's disease, there could be an occult ileosigmoid fistula requiring sigmoid colon resection

Technique

Port Placement

The camera port is placed in a periumbilical position. Whether it is placed superior or inferior to the umbilicus is based on the body habitus and location of the umbilicus. The camera port is best placed at the "top of the dome" when the abdomen is insufflated; in most patients, this could be in the infraumbilical position. However, when the umbilicus is located low in the abdomen (as a result of obesity and in some males), the camera port is best placed in the supraumbilical position. In the majority of cases, this periumbilical port wound is extended around the umbilicus for exteriorization of the colon, resection, and anastomosis.

The port placement is illustrated in Figure 3.1. We favor the blunt Hasson technique (10 mm or 12 mm) for the camera port. The surgeon begins the operation from the left side of the patient using the left lower quadrant and suprapubic ports. The assistant stands to the right of the surgeon, holding the camera and using the left upper port. A monitor near the right shoulder of the patient is used by both operators. After vascular ligation and medial-to-lateral retromesenteric dissection, the surgeon moves to the right of the assistant, using the two left-sided ports, for the hepatic flexure takedown and lateral ligament mobilization. The assistant helps through the suprapubic port.

Operative Steps

The following are the general operative steps in a medial-to-lateral laparoscopic right hemicolectomy:

- Isolation and division of the ileocolic pedicle
- Isolation and division of the right branch of the middle colic vessels
- Separation of the right colon and mesentery from the retroperitoneal fascia in a medial-to-lateral direction
- Dissection of the gastrocolic ligament, takedown of the hepatic flexure and lateral ligament
- Dissection of the ileum and mesentery from the retroperitoneum
- Division of the bowel proximally and distally
- Anastomosis

Ileocolic Pedicle

The patient is placed in a slight Trendelenburg position. The omentum is lifted above the transverse colon, and the distal ileum is moved into the pelvis. The patient is tilted (airplaned) steeply with the right side up, and the small bowel loops are swept to the left of the midline.

The operation starts with the isolation of the ileocolic pedicle. The ileocolic artery is a proximal branch of the superior mesenteric artery that courses just inferior to the third portion of the duodenum. Therefore, the identification of the duodenal sweep through the mesentery as the transverse colon is superiorly retracted is an important initial step in identifying the ileocolic pedicle. Ample tension on this vessel is critical

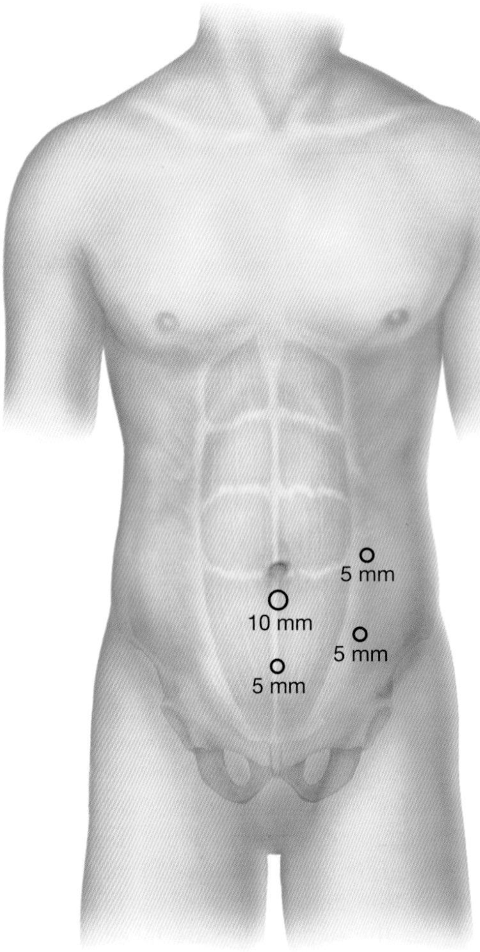

Figure 3.1 The port placement for a medial-to-lateral laparoscopic right hemicolectomy.

in distinguishing it from the superior mesenteric vessels. With traction on the ileocecal region in an anterolateral direction, the ileocolic artery will be seen "bowstringing" through the mesentery (Fig. 3.2). The right colic artery arises from the ileocolic pedicle to supply the hepatic flexure about 90% of the time, and does not need to be separately ligated. In a minority of cases, it will branch from the superior mesenteric artery, superior to the ileocolic pedicle, and will need ligation. Distal in its course, near the ileocecal junction, the ileocolic artery becomes the ileal branch (and accessory ileal branch), which can bleed if injured. Therefore, the dissection of the ileocolic artery should start in the avascular plane between the superior mesenteric vessels and the ileal branch.

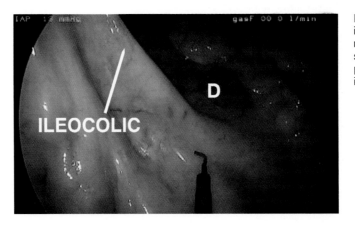

Figure 3.2 The ileocolic pedicle identified through the right colon mesentery. The duodenum (D) should be identified, and the pedicle should travel clearly to the ileocecal junction.

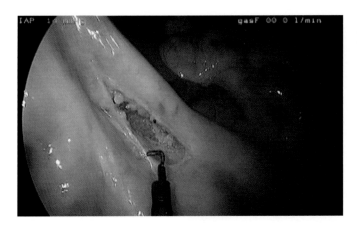

Figure 3.3 Commencing the dissection of the ileocolic pedicle in the avascular plane.

A wide window is made in the peritoneum inferior to the ileocolic pedicle as the retroperitoneal structures are gently swept away in a posterior direction (Fig. 3.3). A mesenteric window is then made on the superior aspect of the ileocolic pedicle, and the pedicle should be isolated adequately to allow for easy vessel division. The surgeon should clearly identify the duodenum to avoid injury (Fig. 3.4).

The division of the ileocolic pedicle can be performed using vessel sealing energy devices, laparoscopic staplers, or clips. The level of division of this vessel will depend on the surgical indication. For malignancy, this pedicle should be proximally divided so as to maximize the lymph node harvest (Fig. 3.5). In cases of Crohn's disease where the mesentery may be thickened, the vessel is divided where it is soft (usually more proximal than distal).

Right Branch of the Middle Colic Vessels
The next series of maneuvers will assist in the identification of the middle colic vessels. First, the previously cut leaf of the peritoneum overlying the duodenum is lifted (it would have been divided during the isolation of the ileocolic pedicle). The duodenum and head of pancreas are then swept posteriorly and separated from the right side of the middle colic vessels (Fig. 3.6). This step must be performed carefully and gently, as excessive force will cause a rip in the pancreaticoduodenal or gastroepiploic vein, resulting in significant hemorrhage. This dissection proceeds deeper and in a cephalad direction, until the transverse colon is separated from the duodenum.

Once there is adequate space to the right of the middle colic vessels, the middle colic pedicle is anteriorly lifted using two points of retraction, one to the right and one to the left of the pedicle (Fig. 3.7). This maneuver is critical in the identification of the right and left branches of the middle colic vessels. The goal of the procedure is to divide the right branch of the middle colic vessels to harvest the lymph nodes draining the hepatic flexure and proximal transverse colon. The middle colic artery supplies the transverse colon and arises from the superior mesenteric artery at the inferior base of the pancreas.

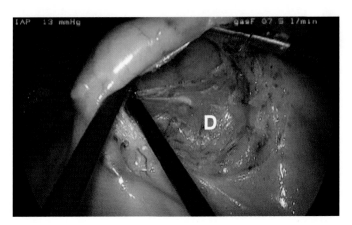

Figure 3.4 The dissection of the ileocolic pedicle with the duodenum preserved. D = duodenum.

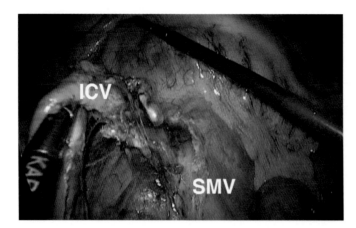

Figure 3.5 Proximal lymphadenectomy of the ileocolic pedicle. The ileocolic vein (ICV) is seen branching from the superior mesenteric vein (SMV), with the enlarged lymph nodes at the root of the ileocolic vessel cleared toward the specimen.

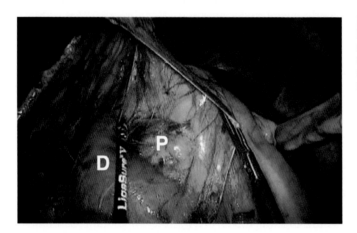

Figure 3.6 The duodenum (D) and head of pancreas (P) are swept away from the transverse mesocolon. Gentle blunt dissection is critical to avoid avulsion of veins at the head of the pancreas.

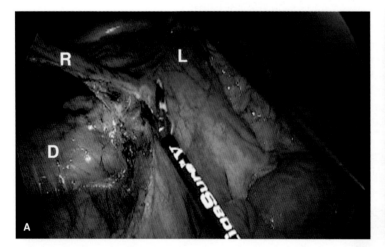
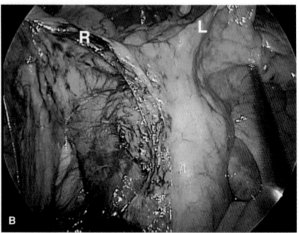

Figure 3.7 **A,B** Two examples of the exposed transverse mesocolon. Identify the right (R) and left (L) branches of the middle colic vessels with adequate two point retraction. D = duodenum.

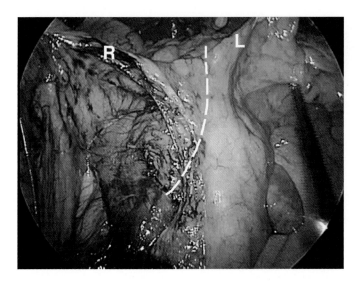

Figure 3.8 The dissection line to identify the origin of the right branch of the middle colic vessels (R).

There may be one, two, or three branches off the superior mesenteric artery, and the classic Y-shaped single trunk occurs in less than 50% of cases. An imaginary line is created from the base of the middle colic vessels toward the anticipated transection point of the transverse colon (Fig. 3.8). The peritoneum of the transverse mesocolon is then divided along this line. The takeoff of the right branch is then identified and divided at its origin (Fig. 3.9). In addition to the middle colic vessels, one will encounter a vein from the head of the pancreas to the hepatic flexure (the right colic vein, located just to the right of the middle colic vessels). This vein is isolated and divided, taking care not to injure the right gastroepiploic vein, which is its adjacent branch running on the surface of the pancreas toward the stomach (Fig. 3.10).

Retromesenteric Dissection

The right colon mesentery is then separated from the retroperitoneum in a medial-to-lateral direction. With the cut edge of the right colon mesentery retracted anteriorly, the retroperitoneal fascia, or white line of Toldt, is identified at its medial aspect, and bluntly separated from the mesentery. This is essentially avascular, and this retromesenteric dissection is taken underneath the hepatic flexure and the ascending colon to the lateral abdominal wall (Fig. 3.11). This dissection should not be carried too far posteriorly, into or underneath Gerota's fascia, and following the retroperitoneal plane of the duodenum more laterally will help maintain this proper plane. At this stage, the hepatic flexure and a thin lateral ligament of the ascending colon act as a natural retractor, keeping the otherwise floppy right colon in place.

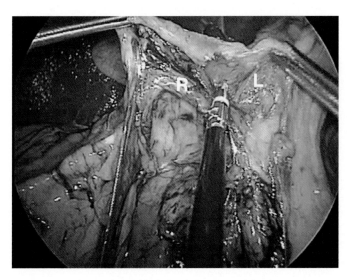

Figure 3.9 Division of the right branch of the middle colic artery at its origin. R = right branch, L = left branch.

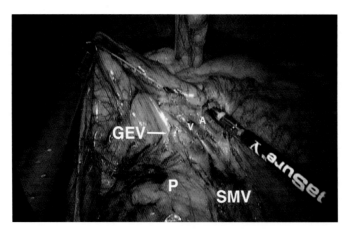

Figure 3.10 A high ligation of the middle colic vessels in locally advanced cancer. This anatomic variant shows an absent right colic vein, with a prominent right middle colic vein (V) that branches from the superior mesenteric vein (SMV). Running together is the right branch of the middle colic artery (A). Both will be ligated where visible. The right gastroepiploic vein (GEV) along the surface of the pancreas must be preserved. P = head of pancreas.

Superior and Lateral Dissection

At the level of the falciform ligament, the gastrocolic ligament is opened. As the transverse colon is inferiorly retracted, the lesser sac is dissected, and the congenital adhesions of the posterior omental leaf and the transverse mesocolon are undone. Adequate traction and tissue triangulation are necessary to identify the correct plane of dissection. Avoiding injury to the right gastroepiploic vessels, the previously dissected retromesenteric plane from the medial approach is then identified. With the transverse colon inferiorly retracted, from left to right, the hepatic flexure is taken down (Fig. 3.12). The lateral ligament of the ascending colon is divided from superiorly as the dissected colon is gradually retracted into the pelvis, until the right psoas muscle and right iliac vessels are identified (Fig. 3.13). The retroperitoneal fascia is preserved, as the mesentery of the ileocecal region is widely dissected from the retroperitoneum. It is often possible to identify the right ureter during this dissection, and this structure should be maintained underneath the intact retroperitoneal fascia if the dissection is properly performed.

Inferior Dissection

The only remaining attachments are from the ileum to the retroperitoneum. The patient is now placed in the steep Trendelenburg position as the dissected right colon is placed back into its original position. The small bowel loops in the pelvis are completely retracted in a superior direction (Fig. 3.14). With the distal ileum retracted anteriorly and superiorly, the ileal attachments to the retroperitoneum are taken down. Strong traction is needed to retract the tissues away from the right iliac vessels and to avoid injury to the right ureter. This dissection is taken laterally around the appendix and cecum, meeting the previous superior dissection (Fig. 3.15). The medial extent of this ileal mobilization is the right iliac vessel; this will ensure adequate reach of the small bowel to the transverse colon for anastomosis.

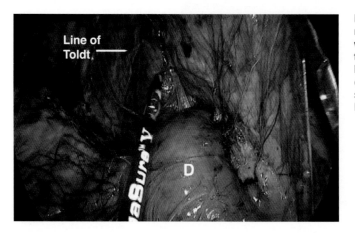

Figure 3.11 Medial-to-lateral retromesenteric dissection. The white line of Toldt is seen from the medial aspect, as this is bluntly separated from the right colon mesentery. A tattoo stains the region of dissection. D = duodenum.

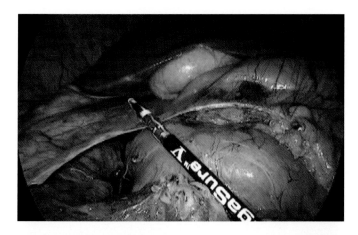

Figure 3.12 Superior takedown of the hepatic flexure. The transverse colon is inferiorly retracted.

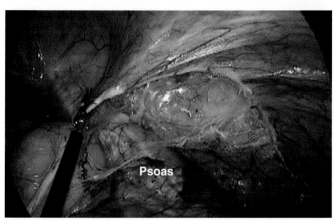

Figure 3.13 The lateral ligament of the right colon is dissected until the right colon is mobilized past the right psoas muscle.

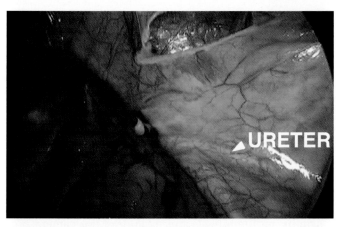

Figure 3.14 The ileum is retracted in a superior direction to expose the mesenteric attachments to the retroperitoneum; the right ureter is visualized and the small bowel is retracted out of the pelvis as much as possible.

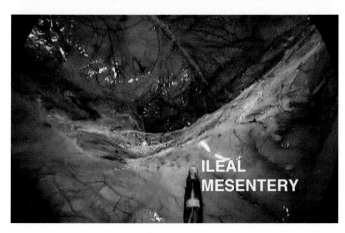

Figure 3.15 The ileal attachments to the retroperitoneum are divided, connecting with the dissection commencing superiorly. Continue this mobilization over the right iliac vessels.

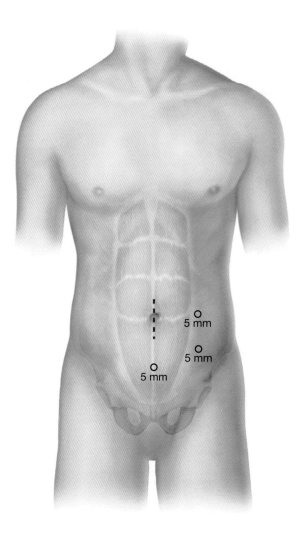

Figure 3.16 A minilaparotomy is usually created for the exteriorization of the specimen, as a superior extension of a vertically placed infraumbilical port wound.

Exteriorization, Bowel Division, and Anastomosis

At this point in time, the intracorporeal dissection is complete, and the right colon is ready for exteriorization, bowel transection, and extracorporeal anastomosis. Using a locking bowel grasper through the left lower abdominal port, the fat of the ileocecal region is grasped for identification through the small incision.

A small incision is now created. Prior to making the incision, however, one must ensure adequate reach of the transverse colon to the proposed incision site; if not, one risks an unnecessarily difficult anastomosis, or undue tension and tearing of the middle colic vessels. This incision is usually periumbilical, and extending the camera port superiorly for 3–6 cm is generally adequate (an incision may need to be larger in cases of obesity or large tumor) (Fig. 3.16).

A wound retractor is placed to avoid a port site recurrence in cases of malignancy. The grasped ileocecal region is brought into view through the small incision, and the dissected right colon is exteriorized and placed in its native configuration (Fig. 3.17). The remainder of the ileal mesentery and marginal artery of the transverse colon are dissected toward the bowel wall. The bowel is divided and an ileocolic anastomosis is created. The type of anastomosis depends on surgeon preference (hand-sewn, stapled functional end-to end, or stapled end-to-side anastomosis) (Fig. 3.18).

The author makes it a practice to leave the ports in and to reinsufflate the abdomen for a "final look" after the minilaparotomy is closed. This assures hemostasis, no twisting of the anastomosis, and no migration of the small bowel into the mesenteric defect.

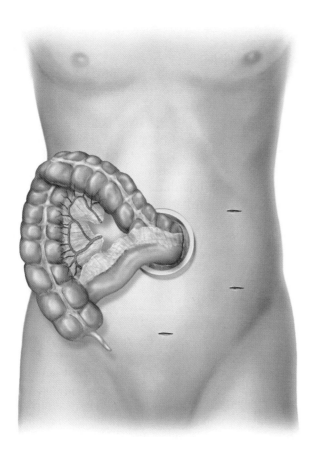

Figure 3.17 The exteriorized right colon anatomically displayed, ready for division and anastomosis.

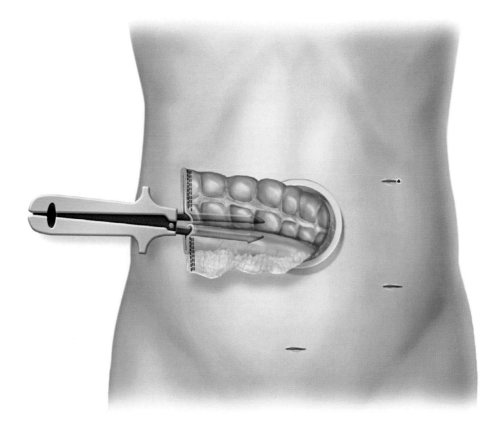

Figure 3.18 A functional end-to-end anastomosis. It is critical to keep the ileum from twisting 360 degrees around its mesentery.

Common Pitfalls and Solutions

Difficulty in the Identification of the Ileocolic Pedicle

The ileocolic artery exists in 100% of anatomic specimens, and always courses underneath the duodenum to the ileocecal area. Make sure that the duodenal sweep is identified through the thinned area of the transverse mesocolon. There is occasionally a congenital fusion of the transverse mesocolon and the right colon mesentery that needs to be undone first. Difficulty in identification of the pedicle mostly results from obesity. If the duodenum is hidden underneath thick fat, start the dissection of the ileocolic pedicle superior to it, and identify the duodenum. The ileocecal region must be placed on enough tension to tent up the pedicle through the thick mesenteric fat. For persistent difficulty, try an inferior approach, where the patient is placed in a steep Trendelenburg position, and the entire small bowel is retracted superiorly. Underneath the ileal mesentery close to the midline, the duodenum should become visible, and from here, the ileal mesentery should be dissected off the retroperitoneum. The ileocolic pedicle will be mobilized from the retroperitoneum and should now be identified readily from the medial approach.

Difficulty in the Dissection of the Middle Colic Vessels

The middle colic vessels need to be retracted away from the retroperitoneal structures using two points of retraction, as vertically as possible. Imagining a "Y" configuration of the middle colic vessels is important. However, due to obesity or short length of the middle colic vessels, this medial approach may be difficult. A superior approach should then be taken. With the transverse colon inferiorly retracted, the gastrocolic ligament should be opened, and the transverse mesocolon dissected free from the posterior leaf of the omentum. The right branch can then be identified and divided from this view, or the transverse colon can be placed back into its original position and a medial approach can be taken. By freeing the posterior attachments of the middle colic vessels, the vessels are effectively elongated, allowing the right branch to be readily identified. If this approach is still not adequate, use the "open book" method. The transverse colon is first divided using an intracorporeal stapler, and the transverse mesocolon is then dissected in an inferior direction toward the bifurcation of the middle colic vessels as the two ends of the colon are separated.

Poor Reach of the Transverse Colon to the Umbilicus

This problem occurs most commonly in obese patients who have a short transverse mesocolon. The options in this setting are to take the dissection of the transverse colon further to the left to increase its reach, or to make a minilaparotomy in the epigastric area close to the distal transection point of the transverse colon. It is simpler to alter the placement of the small incision.

Anastomotic Twisting and Mesenteric Hernia

After the ileal mesentery and ileum are divided, the ileum can be inadvertently twisted 360 degrees during the transverse colon division. Avoid any confusion by placing two stay sutures, one at the end of the ileum and one proximal to it, with the sutures clamped and separated. With this maneuver, it is even possible to place the ileum back into the abdomen without losing its correct orientation in cases where the transverse colon does not exteriorize well through the minilaparotomy.

It is generally not necessary to close the mesenteric defect after a right hemicolectomy. The defect is large, and it is uncommon that a mesenteric hernia develops resulting in incarceration; over time, this defect closes by reperitonealization. In a recent retrospective study of 530 patients, the incidence of complications associated with an unclosed mesenteric defect was 0.8%. By reinsufflating the abdomen after the anastomosis is completed, one can check for mesenteric twisting and small bowel herniation into the mesenteric defect.

POSTOPERATIVE MANAGEMENT

Most patients are safely managed with an accelerated perioperative care pathway, which has helped to reduce the length of hospitalization after both laparoscopic and open colectomy. The main elements of this program are preoperative education, setting of expectations, early oral feeding, and early ambulation. The other potential components of the fast-track approach include epidural anesthesia, opiate-sparing analgesia, limitations of intravenous fluids, gum chewing, and peripheral mu-opioid antagonists.

The orogastric/nasogastric tube should be removed at the time of extubation. Clear liquids are usually started on the first postoperative day, and patients are advanced to a solid diet over the next several days depending on the degree of nausea, distension, and return of bowel function. Patients are discharged home when tolerating an oral diet without significant nausea or distension, abdominal pain, or fever.

 # COMPLICATIONS

A 2009 comparison of laparoscopic and open colectomy of 8,660 patients utilizing the American College of Surgeons' National Surgical Quality Improvement Program showed that the use of laparoscopy decreased the incidence of risk-adjusted complications compared to open surgery. The overall complication rate for patients undergoing laparoscopic ileocolectomy was 15% compared with 24% for open ileocolectomy ($P < 0.05$). The rates of specific complications after laparoscopic ileocolectomy were: sepsis (4–5%), wound complications (8%), cardiopulmonary complications (3%), vascular complications (1.5%), and neurologic/renal complications (3–4%).

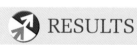 # RESULTS

Patient recovery after laparoscopic colon resection differs in accordance with the postoperative management pathway used, and as a consequence, even randomized prospective studies may report a wide range of results. Thus, a recent prospective multicenter observational study of 148 patients was performed to determine the "benchmark" of recovery when patients undergoing laparoscopic right and left colectomy were treated with a standardized accelerated postoperative care pathway. The results specific to laparoscopic right colectomy were as follows: a conversion rate of 15%, mean time to gastrointestinal recovery (passing stool and tolerating solid food) of 4.2 days, and mean time to discharge order written of 4.5 days. Prolonged postoperative ileus occurred in 10.1% of patients, with 4.7% requiring a nasogastric tube. The readmission rate was 2%.

Regarding the oncologic outcomes of laparoscopy to treat colon cancer, its equivalency to open surgery was published in the Clinical Outcomes of Surgical Therapy Study Group (COST) trial, the large multi-institutional randomized prospective trial of 872 patients. Recently, the 3 year disease-free survival data was published from the European Colon cancer Laparoscopic or Open Resection (COLOR) trial (n = 1,076), which also revealed equivalent oncologic results between laparoscopy and open surgery.

 # CONCLUSION

The medial-to-lateral laparoscopic right hemicolectomy allows for high quality surgery that abides by oncologic principles, including early high ligation of mesenteric vessels. The lateral attachments act as an excellent natural bowel retractor facilitating this approach. The surgical exposure is somewhat reversed as compared with open surgery, where a lateral mobilization is commonly performed, and surgeons will need to relearn the vascular anatomy and their relationship to the retroperitoneal structures to be able to perform a safe operation. However, even for those beginning laparoscopic colectomy, this operation will likely be one of the first to be attempted and learned.

Suggested Readings

Belimoria KY, Bentrem DJ, Merkow RP, et al. Laparoscopic-assisted vs. open colectomy for cancer: comparison of short-term outcomes from 121 hospitals. *J Gastrointest Surg* 2008;12:2001–9.

Cabot JC, Lee SA, Yoo J, Nasar A, Whelan RL, Feingold DL. Long-term consequences of not closing the mesenteric defect after laparoscopic right colectomy. *Dis Colon Rectum* 2010;53(3):289–92.

Colon Cancer Laparoscopic or Open Resection Study Group. Survival after laparoscopic surgery versus open surgery for colon cancer: long-term outcome of a randomized clinical trial. *Lancet Oncol* 2009;10:44–52.

Delaney CP, Marcello PW, Sonoda T, Wise P, Bauer J, Techner L. Gastrointestinal recovery after laparoscopic colectomy: results of a prospective, observational, muticenter study. *Surg Endosc* 2010;24(3):653–61.

Fleshman J, Sargent DH, Green E, et al.; for the Clinical Outcomes of Surgical Therapy Study Group. Laparoscopic colectomy for cancer is not inferior to open surgery based on 5-year data from the COST Study Group trial. *Ann Surg* 2007;246:655–62.

Kennedy GD, Heise C, Rajamanickam V, Harms B, Foley EF. Laparoscopy decreases postoperative complication rates after abdominal colectomy: results from the National Surgical Quality Improvement Program. *Ann Surg* 2009;249(4):596–601.

Liang JT, Lai HS, Lee PH. Laparoscopic medial-to-lateral approach for the curative resection of right-sided colon cancer. *Ann Surg Oncol* 2007;14:1878–79.

Slim K, Vicaut E, Launay-Savary MV, Contant C, Chipponi J. Updated systematic review and meta-analysis of randomized clinical trials on the role of mechanical bowel preparation before colorectal surgery. *Ann Surg* 2009;249(2):203–209.

4 Laparoscopic Lateral to Medial

Joseph B. Petelin

 ## INDICATIONS/CONTRAINDICATIONS

Laparoscopic surgery of the right colon may be indicated for a variety of reasons including uncorrectable bleeding localized to the right colon, unresectable masses of the right colon (polyps, submucosal tumors), adenocarcinoma of the right colon, tumors of the appendix or ileocecal region, cecal bascule, volvulus of the right colon, and inflammatory bowel disease of the ileum and ascending colon.

Laparoscopic right colon surgery (LRCS) may be contraindicated in some situations including patient instability precluding general anesthesia, uncorrectable coagulopathy, severe intra-abdominal adhesions, intestinal obstruction with severe distention, and inability of the surgeon to effectively and efficiently perform laparoscopic colonic surgery. The last item is quite probably the most important. It implies that the surgeon should not attempt LRCS unless he or she is able to perform a resection of the disease process (including adequate margins and nodal harvest in cases involving malignancy) in a timely manner.

 ## PREOPERATIVE PLANNING

General patient preparations, as for any general surgery operation, are routine and described elsewhere. Special preparations for right colon surgery usually include mechanical and antibiotic bowel preparation; specific aspects of these preparations are described elsewhere. In some cases, however, these preparations may be altered.

The patient should be informed of (a) the options for the approach laparotomy or laparoscopy and (b) the potential for conversion from a laparoscopic approach to an open approach if deemed appropriate by the surgeon. The author also believes that the patient should be apprised of the surgeon's training and experience with laparoscopic colectomy. There is a well-documented learning curve (1).

Recent studies suggest that surgeons with little experience and infrequent use of advanced laparoscopic techniques might benefit from a preoperative "warm up" emphasizing laparoscopic instrument handling, suturing, and knot tying.

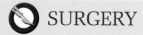 SURGERY

Positioning: Patient and Personnel

The patient is usually placed in the supine position. He or she must be secured safely to the operating table in order to prevent sliding when the table is rotated or moved from a Trendelenburg to a reverse-Trendelenburg position. A Foley urinary catheter is placed in order to keep the bladder decompressed. Although the author does not routinely use ureteral stents, some surgeons may prefer them, and they certainly may be appropriate for use in appropriately selected settings including large tumors, phlegmons, abscesses, and reoperative surgery.

The surgeon stands on the patient's left side. If a human camera holder is used, he or she is positioned on the left side. However, if a surgical assistant is used, he or she is preferentially located on the left side as well; although, for spatial considerations the assistant may be required to be located on the right side of the patient. This presents a problem for the assistant because his or her retina is opposite to that of the camera "retina"—a CCD (charge coupled device) or CMOS (complementary metal oxide semiconductor) chip; this scenario is similar to looking into a mirror and results in significant difficulty with accurate instrument manipulations (Fig. 4.1).

Equipment

Standard laparoscopic equipment is obviously necessary for performance of laparoscopic right colectomy. High definition (HD) cameras and monitors enhance the visualization

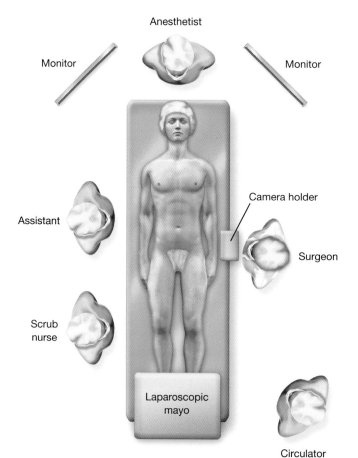

Figure 4.1 Patient and personnel positions.

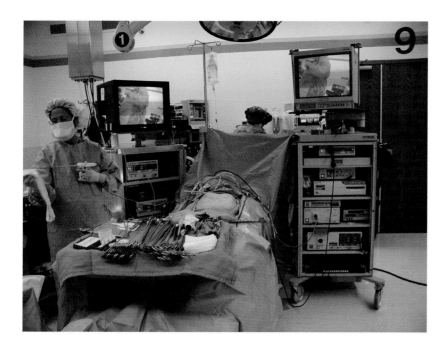

Part I: Right Colon

Figure 4.2 Room setup with patient and equipment.

of the anatomical detail encountered during the laparoscopic portion of the procedure. A straight zero degree scope is used by the author, but many others prefer a 30-degree angled laparoscope.

Laparoscopic scissors, clips, staplers, and sutures are commonly used. Over the past decade, a variety of "energy-applying" devices have dramatically improved surgeons' ability to perform dissection of the mesentery and retroperitoneum. These include unipolar and bipolar radio frequency (RF) coagulating and cutting instruments, and ultrasonic coagulating devices. The wide variety of choices available demands that the surgeon become familiar with his or her selected device(s) prior to starting the operation. The actual setup is illustrated in Figure 4.2.

Because even the antibiotically prepped colon harbors at least some bacteria, it is wise to provide abdominal wall wound protection either by placing the specimen in a plastic bag or covering the wound edges with protective materials prior to removal of the colon from the peritoneal cavity (Fig. 4.3).

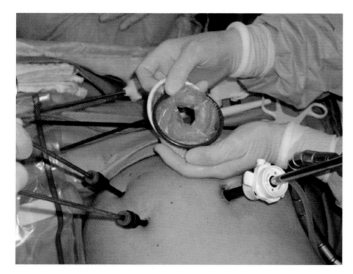

Figure 4.3 Wound protective sleeve.

Technique

General Comments About the Lateral-to-Medial Approach

Each surgeon has a preference for his or her approach to right colon surgery through a laparotomy approach. Laparoscopy has not changed those preferences, and there are strong proponents for each approach. So, the author believes that a laparoscopic right colectomy can be safely and efficiently performed by either a medial-to-lateral or a lateral-to-medial approach. This treatise is not intended to argue the case for either approach, but rather to describe the concepts and maneuvers involved in the lateral-to-medial approach.

That being said, the author prefers the lateral-to-medial approach because it allows the surgeon to identify one of the most important structures related to laparoscopic right colectomy—the right ureter—early in the case before any potentially difficult and/or dangerous mesenteric dissection is initiated. In his opinion, this method significantly reduces the stress that the surgeon may have while performing the dissection. Instead of worrying about *"where is that ureter?"* the surgeon can use that "extra brain power" to focus on the most appropriate extent of the dissection. (Consider the alternative wherein the right ureter is not identified early in the medial-to-lateral dissection, and the surgeon is required to continuously use at least "some" computational energy to be concerned about its whereabouts.) The lateral-to-medial approach is also consistent with the so-called "classical" approach to right colectomy used in open surgery by many surgeons. In fact, when laparoscopic right colectomy was first developed it was the preferred method used by most surgeons (2–5). A decade later reports describing the medial-to-lateral approach surfaced; reasons for this have been debated but this is not the subject of this material (6,7).

Port Placement

Just as with open surgery and surgeon preferences for incisions, port placement in laparoscopic surgery incites vigorous discussions, preferences, and debates regarding the "best" location for, and number of ports placed for LRCS. So, whereas there are a number of options for port placement, the author will present the port configuration that he has come to prefer after performing hundreds of laparoscopic right colon operations.

The initial port—for insufflation and initial laparoscopic scope placement–is placed near the umbilicus. It is placed through a small incision either superior or inferior to the umbilicus so that its extension, later in the case—for specimen extraction—presents an acceptable wound for closure. Some authors prefer a more lateral left abdominal placement for the scope, and the author would not argue with the appropriateness of that location for the scope. However, a midline extraction site for the specimen still seems to be best, and preferred by most laparoscopic surgeons.

The author usually prefers only two additional ports, although more ports may be added according to surgeon preference and needs. A 5 mm port (used for the surgeon's left hand instrument) is placed in the right lower quadrant, preferentially inferior to the cecum if possible. This position allows "antegrade" dissection of the lateral attachments of the right colon (similar to laparoscopic appendectomy) rather than backhanded movements of the surgeon's left hand while dissecting the lateral attachments of the colon.

The second 5 mm accessory port is placed in the upper abdomen, either in the midline or in the left upper quadrant. This port is used for the dissecting, cutting, clipping, stapling, and coagulating instruments that the surgeon uses with his or her right hand. If additional ports are required or preferred, they are most often placed in either the right upper or left upper quadrant as necessary. These extra ports are usually used to provide added exposure for the dissection of the omentum and/or mesentery.

While in most cases the camera/scope assembly can be kept in the periumbilical port, it can be moved to any of the existing ports to provide better visualization of the anatomy. Some surgeons prefer to move it to an inferior port when dissecting the lateral and mesenteric tissues, and move it to a superior position when dissecting the hepatic flexure of the colon (Fig. 4.4).

Figure 4.4 Port placement.

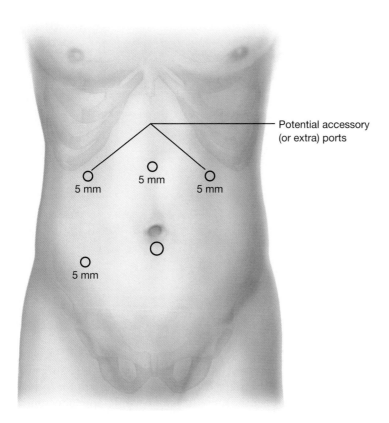

Potential accessory
(or extra) ports

5 mm   5 mm   5 mm

5 mm

Abdominal Exploration

Prior to any maneuvers to dissect the right colon, a general inspection of the abdomen is performed. This step is especially important in treating malignancy. Examination of the peritoneal surfaces and liver are paramount. The location of the primary pathology is identified either by visualizing an India ink mark (reoperatively placed by colonoscopy), a mass effect, or an inflammatory effect. The relative mobility or fixation of the colon is also important to note.

Camera Control

As previously mentioned, laparoscopic camera control may be performed by a human assistant. However, this is inherently inefficient at best, and generally very cumbersome. Ideally it would be best if the surgeon could control the view that he or she wants to see, just as in open surgery without having to direct another person to provide it. With image-based surgery, such as video laparoscopy, this would require the surgeon to somehow have real time control of the scope and camera. While this may be accomplished with high-level robotic camera control systems, such as the DaVinci™ system, the cost, cumbersome spatial requirements, and limitations of viewing angles limit their usefulness to some extent at this point in time.

Alternative simple and inexpensive mechanical systems, employing articulated semi-rigid joints, have been used to control the camera/scope assembly for over two decades by the author and others. These units provide a stable camera view, without jitter or erratic movements by a human, but do require the surgeon to effect movement of the mechanism to change the field of view. While this may seem complicated at first glance, in most cases, with a little practice, the surgeon can move the camera with little effort, and move it simultaneously while manipulating other instruments (Fig. 4.5).

Mobilizing the Colon from its Lateral and Superior Attachments

So this is the essence of the lateral-to-medial approach versus the medial-to-lateral approach to LRCS. Laparoscopic right colectomy evolved from laparoscopic appendectomy. In

Figure 4.5 Mechanical camera holder setup.

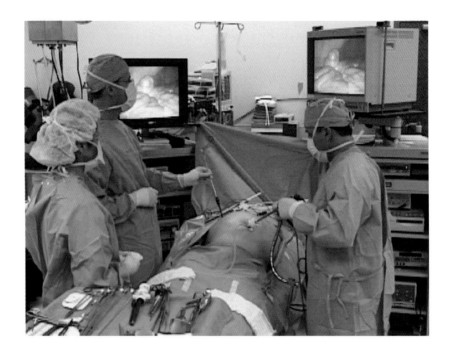

mobilizing the cecum for treatment of retrocecal appendicitis, surgeons realized that the ability to mobilize the entire right colon from a lateral approach (via the right gutter) seemed to make a lot of sense. As with laparoscopic appendectomy, the operating table is rotated to the left so that the right side of the patient is elevated with respect to the left side. The dissection is begun either from the area inferior to the cecum and proceeds superiorly, or begins at the hepatic flexure and proceeds inferiorly. Most commonly, the author proceeds from the cecum superiorly. The white line of Toldt is incised and as the cecum is rotated medially, the right ureter is identified at the pelvic brim as it crosses the iliac artery bifurcation. The ureter ascends from the pelvis superiorly and lateral to inferior vena cava and medial to the gonadal vessels until it crosses the gonadal vessels in its more superior position. The duodenum is identified medially as the dissection proceeds superiorly. The location of the ureter and the duodenum should be rechecked repeatedly throughout the procedure (Fig. 4.6).

Figure 4.6 Lateral dissection.

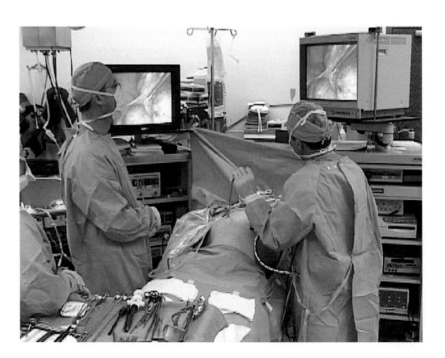

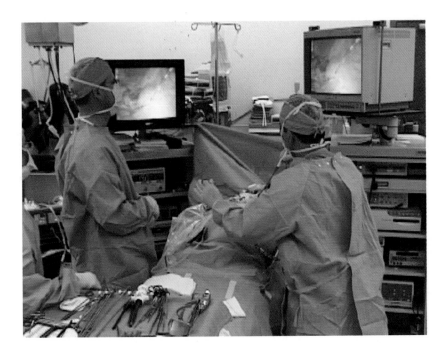

Figure 4.7   Scoring the mesentery.

Mobilizing the Hepatic Flexure and Proximal Transverse Colon

As the hepatic flexure is approached the author has found it helpful to transfer the focus of dissection from the right gutter to the area around the right side of the transverse colon. Altering the operating table to a reverse Trendelenburg position facilitates visualization while the scope is kept in the periumbilical port. Alternatively, the scope may be moved to a more superior location, but this requires altering the port that is used for the right-handed instrument. The hepatocolic and gastrocolic ligaments are divided. In most cases, unless it is involved with encasement by tumor, the omentum is freed from the proximal transverse colon. The posterior attachments of the colon around the hepatic flexure are then divided. This takes time and patience. After this is completed the right colon should be mobilized enough to proceed with the mesenteric dissection.

Mesenteric Dissection

The right colon is displaced laterally and somewhat anteriorly to display its mesentery. Positioning the operating table somewhere between a supine and left lateral decubitus position reveals the optimal visualization of the mesentery and its base. The peritoneal surface of the mesentery is scored with the unipolar RF device to delineate the "line" of dissection. This is important because without it the intended line of dissection becomes difficult to discern as the actual dissection is performed (Fig. 4.7).

The base of the mesentery is incised and the root vessels, ileocolic and right colic, are secured and divided. This can be accomplished with clips and scissors or with energy-applying devices such as the bipolar ones described previously. The remainder of the mesentery is controlled and divided most commonly with these advanced energy-delivering devices. Occasionally it is better to incise the mesentery more distally (closer to the ileum than the mesenteric root) first in order to get enough mobility to secure and divide the mesenteric root closer to its source. The remainder of the mesenteric dissection proceeds superiorly toward the distal line of intestinal resection in the transverse colon. In some cases the right branch of the middle colic vessels must be divided (Fig. 4.8).

Colonic Division and Anastomosis

The decision at this point is whether to extend the periumbilical incision, extract the colon and ileum, and perform the intestinal division and anastomosis on the surface of the abdomen or perform it all laparoscopically. The author usually prefers to do this part of the operation externally because it is usually somewhat faster and because an

Figure 4.8 Mesenteric dissection.

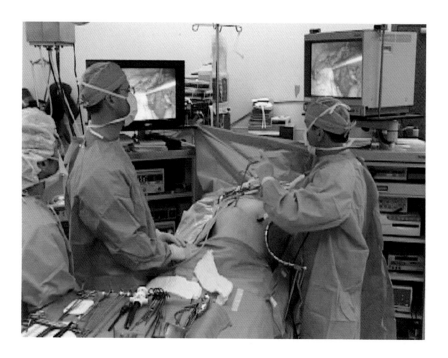

incision in the abdominal wall to remove the specimen will be required anyway. This does not, however, mean that an "extraction" incision in the abdominal wall 7 in. in length should allow the surgeon to claim that the procedure was still a laparoscopic procedure or even a laparoscopic-assisted procedure. In either instance the intestine is usually divided proximally and distally with automated staplers. The specimen is removed from the operative site and the anastomosis is then performed according to the surgeon's preference, either end-to-end or side-to-side, stapled or sutured.

Closure of the Mesentery

The topic of mesenteric closure has become controversial over the past decade, especially in regard to laparoscopic colectomy. Whereas some surgeons routinely close the mesentery when a colectomy is performed via laparotomy, some do not. The same controversy exists when the procedure is laparoscopically performed. The author believes that each surgeon should treat the mesentery with his or her preferred approach, and it should be consistent between approaches. If a surgeon usually closes it when an open approach is used, the making excuses for not closing it when a laparoscopic approach is used is not acceptable in the author's opinion. In my opinion, it should always be closed. Internal herniation and small bowel obstruction are known complications of mesenteric defects left open (8).

During a laparoscopic right colectomy, the author usually closes the base of the mesentery and extends the closure as peripherally as possible while laparoscopy is still be performed. This should help to ensure that the mesentery does not become twisted before the intestinal anastomosis is performed. The remainder of the peripheral closure can be performed while the intestine is exteriorized on the surface of the abdomen if necessary. Alternatively, the entire mesentery can be closed while the intestine is exteriorized. The latter approach usually requires a somewhat larger abdominal wall incision in order to reach the root of the mesentery, and according to author's experience is more cumbersome.

Abdominal Wall Closure

Any abdominal wall incision or port site 10 mm or larger should be closed at the fascial level, even if so-called "expanding" ports are used. Otherwise, abdominal wall hernias may develop (Fig. 4.9).

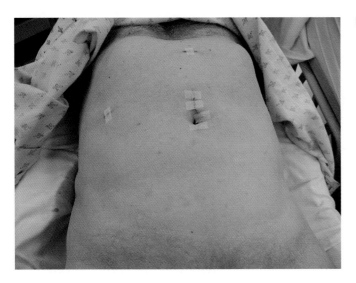

Figure 4.9 Completed wound closure.

 POSTOPERATIVE MANAGEMENT

One of the most impressive aspects of the patient's course after laparoscopic right colectomy is the lack of prolonged ileus in most cases. Patients, according to author's practice, do not usually require postoperative nasogastric decompression. In fact, in most cases, the author does not restrict oral intake unless preoperative or intraoperative indicators, such as severe distention or peritoneal contamination, predict a longer return of normal intestinal function.

Patients usually require much less parenteral and oral analgesics than their counterparts who undergo right colectomy by laparotomy. This probably results in less ileus and certainly allows them to ambulate and resume relatively normal preoperative activities sooner.

 COMPLICATIONS

Major and minor complications associated with open right colectomy and those associated with other types of laparoscopic colectomy are similar to those encountered with laparoscopic right colectomy. These include atelectasis, phlebitis, deep vein thrombosis, pulmonary embolus, hernia, prolonged ileus, bowel obstruction, anastomotic dehiscence, trocar injury, and abscess. Wound complications may be slightly less common with the laparoscopic approach.

 RESULTS

Operative time for laparoscopic right colectomy is usually somewhat longer than that for open right colectomy and ranges from approximately 1½ to 3½ hours. With increased surgeon experience shorter times are obtained. In experienced hands the quality of tissue dissection and the extent of surgical resection, including mesenteric lymph node harvest, are equivalent to or better than that achieved via laparotomy. Length of stay for patients is usually considerably less than that associated with open colectomy—3–5 days versus 5–7 days. Return of intestinal function is generally much more rapid after laparoscopic right colectomy, with patients being able to tolerate a regular diet within 3 or 4 days in most cases. Narcotic analgesic requirements are usually significantly less after laparoscopic right colectomy than after its open counterpart; this is most likely due to less surgical trauma to the abdominal wall typically seen with the laparoscopic approach. The smaller incisions also provide a nicer cosmetic appearance. All of these benefits lead to much faster mobilization of the patient and a quicker return to prehospitalization activities (9–11).

✦ CONCLUSIONS

Laparoscopic right colectomy employing the lateral-to-medial approach (and the medial-to-lateral approach for that matter) provides significant advantages to the patient. It is a much more difficult procedure than a right colectomy via laparotomy, and requires extensive training in advanced laparoscopic techniques. It is the opinion of the author that it cannot be learned in a weekend course or even a series of weekend courses. In most cases, a concentrated training experience in a minimally invasive surgical fellowship is required to achieve competency. The benefits to patients clearly make this effort worthwhile.

References

1. Jacobs M, Verdeja JC, Goldstein HS. Minimally invasive colon resection (laparoscopic colectomy). *Surg Laparosc Endosc* 1991;1:144–150.
2. Fowler DL, White SA. Laparoscopy-assisted sigmoid resection. *Surg Laparosc Endosc* 1991;1(3):183–188.
3. Elftmann T, Nelson H, Ota D, et al. Laparoscopic-assisted segmental colectomy: surgical techniques. *Mayo Clin Proc* 1994; 69:825–833.
4. Young-Fadok TM, Nelson H. Laparoscopic right colectomy—five step procedure. *Dis Colon Rectum* 2000;43:267–273.
5. Li JCM, Hon SSF, Ng SSM, et al. The learning curve for laparoscopic colectomy: experience of a surgical fellow in an university colorectal unit. *Surg Endosc* 2009;23:1603–1608.
6. Senagore AJ, Delaney CP, Brady KM, Fazio VW. Standardized approach to laparoscopic right colectomy: outcomes in 70 consecutive cases. *J Am Coll Surg* 2004;199:675–679.
7. Rotholtz NA, Bun ME, Tessio M, et al. Laparoscopic colectomy: medial versus lateral approach. *Surg Laparosc Endosc Percutan Tech* 2009;19(1):43–47.
8. Nagata K, Tanaka J, Endo S, et al. Internal hernia through the mesenteric opening after laparoscopy-assisted transverse colectomy. *Surg Laparosc Endosc Percutan Tech* 2005;3(15):177–179.
9. Lacy AM, Garcia-Valdecasas JC, Delgado S, et al. Laparoscopy-assisted colectomy versus open colectomy for treatment of nonmetastatic colon cancer: a randomized trial. *Lancet* 2002;359: 2224–2229.
10. Clinical Outcomes of Surgical Therapy Study Group. A comparison of laparoscopically assisted and open colectomy for colon cancer. *N Engl J Med* 2004;350(20):2050–2059.
11. Young-Fadok TM, Fanelli RD, Price RR, Earle DB. Laparoscopic resection of curable colon and rectal cancer: an evidence-based review. *Surg Endosc* 2007;21:1063–1068.

5 Robotic Resection

Leela M. Prasad and Sonia L. Ramamoorthy

 INDICATIONS/CONTRAINDICATIONS

The introduction of laparoscopy to colorectal surgery has created a paradigm shift in the approach to colectomy both for malignant and benign disease. The advantages of minimally invasive surgery over the traditional open approach are clearly evident when short- and long-term patient outcomes are compared. Trials designed to show oncological equivalence have demonstrated that there is no disadvantage in using laparoscopy for cancer patients (1).

Robot-assisted surgery is being increasingly utilized in a number of surgical specialties. Early reports in the United States have demonstrated the safety and feasibility of robot-assisted colectomy using the da Vinci system (2,3). Over the course of the past 5 years, robotic colorectal surgery has increased in popularity, particularly for pelvic procedures. However, the advantage of robotic assistance in a standard colectomy is still unclear (4). In this chapter, the surgical technique pros and cons and outcomes of robot-assisted right hemicolectomy will be discussed.

Advantages of the Robotic Approach

The potential advantages of robotic surgery include improved visualization, tremor filtration, motion scaling, and seven degrees of freedom provided by the robot's unique endowristed instruments. Surgeon comfort is facilitated by the ergonomically designed console and the robotic camera that is surgeon controlled can be zoomed-in to provide high magnification. With the many advantages of the system, technically challenging tasks such as intracorporeal suturing and vessel ligation are made easier. A hand-sewn intracorporeal anastomosis that is extremely challenging when laparoscopically performed is now possible with the robot.

The high definition, 3D imaging of the robotic system improves visualization and surgeon accuracy. Whether this ever translates into improved oncological outcomes with high vascular pedicle ligation, improved node retrieval, and negative radial margins remains to be seen. An important advantage unique to the robotic system is the ability of the surgeon to control three individual instrument arms. This enables the third arm to be placed in a position of fixed and stable retraction while the other two arms are used for precise retraction and dissection at the plane of dissection.

Drawbacks of the Robotic Approach

Haptic Feedback

In the transition from open to laparoscopic surgery, tactile sense was compromised. However, with experience and better instrumentation these challenges are gradually being overcome. Robotic surgery offers even less haptic feedback and therefore the surgeon must "learn" appropriate grasping pressures so as to avoid damage to the bowel and other structures. Much of that feedback relies on the lines of tissue tension upon which the extent of retraction and force applied on the tissues must be based. The three-dimensional imaging does go a long way in recognizing these visual cues (5). Initially developed as a platform for cardiac surgery, the robotic system is limited in the range of available instruments for surgery on the bowel. New instruments for the robotic arms are slowly evolving as the utilization of robotic assistance increases across different surgical specialties. Figure 5.1 depicts the tissue graspers currently available for colorectal surgery.

Cost

There is much debate over the costs of robot-assisted surgery. In a study by Delaney et al. (3), a direct comparison of robot-assisted with laparoscopic colectomy was performed using case matched controls. The authors concluded that although a robot-assisted colectomy was safe and feasible, the additional cost was a matter of concern. A similar study by Rawlings et al. (6) confirmed the safety and efficacy of robotic colectomy but reported similar findings of a longer operative time and a higher cost. We recently conducted a cost analysis in a series of 40 consecutive robotic right hemicolectomies and compared it to the cost associated with a laparoscopic right colon resection (7). The initial investment to procure the robot as well as the maintenance and ongoing costs for the robot was also considered. Costs associated with a robotic procedure were higher in every cost category.

Figure 5.1 Bowel graspers for the da Vinci robot.

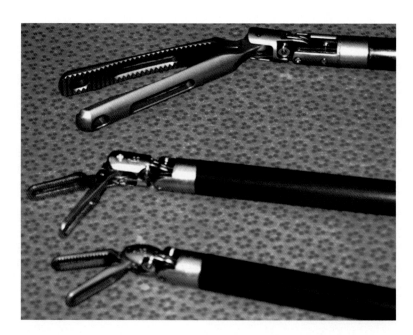

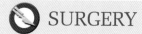 SURGERY

Setup and Preparation

The entire robotic system is a bulky apparatus consisting of the robotic cart, the vision cart, and the surgeon's console, which can take up a significant amount of space in the operating room (OR). Selecting an OR of sufficient size and establishing dedicated ORs for robotic surgery limit frequent transportation of the entire apparatus from one room to another. The robot, the anesthesia trolley, the mayo stand, and the operating table should be positioned before the patient is brought into the OR. As the robotic cart is used in different positions for different procedures, the setup of the OR may differ for each procedure. Figure 5.2 demonstrates a possible OR setup for a right hemicolectomy.

On average, each robotic instrument can be used up to ten times, but this can vary with the type of instrument used. The validity of the required robotic instruments must be verified before the procedure to limit intraoperative delays. Draping the robotic arms with the specially crafted disposable drapes and calibration of the robotic camera are other aspects of robot setup that must be performed by the scrub

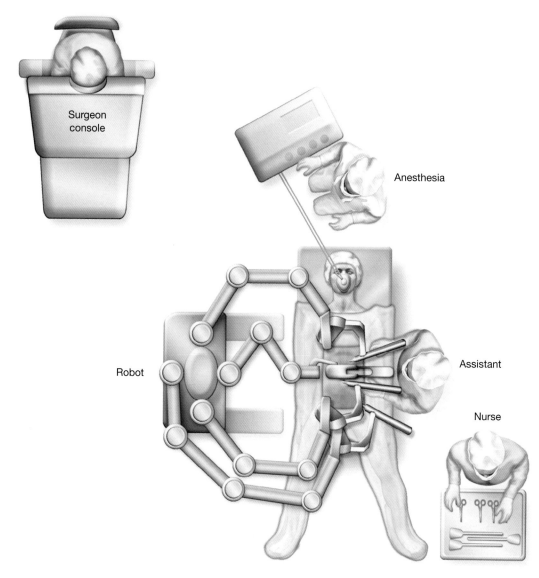

Figure 5.2   Operating room setup for robotic right hemicolectomy.

nurse. Significant time can be saved by using an OR nursing team trained in the setup and functioning of the robot.

Patient Positioning

For a right hemicolectomy, either a supine or lithotomy position can be used. Lithotomy allows for some excursion of the robot arms between the legs if needed, although this must be weighed against the interference from the stirrups that are used for lithotomy positioning. Since access to the perineum is not necessary for right colectomy, the split-leg stirrups are optimal when a lithotomy position is chosen. Both arms are tucked in beside the patient and the patient is secured to the operating table using a suction operated bean bag. Careful attention should be paid to protecting pressure points with adequate padding to avoid postoperative neuropathy. Additional shoulder harnesses are placed to support the patient when placed in the Trendelenburg position. Patient positioning is tested for security before the operative site is prepped and draped to enable changes to be made if required.

The robot is brought in from the right side, and the bedside assistant and scrub nurse are on the patient's left. Once the robot is docked, the patient position cannot be altered without undocking the robot.

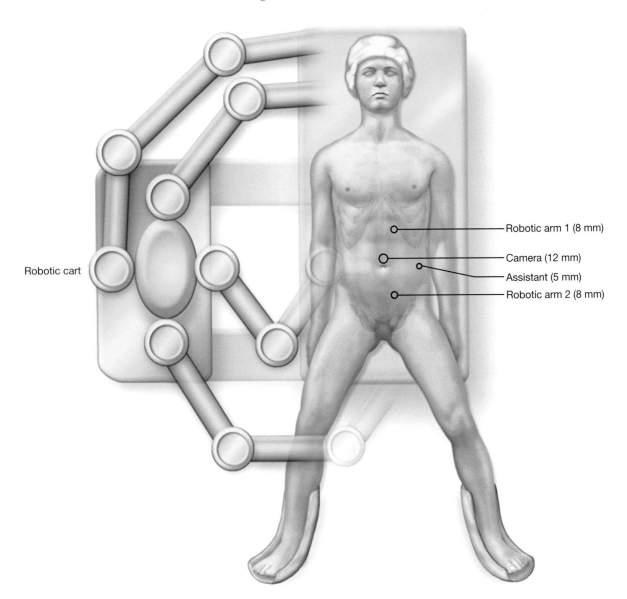

Figure 5.3 Robotic port placement (three robotic ports).

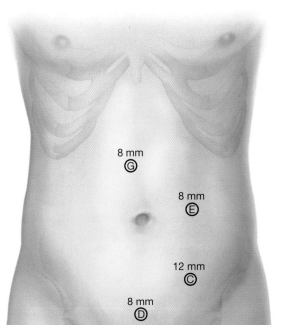

Figure 5.4   Robotic port placement (four robotic ports).

PORTS

G. Grasper

E. Energy device

C. Camera

D. Dissector

Port Placement

Port placement is vital for any robotic procedure as slight errors in port position can cause external arm collisions that can significantly reduce the intraabdominal range of movement of the robotic instruments. We routinely use just two of the three robotic instrument arms for the procedure and the port configuration is as depicted in Figure 5.3. Alternatively, the procedure can be performed using all four robotic arms as shown in Figure 5.4. We prefer to use three ports for the robot and one for the assistant, using a total of four ports that is similar to the port configuration for a laparoscopic right colon resection. When using four robotic arms, a fifth port is necessary if bedside assistance is required. Most series (Table 5.1) use the three-arm approach for a right hemicolectomy with extracorporeal anastomosis. Engagement of the fourth arm can be advantageous when performing an intraperitoneal anastomosis.

If use of a stapling device is anticipated, one robotic cannula can be inserted through a standard 12-mm laparoscopic port (Fig. 5.5). To insert the stapler, the robotic arm is undocked and the cannula is removed.

Procedure

Pneumoperitoneum is first established using the Veres needle or the Hassan Technique, and the port for the camera is inserted. The remaining ports are then inserted under vision and a diagnostic laparoscopy is performed using standard laparoscopic technique. As the robotic arms have a limited range of movement it is beneficial to retract

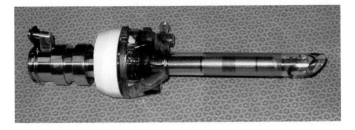

Figure 5.5   Placement of a robotic 8-mm trocar within a standard 12-mm trocar allows for ease of docking and undocking when use of an endostapling device is anticipated.

the small bowel and expose the terminal ileum and ascending colon using laparoscopic instruments, before docking the robot. Accordingly, the patient is placed in a steep Trendelenburg position with a 15–20 degree left tilt and the small bowel is displaced from the pelvis and placed in the left upper quadrant.

The robot is then positioned on the right side of the patient and docked onto the ports. Either a lateral-to-medial or medial-to-lateral approach is feasible for ascending colon mobilization.

Lateral-to-Medial Approach
A bipolar fenestrated grasper is used in robotic arm one through the epigastric port and the hook cautery is used in robotic arm two through the infraumbilical port. The cecum is grasped and retracted medially and the peritoneum is incised in the right paracolic gutter along the line of Toldt. This maneuver opens the avascular retroperitoneal plane that is developed lateral to medial till the second portion of the duodenum is encountered. The right ureter and gonadal vessels are visualized and preserved. Traction by the assistant on the cecum during this part of the dissection aids in visualization (Fig. 5.6A–D).

Medial-to-Lateral Approach
The cecum is grasped by the assistant and laterally retracted to tent up the ileocolic pedicle. Using the hook cautery in robotic arm one and the bipolar fenestrated grasper in robotic arm two, the ileocolicpedicle is dissected and isolated. This is then divided

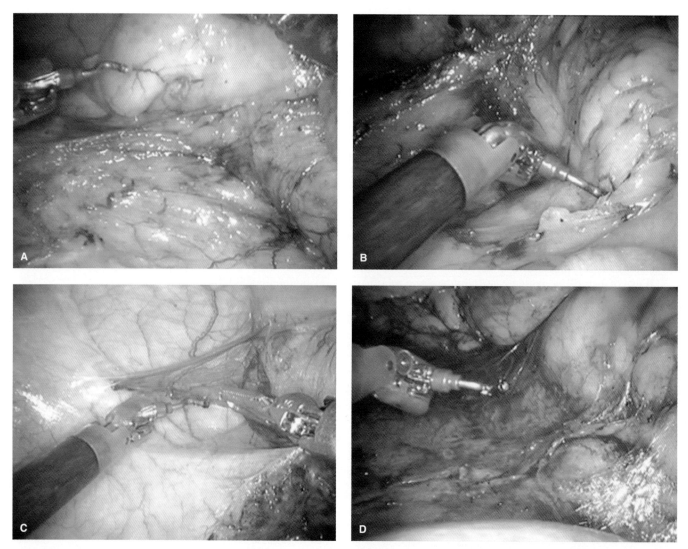

Figure 5.6 **A**. Release of the peritoneal reflection beginning at the appendix. **B**. Lateral-to-medial mobilization. **C**. Dissection proceeding superiorly to the hepatic flexure. **D**. Colon mobilized medially till the third portion of the duodenum.

by the assistant using an appropriate energy device inserted through the assistant port. The retroperitoneal avascular plane is developed to identify the second portion of the duodenum medially. Dissection is carried out in this plane, medial to lateral, to mobilize the ascending colon. The cecum is then retracted medially and the peritoneum is incised along the line of Toldt in the right paracolic gutter to complete the medial-to-lateral mobilization of the ascending colon (Fig. 5.7A–E).

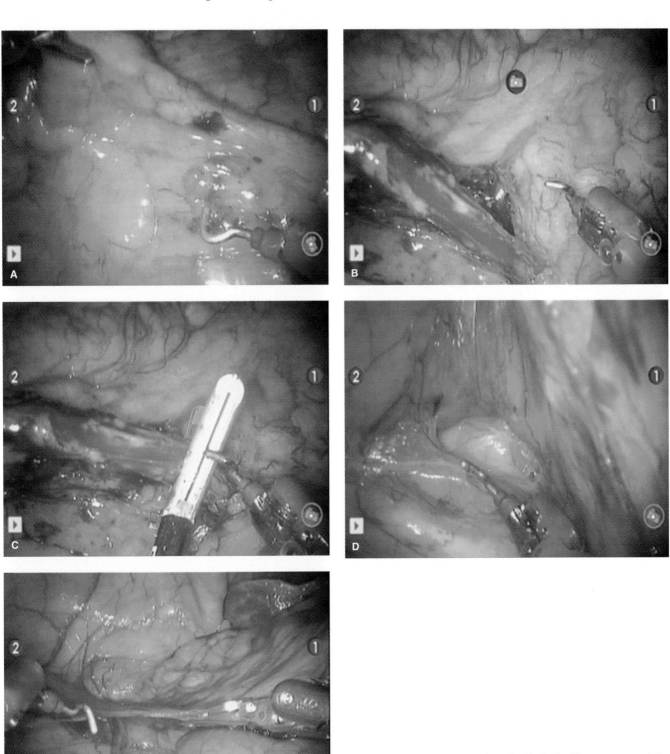

Figure 5.7 **A**. The cecum is retracted with the Cadiére graspers and the ileocolic vessels are identified. **B**. Isolation of the Ileocolic pedicle and identification of the duodenum. **C**. Ligation of the ileocolic pedicle with an energy source, or stapler. **D**. Dissection of the mesentery off the retroperitoneum toward the hepatic flexure. **E**. Division of the lateral peritoneal reflection.

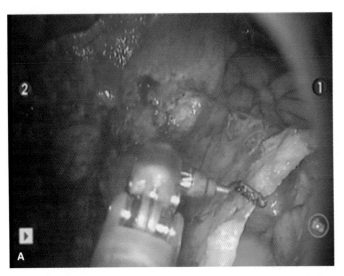 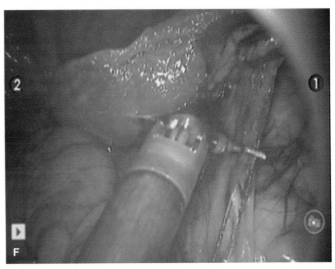

Figure 5.8 A. Division of gastrocolic omentum and mobilization of the proximal transverse colon. **B**. Hepatic flexure mobilization.

Attention is then directed to the mobilization of the hepatic flexure. It often helps to place the patient in a reverse Trendelenburg position for this part of the procedure as this displaces the transverse colon inferiorly. However, the robotic arms need to be undocked from the ports for this change in patient position. The gastrocolic omentum is then divided using the harmonic grasper in robotic arm one to enter the lesser sac. Dissection is then carried toward the hepatic flexure to disconnect the omentum from the proximal transverse colon. The hepatocolic ligament is then divided and the hepatic flexure is retracted medially to divide the final attachments to the retoperitoneum (Fig. 5.8A–B).

The incision for the camera port is then superiorly extended to create a small midline, minilaparotomy through which the specimen is exteriorized. Bowel transection and a standard side-to-side stapled ileocolic anastomosis can then be performed using open techniques. When using a lateral-to-medial approach, the vascular pedicles can be divided intracorporeally although the location of the minilaparotomy gives direct access to the root of the vascular pedicles making extracorporeal vascular pedicle division very easy.

Although the robot does enable one to perform an intracorporeal hand-sewn anastomosis, the technique of a totally robotic hand-sewn intracorporeal ileocolic anastomosis is still being evaluated for safety and efficacy. Data on the complications and anastomotic leaks associated with this technique are necessary before it can be adopted as an acceptable standard of care.

RESULTS

The safety and feasibility of robotic assistance in right hemicolectomy has been demonstrated in a number of published reports (Table 5.1). However, no report was able to demonstrate an objective advantage for the robot over conventional laparoscopy. Moreover, the use of the robot is associated with a longer operating time and a higher cost, questioning the role of the robot in this procedure.

The potential benefit of robotic assistance is probably most appreciated in pelvic procedures, where the confined surgical field makes retraction and precise dissection cumbersome and time-consuming. The seven degrees of freedom, superior visualization, and stable third arm retraction of the robot are distinctly advantageous in this setting. From a colorectal standpoint, rectal resections appear to be most suited for robotic assistance. However, performing a total mesorectal excision (TME) for cancer is

TABLE 5.1	Reported Robotic Case Series with Right Hemicolectomy		
Author (year)	**No. of cases**	**Type (number of cases)**	**Outcome (robot vs. laparoscopic)**
Delaney et al. (2003) (3)	6	Right (2), sigmoid (3), rectopexy (1)	Time: 165 min vs. 108 min Complications, LOS, EBL: NS
Anvari et al. (2004) (8)	10	Right (5), left (2), LAR (2), subtotal (1)	Time: 155.3 min vs. 94.4 min Complications, LOS, EBL: NS
D'Annibale et al. (2004) (9)	53	Right (10), left (28), LAR (10), APR (1), total colectomy (2), Hartmann (1), rectopexy (1)	Time: 240 min vs. 222 min Complications, LOS, EBL: NS
Spinoglio et al. (2008) (10)	50	Right (18), left (10), LAR (19), APR (1), transverse colectomy (1), total colectomy (1)	Time: 383 min vs. 266 min Complications, LOS: NS
Rawlings et al. (2007) (6)	30	Right (17), sigmoid (13)	Right hemicolectomy: Time: 218.9 min vs. 169.2 min LOS, EBL: NS
deSouza et al. (2010) (7)	40	Right (40)	Time: 158.9 min vs. 118 min Complications, LOS, EBL: NS

APR, abdominoperineal resection; EBL, estimated blood loss; LAR, low anterior resection; LOS, length of stay; NS, no significant difference.

Part I: Right Colon

a challenging procedure and a robotic TME is therefore best attempted in the later half of the learning curve.

A right hemicolectomy on the other hand is a relatively easy procedure and can be performed with just two robotic instrument arms. In addition, conversion to either the open or laparoscopic approach can easily be achieved should the need arise. The procedure is therefore an excellent learning tool and is ideally suited to begin clinical experience with the robot. Once the basic techniques of robotic surgery have been acquired, more advanced procedures can be attempted.

An intracorporeal hand-sewn anastomosis though technically challenging with conventional laparoscopy is now made easier with the three-dimensional imaging and endowristed movement of the robot. With an intracorporeal anastomosis, the specimen could be extracted through a Pfannenstiel incision that is associated with fewer complications and a significantly lower hernia rate. However, the optimal technique for a robotic hand-sewn intracorporeal anastomosis is still being developed and results on the complications and leak rates associated with this technique are still awaited.

Single incision laparoscopic surgery is a fairly recent concept that is being extensively investigated. Of all the colorectal procedures, a right colon resection appears most suited for single incision laparoscopy. However, the crossing of laparoscopic instruments in this technique places the instrument controlled by the surgeon's right hand on the left side of the screen and vice versa. This can be quite difficult to get accustomed to and is usually associated with a steep learning curve. The robot on the other hand is capable of switching masters, and control of the instrument on one side of the visual field can be assigned to the ipsilateral hand although the instruments are crossed. This feature of the da Vinci robot has significant potential in single incision surgery. The feasibility of a robot-assisted single incision right hemicolectomy is currently being evaluated and an initial report on the early experience with this technique has recently been published (11).

CONCLUSIONS

The da Vinci robotic system offers numerous technological advances to the minimally invasive surgeon and is being increasingly used in a wide variety of colorectal procedures. Although a robot-assisted right hemicolectomy has been shown to be safe and feasible, no definite advantage for the robot has been demonstrated in this procedure at this stage. However, a right hemicolectomy serves as an effective learning tool to acquire the basic skills in robotic surgery before progressing to more challenging procedures. Robotic assistance greatly facilitates intracorporeal suturing and a hand-sewn, intracorporeal anastomosis is now simplified with the robot though the results of this technique are still awaited. Single incision surgery is a relatively new surgical approach and the robot shows great potential in this field. The future will surely see more advanced versions of the robotic surgical system and a greater utilization of robotic assistance in routine surgical practice.

Acknowledgment

The authors' wish to thank Ashwin L. deSouza, M.D., for his help with the preparation of the manuscript.

Recommended References and Readings

1. Fleshman J, Sargent DJ, Green E, et al.; for The Clinical Outcomes of Surgical Therapy Study Group. Laparoscopic colectomy for cancer is not inferior to open surgery based on 5-year data from the COST Study Group trial. *Ann Surg* 2007;246(4):655–62.
2. Weber PA, Merola S, Wasielewski A, Ballantyne G. Telerobotic-assisted laparoscopic right and sigmoid colectomies for benign disease. *Dis Colon Rectum* 2002;45:1689–96.
3. Delaney CP, Lynch AC, Senagore AJ, Fazio VW. Comparison of robotically performed and traditional laparoscopic colorectal surgery. *Dis Colon Rectum* 2003;46:1633–39.
4. Wexner SD, Bergamaschi R, Lacy A, et al. The current status of robotic pelvic surgery: results of a multinational interdisciplinary consensus conference. *Surg Endosc* 2009;23:438–43.
5. Hagen ME, Meehan JJ, Inan I, Morel P. Visual clues act as a substitute for haptic feedback in robotic surgery. *Surg Endosc* 2008;22(6):1505–8.
6. Rawlings AL, Woodland JH, Vengunta RK, Crawford DL. Robotic versus laparoscopic colectomy. *Surg Endosc* 2007;21:1701–8.
7. deSouza AL, Prasad LM, Park JJ, et al. Robotic assistance in right hemicolectomy: is there a Role? *Dis Colon Rectum* 2010;53(7):1000.
8. Anvari M, Birch DW, Bamehriz F, et al. Robotic-assisted laparoscopic colorectal surgery. *Surg Laparosc Endosc Percutan Tech* 2004;14(6):311–5.
9. D'Annibale A, Morpurgo E, Fiscon V, et al. Robotic and laparoscopic surgery for treatment of colorectal diseases. *Dis Colon Rectum* 2004;47(12):2162–8.
10. Spinoglio G, Summa M, Priora F, et al. Robotic colorectal surgery: first 50 cases experience. *Dis Colon Rectum* 2008;51:1627–32.
11. Ostrowitz MB, Eschete D, Zemon H, DeNoto G. Robotic-assisted single incision right colectomy: early experience. *Int J Med Robot* 2009;5(4):465–70.

6 Hand-Assisted Right Hemicolectomy

Christine M. Bartus, Deborah R. Schnipper, and Jeffrey L. Cohen

Introduction

Hand-assisted laparoscopic (HAL) surgery involves the intra-abdominal placement of a hand through a minilaparotomy incision while pneumoperitoneum is maintained. The HAL approach is thought to facilitate colonic mobilization while maintaining the benefits of laparoscopic surgery. Laparoscopic colectomy lends itself to hand-assisted techniques. Most surgeons make an abdominal incision near the end of a laparoscopic-assisted colectomy to extract the specimen. This incision is often utilized to divide the mesentery or to fashion the anastomosis. Supporters of the hand-assisted technique believe that the hand should be placed through the wound to facilitate dissection and mobilization of the colon. By 1992, a number of surgeons began to make this incision early in the operation to facilitate dissection and return tactile sensation to the procedure. The hand can be used, similar to an open procedure, to palpate organs or tumors, reflect structures atraumatically, retract sutures, identify vessels, dissect bluntly, and to provide finger pressure to bleeding points while proximal control is obtained. The development of new sleeveless hand-assisted devices provides for hand exchanges without the loss of pneumoperitoneum, thus, allowing the operation to proceed without interruption. In addition, these devices protect the wound, act as a retrieval site for the specimen, and serve as the portal for construction of the extra-corporeal anastomosis (1).

Randomized trials by the HALS Study group (2,3) and by Targarona et al. (4) demonstrated that HAL resection provides similar results to traditional laparoscopic colectomy with fewer conversions. Kang et al. (5) performed a study comparing hand-assisted versus open colectomy and showed that the hand-assisted approach resulted in shortened postoperative ileus, shortened length of stay, and smaller incision size with no difference in operative time or complications. A multicenter randomized prospective study group showed that hand-assisted left and total colectomy takes less time than laparoscopic and results in equivalent short term outcomes (6).

The procedures that can potentially benefit most from the hand-assisted technique are those operations that already require the creation of a minilaparotomy for their completion. More specifically, hand-assisted right hemicolectomy for cancer or benign disease involves extracorporeal bowel division and creation of the anastomosis after complete mobilization of the bowel. The approach was developed to balance the competing demands of optimizing patient benefits and simplifying the procedure, such that it may be more readily taught and learned. A completely laparoscopic approach, with creation of an intracorporeal anastomosis, still requires an extraction incision to remove the specimen and risks spillage of bowel contents, takes longer, costs more (uses more stapler reloads), and is technically more demanding with no demonstrated benefit to the patient. Thus, HAL right hemicolectomy will be described here as a viable and safe alternative to open right hemicolectomy.

INDICATIONS

Accepted indications for laparoscopic colectomy include most benign colonic diseases, such as colorectal polyps, rectal prolapse, diverticular disease, inflammatory bowel disease, intestinal stomas for diversion, volvulus, and symptomatic colonic lipomas. Right hemicolectomy is also performed for acutely bleeding angiodysplastic lesions that cannot be controlled with nonoperative therapy. More recently, data has emerged to support the use of laparoscopic techniques for malignant colonic disease, in addition to adenocarcinoma of the appendix.

Laparoscopic sigmoid resection remains the leading indication for minimally invasive colon resection for benign disease. Inflammatory bowel disease, both Crohn's disease and ulcerative colitis, can be laparoscopically treated. For example, the majority of reports have shown that laparoscopic total colectomy and laparoscopic proctocolectomy with and without ileoanal pouch construction are technically feasible and share the same advantages of minimally invasive surgery as segmental colon resection. Laparoscopic proctocolectomy has been performed in the elective setting, but several groups have performed laparoscopic total colectomy for acute unresolving colitis in the urgent setting. Neither procedure is recommended for the patient with toxic colitis.

Early in the history of laparoscopic resection of colon cancer, there was controversy related to the phenomenon of cancer implants at incision sites. However, subsequent extensive data from numerous large randomized controlled trials have supported the safety of minimally invasive approaches. Oncologic techniques must not be compromised by laparoscopic resection for colon cancer. Standard principles must be adhered to with the laparoscopic technique, including acceptable proximal and distal resection margins based upon the area supplied by the named feeding vessel, mesenteric lymphadenectomy containing a minimum of 12 lymph nodes and ligation of the primary feeding vessel at its base (7).

PREOPERATIVE PLANNING

Prior to any surgery, a definitive diagnosis should ideally be established. Colonoscopy, barium enemas, and computed tomography scanning aid in the establishment of a diagnosis. The specific choice of modality should be tailored to the individual patient presentation. With the exception of the ileocecal valve, much of the colon displays indistinct geography. Due to the lack of easily identifiable landmarks, India ink tattooing may be used to mark lesions located in segments of bowel remote from the ileocecal valve (1). The ink is injected into the submucosa in three or four quadrants around the lesion. Other options for localization involve the placement of metallic clips or intraoperative endoscopy. If clips are placed, immediate postoperative abdominal X-rays or intraoperative imaging with laparoscopic ultrasound or fluoroscopy should be utilized to locate the clips. This procedure is less frequently used, as the presence of an experienced radiologist and/or endoscopist is required.

Patient selection is a key component of preoperative planning. Patients with a history of severe cardiopulmonary disease, hepatic disease, coagulopathy, and significant respiratory compromise should not be considered for laparoscopic colectomy. Obesity and the distribution of intra-abdominal fat may preclude laparoscopic resection. In addition, the presence of extensive intra-abdominal adhesions favors open procedures. Patients with larger tumors or lesions are less likely to be candidates for minimally invasive procedures as larger specimens necessitate larger incisions for specimen removal. Prior to any laparoscopic operation, both the surgeon and the patient must be cognizant of the possibility of conversion to a standard laparotomy.

Standard bowel preparation should be provided, in addition to an epidural catheter or a patient controlled analgesic device for postoperative pain control. Perioperative guidelines address the use of bowel preparation, prophylactic antibiotics, blood cross-matching, and thromboembolism prophylaxis (8). These aspects do not differ markedly between the laparoscopic and open approach. An empty colon facilitates manipulation of the bowel with laparoscopic instruments. Preoperative use of large volume mechanical bowel preparations may leave fluid filled loops of small bowel that are more difficult to handle with laparoscopic instruments. A smaller volume preparation or a large volume preparation followed by laxatives may reduce the volume of residual intraluminal fluid. Alternatively, ileocolic anastomosis is safe in unprepared bowel, provided the patient's condition is reasonable.

More specifically, for malignant disease, preoperative staging, assessment of resectability, and a determination of the patient's operative risk should be made. The entire colon must be evaluated for synchronous lesions. The laparoscopic approach requires accurate localization of the tumor to a specific segment of colon, because even a known tumor may not be visualized from the serosal aspect of the bowel during laparoscopy. Failure of preoperative localization provides for the removal of the wrong segment of bowel (9,10). To ensure accurate preoperative staging with the laparoscopic approach, the liver should be evaluated with computed tomography with intravenous contrast, ultrasound, or magnetic resonance imaging. Due to the limitations in tactile sensation associated with laparoscopy, these studies should be preoperatively performed. Alternatively, intraoperative laparoscopic ultrasonography enables the surgeon to evaluate the liver at the time of colonic resection.

PROCEDURE

Positioning of Patient and Operative Team

The patient is placed supine or in Lloyd Davis position on the operating table. A restraining device should be employed to minimize the risk of patient falls during position manipulation. Pneumatic compression stockings are placed to reduce the risk of deep vein thrombosis. After induction of general anesthesia, a foley catheter and an orogastric or nasogastric tube may be placed. The left arm is tucked and the abdomen is prepped and draped in the usual sterile fashion. The surgeon, an assistant, and/or a camera operator stand on the patient's left. If there is an additional first assistant, he or she may stand on the patient's right side. Monitors are placed at the patient's shoulder level on either side (9) (Fig. 6.1).

Placement of Trocars and Exploration of Abdomen

Port placement may vary slightly depending upon surgeon preference and patient anatomy. First, a 10–12 mm trocar is placed in either the supraumbilical or infraumbilical position. The procedure involves either a cut down technique with placement of a blunt trocar or the use of a Veress needle. Pneumoperitoneum is created using standard technique and is maintained at 12–15 mmHg by an automatic CO_2 insufflator. A 10 mm

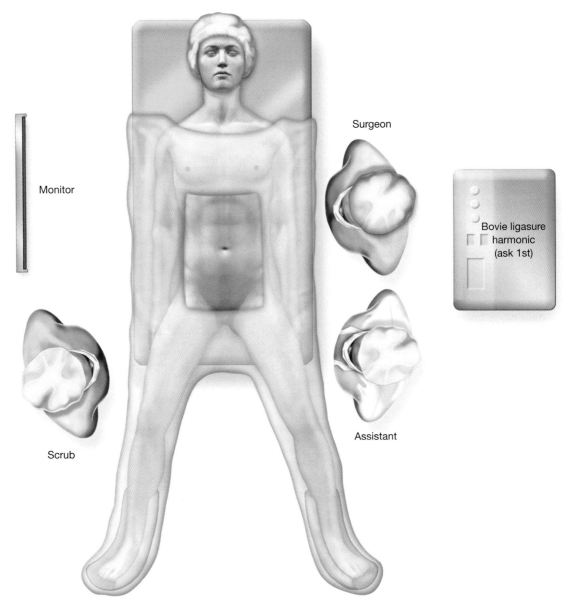

Figure 6.1 Positioning for HAL right colectomy.

30 degree laparoscope is inserted through a supraumbilical port and initial diagnostic laparoscopy is performed. The peritoneal cavity is examined for adhesions such that a conversion decision is made early. The liver and peritoneal surfaces are explored. Reasons to convert to open include massive adhesions, small bowel fixed in the pelvis, extensive right upper quadrant scarring, bulky disease, unusual anatomy, or unexpected findings. The site for hand port placement is then selected and marked on the skin. The most common site for the incision is an infraumbilical transverse or vertical midline incision. The size of the incision is usually the same size as that of the surgeon's glove. A 5–10 mm port is inserted in the left lower abdomen for the camera and an epigastric or left upper abdomen 5 mm port is placed for dissection, which facilitates separation of the omentum from the transverse colon. The previously inserted midline port may be utilized for dissection. A minilaparotomy is created at the marked site and the peritoneal cavity is entered. The lower ring of the base retractor is inserted into the peritoneal cavity, while ensuring that no bowel is trapped between the device and the anterior abdominal wall (Fig. 6.2).

Sites of incision and port placement. All measurements are in millimeters (6,7).

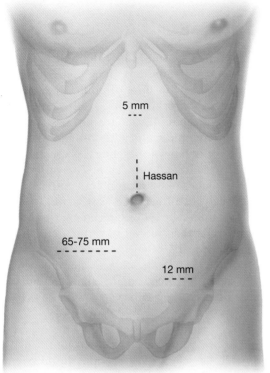

A

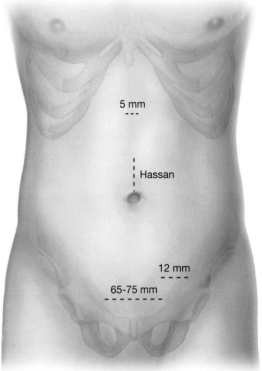

B

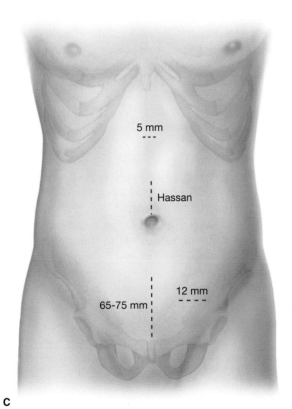

C

Figure 6.2 Hand port options for HAL right colectomy: **A.** Infraumbilical transverse incision. **B.** Periumbilical midline incision. **C.** Lower midline incision.

Mobilization of Ascending Colon and Division of the Mesenteric Vessels

Lateral-to-Medial Approach

The patient is placed in Trendelenburg, right side up. Utilizing the lateral-to-medial approach, the cecum and terminal ileum are mobilized along the right paracolic gutter by incising the patietal peritoneum at the white line of Toldt. Frequently adhesions must be sharply lysed along the right pelvic brim to the terminal ileal mesentery. In doing this, the colon is mobilized toward the midline. This process is continued moving toward the hepatic flexure using a harmonic scalpel. The proper plane of dissection lies between the retroperitoneal fat and the bowel mesentery. Dissection in this plane prevents injury to the ureter, gonadal vessels, and vena cava. This approach is used for many open procedures, and therefore, planes of dissection are familiar to most trainees (1). The duodenum must be definitively identified and care should be taken not to elevate it along with the colonic mesentery in the region of the hepatic flexure. To mobilize the hepatic flexure, the patient is then placed in reverse Trendelenburg, with right side tilted up. The greater omentum is dissected free from the transverse mesocolon along with any gastrocolic attachments. Mobilization is continued from the mid-transverse colon to complete the previously entered plane along the ascending colon. At this point, the mesentery can be divided using either a stapling device or an energy source.

Medial-to-Lateral Approach

Should the medial to lateral approach be selected, dissection would commence with the identification of the ileocolic artery. Once this is isolated, it is divided using either energy source or stapler, and the mesentery is lifted to expose the retroperitneum. These attachments are then dissected laterally. Once the retroperitoneal landmarks are clearly identified, the remaining mesentery is divided. The mesenteric vessels can be divided either intracorporeally with an energy source or an endoscopic linear cutting stapler or extracorporeally in any manner desired though the hand access port (8). The terminal ileum and right colon are then mobilized off the lateral sidewall attachments using the Harmonic scalpel or electrocautery. The transverse mesocolon is freed from the omental attachments in a matter similar to the lateral to medial approach. Finally, the remaining hepatocolic attachments are divided.

Completion of the Anastomosis and Closure

The mobilized colon is then delivered though the hand port. The bowel and any remaining vessels are divided and a standard side to side anastomosis completed using either a stapled or hand-sewn technique. The mesenteric defect need not be closed routinely. The anastomosis is returned to the peritoneal cavity followed by warm saline irrigation. The fascia is then closed and the option exists at this point to reinsufflate to confirm hemostasis and bowel positioning. Following re-examination laparoscopically, trocars are removed under direct visualization. The larger port sites are closed at the fascial level and all skin incisions are irrigated and closed at the subcuticular level with absorbable sutures. Local anesthesia is infiltrated into each of the wounds at closure.

 POSTOPERATIVE CARE

Postoperative care is similar to that of patients who have undergone open right hemicolectomy, except that a shorter recovery period may be anticipated. Patients are often started on clear liquids on the evening of surgery and maintained on epidural or parenteral analgesia until adequate oral intake is achieved. Enteral feeding is advanced on an individual basis and patients are ready for discharge when tolerating a regular diet and when pain is well controlled with oral pain medication. Hospital stays generally range from approximately 3–4 days.

COMPLICATIONS

Since the critical portions of the HAL and open techniques are the same, the complications remain similar. These potential complications include vessel injuries, enterotomies, strictures, leaks, abscess, fistulae, sepsis, and obstruction. In response to previous concerns regarding the safety of laparoscopic resection of colon cancer with regard to recurrence at port sites, multi-institutional studies have provided data in support of the safety and efficacy of laparoscopic assisted colectomy with respect to complications, time to recurrence, disease free survival, and overall survival (9).

 CONCLUSIONS

HAL right colectomy is a safe and effective alternative to open colectomy. Laparoscopic colectomy for cancer is no longer a controversial topic. Multicenter national studies have confirmed that oncologic outcomes are at least equivalent to the open approach and are not compromised by the laparoscopic approach. There is evidence that due to the reduction of surgical stress afforded by laparoscopic surgery, the immune response is impaired to a lesser extent. Some studies have shown that depressions of the cell-mediated immune response is less pronounced after laparoscopic than after open operations (10). This coupled with the decreased operative time and decreased length of hospital stay, further minimizes the impact on the patient and enhances the benefit of hand-assisted technique.

Recommended References and Readings

1. Chung CC, Chung Kei Ng D, Wen Chieng Tsang, et al. Hand-assisted laparoscopic versus open right colectomy: a randomized controlled trial. *Ann Surg* 2007;246:728–33.
2. HALS Study Group. Hand-assisted laparoscopic surgery vs. standard laparoscopic surgery for colorectal disease: a prospective randomized trail. *Surg Endosc* 2000;14:896–901.
3. Litwin D, Darzi A, Jakimowicz J, et al. Hand-assisted laparoscopic surgery (HALS) with the HandPort system: initial experience with 68 patients. *Ann Surg* 2000;231:715–23.
4. Targarona EM, Gracia E, Garriga J, et al. Prospective randomized trial comparing conventional laparoscopic colectomy with hand-assisted laparoscopic colectomy. *Surg Endosc* 2002;16:234–39.
5. Kang JC, Chung MH, Yeh CC, et al. Hand-assisted laparoscopic colectomy vs. open colectomy: a prospective randomized study. *Surg Endosc* 2004;18:577–81.
6. Marcello P, Fleshman J, Milsom J, et al. Hand-assisted laparoscopic vs. laparoscopic colorectal surgery: a multicenter, prospective, randomized trial. *Dis Colon Rectum* 2008;51:818–28.
7. Chew SSB, Adams WJ. Laparoscopic hand-assisted extended right hemicolectomy for cancer management. *Surical Ensocopy* 2007;21:1654–56.
8. Young-Fadok TM. Laparoscopic right colectomy. *Operative Techniques in General Surgery* 2005; 7(1):15–22.
9. Baca I, Perko Z, Bokan I, et al. Technique and survival after laparoscopically assisted right hemicolectomy. *Surg Endosc.* 2005;19:650–55.
10. Nelson H, Sargent DJ, Wieand HS, et al. A comparison of laparoscopically assisted and open colectomy for colon cancer. *NEJM* 2004;350:2050–59.

7 Open Medial-to-Lateral

Jorge A. Lagares-Garcia and Paul R. Sturrock

 ## INDICATIONS/CONTRAINDICATIONS

Segmental colectomy is performed to treat benign or malignant conditions of the colon. Left sided colectomy is performed as a single procedure or as a step in a complex resection such as total abdominal colectomy. The steps of the colectomy have been determined for over a century of medicine, with the most common description being the lateral-to-medial approach. However, Turnbull championed the medial-to-lateral approach as part of the "no touch" technique. Whether it is performed for benign or malignant disease, the steps are simple. The surgeon can rapidly control the vascular pedicle of the segment to be resected and proceed with the dissection. Full identification of vital structures avoids early injury.

Current indications for colon resection are displayed in Table 7.1. Strong consideration should be given to performing an open colectomy for patients who have a contraindication to laparoscopic surgery.

Debate exists in the literature regarding the optimal approach to left sided colectomy, and the proponents of medial-to-lateral approach describe this technique as more adequate when colonic pathology is lateral or adherent to the abdominal wall. This approach allows an easier access to the lateral structures (iliac vessels, ureter, renal pelvis, inferior mesenteric vein, ligament of Treitz, and splenic pedicle) through the mesenteric window.

 ## PREOPERATIVE EVALUATION

A thorough history and physical examination should be performed prior to any procedure. Special emphasis must be placed on premorbid cardiac and pulmonary disease. Also, it is important to obtain a history of any prior abdominal surgery and, if available, operative reports should be reviewed to aid in the planning of the procedure. Auxiliary studies that help complete the preoperative assessment vary depending on the underlying pathology. Whenever possible, a colonoscopy should be performed to assist in the

TABLE 7.1	Indications for Colon Resection	
Colon cancer		Inflammatory bowel disease
Endoscopically unresectable polyp		Gastrointestinal bleeding
Diverticular disease		Diverticular
Ischemic colitis		Arteriovenous malformation
Trauma with perforation		Miscellaneous
Endoscopic iatrogenic colon injury		

diagnosis and to detect any underlying synchronous processes that may alter the surgical approach. Colonoscopy also allows for tattooing of pathologic lesions to aid in operative identification. Computed tomography scanning of the abdomen and pelvis can be helpful in both benign and malignant conditions, either to identify the extent of disease or to discover the presence of intra-abdominal metastases, which also can affect the operative plan. Baseline biochemical studies should include a complete blood cell count, carcinoembiogenic antigen when malignancy is suspected, liver profile, and coagulation studies.

Preoperative anesthesia consultation should be obtained and a chest X-ray and preoperative electrocardiogram is routinely recommended. Most of the institutions have protocols regarding the performance of these tests based on age and associated risk factors.

If cardiac or respiratory comorbidity needs to be further assessed, preoperative cardiac stress test, cardiac catheterization, and pulmonary function tests may be indicated at the request of the consulting specialist.

Once the patient has been medically cleared, discussion is undertaken regarding the procedure, risks, benefits, and alternatives of the surgery and informed consent is obtained.

SURGERY

Patient Preparation

It is routine in the authors' practices to avoid mechanical and antibiotic oral bowel preparation. The patient must remain NPO for at least 6 hours prior to the procedure; this timeline may vary depending on the preferred practice of the anesthesia staff. In patients with intestinal obstruction, it is normally recommended and preferred by the anesthesia team to have a nasogastric tube inserted with decompression of the upper intestinal tract to minimize the risk of aspiration during induction of anesthesia. The morning of the procedure, the patient is instructed to perform two enemas and a chlorhexidine based soap shower.

Recent studies have shown that the use of intraoperative bispectral index guided general anesthesia on recovery in patients after colon resection resulted in earlier extubation and shorter recovery unit length of stay. This method translated into a reduction by 23% in the cost of anesthetic and also a decrease in intra- and postoperative hypotension.

After consultation with anesthesia, patients may elect for placement of an epidural catheter for postoperative pain control. In the authors' practice, we have not found significant differences in postoperative recovery in those who have had an epidural compared to patients who have not, so we routinely leave this decision up to the patient. The authors do recommend epidural placement in patients who have a low pain threshold or who have been receiving chronic narcotics, as these patients can be predicted to find it difficult to control pain after a laparotomy.

Within an hour of incision time, a prophylactic dose of antibiotic is given by anesthesia. This could be a second generation cephalosporin in an appropriately weight-based dosage. Alternatively, we have used a combination of ciprofloxacin and metronidazole if the patient has a penicillin or cephalosporin allergy. Intraoperative re-dosing of antibiotic is done at 4-hour intervals in the event of a long operative case.

Equipment

Adequate review of the equipment needed for open colectomy prior to the procedure is always recommended to avoid intraoperative delays due to the lack of equipment. All surgeons should have a preference list of equipment for each abdominal operation. Exposure during the performance of a colectomy is basic, and routinely employs the principles of triangulation for the dissection. The authors routinely use Bookwalter™ retractor (Raynham, MA, USA) for any abdominal operation. This equipment was originally idealized by Dr. John R. Bookwalter in 1964 after falling asleep during an operation while holding a retractor.

Patients in whom an extended resection of the rectum or pelvic floor is necessary at the performance of the left colectomy, we routinely have available in the operating theater a St. Mark's pelvic retractor with a 15 degree angle at the tip and a lip at the end of the blade.

To expedite the dissection and vessel ligation, we routinely use the LigaSure 10 mm diameter Impact™ (Valleylab, Boulder, CO, USA) and the electrocautery. However, other dissection devices such as the Harmonic Wave® (Ethicon Endo-Surgery Inc, Cincinnati, OH, USA) may be used for the dissection and the vessel coaptation during the procedure. All of these devices are obviously dependent on hospital availability and cost.

Patient Position and Protective Devices

The patient is routinely positioned in the modified lithotomy position to allow access to the perineum for passing a surgical stapler, and for the operating surgeon or an assistant to stand between the patient's legs during periods of difficult dissection. The authors' preference is to use Yellowfin® stirrups (Allen®, Acton, MA, USA) (Fig. 7.1). There are significant advantages of this system in the boot design; it decreases the pressure under the peroneal fossa and the superficial peroneal nerve, allows for a significant lithotomy and abduction range of the hip with a squeeze grip handle. The boot configuration is thus much safer than the traditional Lloyd-Davies stirrups.

The authors advocate about 5–7 cm of the perineum to be below the surgical table after the patient has been placed in the stirrups, with support of a jelly pad underneath the sacroiliac joint.

The arms may be tucked or extended on arm bands. There are some difficulties in tucking the arms in wide patients, and the locking system for the Bookwalter™ arising from the rails of the table may compress the arm. Extended arms may also injure the brachial plexus if there is too much abduction of the shoulder. We routinely position

Part II: Left Colon

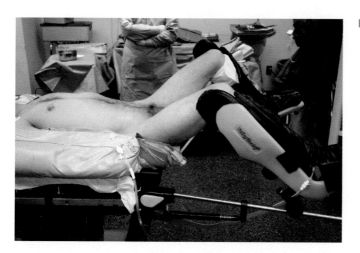

Figure 7.1 Patient positioning.

at 90 degrees or less from the body. All areas of pressure must be padded to avoid pressure necrosis and nerve damage (Fig. 7.1).

Abdominal Entry and Exploration

The authors routinely incise the patients with the electrocautery in the cutting setting. The preferred incision for laparotomy is the midline as it allows access to the entire abdominal cavity and it eases the application of the Bookwalter™ retractor. The dissection is carried down through the *linea alba* with the cautery device. In patients with previous laparotomies or midline incisions, dissection clamps are used to separate the underlying peritoneum from the fascia. The peritoneum is incised with scissors or a scalpel and the abdominal cavity is entered. All adhesions are sharply dissected to allow full exposure of the abdominal cavity.

Inspection and palpation of all internal organs is done with special attention to the liver lobes for metastatic disease; the nasogastric tube placement is confirmed. The peritoneal surface of the abdominal cavity and pelvic floor and organs are also inspected.

Exposure of the abdominal cavity is accomplished with right angle abdominal wall retractors on the Bookwalter™. With an assistant retracting the colon laterally, an abdominal pad is placed wide open to encircle the small intestines and position them in the right upper quadrant of the abdomen. This maneuver allows full exposure of the left colon, sigmoid, and upper rectum. The inferior mesenteric artery (IMA) will be located on the anterior surface of the aorta below the third portion of the duodenum (Fig. 7.2).

Technique of Medial-to-Lateral Mobilization Starting at the Sacral Promontory

The peritoneum is incised with the electrocautery at the sacral promontory on the right side with left and outwards retraction of the rectosigmoid junction. The incision is extended to the ligament of Treitz. In most patients, this maneuver will expose the areolar plane over the presacral area and anterior to the aorta and common iliac arteries. The vascular pedicle is easily identified and cranial dissection is performed with electrocautery to the IMA origin (Fig. 7.3). Lateral structures at the level of the promontory are recognized including the left iliac artery, gonadal vessel, and left ureter. These structures can be tracked upwards and left intact in the retroperitoneum, thus avoiding injury during the ligation of the vascular pedicles. The bifurcation of the parasympathetic plexus is identified and is preserved.

The pedicle of the IMA is then divided with the sealing device proximal to the origin of the left colic vessel. Alternatively, this step may be undertaken with a clamp-and-tie technique using a suture ligature on the patient side of the vessel. Care must be

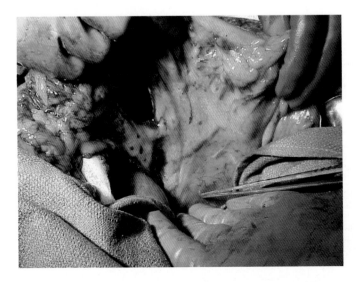

Figure 7.2 Left colectomy: medial-to-lateral approach (courtesy Dr. Neil Hyman).

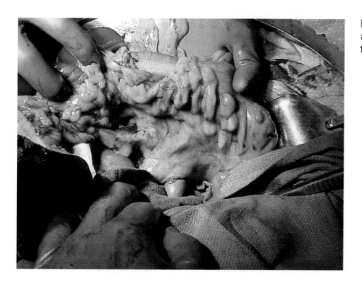

Figure 7.3 Medial-to-lateral approach Left Colectomy (Courtesy Dr. Neil Hyman).

taken to avoid damage to the parasympathetic plexus at the origin of the IMA. If a left colectomy is planned, the left colic artery can be divided at its origin. The entire lymphovascular pedicle allows proper staging. The anatomic planes are followed in a cephalad direction until the inferior mesenteric vein (IMV) is identified, and then isolated and divided.

At that point, the entire medial aspect of the colon has been freed and the lateral dissection is performed above Gerota's fascia, the tail of the pancreas, and tip of the spleen. The dissection is extended laterally to the paracolic gutter.

Lateral incision of the line of Toldt allows full mobilization of the left segment of the colon to the level of the splenic flexure.

Technique of Medial-to-Lateral Mobilization Starting at the IMV

The left colon is retracted at the level of the ligament of Treitz where the IMV is easily isolated, ligated, and divided. In that plane, areolar tissue is dissected laterally and caudally until the IMA pedicle is found on the anterior surface of the aorta. This pedicle is also ligated and the dissection is continued to the level of the pelvic inlet medially and laterally. Identification and preservation of the retroperitoneal structures is important.

Lateral release of the colonic attachments, beginning at the pelvic brim, is carried to the level of the splenic flexure.

This maneuver is especially helpful when the pathology is located high in the splenic flexure or significant bulky disease complicates the dissection in a lateral-to-medial approach.

Splenic Flexure Takedown

Retrospective studies have reported a higher incidence of iatrogenic splenic injuries during open colectomy when compared to laparoscopic approach (0.24 vs. 0%, respectively). Our preference is to approach the spleen with the patient in reverse Trendelenburg position. The Bookwalter™ retractor is repositioned with the center of the oval ring toward the left upper quadrant. The intestinal contents are packed to the right lower quadrant using the large retracting blade and an abdominal laparotomy pad or a towel with radiopaque marker and two short blades in the left upper quadrant of the incision to triangulate.

The operating surgeon stands between the legs. The distal transverse colon is mobilized from the omentum, through the gastrocolic omentum if necessary, to enter the lesser sac and expose the posterior surface of the stomach. The lateral dissection of the areolar plane is performed with the electrocautery or the vascular sealing devices since there may be a middle size vessel involved in the planes. Many times, this area has significant congenital or acquired adhesions that cause difficulties with the approach of the splenic flexure from the lateral approach. The method of approaching the splenic flexure from the medial aspect decreases the tension placed over the gastrosplenic ligament and vascular pedicle, as well as the capsule of the spleen. Therefore, the likelihood of splenic damage is greatly decreased.

The posterior areolar plane is developed all the way to the lateral attachment of the line of Toldt. The splenic flexure is then peeled, medial to lateral, from the tail of the pancreas, Gerota's fascia, and retroperitoneal structures.

Care must be taken to avoid excessive traction that may injure the marginal artery of Drummond in the mesentery of the splenic flexure that will be needed to supply the portion of colon intended for anastomosis or colostomy. Once the transverse colon is mobilized, the left branch of the middle colic artery is taken at its origin, which normally allows full mobilization of the transected colon to the level of the pelvis. The distal left colon or sigmoid or rectum can be divided with a transverse stapler at the desired level appropriate for the disease process. The mesenteric vessels can be sealed or ligated as the mesentery is divided at right angles to the point of bowel transection.

Anastomosis

The authors preference is to use a circular stapler, employing a 2/0 prolene purse-string to secure the anvil of the stapler in the proximal end of the colon. The stapler is passed through the anus and guided up to the stapled end of the colon or rectum. After firing the stapler, the anastomosis is inspected with a rigid proctoscope, air is insufflated with the proximal bowel occluded, and the anastomosis submerged in saline to inspect for bubbling—the so-called "leak test." In the event of a positive test, the anastomosis can be reinforced with sutures or occasionally may need to be resected and re-performed. The authors do not routinely perform a diverting ileostomy for elective cases, although diversion is always an option.

Another alternative is to perform a hand-sewn anastomosis. The authors use a 2/0 PDS in a single running layer using two sutures starting at the mesenteric at the bowel and proceeding in opposite directions to reach the antimesenteric surface. The anterior portion of the anastomosis is imbricated.

 POSTOPERATIVE MANAGEMENT

After the patient has been stable in the recovery room and transferred to the regular surgical floor, sips of clear noncarbonated liquids are started. Sequential compression devices must be worn at all times while the patient is in bed. In addition, heparin 5,000 units subcutaneously three times daily or Lovenox® 40 mg once daily is administered to the patient. The patient should ambulate six times each daily. If the patient does not have an epidural catheter, a hydromorphone or morphine patient controlled analgesia pump is routinely used. Ketorolac is given as supplemental analgesia for 3 days starting the first postoperative day. Normal renal function and a low risk of bleeding are required.

The incentive spirometer must be used and titrated to patient's pulmonary volumes hourly while awake.

Early feeding in open colectomy has been reported with overall oral intake intolerance in 13% of the patients, 8% being immediately postoperatively and 5% requiring readmission for emesis. Males are significantly more prone to oral intake intolerance and the use of metoclopramide does not improve the rate.

In certain institutions, the creation of fast-track recovery programs has reported improvement in outcomes and a high rate of compliance by nursing and physician staff. Fast-track programs such as the German Multicenter Quality Assurance Program have shown that the use of epidural analgesia, nonopioid analgesia, restriction of intraoperative fluids, and early oral feeding and mobilization can shorten hospital stay with an acceptable morbidity of 13% and mortality of 0.4%. Readmission is only needed in 4% of the patients.

Not only does this approach seem to be beneficial for the patient but also results in significant cost saving for the institution with a decrease in length of hospital stay by 2 days and almost $2,000 in savings per patient.

Surgical dressings are removed on postoperative day 2 and the patient is allowed to shower after the third day pat drying the wound.

As the return of bowel function begins with the passage of flatus, the diet is advanced to regular and the pain medication is switched to oral. Discharge planning is done for home with or without home nursing evaluations, or, if needed, to skilled nursing facility or nursing home.

 # COMPLICATIONS

A list of early and late complications is included in Table 7.2. Patients undergoing left colectomy are at risk for the same postoperative complications as for any open abdominal operations. Deep vein thrombosis and pulmonary embolism may result from a prolonged sedentary state. This complication can be minimized through early ambulation and chemical DVT prophylaxis mentioned earlier. Atelectasis and subsequent pneumonia can occur from the shallow breathing secondary to incisional pain. Adequate pain control and aggressive incentive spirometry are used to stave off this process. Cardiac complications such as myocardial infarction or congestive heart failure are best minimized through preoperative optimization of cardiac risk factors, judicious perioperative fluid monitoring, and beta-blockade when appropriate.

In-hospital complications specific to performance of left colectomy include postoperative ileus, surgical site infection, wound dehiscence, anastomotic leak with intra-abdominal abscess formation, unrecognized ureteric injury, staple line hemorrhage, urinary retention, urinary tract infection, and *Clostridium difficile* colitis. In-hospital and 30-day mortality should be less than 1% in elective cases. The duration and severity of postoperative ileus is limited by the use of fast-track protocols. The early removal of urinary catheters can reduce or eliminate urinary tract complications. Surgical site infection is treated with opening of the wound and local wound care. Perioperative antibiotics are discontinued on postoperative day 1, thus reducing the risk of *C.difficile* colitis infection. Unrecognized injury to the ureter requires reoperation with repair over a stent or resection and reimplantation of the ureter. It is highly recommended to enlist the assistance of a urologist to appropriately deal with a ureteric injury. Hemorrhagic complications can often be conservatively treated and will resolve on their own. Occasionally, endoscopic evaluation of the anastomosis with clip application for hemostasis is necessary. If an anastomotic leak or abscess is discovered and the patient is stable, conservative treatment with antibiotics and interventional radiologic drainage of the fluid collection may obviate a return trip to the operating room. Unstable patients or those with peritonitis require operative re-exploration with repair or resection of the anastomosis. In these circumstances, a colostomy or ileostomy is usually mandated.

TABLE 7.2

Early complications of left colectomy	Late complications of left colectomy
Deep venous thrombosis/pulmonary embolus	Incisional hernia
Atelectasis/pneumonia	Recurrence of disease
Myocardial infarction	Anastomotic stricture
Congestive heart failure	Sexual/urinary dysfunction
Staple line hemorrhage	Bowel obstruction
Anastomotic leak/abscess formation	
Surgical site infection	
Wound dehiscence	
Unrecognized ureteric injury	
Urinary retention/urinary tract infection	
Death	

Part II: Left Colon

Long-term complications of left colectomy vary with the indication for surgery. All patients undergoing open left colectomy are at risk for postoperative adhesion formation and bowel obstruction. Often this condition can be managed conservatively, but a minority of patients may require reoperation with adhesiolysis. Incisional hernia may occur as a long-term manifestation of surgical site infection or wound dehiscence and can be treated with operative hernia repair if the patient is a candidate for elective surgery. Anastomotic stricture formation may result as a technical complication of surgery, either due to ischemia at the anastomosis or the use of a smaller caliber stapler. Stricture can often be overcome with the use of stool bulking agents or endoscopic balloon dilation. In rare cases, operative resection of the anastomosis may be required. Sexual dysfunction may result if injury to the autonomic nerve plexus occurs at the initial operation. This is best avoided by meticulous dissection during the primary surgery. In patients with colon cancer as an indication for surgery, locoregional recurrence may cause pain or obstructive symptoms. Likewise, recurrence of Crohn's disease can cause stricture formation or bowel obstruction. These patients should be treated on the basis of their symptoms.

 RESULTS

The long-term results of open left colectomy have improved over time with the development of newer and better technologies. The procedure has been performed for decades with an acceptably low mortality rate (~1% in experienced groups) and minimizing the above mentioned complications.

The use of alvimopan has been prospectively shown to decrease the postoperative ileus. Bell et al. performed an economic analysis of the North American phase III efficacy trials in which the drug showed an 18 hour shorter recovery time in comparison to the placebo arm. The hospital length of stay was reduced by a full day and the rate of postoperative ileus in the alvimopan was 19% in comparison to the placebo arm. These results translated to $879 savings per patient in the study arm.

CONCLUSIONS

Although the performance of open left colectomy has a significant prolonged recovery and length of stay, clinically sound "fast-track" protocols may improve the outcome without compromising patient safety.

Suggested Readings

Bell TJ, Poston SA, Kraft MD, et al. Economic analysis of alvimopan in North American phase III efficacy trials. *Am J Health-Syst Pharm* 2009;66:1362–68.

Braumann C, Guenther N, Wendling P, et al. Multimodal perioperative rehabilitation in elective conventional resection of colonic cancer: results from the German multicenter quality assurance program 'fast-track colon II'. *Digest Surg* 2009;26(2):123–29.

Chan MKY, Law WL. Using of chewing gum in reducing postoperative ileus after elective colorectal resection: a systematic review. *Dis Colon Rectum* 2007;50:2149–57.

Di Fronzo AL, Cymerman J, O'Connell TX. Factors affecting early postoperative feeding following elective open colon resection. *Arch Surg* 1999;134(9):941–46.

Franklin ME, Trevino JM, Whelan RL. Laparoscopic right, left, low anterior, abdominoperineal and total colon resections. In: Fischer JE, Bland KI, eds. *Mastery of Surgery*. 5th ed. Philadelphia: Lippincott Williams & Wilkins, 2007:1490–509.

Gendall KA, Kennedy RR, Watson AJ, et al. The effect of epidural analgesia on postoperative outcome after colorectal surgery. *Colorectal Dis* 2007;9(7):584–98.

Guenaga KF, Matos D, Castro AA, et al. Mechanical bowel preparation for elective colorectal surgery. *Cochrane Database Syst Rev* 2005;CD001544.

Malek MM, Greenstein AJ, Chin EH, et al. Comparison of iatrogenic splenectomy during open and laparoscopic colon resection. *Surg Laparosc Endosc Percutan Tech* 2007;17(5):385–87.

Mayer J, Boldt J, Schellhaa A, et al. Bispectral index-guided general anesthesia in combination with thoracic epidural analgesia reduces recovery time in fast-track colon surgery. *Anesth Analg* 2007;104(5):1145–49.

Schuster R, Grewal N, Greaney GC. Gum chewing reduces ileus after elective open sigmoid colectomy. *Arch Surg* 2006;141(2):174–76.

Senagore AJ, Fry R. Surgical management of colon cancer. In: Wolff BG, Fleshman JW, Beck DE, et al., eds. *The ASCRS Textbook of Colon and Rectal Surgery*. New York: Springer, 2007:395–04.

Slim K, Vicaut E, Launay-Savary MV, et al. Updated systematic review and meta-analysis of randomized clinical trials on the role of mechanical bowel preparation before colorectal surgery. *Ann Surg* 2009;249:203–09.

Stephen AE, Berger DL. Shortened length of stay and hospital cost reduction with implementation of an accelerated clinical care pathway after elective colon resection. *Surgery* 2003;133(3):277–82.

8 Open Left and Sigmoid Colectomy

James W. Fleshman and Matthew G. Mutch

INDICATIONS

The most common indication for a left colectomy or left and sigmoid colectomy is colon cancer. However, sigmoid and left colon diverticulitis most certainly rank a close second. The anatomic considerations for performing a left colectomy versus a left and sigmoid colectomy are influenced by the position of the tumor or the inflammation. The blood supply to the left colon arises from arcades coming from the middle colic pedicle around the splenic flexure from the marginal artery of Drummond. The distal blood arises from the inferior mesenteric artery via the left colic ascending branch. The sigmoidal branch is also derived from the inferior mesenteric artery. It is imperative in a cancer procedure to remove all of the vascular and lymphatic drainage. Therefore, removing the entire sigmoid and left colon is sometimes necessary. Diverticulitis requires only that the entire sigmoid be removed and the anastomosis be performed between soft proximal colon and normal rectum with no sigmoid left behind.

There are essentially no contraindications to left colectomy unless the patient is unable to undergo general anesthetic. The left and sigmoid colons are easily sacrificed and should not be considered other than a sewer pipe transmitting the stool from the transverse colon to the rectum.

PREOPERATIVE PLANNING

Patients usually benefit from a mechanical bowel preparation to reduce the burden of the stool, especially in a laparoscopic case. However, in an open colectomy, the need for a full mechanical bowel preparation is probably based on surgeon's preference. There is adequate data to suggest that a left colon resection can be performed in the setting of an emergency without preparation and certainly in elective surgery with no preparation. The presence of dense adhesions along the left gutter or severe inflammation around the ureter may be an indication for cystoscopy and ureteral stent placement at the beginning of the operation.

- It is unusual to require proximal diversion after a left colectomy; but if the plan is in anyway to include a stoma, the preoperative marking of the site can improve the outcomes of the patient.
- In the case of a patient with a left colon cancer, preoperative CT scan provides adequate staging. Full colonoscopy should be performed if at all possible to clear the rest of the colon of other disease.
- The patient should be informed of the postoperative bowel function expected after segmental resection of the left and/or sigmoid colon. Bowel function is somewhat less than normal and usually results in multiple bowel movements that occur rapidly with possible urgency, depending on the patient's age.
- Antibiotic and deep venous thrombosis (DVT) prophylaxis are essential for reducing wound infection and venous thromboembolic occurrence.
- Colonoscopic tattooing of the lesion will assist in identification of the neoplastic disease.

POSITIONING

- The patient is placed in lithotomy position using the Allen's stirrups with sequential compression devices in place, bladder catheter in place, and the rectum is irrigated to clear the rectum of any solid stool. The arms are placed with the left arm extended and the right arm tucked to allow an overhead Mayo stand placed for draping.

TECHNIQUE

- The abdomen is entered through a vertical midline incision from xiphoid to pubis and the Bookwalter retractor is placed for exposure and opened widely. The small bowel is retracted to the right upper quadrant and upper midline.
- An incision is made at the base of the lateral aspect of the left colon mesentery along the white line of Toldt with the left colon retracted medially and anteriorly (Fig. 8.1). The incision is extended from the pelvis to the left upper quadrant. The exposed areolar tissue plane allows dissection anterior to the retroperitoneum. Blunt dissection frees the left colon from the retroperitoneum and exposes the ureter and gonadal vessels

Figure 8.1 Expose the left ureter and gonadal vessels and push posteriorly.

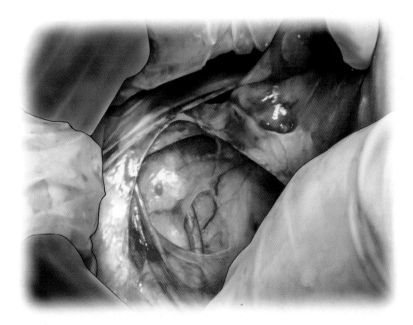

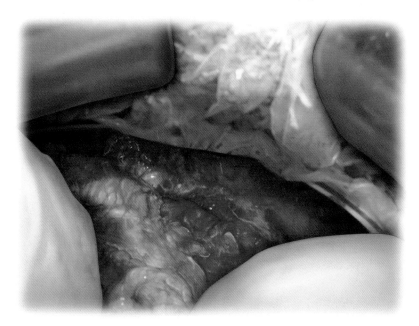

within the retroperitoneum. The blunt dissection is carried medially to the base of the aorta and cephalad to the splenic flexure level, freeing the left colon from the anterior surface of the kidney (Fig. 8.2).

- An incision is made on the peritoneal attachments of the splenic flexure using the finger as a guide, incising lateral to medial to release the splenic flexure from the undersurface of the tip of the spleen, the lateral aspect of the abdominal cavity, and the anterior surface of the kidney. The tip of the spleen is freed from the splenic flexure, releasing the multiple congenital adhesions and incising the omental attachment to release the splenic flexure toward the midline (Fig. 8.3). The attachments of the splenic flexure to the undersurface of the tail of the pancreas and the retroperitoneum are incised all the way to the midline toward the duodenum at the ligament of Treitz.

- The omental attachments to the anterior surface of the transverse colon are incised releasing the splenic flexure from the left upper quadrant. The omental attachments to the transverse colon are incised all the way to the middle of the transverse colon or to the right colon itself (Fig. 8.4).

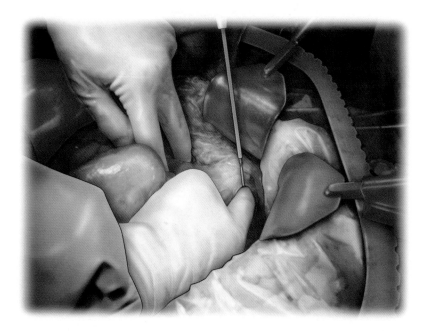

Figure 8.3 Release lateral attachments of splenic flexure anterior to left kidney.

Part II: Left Colon

Figure 8.4 Release omentum from antimesenteric surface of transverse colon all the way to right.

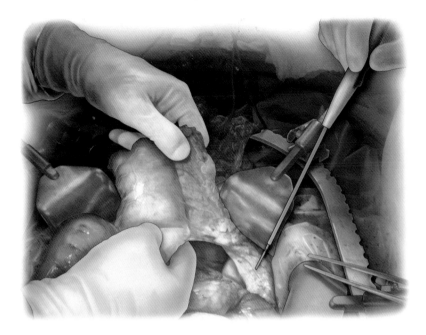

- The left colon is lifted from the abdomen and is pulled to the patient's left, exposing the medial aspect of the left colon mesentery over the aorta. The inferior mesenteric artery is encountered at the level of the aorta just above the bifurcation of the common iliac artery. The inferior mesenteric vein (IMV) is identified at the level of the ligament of Treitz at the base of the mesentery of the left colon above a window of clear peritoneum along the anterior surface of the aorta (Fig. 8.5). The inferior mesenteric artery and vein are isolated at their origins and divided between ties.
- The left colon is stretched all the way to the pelvis bringing the splenic flexure to near the pelvic brim. This allows the left colon to be evaluated for point of transection,

Figure 8.5 The IMV is identified at the level of the ligament of Treitz at the base of the mesentery of the left colon above a window of clear peritoneum along the anterior surface of the aorta.

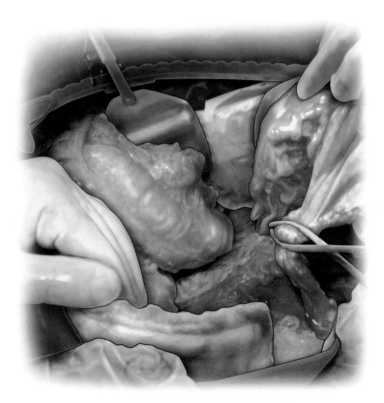

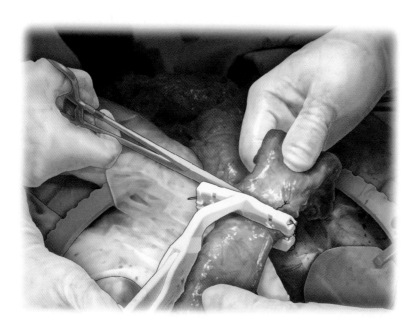

Figure 8.6 Place a purse string on the proximal aspect of the proximal margin and transect the bowel between purse strings and clamp.

removing adequate proximal and distal margins for the lesion. A purse-string instrument is used to place a purse string, or a hand-sewn purse string is placed at the site of transection after dividing the mesenteric vessels. The purse string is placed so that adequate blood supply is available and there is no tension or twist (Fig. 8.6).

- For a stapled circular anastomosis, the circular stapler anvil and shaft are secured in the proximal purse string and reinforced with ties as needed to complete the donut around the base of the shaft of the stapling instrument head.
- The sigmoid or rectum is transected at the level of the sacral promontory using either a linear cutter stapler or a transverse linear stapler to create the transverse staple line. The circular stapler itself is then introduced through the anal canal to the level of the transverse staple line and the post is inserted and extended through the midportion of the rectal stump at the midportion of the transverse staple line.
- The left colon is brought into the pelvis without twist. The stapler is then reconnected and closed under direct vision maintaining good orientation with the mesentery of the left colon directed posteriorly (Fig. 8.7).

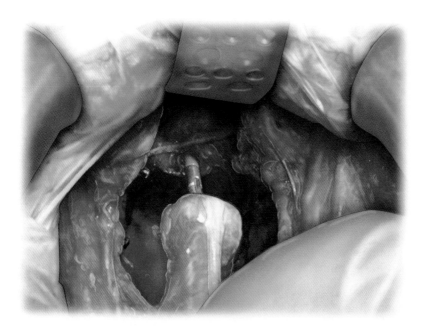

Figure 8.7 Reconnect the stapler and create a double-stapled end-to-end circular anastomosis.

- The anastomosis can be checked by insufflating air through a rigid proctoscope, with the bowel proximal to the stapled anastomosis occluded and the pelvis filled with saline, to create an underwater test. Any bubbles seen would indicate a leak at the staple line and should be oversewn with Lembert sutures of 3–0 absorbable suture.
- The abdomen is then closed after irrigation and returning the small bowel in a gentle S-shaped curves and covering them with adhesion barrier.

 # POSTOPERATIVE MANAGEMENT

- Patients are ambulated early.
- IV fluid replacement maintains a urine output of greater than 30 ml/hour.
- Nasogastric decompression is not required unless the patient becomes nauseated. Within 24–48 hours most patients will tolerate clear liquids and the diet can be advanced as tolerated.
- Patients should be given 24 hours of prophylactic antibiotic coverage, incentive spirometry, DVT prophylaxis, and encouraged to ambulate as much as possible during the early time period.
- Usual hospital stay after an open left colectomy is 4–5 days, or less when placed on a fast-tracking post-op regimen.
- Post-op analgesia is usually managed with patient-controlled analgesia followed by switch to oral analgesics.

 # COMPLICATIONS

- The most feared complication is the anastomotic leak. The anticipated leak rate for a routine left and sigmoid colectomy with colorectal anastomosis is less than 4%. The anastomotic leak can be managed conservatively with percutaneous drainage of fluid collection if it is walled off and contained. Only when there is frank peritonitis and diffuse fecal contamination, reexploration and takedown of the anastomosis and end colostomy are required.
- Deep venous thrombosis should only occur in less than 1% of patients if the patient received mechanical and chemoprophylaxis during the operation. However, heightened awareness of the possibility of lower extremity DVT and pulmonary embolism will usually prevent death. Early anticoagulation with either Enoxaparin or Heparin will allow dissolution of the clot by autothrombolysis. Only if the patient continues to throw clots would an inferior vena cava filter become necessary.
- Surgical site infection will be a more common complication. Because the open left colectomy is a contaminated of clean contaminated case, a wound infection can be expected in up to 8% of patients. Strict attention to avoidance of spillage and wound protection can theoretically reduce the contamination of the surgical site. Local management of the wound is essential with opening and packing or placement of vacuum-assisted therapy if a deep subcutaneous wound infection occurs.
- Urinary tract infections (UTIs) are a side effect of a long-term indwelling bladder catheter. For this reason, early removal of the catheter after close monitoring of fluid status is no longer needed to prevent UTI. Recognition of ureteral injury may be facilitated by observation of a drain left in the pelvis. Should the volume increase rapidly, a creatinine level can be obtained on the drainage. A fluid creatinine level that is higher than the serum creatinine level would indicate a leak from the urinary tract itself into the abdomen, such as caused by ureteral injury or bladder injury.
- In-hospital pneumonia after abdominal surgery can almost entirely be avoided by encouraging a routine and barometer use and early ambulation. Patients who smoked heavily all of their life succumb to the inevitable atelectasis and may develop pneumonia.

Postoperative ileus is not uncommon after an open operation. Even so, the patient can be treated without a nasogastric tube and can undergo an early trial of liquids after surgery. However, if the patient becomes nauseated and does not respond to intravenous antiemetics, the patient should be placed on bowel rest and a nasogastric tube considered. Ileus can be expected in 10–25% of patients.

RESULTS

The use of lateral to medial left colectomy should still be considered the standard of care because of the known anatomic relationships and the ability to develop avascular planes and perform anatomic resection of the left colon and sigmoid. The use of the lateral to medical approach makes wedge resection or small segmental resection unnecessary because the anatomic relationships are well seen and a colorectal anastomosis can be accomplished without compromising on cure, especially in cancer cases. Local recurrence after a lateral to medial left colectomy for a Stage I through III colon cancer should be less than 1%. Wide resection of the lymphatics and removal of all adherent retroperitoneal or abdominal wall tissues should remove all possibility of local recurrence. The most common cause of local recurrence then is lymphatic spread to adjacent periaortic lymph node change.

CONCLUSION

The use of an open to lateral medical left colectomy should be the basic approach to left-sided colonic disease. Any surgeon performing laparoscopic or robotic resection should be capable of performing an open lateral to medical left colectomy exposing known avascular anatomic planes and transecting vessels at their origin. A low rate of complications and good long-term outcomes should be possible in these patients.

Suggested Readings

Adachi Y, Sato K, Kakisako K, et al. Quality of life after laparoscopic or open colonic resection for cancer. *Hepatogastroenterology* 2003;50(53):1348–51.

Seitz G, Seitz EM, Kasparek MS, et al. Long-term quality-of-life after open and laparoscopic sigmoid colectomy. *Surg Laparosc Endosc Percutan Tech* 2008;18(2):162–7.

Part II: Left Colon

9 Laparoscopic Medial-to-Lateral

Jonathan Efron and Michael J. Stamos

●●● INDICATIONS

The indications for laparoscopic left colectomy performed either by a medial-to-lateral approach or a lateral-to-medial dissection are diverse, including both malignant and benign conditions. Early in the history of laparoscopic colectomy, controversy existed as to the safety and feasibility of laparoscopic colectomy for cancer. This was secondary to early recurrence rates, primarily port site recurrences, which surgeons feared may be secondary to the technical aspects of laparoscopic colectomy, such as the pneumoperitoneum. Several prospective, randomized trials, however, have demonstrated equivalent recurrence and long-term survival rates between laparoscopic and open colectomies performed for cancer (1–3). Currently, malignancy is considered an optimal indication for laparoscopic colectomies. Some relative contraindications for performing a laparoscopic colectomy for cancer include T4 cancers with extensive involvement of other abdominal organs, or tumors that are greater than 8 cm in diameter.

Most benign conditions also lend themselves to laparoscopic resection by a medial-to-lateral approach. These reasons include diverticulitis, inflammatory bowel disease, and polyps. In complicated diverticulitis or Crohn's disease with an associated pericolonic abscess, the medial approach may allow early identification of the ureter and iliac vessels, allowing for a safer lateral dissection in the inflamed tissue. Conversely, if the intestinal mesentery is significantly thickened from Crohn's disease, approaching the dissection laterally may avoid injuring the mesentery preventing excess bleeding or the formation of a mesenteric hematoma. Dividing thickened Crohn's mesentery is difficult with either vessel sealing devices or intracorporeal staplers and this may limit the ability of the surgeon to perform a medial-to-lateral dissection as division of the inferior mesenteric vessels may not be possible. Similarly, conditions such as sigmoid volvulus and rectal prolapse generally require minimal sigmoid mobilization and therefore are not well served by a medial-to-lateral approach with high ligation of the inferior mesenteric vessels.

When approaching a laparoscopic colectomy, standardizing the surgical technique helps to facilitate the operation. Standardization facilitates the procedure, allowing it to be performed in a quick and efficient manner, decreases surgeon frustration, and decreases operative time. Each step must have specific targets and those targets should be reached in a timely fashion. If the surgeon is not meeting those goals and the operation is failing to progress, early conversion is advocated and may reduce the risk of intraoperative complications. Just as standardization facilitates performing the procedure, instituting standardized preoperative and postoperative care pathways have shown to be safe and cost effective, reducing length of stay and decreasing hospital costs (3–6).

PREOPERATIVE PLANNING

Preoperative preparation prior to laparoscopic colectomy includes ensuring that the patient's medical comorbidities are well controlled and that he or she is an acceptable candidate for surgery. Preoperative teaching of the patient and family should include instructions on the patient's postoperative responsibilities. These include early eating and ambulation, use of incentive spirometers, and expectations for early discharge. Implementing a fast-track protocol reduces hospital length of stay with similar morbidity and low readmission rates to patients treated off protocol (7–9).

Bowel preparation is a controversial practice for left colectomy that may still be initiated. Multiple prospective randomized studies have been performed examining the outcome of elective colonic resections with and without bowel preparation. Most authors have shown no difference in complication rates between the two groups, including anastomotic leak rates, whereas some investigators have shown a higher rate of wound infections in the patients who have received a bowel preparation (10,11). Recent large studies have again failed to show the necessity of routine bowel preparation (12–14). Patients who may require intraoperative colonoscopy for localization of polyps or tumors during the surgery will require mechanical bowel preparation. It is also the practice of the authors to prepare the patients with a mechanical bowel preparation if proximal fecal diversion is planned after completing the colectomy and anastomosis. If no mechanical oral preparation is used for a laparoscopic left colectomy, the patient should perform two disposable phosphate enemas before entering the operating room to allow unimpeded transanal passage of a circular stapler.

Final preoperative preparation includes instillation of intravenous antibiotics and administration of subcutaneous heparin. Sequential compression stockings should also be used. Placement of an epidural catheter is advocated by some surgeons for postoperative pain management to limit postoperative narcotic intake and to enhance recovery. Epidural placement should be performed in the preoperative area in addition to ensuring that adequate intravenous access is obtained prior to positioning the patient in the operating room as both arms will be tucked at the patient's side during the operation. Keeping the patient warm in the preoperative area will help maintain core body temperature during the procedure.

Procedure

Preparation for the operation continues upon entry to the operating room. After placement of intravenous lines and epidural catheter if utilized, the patient is then induced under general anesthesia. The patient is placed in the modified lithotomy position with carefully padded Allen stirrups and with thigh high sequential compression stockings utilized. Positioning of the patient in the operating room should include tucking of the right (or both) arm(s) by the patient's side to allow full access to that side of the patient, since the conduct of the operation has the operating surgeon and assistant standing on the right side and also intermittently between the legs to facilitate splenic flexure mobilization.

The monitors should be positioned so that they are available near the left shoulder of the patient as well as the left hip area for maximal viewing capability of this multiquadrant operation. The patient needs to be not only carefully padded to avoid any pressure injuries, but also carefully secured to the bed to allow extreme positioning changes during the operation. In particular, steep Trendelenburg position is utilized and therefore gel pads placed above the shoulder or some other method of securing the patient (beanbag) are essential. In addition, these pads or beanbags must be thoroughly secured to the table. It is the practice of the authors to test the secure positioning of the patient prior to prepping and draping by moving the bed into extreme left side up position, and extreme Trendelenburg position prior to draping so that any potential issues regarding patient movement can be corrected before beginning the operation. This time is well spent and should not be disregarded. Following this positioning, the patient's abdomen is prepped and draped extending over to the anterior axillary lines laterally and up to the rib cage superiorly and inferiorly down to and including the pubic area.

After draping, primary abdominal insufflation is typically obtained using a Veress needle technique. The primary insufflation site is placed off of the midline, generally two finger breadths lateral to and above the umbilicus in the right upper quadrant. This position may vary based on any prior surgery or expected adhesions in the abdominal cavity. Once insufflation is obtained, a 5 mm trocar is placed at that site and then two additional trocars are placed, one 5 mm size in the epigastric area just slightly to the left of midline and a 12 mm trocar in the right lower quadrant just medial and slightly superior to the anterior superior iliac spine. If necessary, a fourth 5 mm trocar can be placed in the left lower quadrant lateral to the rectus muscle, and this fourth trocar site can then be utilized for a muscle splitting incision for extraction of the specimen and insertion of the circular stapling anvil if utilized.

In the case of a cancer diagnosis, the initial steps are to perform a staging laparoscopy by first placing the patient in reverse Trendelenburg position to evaluate the liver and peritoneal surface and then returning to a slight Trendelenburg to evaluate the rest of the abdominal peritoneal cavity and the pelvis.

To begin the left colon mobilization, the patient is placed in steep Trendelenburg with slight left side up tilt and the small intestine is mobilized out of the pelvis. Not infrequently there are adhesions of the terminal ileum or cecal region to the right pelvic region that restrict mobility of the small bowel. These adhesions should be divided to ensure that the small bowel is fully mobilized and out of the pelvis and therefore not obscuring the view.

At this time any attachments of the sigmoid colon to the left pelvis or lateral pelvic side wall are appreciated. The mesosigmoid is grasped near its mid to distal portion using an atraumatic grasper and the colon is allowed, if mobile, to flip behind the mesentery out of the view of the operating surgeon. A grasper, placed through the epigastric trocar elevates the mesosigmoid anteriorly towards the anterior abdominal wall. It can be moved slightly from right to left to identify the plane of dissection behind the mesocolon just at or above the sacral promontory. The iliac vessels are often visualized at this time through the retroperitoneal surface and in a thin patient the right ureter may also be obvious. Dissection is commenced in this plane behind the mesosigmoid and above the sacral promontory but caudal to the inferior mesenteric artery (IMA) origin. The IMA is usually obvious because when the mesosigmoid is grasped and elevated anteriorly, it typically tents up and is quite prominent as the dissection continues.

The peritoneum overlying the dissection plane is scored along the sacral promontory into the pelvis and also cephalad toward the IMA. Establishing this dissection plane is an essential first step.

Dissection should be anterior to the iliac vessels and to the hypogastric nerves, which are typically easily seen through this plane. Once this dissection plane is established, blunt dissection using an atraumatic instrument is often possible to begin the dissection and to establish this tissue plane. The left ureter should now be identified, and the dissection plane, once the posterior aspect of the mesocolon is reached, should actually be in an anterior angled direction. If the dissection plane wrongly continues in a posterior angled direction, the left ureter will be elevated and placed at risk for injury. If the ureter cannot be quickly and easily identified, the most likely conclusion is that it has indeed been elevated along with the mesocolon. Once the ureter is identified and traced, dissection is continued on the peritoneal surface, scoring and dissecting out the IMA and vein. The clear area cephalad toward the IMA and vein within the mesentery of the mesosigmoid is identified and the vessels themselves are then freely mobile off the retroperitoneum. The artery is then divided either utilizing a bipolar energy device or other techniques including clips and/or staples. The vein can be divided at the same time or individually at this same location, or in the case of a planned low anastomosis, the vein may be preferentially divided at the level of the pancreas at a later time.

The IMA division allows free mobility of the mesosigmoid off the retroperitoneum so that dissection can continue in this medial-lateral plane all the way to the posterior-lateral edge of the sigmoid and then up behind the descending colon. The dissection continues in this plane both cranially and caudally deep into the pelvis. Upon completion of this dissection, the colon is then grasped on its medial aspect and lateral incision of the peritoneal attachments is commenced usually using sharp dissection technique with a scissor. Typically, the retroperitoneum behind the lateral aspect of the sigmoid and descending colon is stained a purplish color, which is useful to identify the correct tissue plane. This staining is from the previous medial-lateral retroperitoneal dissection. This lateral incision is continued both cranially including the splenic flexure and caudally down into the true pelvis. The proximal line of resection is then selected based largely on the mesenteric blood supply and location of pathology (e.g., tumor), but may also be determined by the quality of the sigmoid colon and the presence or absence of previous radiation therapy. In a case of diverticular disease affecting the sigmoid colon or in the face of previous radiation therapy, the authors prefer a descending colon to rectal anastomosis. This obviously may affect the degree of splenic flexure mobilization necessary to result in a tension-free anastomosis.

Splenic flexure mobilization begins by putting the patient into a slight reverse Trendelenburg position with left side elevated. The omentum is grasped and elevated cranially to identify the transverse colon and then the splenic flexure is mobilized either by a continuation of the lateral approach as would commonly be done with an open operation, or with a medial-lateral approach starting from the lesser sac entered by a tissue plane identified between the omentum and the transverse colon and then extended over laterally from that direction. Alternatively, the splenic flexure can be mobilized from posterior by going into the retroperitoneal tissue plane behind the mesocolon extending up towards the spleen. This maneuver is utilized only infrequently but can be quite useful, but mandates the use of a 45-degree angled or flexible tip laparoscope.

Once the splenic flexure is fully mobilized, the proximal site of planned resection is grasped and brought down into the pelvis to insure that there is adequate mobility for a tension-free anastomosis at the distal planned line of resection. If mobility is not adequate, it may require further division of the inferior mesenteric vein at the level of the pancreas, if not already conducted.

At this point the patient is placed back into Trendelenburg position and the distal line of resection is then chosen, either based on anatomic landmarks or on endoscopic confirmation in the case of a neoplasm. Tattooing is of some value but cannot be fully relied on because of the nonspecificity of the exact location when dealing with rectal neoplasms and anticipated margins of 2 cm or even less. The authors strongly prefer CO_2 insufflation for their intraoperative colonoscopy for localization and confirmation of margins to avoid troubling colonic dilation, which can impair the conduct of the remainder of the operation.

 ## POSTOPERATIVE MANAGEMENT

While every patient is different and has specific needs, standardization of postoperative management is possible, and as mentioned above, decreases length of stay and may enhance patient satisfaction. Preoperative education of the patient is essential. This preoperative teaching is easily performed with supplementary booklets or videos and should be part of the patient's preoperative preparation. Education of the nursing staff caring for the patient is also required.

Many of the practices implemented in fast-track protocols aim to decrease postoperative ileus. With rapid recovery of gastrointestinal function, patients can transition to oral diet and hydration, oral pain medication, and early discharge (15). Reviewed below are the currently available methods for enhancing early gastrointestinal recovery and may be instituted in a "fast track" after laparoscopic colectomy.

Epidural Anesthesia

Multiple prospective randomized clinical trials have examined the efficacy of epidural anesthesia on postoperative ileus. All have shown some significant effects reducing either time to first bowel movement or flatus. Maron et al. summarize these results in their review on postoperative ileus (16). A key step in ensuring the effectiveness of epidurals is to make sure they are positioned appropriately for the specific operative procedure performed. Colectomies generally require a mid thoracic placement to ensure the entire incision and upper abdomen is included in the distribution of the epidural's effectiveness. Reviewing the literature also implies that bowel function resumes earlier with the use of local anesthetics as opposed to epidurals using opioids or a mixture of both opioids and local anesthetics. Jorgensen et al. in a recent Cochrane review determined that local epidurals when compared to systemic opioids reduced the length of postoperative ileus by 36 hours. Similarly they reduced postoperative ileus by 24 hours when compared to opioid epidurals (17). The placement and management of epidural catheters requires a dedicated anesthesia service and pain management team. When not working, they need to be removed or repositioned. Postoperative hypotension can be associated with a well function epidural catheter. This may result in overly aggressive fluid resuscitation of patients if not recognized as a potential side effect.

Gum Chewing

In 2002 Asoa first reported on the effect of gum chewing on postoperative ileus. They randomized 19 patients to either chew gum or not. The gum chewing group had a significantly shorter length of time to passage of flatus; however, there was no significant difference in the length of stay (18). In 2006 Scuster et al. (19) randomized 34 patients. They found a significantly shorter length of time to flatus, bowel movement, and a 2-day reduction in hospital stay. The same year, Matros et al. (20) randomized 66 patients to either sips of water, gum chewing, or use of an acupuncture bracelet. There was no difference in passage of flatus, bowel movement, or time to discharge. Multiple studies have been performed examining the effect of gum chewing, but recently two meta-analysis have been published. De Castro et al. (21) described five randomized trials including a total of 158 patients. The gum-chewing patients had a shorter time to flatus (20 hours) and bowel movement (29 hours). There was no difference in length of stay. Purkayastha et al. (22) also found a reduction in time to passage of first flatus and bowel movement. When they eliminated patients with stomas from the analysis they also found a significant reduction in length of stay. Gum chewing is a cheap and effective technique that can be initiated to enhance bowel recovery with minimal risk to the patient.

Nasogastric Tubes

Nasogastric (NG) tubes have been shown to increase patient's length of stay after colectomy and decrease overall recovery from elective surgery. Their routine use has also been questioned in emergent procedures. St Peter et al. (23) recently examined all children undergoing surgery for perforated appendicitis from 1999 to 2004. They found 105 patients with NG tubes and 54 without. Those with tubes had a significantly longer time to first oral intake (3.8 days vs. 2.2 days). Length of stay was 6.0 days in the NG group and 5.6 days in the non-NG group. Their conclusion was that there was no benefit from the use of NG tubes and their routine use in emergent operations is not recommended. Despite the lack of evidence for the routine use of NG tubes, they continue to be utilized routinely by colorectal surgeons. A recent survey by Roig et al. (24) of Spanish colorectal surgeons demonstrated that 22% utilize them routinely. At this point in time there is no evidence for the use of routine NG tubes for either elective or emergent operations.

Laxatives and Lidocaine

Several medications have shown some promise with respect to preventing postoperative ileus, but there is still little objective evidence that they are beneficial. Oral laxatives have shown some benefit in primary studies, but no randomized data are available to confirm their effectiveness (15). Similarly, prokinetic drugs such as metoclopramide have never been shown to decrease the time of postoperative ileus.

The effects of intravenous lidocaine on postoperative ileus, however, have been studied in several randomized prospective trials. Marret et al. (25) recently performed a meta-analysis on eight prospective, double-blinded, randomized controlled trials that included a total of 161 patients receiving lidocaine and 159 controls. These studies demonstrated a significant benefit from the lidocaine with a reduction in the duration of the ileus, decreased length of stay, and improved pain scores. The authors conclude that intravenous lidocaine, initiated during surgery and continued postoperatively improves patient rehabilitation and decreases length of stay.

Countering the Systemic Effects of Narcotics

The systemic effects of opioids are well known to prolong postoperative ileus. There are currently two strategies for decreasing these systemic effects. One is to decrease the overall need for peripherally administered narcotics by utilizing anti-inflammatory medications or by utilizing some of the methods already discussed, such as local epidural catheters and intravenous administration of lidocaine. The other is by the administration of mu-opioid receptor antagonists, alvimopan being the currently available oral agent in this class of medication. The use of nonsteroidals, such as ketorolac, has been shown to decrease opioid requirements along with postoperative nausea and vomiting (26). There does not seem to be an increased risk of postoperative bleeding associated with the use of ketorolac (27); however, care should be taken in administering the drug to patients with renal insufficiency.

Local anesthetic preperitoneal pain pumps have been shown to decrease narcotic requirements and improve overall pain control; however, there is no clear data on reduction of postoperative ileus. Beaussier et al. (28) have shown a reduction in the length of stay with decreased narcotic requirements and improved pain control with a 48 hour preperitoneal pain pump administering local anesthetic in a randomized, double-blinded study in patients undergoing colonic resection. This method does appear safe and effective; however, the risk of increased wound infections in patients undergoing colectomy and placement of a preperitoneal pump remains to be clearly identified.

The safety and efficacy of the peripherally acting mu-opioid receptor antagonists have been examined in six large placebo controlled trials. The available products are the orally administered alvimopan or the systemically administered methylnaltrexone. Phase III studies on alvimopan have clearly shown that a dose of 12 mg initiated and continued postoperatively decreases postoperative ileus by 12–18 hours as compared to controls, and enhances gastrointestinal (GI) recovery in various patient populations (29,30). While a 12–18 hour reduction in time to GI function does not seem awe inspiring, these same studies have shown a significant reduction in the postoperative ileus related morbidity (having to treat 12 patients to reduce morbidity in one), including significantly reducing the need for NG tube insertion, reduction in prolonged hospital stay as a consequence of postoperative ileus, and a significant reduction in the readmission rates for postoperative ileus (1). The most recently published data by Ludwig et al. demonstrated that alvimopan significantly reduced hospital length of stay by 1.4 days, and enhanced GI recovery in patients who were incorporated into a standardized GI recovery plan (30).

The benefit of alvimopan has been clearly shown in multiple randomized trials and the drug has been approved for widespread use by the Federal Drug Administration (FDA), however, more data is needed to clearly define if alvimopan accelerates postoperative GI function and reduces length of stay as compared to standardized fast-track postoperative recovery programs. Cost benefit studies are also required given the significant expense of the medication.

Standardized Postoperative Management

Early oral feeding, early ambulation, standardized postoperative antiemetic agents, and limiting excessive fluid administration postoperatively have all been shown to enhance early GI recovery (7). Each of these items is usually incorporated into standardized postoperative care, or fast-track plans. These perioperative care plans have shown significant improvement in postoperative prevention of ileus and decreasing length of stay. For open colonic surgery, this equates to a decrease in length of stay by 2 days. Other commonly included tactics include elimination of NG tubes and limiting narcotic intake with the use of non-steroidal antiinflammatory agents (NSAIDs) and epidural catheters for pain control.

The ultimate goal of any standardized postoperative care protocol is to reduce postoperative complication rates, enhance recovery, and reduce costs to the health care system. The techniques and medications discussed above may be incorporated into a protocol to allow for this enhanced recovery. While more study is required for some of the newer drugs and interventions, most are cheap, low risk interventions for the patient that are effective in enhancing GI recovery.

Recommended References and Readings

1. Guillou PJ, Quirke P, Thorpe H, et al. Short-term endpoints of conventional versus laparoscopic-assisted surgery in patients with colorectal cancer (MRC CLASICC trial): multicentre, randomized controlled trial. *Lancet* 2005;365:1718–26.
2. Jayne DG, Guillou PJ, Thorpe H, et al. Randomized trial of laparoscopic-assisted resection of colorectal carcinoma: 3-year results of the UK MRC CLASSIC trial group. *J Clin Oncol* 2007;25:3061–68.
3. Nelson H, Sargent DJ, Wieand HS, et al. Clinical outcomes of surgical therapy study group of the laparoscopic colectomy trial: a comparison of laparoscopically assisted and open colectomy for colon cancer. *N Engl J Med* 2004;350:2050–59.
4. Schwandner O, Farke S, Fischer F, Eckmann C, Schiedeck TH, Bruch HP. Laparoscopic colectomy for recurrent and complicated diverticulitis: a prospective study of 396 patients. *Arch Surg* 2004;389(2):97–103.
5. Senagore AJ, Duepree HJ, Delaney CP, Dissanaike S, Brady KM, Fazio VW. Cost structure of laparoscopic and open sigmoid colectomy for diverticular disease: similarities and differences. *Dis Colon Rectum* 2002;45(4):485–90.
6. Senagore AJ, Duepree HJ, Delaney CP, Brady KM, Fazio VW. Results of a standardized technique and postoperative care plan for laparoscopic sigmoid colectomy: a 30-month experience. *Dis Colon Rectum* 2003;46(4):503–09.
7. Vlug MS, Wind J, Van Der Zaag E, Ubbink DT, Cense HA, Bemelman WA. Systematic review of laparoscopic vs. open colonic surgery within an enhanced recovery programme. *Colorectal Dis* 2009;11(4):335–43.
8. Polle SW, Wind J, Fuhring JW, Hofland J, Gouma DJ, Bemelman WA. Implementaion of a fast-track perioperative care program: what are the difficulties? *Dig Surg* 2007;24(6):441–49.
9. Schwenk W, Gunther N, Wendling P, et al; Fast track Colon II Quality Assuance Group. "Fast-track" rehabilitation for elective colonic surgery in Germany-prospective observational data from a multi-centre quality assurance programme. *Int J Colorectal Dis* 2008;23:93–99.
10. Guenaga KF, Matos D, Castro AA, Atallah AN, Willie-Jorgensen P. Mechanical bowel preparation for elective colorectal surgery. *Cochrane Database Syst Rev* 2005;25(1):CD001544.
11. Slim K, Vicaut E, Panis Y, Chipponi J. Meta-analysis of randomized clinical trials of colorectal surgery with or without mechanical bowel preparation. *Br J Surg* 2004;91(9):1125–30.
12. Slim K, Vicaut E, Launay-Savary MV, Contant C, Chipponi J. Updated systematic review and meta-analysis of randomized clinical trials on the role of mechanical bowel preparation before colorectal surgery. *Ann Surg* 2009;249(2):203–09.
13. Jung B, Pahlman L, Nyström PO, Nilsson E; Mechanical Bowel Preparation Study Group. Multicentre randomized clinical trial of mechanical bowel preparation in elective colonic resection. *Br J Surg* 2007;94(6):689–95. Mechanical bowel preparation for elective colorectal surgery: a multicentre randomised trial.
14. Contant CM, Hop WC, van't Sant HP, et al. Mechanical bowel preparation for elective colorectal surgery: a multicentre randomised trial. *Lancet* 2007;370(9605):2112–17. Erratum in: Lancet. 2008;371(9625):1664.
15. Kehlet H. Postoperative ileus–an update on preventive techniques. *Nat Clin Pract Gastroenterol Hepatol* 2008;5(10):552–58.
16. Maron DJ, Fry RD. New therapies in the treatment of postoperative ileus after gastrointestinal surgery. *Am J Ther* 2008;15(1):59–65.
17. Jorgensen H, Wetterslev J, Moiniche S, Dahl JB. Epidural local anaesthetics versus opioid-based analgesic regimens on postoperative gastrointestinal paralysis, PONV and pain after abdominal surgery. *Cochrane Database Syst Rev* 2000(4):CD001893.
18. Asao T, Kuwano H, Nakamura J, Morinaga N, Hirayama I, Ide M. Gum chewing enhances early recovery from postoperative ileus after laparoscopic colectomy. *J Am Coll Surg* 2002;195(1):30–32.
19. Schuster R, Grewal N, Greaney GC, Waxman K. Gum chewing reduces ileus after elective open sigmoid colectomy. *Arch Surg* 2006;141(2):174–76.
20. Matros E, Rocha F, Zinner M, et al. Does gum chewing ameliorate postoperative ileus? Results of a prospective, randomized, placebo-controlled trial. *J Am Coll Surg* 2006;202(5):773–78.
21. de Castro SM, Van Den Esschert JW, van Heek NT, et al. A systematic review of the efficacy of gum chewing for the amelioration of postoperative ileus. *Dig Surg* 2008;25(1):39–45.
22. Purkayastha S, Tilney HS, Darzi AW, Tekkis PP. Meta-analysis of randomized studies evaluating chewing gum to enhance postoperative recovery following colectomy. *Arch Surg* 2008;143(8):788–793.
23. St Peter SD, Valusek PA, Little DC, Snyder CL, Holcomb GW III, Ostlie DJ. Does routine nasogastric tube placement after an operation for perforated appendicitis make a difference? *J Surg Res* 2007;143(1):66–69.
24. Roig JV, Garcia-Fadrique A, Garcia Armengol J, et al. Use of nasogastric tubes and drains after colorectal surgery. Have attitudes changed in the last 10 years? *Cir Esp* 2008;83(2):78–84.

25. Marret E, Rolin M, Beaussier M, Bonnet F. Meta-analysis of intravenous lidocaine and postoperative recovery after abdominal surgery. *Br J Surg* 2008;95(11):1331–38.
26. Marret E, Kurdi O, Zufferey P, Bonnet F. Effects of nonsteroidal antiinflammatory drugs on patient-controlled analgesia morphine side effects: meta-analysis of randomized controlled trials. *Anesthesiology* 2005;102(6):1249–1260.
27. Marret E, Flahault A, Samama CM, Bonnet F. Effects of postoperative, nonsteroidal, antiinflammatory drugs on bleeding risk after tonsillectomy: meta-analysis of randomized, controlled trials. *Anesthesiology* 2003;98(6):1497–1502.
28. Beaussier M, El'Ayoubi H, Schiffer E, et al. Continuous preperitoneal infusion of ropivacaine provides effective analgesia and accelerates recovery after colorectal surgery: a randomized, double-blind, placebo-controlled study. *Anesthesiology* 2007;107(3):461–468.
29. Senagore AJ, Bauer JJ, Du W, Techner L. Alvimopan accelerates gastrointestinal recovery after bowel resection regardless of age, gender, race, or concomitant medication use. *Surgery* 2007;142(4):478–486.
30. Ludwig K, Enker WE, Delaney CP, et al. Gastrointestinal tract recovery in patients undergoing bowel resection: results of a randomized trial of alvimopan and placebo with a standardized accelerated postoperative care pathway. *Arch Surg* 2008;143(11):1098–1105.

10 Laparoscopic Lateral-to-Medial

Morris E. Franklin Jr, Guillermo Portillo, and Karla Russek

Introduction

A laparoscopic approach to colon resection has been quoted as showing numerous advantages when compared to similar open procedures including less postoperative pain, reduced ileus, reduced immunosuppression, decreased length of hospital stay, improved cosmesis, and earlier return to normal activities. Numerous reports have shown equal or better survival in cancer patients when a laparoscopic approach is utilized.

Several options of performing laparoscopic colon surgery have been developed, but according to the authors there are three currently accepted techniques. Laparoscopically assisted, in which the dissection is completed all through a laparoscopic approach, but the specimen is extracted by way of an incision, with an extracorporeal anastomosis subsequently performed.

Laparoscopically hand-assisted, where the dissection is hand aided and the specimen is extracted by the hand port or an incision.

Laparoscopic, where all of the dissection, vascular control, bowl resection, and anastomosis are laparoscopically performed, with the specimen being extracted through natural orifices such as the anus or vagina. According to the editors, the laparoscopic approach also includes specimen delivery through either the abdominal wall or a perineal incision.

The authors' preferred method is the totally intracorporeal technique, suitable for left colon resections, including partial resections, sigmoid, and low anterior resections, which may be used in a large number of patients. In cases of right colon resection a totally intracorporeal anastomosis is preferable with a small muscle splitting incision or vaginal extraction.

These techniques allow a more anatomical and physiologic resection. It is well known that surgical trauma modifies and modulates the immunological response; therefore, minimizing trauma to the abdominal wall may enhance the recovery of the patient. We have seen a faster recovery and a diminished number of complications compared to published reports with laparoscopically assisted and hand-assisted laparoscopic surgery.

The purpose of this chapter is to demonstrate and discuss the technical tips that the authors have found to be beneficial in the performance of laparoscopic colorectal surgery.

INDICATIONS AND PATIENT SELECTION

Results from randomized prospective trials have proven that the laparoscopic method, in experienced hands, yields results that are at least equivalent, from an oncologic perspective, to traditional open methods. A laparoscopic approach has become the preferred method for performing colectomy for all benign and malignant conditions.

Accurate preoperative tumor localization is an important consideration when planning a successful laparoscopic colectomy for malignancy. Patients can undergo colonoscopy, when possible, the day prior to surgery, obviating the need for two separate bowel preparations; the lesion can be marked with tattoo ink. At the time of surgery, the air that was insufflated during colonoscopy will have been evacuated, thus colonic distension should not pose a problem during the procedure. While endoscopic localization of right-sided tumors may be ascertained if the lesion is visualized within sight of the ileocecal valve, there is no comparable landmark when dealing with transverse colon or left-sided lesions.

India ink and other nonchemically carbon-based inks are the most common agents used. Intraoperative colonoscopy should be performed if the tattoo cannot be seen or if the surgeon is not confident with the localization as is described elsewhere in this chapter. Pre operative barium enema can also be extremely useful in localization of specific lesions and is used routinely in our practice.

SURGERY

Port Placement

Pneumoperitoneum is achieved by a Veress needle placed in the right side, right upper quadrant, right mid flank outside of rectus sheath. There are many different port site arrangements utilized for laparoscopic left and sigmoid colectomy. The patient's body mass index and abdominal breadth should be taken into consideration when choosing port locations; target quadrants should be identified and the ports placed to assure adequate access. When placing the right lower quadrant port to accommodate the endoscopic stapler, the surgeon must consider the angle that the stapler will achieve coming across the rectosigmoid. Similarly, instruments introduced through the left-sided port(s) should reach to the splenic flexure and also allow retraction of the sigmoid colon mesentery deep in the pelvis. As with other advanced laparoscopic procedures, working ports should be triangulated to the operative field to avoid sword fighting of the instruments and to accommodate two-handed dissection.

Depending on the availability of and the need for a second assistant to hold the laparoscope, a 4-port or a 5-port setup is utilized. Once port placement is completed, the operation commences.

Surgical Technique

The initial maneuver is mobilization of the sigmoid and visualization of the left ureter. In the lateral-to-medial approach, the peritoneum is first incised with a steady dissection of the sigmoid colon and the high portion of the rectum toward a medial direction, with care taken to avoid injury to the external iliac artery, vein, and nerves. Mobilization of the sigmoid should be performed until the ureter is identified and the peritoneum has been incised to the level of middle hemorrhoidal vessels. If the vessels can be readily identified on the left they can be ligated. It is important to remember that the ureter can easily be confused with the superior rectal artery and we feel each should be identified before incision. With the sigmoid colon on anterior stretch, the peritoneum is incised on the right of the rectosigmoid mesentery. This maneuver establishes a window through which the left ureter is identified. Laparoscopically, this step is quite easy and frequently the CO_2 will help establish this dissection plane. Following this phase, the inferior mesenteric artery and vein are identified 3–5 cm above the iliac bifurcation and can be ligated at the highest level possible. We recommend separate division of the artery and vein with either a bipolar cutting device or ligation with 10 mm clips and then followed by division and application of polydoioxane pre-tied endoloop. The artery should never be incised in one cut; rather, the artery should be partially incised, checked for residual back flow, or additional bleeding. If such bleeding occurs, additional clips and/or ligation may be applied as needed. With intracorporeal knot tying skills, the vessels may also be quite economically ligated with sutures.

The inferior mesenteric vein is often adjacent to the artery and as such care should be taken to identify this structure. In case of colon cancer the inferior mesenteric vein may be traced to its origin at the splenic vein or at least to the ligament of Treitz, and ligation and division performed at this point. Care should be taken to avoid injury of the ureter in this ligation. We perform splenic flexure mobilization in almost every patient, to help prevent tension on the anastomosis. The patient should be placed in reverse Trendelenburg position with the left side rolled up. Mobilization of the splenic flexure is easier to perform laparoscopically than during open surgery because of the excellent visualization and identification of anatomical structures with the laparoscope. We use three approaches for splenic flexure mobilization, lateral-to-medial, medial to lateral, and retroperitoneal approach.

After complete dissection of the proximal portion of the colon, the point at which resection is to be performed should be determined by intraoperative colonoscopy and the pericolonic tissue in this area cleaned circumferential for a distance of 1–2 cm. If an endoloop is to be used to secure the head of the circular stapler, at least 2 cm should be used. If an Endo-GIA is to be used, a lesser amount of dissection will be needed. If a totally intracorporeal anastomosis is to be performed, we recommend using Endo-GIA or sharp dissection to divide the colon at the predesignated site proximally and distally. Each end can be controlled with a prettied Endoloop, if using sharp dissection, to prevent tumor or fecal spillage.

Before the division of the colon, an on-the-table colonoscopy can be preformed to ensure and determine adequate margins, as well as to ascertain complete cleanliness of the colon. The colon is frequently irrigated with diluted Betadine as an additional precaution. Before the colon is insufflated, the proximal bowel should be clamped with a laparoscopic Bulldog Glassman clamp (Klein Surgical, San Antonio, TX, USA) or with an externally held conventional 10 mm instrument to prevent distension of the proximal colon and potentially the small bowel. The distal line of resection should be accurately determined with the colonoscope. After division of the distal portion of the colon, the rectum is left open. The distal segment of the resected colon should be encircled with a prettied Endoloop and the entire specimen placed in an impermeable bag for subsequent removal. If the specimen is not too large, the anus can be dilated with two fingers. Most specimens up to 6 or 7 cm in diameter can be readily removed with transanal route. If a laparoscopically assisted anastomosis is to be performed, the lower abdominal incision can be extended or a Pfannenstiel type incision can be made to remove the specimen at this point of time. If the specimen does not fit through the anus and an intracorporeal anastomosis is to be performed, the bagged specimen can now be placed in the left upper quadrant and stored until the anastomosis is completed.

For laparoscopic assisted anastomosis, the proximal end of the colon should be brought through the abdominal wall, a purse-string suture applied and the anvil inserted, followed by the closure of the purse-string suture. Meticulous attention to detail is imperative for the successful completion of this portion of the procedure and care must be taken to leave a small rim of tissue rather than a large rim that can interfere with the mechanics of the end-to-end stapler. An Endo-GIA, if not previously used to divide the distal portion of the colon, can now be used to close the distal portion of the colon and the stapler spike brought through the closed rectum. The head and anvil of the stapler can be joined and the anastomosis completed. It is strongly recommended that the tissue between the head and the anvil of the stapler be carefully inspected to ensure that adjacent tissue such as fallopian tube or ureter has not been incorporated into the staple line.

If a totally intracorporeal anastomosis technique is to be used, the anvil should be introduced through the rectum either on the head of the stapler or on a separate introducing device. The anvil can be stored in the right or left iliac fossa for subsequent insertion into the proximal colon and the distal rectum can be stapled with an Endo-GIA 60 or similar stapling device. The anvil can now be inserted into the proximal portion of the colon and a second line of staples applied across the open end with subsequent protrusion and extraction of the point of the anvil through the staple line or adjacent to the staple line. Care should be taken using this technique to avoid losing the anvil in the proximal colon. The laparoscopic bulldog Glassman clamp works very well for this procedure. A secondary technique is that of application of prettied loop preferably of a strong suture such as (polydioxanone) suture (PDS), around the anvil again insuring an adequate rim of tissue. Excising all redundant tissue affords a good mechanical working of the stapler.

After securing the anvil in the proximal colon and bringing it into the pelvis, the two parts are joined. Again care is taken to circumferentially inspect the staple line to ensure that additional extraneous tissue is present. After firing, the stapler is removed, and a colonoscopy is performed exerting pressure into the rectum to test the anastomosis and directly visualize the anastomosis internally. Most leaks can be controlled with a simple suture; however, a protective ileostomy can be performed and brought out through a 10-mm trocar site if there is any doubt to the integrity of the anastomosis.

A drain is not routinely left in the pelvis, but the entire area is irrigated with saline, as well as 3.5% betadine solution in the case of carcinoma. All ports are then irrigated with the dilute betadine solution as well. The trocar sites are individually closed with 0 Vicryl using a suture passer (Carter-Thomason® [Louisville Laboratories Inc., Louisville, KY, USA]). The abdominal cavity and pelvis are then irrigated with same solution and completely suctioned before finishing the procedure.

POSTOPERATIVE MANAGEMENT

We use standard agents in the postoperative period including perioperative antibiotics that cover colon flora such as cefotaxime, metronidazole, or cefepime. Intravenous fluid is required to maintain urine output of 1 ml/kg/hr. A nasogastric tube may or not be left in place depending on the manipulation of the bowel, number of adhesions, length of the surgery, age of the patient, and other factors. Additional medications include analgesia in an amount to maintain good pain control as well as medication for the undesirable postoperative nausea. Other preoperative medications such as antihypertensives and diabetic and cardiac medications are continued in the postoperative period.

We recommend waiting at least 6 hours to start oral intake, but in elderly patients the waiting time may extend to 12 hours, however, most patients will tolerate clear liquids the next day. The indication for a full diet is passage of gas or stool.

The patient's progress determines the disposition of the patient; the requisites for a satisfactory discharge include the patient being able to tolerate a solid food diet and regular bowel movements, well controlled comorbidities afebrile for at least 24 hours, satisfactory ambulation and pain control, healing wounds clean. All drains should also be removed. In the authors' experience, this time period averages 3.5 days in patients less than 50 years of age and 5.5 days in patients over 50 years of age for most colon surgeries.

Timing for return to normal activity is loosely determined depending on the individual practitioner. Most of the patients are able to return to normal activity within 14 days. We do not recommend returning to work any sooner than 5–10 days after surgery unless the patient has a sedentary occupation. Most patients are able to tolerate returning to full activity and/or work within 7–10 days. Some patients who have particular problems may not be able to return to work earlier than 2 weeks. Patients with very heavy labor-related occupations require at least 10 days to 2 weeks before they can return to full, unrestricted work activities.

It is very important to advise the patients about fecal urgency and frequency; to help diminish this, we recommend the use of bulky or high fiber supplements.

Laparoscopic left colon resection is a feasible and safe procedure. It should be performed by experienced surgeons to assure the best results. It is important to recognize the different anatomical aspects it presents compared to open surgery.

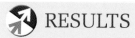

RESULTS

Left colon: Totally Intracorporeal Anastomosis Results

From January 1996 to December 31, 2006, 1,063 laparoscopic colon resections involving left colon, sigmoid, or rectum were performed at the Texas Endosurgery Institute, and prospectively analyzed.

Six hundred and four laparoscopic left-colon resections were completed with transanal specimen extraction (62%). The average operating time was 152 minutes for transanal extraction and 170 minutes for the laparoscopically assisted group. The average estimated blood loss was 94 cc for transanal extraction, but was 204 cc for the laparoscopically assisted group. Anastomotic leak occurred once in the transanal extraction group and seven times in the laparoscopically assisted group ($P = 0.01$). Abdominal abscess requiring intervention occurred once in the transanal extraction group and four times in the laparoscopically assisted group ($P > 0.05$). Incisional hernia was noted once in the transanal extraction group and six times in the laparoscopically assisted group ($P = 0.01$). Postoperative wound infections occurred once in the transanal extraction group and six times in the laparoscopically assisted group ($P = 0.01$). No permanent incontinence was observed, although transient incontinence was noted in 14 of the 664 patients in the transanal extraction group (2%) but in none of did not occur in the laparoscopically assisted group ($P = 0.01$). Transanal extraction was associated with less blood loss and a shorter operative time.

Suggested Readings

American Society of Colon and Rectal Surgeons. Position statement on laparoscopic colectomy for curable cancer. *Dis Colon Rectum* 2004;47:A1.

Bergamaschi R, Arnaud JP. Intracorporeal colorectal anastomosis following laparoscopic left colon resection. *Surg Endosc* 1997;11:800–01.

Bokey EL, Moore JWE, Keating JP, et al. Laparoscopic resection of the colon and rectum for cancer. *Br J Surg* 1997;84:822–25.

Chen HH, Wexner SD, Weiss EG, et al. Laparoscopic colectomy for benign colorectal disease is associated with a significant reduction in disability as compared with laparotomy. *Surg Endosc* 1998;12:1397–400.

Clinical Outcomes of surgical therapy Study Groups. A Comparison of laparoscopically assisted and open colectomy for colon cancer. *NEJM* 2004;350(20):2050–59.

Cohen SM, Wexner SD. Laparoscopic colorectal resection for cancer: the Cleveland Clinic Florida experience. *Surg Oncol* 1993;2(Suppl 1):35–42.

Dunker MS, Stiggelbout AM, van Hogezand RA, et al. Cosmesis and body image after laparoscopic-assisted and open ileocolic resection for Crohn's disease. *Surg Endosc* 1998;12:1334–40.

Feingold DL, Addona T, Forde KA, et al. Safety and reliability of tattooing colorectal neoplasms prior to laparoscopic resection. *J Gastrointest Surg* 2004;8:543–46.

Fielding GA, Lumley J, Nathanson L, et al. Laparoscopic colectomy. *Surg Endosc* 1997;11:745–49.

Fowler DL, White SA. Laparoscopy-assisted sigmoid resection. *Surg Laparosc Endosc* 1991;1:183–88.

Franklin ME Jr, Berghoff KE, Arellano PP, et al. Safety and efficacy of the use of bioabsorbable seamguard in colorectal surgery at the Texas Endosurgery Institute. *Surg Laparosc Endosc Percutan Tech* 2005;15(1):9–13.

Franklin ME, Kazantsev GB, Abrego D, Diaz-E JA, Balli J, Glass JL. Laparoscopic. surgery for stage III colon cancer: long-term follow-up. *Surg Endosc* 2000;14:612–16.

Franklin ME, Ramos R, Rosenthal D, Schussler W. Laparoscopic colonic procedures. *World J Surg* 1993;17:51–56.

Franklin ME, Rosenthal D, Abrego-Medina D, et al. Prospective comparison of open vs. laparoscopic colon surgery for carcinoma: five-year results. *Dis Colon Rectum* 1996;39:S35–S46.

Franklin ME, Rosenthal D, Norem RF. Prospective evaluation of laparoscopic colon resection versus open colon resection for adenocarcinoma. *Surg Endosc* 1995;9:811–16.

Greznlee RT, Murray T, Bolden S, et al. Cancer statistics, 2000. *CA Cancer J Clin* 2000;50:7–33.

Jacobs M, Verdeja G, Goldstein D. Minimally invasive colon resection. *Surg Laparosc Endosc* 1991;1:144–50.

Khalili TM, Fleshner PR, Hiatt JR, et al. Colorectal cancer: comparison of laparoscopic with open approaches. *Dis Colon Rectum* 1998;41:832–38.

Kockerling F, Reymond MA, Schneider C, et al. The Laparoscopic Colorectal Surgery Study Group. Prospective multicenter study of the quality of oncologic resections in patients undergoing laparoscopic colorectal surgery for cancer. *Dis Colon Rectum* 1998;41:963–70.

Kockerling F, Rose J, Schneider C, et al. Laparoscopic Colorectal Surgery Study Group (LCSSG). Laparoscopic colorectal anastomosis: risk of postoperative leakage: results of a multicenter study. *Surg Endosc* 1999;13:639–44.

Kockerling F, Schneider C, Reymond MA, et al, Laparoscopic Colorectal Surgery Study Group (LCSSG). Early results of a prospective multicenter study on 500 consecutive cases of laparoscopic colorectal surgery. *Surg Endosc* 1998;12:37–41.

Lacy AM, Garcia-Valdecasas JC, Delgado S, et al. Postoperative complications of laparoscopic-assisted colectomy. *Surg Endosc* 1997;11:119–22.

Lord SA, Larach SW, Ferrara A, et al. Laparoscopic resections for colorectal carcinoma: a three-year experience. *Dis Colon Rectum* 1996;39:148–54.

MacRae HM, McLeod RS. Handsewn vs. stapled anastomoses in colon and rectal surgery: a meta-analysis. *Dis Colon Rectum* 1998;41:180–89.

Monson JRT, Darzi A, Carey PD, Guillou PJ. Prospective evaluation of laparoscopic-assisted colectomy in an unselected group of patients. *Lancet* 1992;340:831–33.

Phillips EH, Franklin M, Carroll BJ, et al. Laparoscopic colectomy. *Ann Surg* 1992;216:703–07.

Puente I, Sosa JL, Sleeman D, et al. Laparoscopic assisted colorectal surgery. *J Laparoendosc Surg* 1994;4(1):1–7.

Schlachta CM, Mamazza J, Seshadri PA, et al. Defining a learning curve for laparoscopic colorectal resections. *Dis Colon Rectum* 2001;44:217–22.

Stocchi L, Nelson H. Laparoscopic colectomy for colon cancer: trial update. *J Surg Onc* 1998;68:255–67.

Whelan RL. Laparotomy, laparoscopy, cancer, and beyond. *Surg Endosc* 2001;15:110–15.

Ziprin P, Ridgway PF, Peck DH, Darzi AW. The theories and realities of port-site metastases: a critical appraisal. *J Am Coll Surg* 2002; 195:395–408.

11 Robotic Left Colon and Rectal Resection

Leela M. Prasad and Slawomir Marecik

 ## INDICATIONS/CONTRAINDICATIONS

Since the first laparoscopic cholecystectomy in the United States in 1988, the evolution of surgical technique has seen a minimally invasive revolution! Laparoscopic surgery is now accepted as a standard of care for colonic resections and is being increasingly offered to patients requiring a rectal resection. Despite its widespread use, laparoscopic surgery poses significant technical challenges to the colorectal surgeon. This is probably why the majority of colorectal procedures in the United States are still being performed through the traditional open approach.

The technical advantages of the Da Vinci® Robotic system (Intuitive Surgical, Sunnyvale, CA, USA) with true three-dimensional imaging, tremor filtration, a stable camera platform, and endowristed movements have attempted to overcome the technical limitations of current laparoscopic instrumentation. These advantages have the potential to benefit patients in terms of possible better oncological and functional outcomes. The surgeon also stands to benefit from the improved ergonomics of the robot that can now avoid the abnormal posturing and hand configuration associated with laparoscopic surgery.

Right at the outset, it should be mentioned that robotics in surgery is a new technology, and the experience with its use in colorectal surgery is probably less, as compared to its use in other surgical fields. At the same time different groups working independently have confirmed the safety and feasibility of robotic assistance in a number of colorectal procedures. At present, there exist a number of colorectal applications of the robot, each with its unique cart position and port placement. This presents a number of options to the colorectal surgeon to suit various patient populations and tumor locations. The purpose of this chapter is to present under one head the various options for robotic assistance in left colon and rectal resections.

It is presumed that the reader is familiar with the parts and setup of the Da Vinci robot, and is proficient with its basic positioning and functioning. This chapter focuses on elaborating the specific cart positions, port placements, and surgical steps essential for robot-assisted left colon resections. As there is no substitute for mentored surgical training, a study of the surgical techniques presented here probably requires initial mentoring for the colorectal surgeon new to robotic technology.

In an attempt to present systematically to the reader the different surgical techniques, the left colon and rectum have been addressed in different chapters. Quite often, resection of the left colon involves mobilization of the upper rectum and a rectal resection always requires mobilization of the left colon to some extent. To maintain some degree of continuity and to enable a comprehensive presentation of the principles of robotic colorectal surgery, some details of robotic rectal dissection have been included here as well.

Finally, it should be appreciated that robotic technology as a whole is rapidly evolving. The Da Vinci Robot itself is in its second version with longer and more maneuverable arms, better ergonomics, and high definition imaging. It is possible that as robotic technology evolves, the techniques presented here might give way to new and better applications of the robot. The need for more precise and ergonomic surgical instruments constantly drives technology to develop better and more efficient tools. It is important to always keep in perspective the primary goal, that is, a better and safer patient care, when evaluating and using these new technologies.

Robot-Assisted Surgical Options

A significant limitation of the robotic system is its restricted surgical field for a given cart position. This enables a precise dissection in one quadrant of the abdomen while limiting access to another without shifting the robotic cart. Every change in robotic cart position requires a complete undocking of the robot, moving the cart to a new position and redocking the robot in the required position. This significantly adds to the operating time.

A colon or rectal resection involves a precise dissection of the tumor/diseased area and a sufficient mobilization of the remaining colon to achieve a tension-free anastomosis. This therefore expands the working surgical field to include a number of abdominal quadrants. As the Da Vinci Robot has a limited access with one cart position, a number of different options have been proposed for the optimal use of the robot in a left colon/rectal resection. Options vary from using the robot in one position to shifting the robotic cart three times during a single procedure. To limit the number of changes in cart position, attempts have to be made to restrict the use of the robot for a part of the procedure or to tailor the use of the robot according to the patient's habitus, tumor location or colonic anatomy. All the feasible options of robot-assisted left colon/rectal resection have been presented in this chapter. The final choice on the extent of robotic assistance and the number of cart positions should ideally be made on an individual basis.

The Laparoscopic–Robotic *"Hybrid Procedure"*

The maximal advantage of the robotic system is probably best appreciated in the rectal dissection. The deep retraction along with the precise dissection required to achieve an intact mesorectal envelope while preserving the autonomic nerves is probably what makes a laparoscopic rectal excision for cancer particularly challenging. This technical challenge is more appreciated in the obese, male pelvis, when resecting the mid or low rectal lesion. It is here that the advanced dexterity of the robotic system probably has the potential to offer the greatest benefit.

A rectal resection for cancer requires a total mesorectal excision along with the mobilization of the descending colon, with or without the splenic flexure in order to achieve a tension-free anastomosis. Unlike laparoscopic rectal dissection, laparoscopic mobilization of the descending colon is fairly easily accomplished. The robot could also be effectively used for this mobilization but would probably require a change in cart position. This change in cart position would be more likely when resecting a low rectal tumor, when operating in an obese individual or with a high-riding splenic flexure. These situations would probably expand the surgical field out of the range of the robotic instruments if the position of the robot is not changed.

Taking the "best from both worlds" as it were, a hybrid technique using laparoscopy for the left colon mobilization and the robot for the rectal dissection has been suggested.

This maximizes the advantage of the robot where it is most beneficial, that is, the rectal dissection and overcomes its limitation of a restricted access by using laparoscopic technique for the descending colon mobilization.

The extent of colonic mobilization is largely determined by the level of the lesion and the redundancy of the sigmoid colon. The need for splenic flexure mobilization is often appreciated once the descending colon is completely mobilized. Using laparoscopy for the left colon mobilization provides the flexibility to mobilize a length of colon required to achieve a tension-free anastomosis, which is the main objective. Using the robot for the entire procedure would most likely require more than one cart position if a high-riding splenic flexure and a low rectal lesion have to be addressed during the same procedure. Eliminating the increased time for changing robotic cart positions is an advantage of the hybrid procedure.

Options for Robot-Assisted Left Colon/Rectal Dissection

The following options have been described:

1. Robotic left colon/sigmoid resection
2. Robotic low anterior resection—single cart position
3. Robotic low anterior resection—multiple cart positions
4. Hybrid procedure (laparoscopic left colon mobilization + robotic rectal dissection)
5. Robotic abdominoperineal resection (APR)

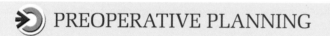

PREOPERATIVE PLANNING

Principles of Robotic Cart Positioning

The robotic cart is always placed on the side of dissection. This enables the robotic arms that arch away from the robotic cart to be directed back toward the site of dissection. Based on this principle, for dissection of the left colon the cart is placed on the left side of the patient, and for a rectal dissection the best position for the robotic cart would be between the patient's legs. As an anterior resection always requires some mobilization of the left colon in addition to the rectal mobilization, a totally robotic anterior resection would theoretically require two cart positions, that is, the position between the legs for the rectal dissection and the robotic cart placed by the patient's left side for the left colon mobilization.

Changing cart positions during the procedure adds significantly to operating time. This is why a position by the patient's left hip has been described to address the rectum as well as the left colon with the robot in one cart position. The left hip position though not ideal for either a rectal dissection or for a left colon mobilization, is an effective compromise and works in a number of patients. However, in patients with a low rectal lesion, or with a high-riding splenic flexure, the left hip position may not provide the required range of movement to the robotic arms. In such cases, shifting the robotic cart between the legs for the rectal dissection and to the left side or even besides the patient's left arm for the splenic flexure is required.

To summarize, there are three robotic cart positions described for the left colon and rectum. Table 11.1 lists these positions with the surgical access provided in each position. Figures 11.1–11.3 graphically depict these positions.

The efficacy of different robotic cart positions also varies with the body habitus of the patient. In a short, thin patient of low body mass index (BMI), the position by the left hip alone might provide adequate access to the pelvic floor as well as the splenic flexure. In a tall patient with a high BMI, this might not be the case and a change in cart position may be required for a totally robotic procedure.

The close proximity of the left hip and left arm positions for the robotic cart makes it easier to sometimes move the patient about the stationary robotic cart instead of moving the cart about the patient. If the rectum, sigmoid, and descending colon are

TABLE 11.1	Available Robotic Cart Positions
Robotic cart position	**Surgical access offered**
Between the legs	Rectum • Upper • Mid • Lower (pelvic floor) Rectosigmoid junction Inferior mesenteric artery pedicle Sigmoid colon
Left hip	Rectum • Upper • Mid • Lower—not in all patients Rectosigmoid junction Inferior mesenteric pedicle (artery and vein) Sigmoid colon Descending colon Splenic flexure—not in all patients
Left side a. Left flank b. Left arm*	Sigmoid colon Inferior mesenteric pedicle (artery and vein) Descending colon Splenic flexure*

*A high-riding splenic flexure may sometimes be inaccessible in the left flank position; in these situations, the robot might have to be shifted to the left arm position. Dissecting a high-riding splenic flexure is probably the only indication of the left arm position.

mobilized with the robot in the left hip position, but the robotic arms do not reach the splenic flexure, the robot can be undocked and the patient rotated around the stationary robotic cart so that the robot is now by the patient's left arm. The splenic flexure can be easily mobilized in this position to complete the colon mobilization. This maneuver may save operative time.

It is important to begin every robot-assisted procedure with a preplanned cart position or a plan to use multiple cart positions. A knowledge of the different cart positions and the surgical access offered by each position is essential in this planning. Careful consideration should be given to the patient's height, BMI, and tumor location. The first step in the preoperative planning of cart positions is to decide whether it is possible to complete the entire procedure in a particular patient with a single position of the robotic cart (Fig. 11.4). This is more likely to be possible in a short, thin patient with a high rectal lesion. As we move to the other end of the spectrum to a tall, obese patient with a low rectal lesion, it is more likely that a change in cart position will be required to complete the procedure robotically. One then has to decide whether to opt for a totally robotic procedure with a change in cart position, or to use the hybrid procedure, reserving the robot for the rectal dissection alone.

As the greatest advantage of the robot is probably for rectal dissection, some centers have adopted the hybrid procedure for all anterior resections irrespective of patient factors. In this procedure, the robot is used for the rectal dissection alone from a position between the patient's legs. This position is the most ideal for rectal mobilization. While the algorithm is clear at the two ends of the spectrum, there is insufficient data at this stage to make any recommendation for patients in between. For this group of patients, any of the three options of a totally robotic procedure with a single cart position, a totally robotic procedure with multiple cart positions, or a hybrid procedure are acceptable.

Due to lack of data at this stage, it is premature to make any evidence-based recommendation on the ideal use of the robot in left colon/rectal resections. However, it has been our experience that the robot offers the greatest benefit for rectal dissection, which is best achieved with the robot placed between the patient's legs. At the time of writing this chapter, we use the hybrid procedure for all low anterior resections.

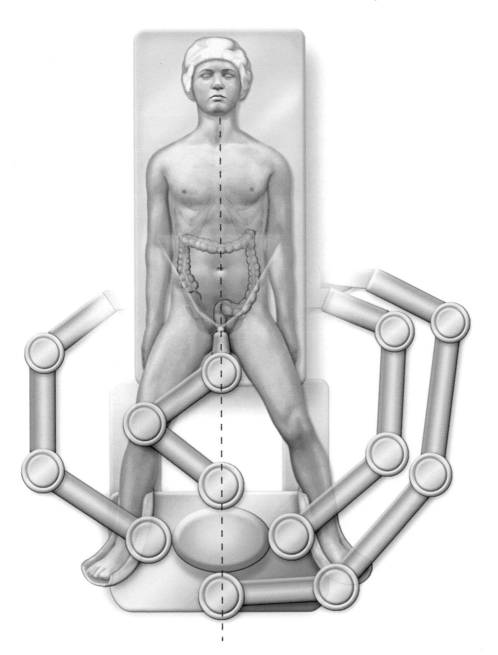

Figure 11.1 Robotic cart between the legs.

![SURGERY icon] **SURGERY**

Patient Positioning

The patient is placed on the operating table in a modified lithotomy position with the legs in Allen stirrups and minimal flexure of the hips. The patient's arms are placed at the side. We use a suction operated bean bag underneath the patient, which is brought up on either side to cradle the patient and support both upper limbs. It is important to place adequate padding between the bean bag and the patient so that there is no contact between the two. We use gel pads beneath the patient and on either side of each arm. Additional foam padding is provided over each shoulder. Care should be taken to ensure that all pressure points and bony prominences are adequately padded and protected.

The bean bag together with the patient is fixed to the operating table with the help of adhesive strapping over the patient's chest. Shoulder supports, fixed to the operating table, are placed against the bean bag, above the shoulders. These support the patient

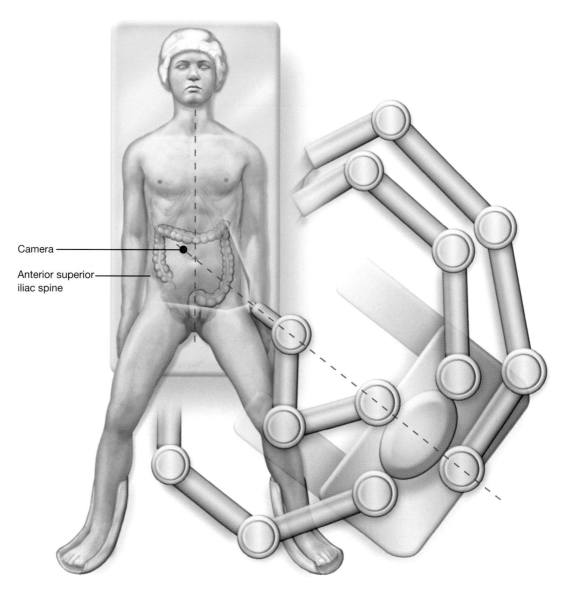

Camera

Anterior superior
iliac spine

Figure 11.2 Robotic cart in left hip position.

when placed in steep Trendelenburg position. This method of immobilization and padding is routine for any minimally invasive resection of the left colon/rectum and is not specific for robotic surgery. However, it should be noted that as the majority of the procedure for a left colon resection is performed with the patient in Trendelenburg position with a left upward tilt, the right side of the patient needs careful attention while padding the pressure points. We routinely use a three-way rectal irrigation tube for a distal rectal washout prior to rectal transection. This is placed at the time of initial positioning.

Operating Room Setup

The operating team consists of the surgeon at the console, a bedside assistant, a scrub nurse, and a circulator. It is necessary for the bedside assistant to have experience with laparoscopic surgery and robotic instrumentation. It is also beneficial for the nursing staff to be familiar with the robotic instruments, setup, and draping. This facilitates a harmonious cooperation between the entire surgical team.

The operating room setup should take into consideration the changes in robotic cart position expected during the procedure. A setup designed to provide the required space around the robotic cart will significantly increase the efficiency in the change in cart position. From Figure 11.5A it can be appreciated that the robotic cart can be moved to

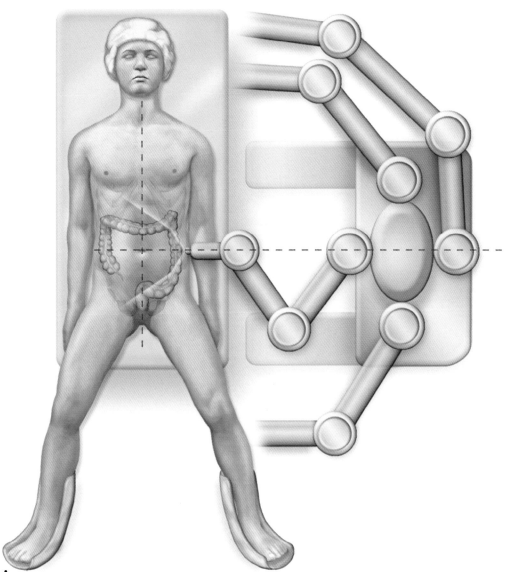

Figure 11.3 A. Robotic cart in left flank position. (*continued*)

A

all three described positions without changing the position of the scrub nurse. If, however, a single cart position between the patient's legs is used, the operating room setup can be accordingly modified (Fig. 11.5B). Two additional points need to be considered here. First, as the assistant stands on the patient's right, there should be at least one monitor available on the patient's left side, preferably over the patient's left shoulder. Second, one of the major roles of the bedside assistant is to clean the robotic laparoscope and replace the scope with another lens, that is, 0 or 30 degree. It is very convenient to have the fluid warmer with the robotic laparoscopes at the left of the bedside assistant. This makes the cleaning and replacement of the lens very quick and efficient.

Instruments

Robotic Instruments

    Camera 0 and 30 degree
    Robotic hook cautery or hot shears
    Fenestrated bipolar grasper or Maryland bipolar forceps
    Cadiére forceps

Figure 11.3 (*Continued*) **B.** Robotic cart in left arm position.

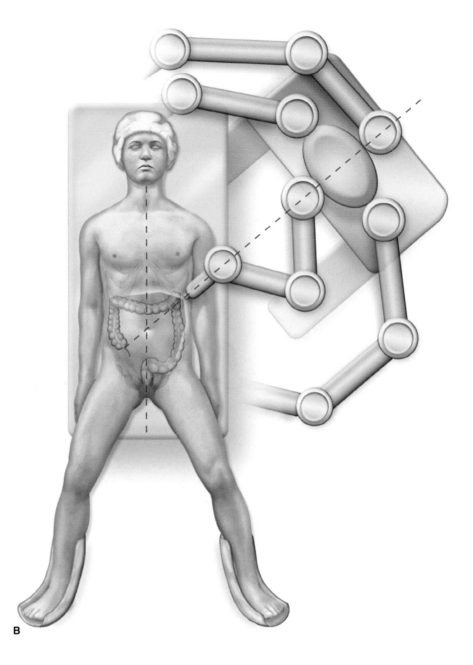

B

Figure 11.4 Preoperative planning of cart position.

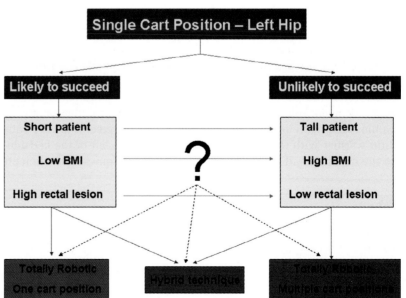

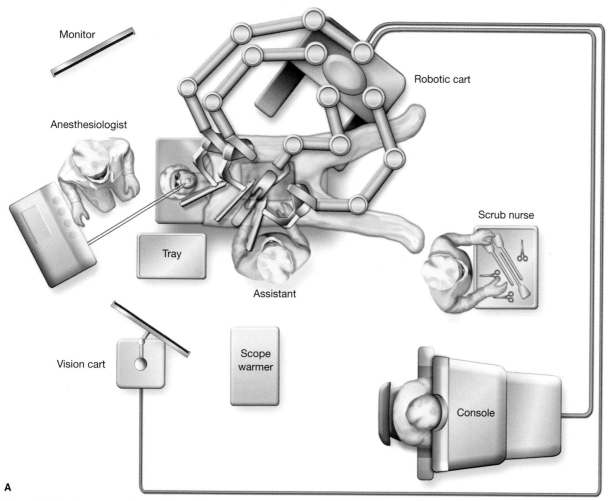

Figure 11.5 **A.** Room setup for cart in left side position. (*continued*)

Laparoscopic Instruments
    Camera 0 degree
    Long bowel grasper (1 or 2)
    Suction irrigator
    Energy device
        Electrocautery (monopolar and bipolar)
        Enseal (5 mm) or LigaSure
        Hand-assist device (optional)

Ports
    12 mm (1 or 2)
    5 mm (1 or 2)
    8-mm robotic cannulas (3 or 4)

Staplers
    Endo GIA, roticulator (OR TA 45 mm)
    EEA
    Automated purse string applicator (1 or 2) (optional)

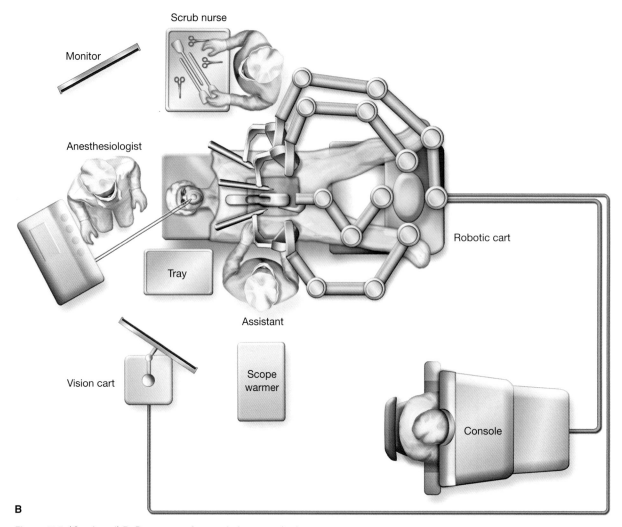

Figure 11.5 (*Continued*) **B.** Room setup for cart in between the legs.

Port Placement

The pattern of port placement in robotic surgery is a little different as compared to laparoscopic port placement on account of a few features unique to robotic surgery. The following factors should be taken into consideration when placing the ports.

1. The external movement of the robotic arms is as important as the internal range of movement offered by the robotic instruments. An ideal port positioning provides the required internal range of movement without external collision. As a working principle, a distance of 10 cm between the ports is optimal to prevent external arm collision.

2. All port positions should be considered on the insufflated abdomen. Port positions marked on the flat abdomen undergo lateral fanning out and superior displacement when the abdomen is insufflated. The lateral displacement of the ports is beneficial in avoiding external arm collisions but the superior displacement can hinder the access of the robotic instruments to the deep pelvis. Ports marked without taking this into consideration may be displaced too superior to enable the robotic instruments to reach the pelvic floor. As described in the procedural details in the following text, it is better to use laparoscopic technique to create the pneumoperitoneum, insert the first port, and perform a diagnostic laparoscopy. The robotic ports can then be accurately positioned.

3. In contrast to a traditional midline port for the camera, the 12-mm port for the robotic camera is frequently placed just to the right of the umbilicus. This is usually done when there are two ports in the left lower quadrant, and one on the right.

Shifting the camera to the right of the umbilicus provides additional room for the two robotic ports on the left.

4. The robotic instrument arms use specially crafted, stainless steel, reusable, 8-mm cannulas. These cannulas can be inserted directly into the abdominal wall at the port sites. Docking the robot onto cannulas already inserted into the abdominal wall is a little difficult, as the robotic arms have to be oriented into the same angle of insertion of the ports. After this has been done a few times it is quite easily accomplished in a short duration of time. However, it might be easier in the beginning of the learning curve to place standard 12-mm cannulas at the port sites and insert the 8-mm robotic cannulas already clipped onto the robotic arms through them. The robotic cannulas are designed to maintain an airtight seal when used with the robotic instruments. However, they come with a reducer that can be capped on the end to enable the ports to be used with 5-mm standard laparoscopic instruments. Using this feature, the robotic cannulas can be inserted right at the beginning of a hybrid procedure and can be used for the initial laparoscopic colonic mobilization.

5. Perhaps the most important point to be remembered is that the patient's position cannot be changed in any way after the robot is docked. This is because docking the robot onto the cannulas in the ports converts them into fixed points. Any subsequent movement of the patient with the robot docked has the potential to cause severe injury.

As there are a number of positions of the robotic cart described for a left colon/rectal resection, it is expected that each cart position should have its unique port configuration. To maintain some degree of uniformity, we have termed the arm with the cautery/hot shears as the "right working arm" and the retracting arm as the "left working arm." Whenever the third instrument arm of the robot is used in any port configuration, it is termed as the "third arm." Using these terminologies, the port configurations for the different robot-assisted options are described in the following text.

Option 1. Robotic Left Colon/Sigmoid Resection

Robotic cart position—single position by the left flank.

The port positions are as depicted in Figure 11.6. If needed, a 12-mm port is used in right lower quadrant for the introduction of the laparoscopic stapler to transect the upper rectum. An optional 8-mm robotic port may be placed in left lower quadrant in the case of a high-riding splenic flexure or an obese individual to facilitate splenic flexure mobilization.

Option 2. Robotic Low Anterior Resection

Robotic cart position—single position by the left hip (Fig. 11.7).

Option 3. Robotic Low Anterior Resection

Robotic cart position—multiple positions (Fig. 11.8).

Option 4. Hybrid Procedure (Laparoscopic Left Colon Mobilization + Robotic Rectal Dissection)

Robotic cart position—single position, between the patient's legs (Fig. 11.9).

The hybrid procedure can be performed with or without a hand-assist device.

The placement of a hand-assist device in the suprapubic position via a Pfannenstiel incision permits the placement of a laparotomy pad in the peritoneal cavity. This maneuver helps in retracting the small bowel and also facilitates rapid drying of the surgical field in the event of any bleeding. The HandPort also serves as the site of specimen extraction. A TA stapler can also be introduced via the HandPort to transect the distal rectum. This method achieves a safe distal margin in comparison to the laparoscopic stapling devices especially in low rectal tumors. The assistant needs to find the most appropriate position for the suprapubic port for effective retraction. This

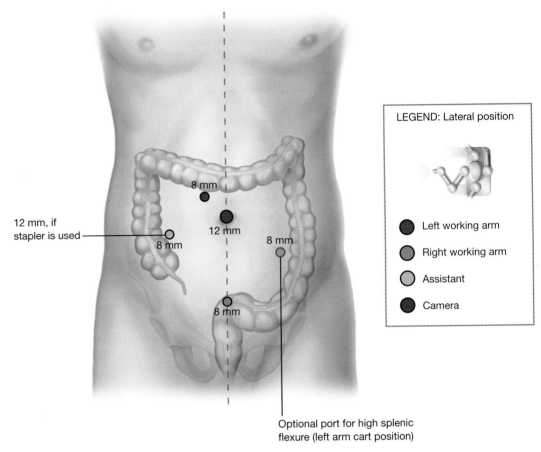

LEGEND: Lateral position

● Left working arm

● Right working arm

○ Assistant

● Camera

8 mm

12 mm

12 mm, if stapler is used

8 mm

8 mm

8 mm

Optional port for high splenic flexure (left arm cart position)

Figure 11.6 Port placement for left colon/sigmoid resection.

goal is not always easily administered as the external movement of the robotic arms, the internal movement of the robotic instruments, and the unique pelvic anatomy in every case need to be considered when introducing this port. Often this requires a process of trial and error. Having a hand-assist device in the suprapubic position enables the suprapubic port to be adjusted as required till the optimal position is identified.

Option 5. Robotic APR

Robotic cart position—single position, between the patient's legs (Fig. 11.10).

After completion of the robotic total mesorectal excision (TME), the robotic cart is removed and the perineal dissection is undertaken at the time of stoma creation. In suitable patients, an APR can also be robotically performed with the robot positioned at the patient's left hip. In such situations, the perineal dissection can be simultaneously undertaken by another surgical team.

Technique

For a single surgical procedure, it is relatively easy to describe the exact surgical steps, as every instrument introduced through each port can be specified. With so many different cart positions and port configurations for a robot-assisted left colon/rectal dissection, the task of presenting a simple and succinct description of the procedure is indeed a difficult one. Keeping this in mind, the port configurations have been presented with a uniform terminology for the robotic arms: the right working arm, the left working arm, and the third arm. Although the port site locations might change with every cart position, the arm configuration as right, left, and third remains the same. The procedure

Upper Left Quadrant Set Up

Pelvic Set Up

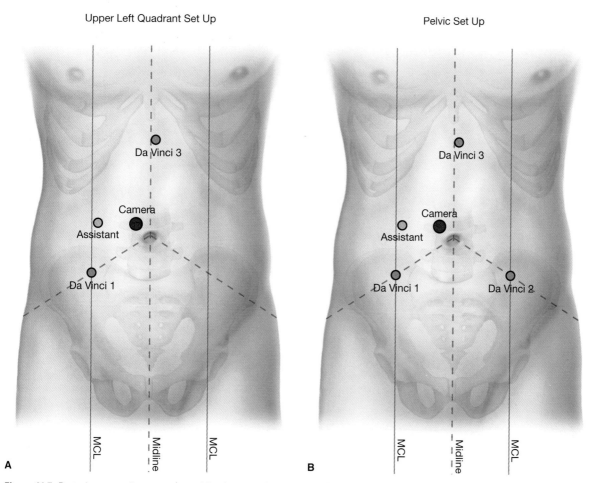

A

B

Figure 11.7 Port placement for one cart position low anterior resection (with permission, *Hellan M, Stein H, Pigazzi A. Totally robotic low anterior resection with total mesorectal excision and splenic flexure mobilization. Surg Endosc 2009;23:447–451*).

described in the following text uses this terminology. The reader is requested to correlate the procedural steps with the port configuration for each cart position by recalling the right working arm, the left working arm, and the third arm in each port placement.

As the extent of bowel mobilization and resection depends on the location of the lesion rectum/sigmoid/descending colon, a complete mobilization of the left colon from splenic flexure till the pelvic floor will not be necessary in all patients. Therefore, the procedural details have been described in three steps:

- Left colon mobilization
- Robotic TME
- Distal rectal transection and anastomosis

A suitable combination of these three steps, given in the preceding text, according to the location of the lesion, will provide the details of the appropriate procedure.

Robot-Assisted Left Colon Mobilization

We prefer the medial-to-lateral approach for a robot-assisted left colon mobilization and this is the technique described here.

The first step is the creation of the pneumoperitoneum. This is done with a Veress needle through the port site for the robotic camera. As explained in the preceding text (principles of port positioning) in some cases, the robotic camera can be placed to the right of the midline. As compared to the periumbilical position, it might be safer and easier to insert the Veress needle via a minute stab incision through the umbilical cicatrix. This minute incision is not seen and does not need any closure at the end of the procedure.

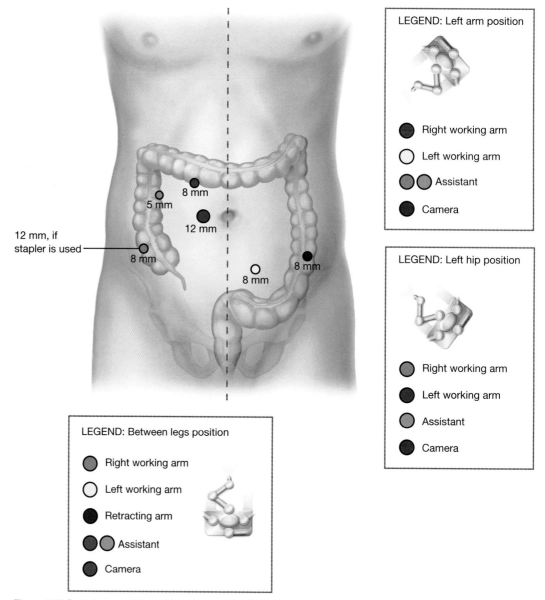

12 mm, if stapler is used

Figure 11.8 Port placement for multiple cart position low anterior resection.

The first port to be inserted is a standard laparoscopic 12-mm port for the robotic camera. The laparoscopic camera is then introduced through this port to perform a diagnostic laparoscopy as well as for the introduction of the remaining ports. As per the selected port site configuration, the remaining ports are introduced under direct visualization (refer to port placement given in the preceding text).

The patient, who has been in supine position till now, is placed in a steep Trendelenburg position with a right tilt. An initial preparation of the surgical field by displacing the small bowel to the right upper quadrant and retracting the omentum superiorly is necessary to enable clear visualization of the left colon. As the robot is not efficient, when large movements transgressing many abdominal quadrants are called for, this initial preparation is best laparoscopically undertaken, using a bowel grasper. This method makes efficient use of the robot, and considerably decreases the operative time. The end point of this initial preparation is to expose the descending and sigmoid colon and the root of the inferior mesenteric vessels.

The robot is then brought up to the patient in the selected cart position and docked onto the robotic ports (refer to principles of cart positioning). The procedure is begun

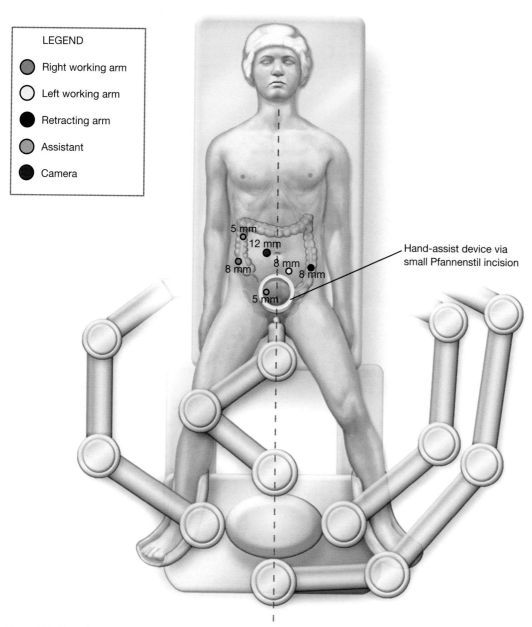

LEGEND

- ○ (grey) Right working arm
- ○ (white) Left working arm
- ● (black) Retracting arm
- ○ (grey) Assistant
- ● (black) Camera

5 mm
12 mm
8 mm   8 mm   8 mm
5 mm

Hand-assist device via
small Pfannenstil incision

Figure 11.9 Port placement in hybrid procedure.

with a bowel grasper in the left working arm and a cautery hook in the right working arm. We use a bipolar fenestrated cautery in the left working arm. This serves as a bowel retractor and can also be sued for accurate hemostasis. The third arm is not essential at this stage but can be used for additional retraction with a Cadiere forceps. The assistant uses a laparoscopic bowel grasper through the assistant port. This can be exchanged for a suction irrigator as required.

The root of the sigmoid mesocolon is retracted anteriorly to identify the inferior mesenteric pedicle. The peritoneum is then incised beneath this vascular pedicle to enter the avascular retroperitoneal plane. The left ureter and gonadal vessels are then identified and reflected posteriorly. The inferior mesenteric artery is dissected to its origin with preservation of the sympathetic nerve plexus. The artery can then be clipped and divided, or divided with an appropriate energy device (or a stapler inserted through the assistant port.) The retroperitoneal plane is then developed in a medial-to-lateral fashion, mobilizing the colonic mesentery from the underlying Gerota's fascia. This mobilized left colon mesentery (avascular peritoneal fold) is then incised along the

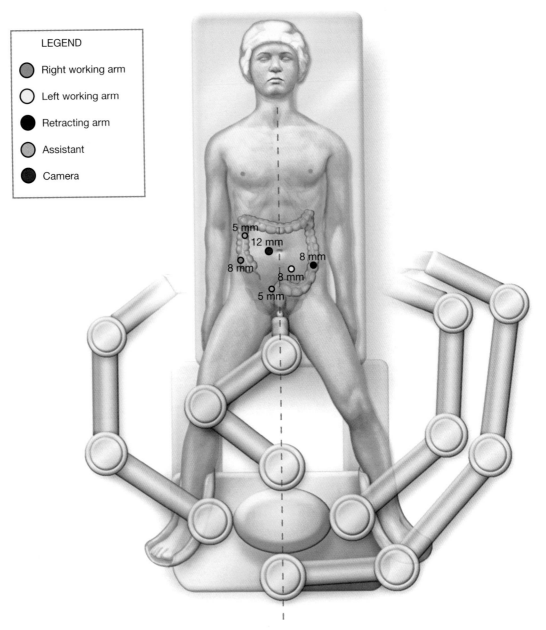

Figure 11.10 Port placement for robotic abdominoperineal resection.

aorta up to the level of the inferior mesenteric vein. The vein is then isolated and divided in a similar fashion as the artery. The last step of the descending and sigmoid colon mobilization is to retract the colon medially and divide the left lateral peritoneal reflection along the line of Toldt.

Most often, mobilizing the splenic flexure requires shifting the patient to a reverse Trendelenburg position. This displaces the transverse colon inferiorly and moves the small bowel to the lower quadrants thus clearing the left upper quadrant. As mentioned before, the robot has to be undocked (the ports have to be detached from the robotic arms and the arms moved away), for every change in patient position. The robotic cart, however, need not be moved, so this maneuver is not as time-consuming as it seems. Undocking the robot, changing the patient position to reverse Trendelenburg, and redocking the robot can be achieved in a couple of minutes.

Splenic flexure mobilization is begun by retracting the omentum anteriorly to suspend the left half of the transverse colon. The right working arm still holds the cautery hook and the left working arm holds the bipolar forceps/bowel grasper. The omentum is then detached from the transverse colon by incising the avascular plane. This maneuver gains access to the lesser sac. If present, the adhesions between the posterior layer of the gastrocolic omentum and the transverse mesocolon can be divided at this stage. The line of omental detachment from the transverse colon is continued to the phrenocolic ligament that is transected to connect with the line of peritoneal division in the left paracolic gutter. The splenic flexure is retracted medially and the remaining attachments are transected. This plane eventually meets the previously dissected retroperitoneal plane to complete the mobilization.

The mobilization described in the preceding text can usually be completed with the robotic cart in one position in the left flank. For the high-riding splenic flexure the robot may need to be repositioned by the patient's left arm. This can be quickly achieved by rotating the patient around the stationary robotic cart. Similarly, the mobilization of the upper rectum if required may need repositioning of the robotic cart by the left hip.

Robotic TME

The technique for creating the pneumoperitoneum and for port insertion is as described in the preceding text for left colon mobilization.

It is possible to perform a robotic TME with the patient in a straight Trendelenburg position with no tilt. However, it is often beneficial to add a slight right tilt to facilitate displacement of the small bowel to the right upper quadrant. Again, as per the selected port configuration, the ports are inserted. It is important to remember that the right lateral assistant port should not be placed too far above the umbilicus. This is to avoid the sacral promontory from obstructing the line of access of the assistant's bowel grasper to the pelvis. The right working arm holds the cautery hook (or cautery sheers) and the left working arm holds the bipolar fenestrated grasper. The third arm is vital for rectal dissection and holds a Cadiere forceps for retraction.

The assistant is positioned on the right side of the patient and holds a long bowel grasper in the left hand and a short suction irrigator in the right. Unlike an assistant in laparoscopic surgery, the assistant here has to work with the robotic arms both outside and inside the patient. The best position for the assistant's right hand is underneath the robotic arms. This provides the best access to the supraumbilical assistant's port (Fig. 11.11).

A successful and accurate TME in any minimally invasive technique depends on the retraction provided. This is especially appreciated in the male pelvis and in the obese patient. The use of a robot with a single assistant provides five working arms (three robotic and two assistant) in addition to the camera at any given time (Fig. 11.12A). Prior to beginning of an actual dissection, the third robotic arm with the Cadiere forceps is positioned at the rectosigmoid junction to provide "macroretraction" (Fig. 11.12B). The camera in panoramic view at this stage helps in positioning the third arm. This arm is then fixed in this position and the camera is zoomed in to visualize only the right and

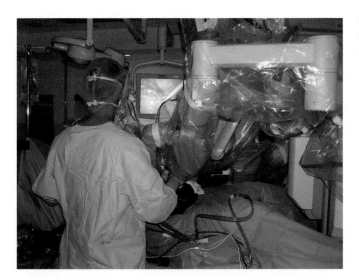

Figure 11.11 Assistant position and access to the suprapubic port.

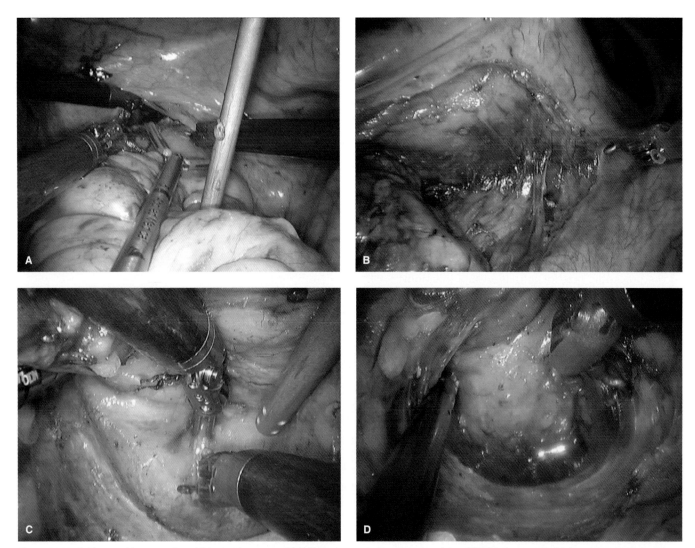

Figure 11.12 **A.** Five working arms (in addition to the camera) available for total mesorectal excision (TME) are controlled by two-person team. **B.** Third robotic arm is retracting the rectosigmoid (macroretraction) opening the presacral space. **C.** Left working arm is providing "microretraction" at the working plane. **D.** Posterior mobilization of mesorectum. (*continued*)

left working arms at the point of dissection. The left working arm can then provide precise "microretraction" at the working plane (Fig. 11.12C). The assistant with the bowel grasper and the suction irrigator supplements this "microretraction." This stable retracting ability of the robot together with the enhanced three-dimensional visualization is the key to a precise TME. As the dissection progresses toward the pelvic floor the Cadiere forceps needs to be distally advanced. The camera may be zoomed out at periodic intervals to facilitate the repositioning of the Cadiere forceps. With the Cadiere forceps positioned for macroretraction, dissection is begun by incising the right leaf of the rectal mesentery at the level of the sacral promontory. This opens the avascular presacral plane. This plane is developed just outside the mesorectal envelope to avoid injury to the presacral venous plexus (Fig. 11.12D). The left working arm retracts the mesorectum anteriorly, and the cautery hook in the right working arm achieves this sharp posterior dissection (Fig. 11.12E). As this plane is developed the hypogastric nerves are identified and preserved (Fig. 11.12F). The presacral avascular plane is best defined in the posterior midline and hence it is important to keep oneself oriented to the midline by the noting position of the sacral promontory. In this manner the dissection is continued in the posterior midline to the pelvic floor. Once the pelvic floor is reached in the posterior midline, the dissection is continued toward the left curving

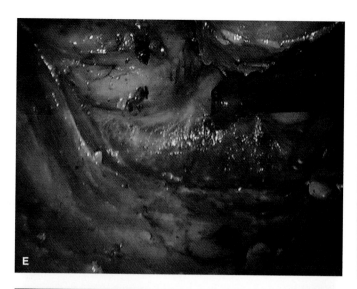

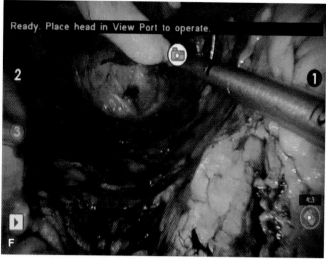

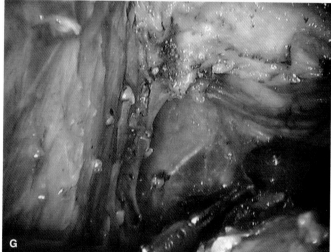

Figure 11.12 (*Continued*) **E.** Posterior mobilization of mesorectum, low pelvic attachments. **F.** Posterior mobilization of mesorectum, patient with BMI of 36. **G.** Posterior mobilization curving to the left at the bottom of the pelvis.

around the mesorectal envelope (Fig. 11.12G). As the view of the robotic system can be zoomed in, very close to the line of dissection, it is possible to inadvertently carry the dissection too far laterally and hit the pelvic sidewall especially on the left. To avoid this, the camera should be zoomed out periodically to orient oneself to the sacral promontory and the midline. Every time the camera is zoomed out, the position of the Cadiere forceps can be evaluated, and advanced down the rectum to maintain a good macroretraction. The next step involves division of the right lateral rectal attachments (Fig. 11.13A). For this the camera is zoomed out and the Cadiere forceps is positioned to retract the rectum anteriorly and to the left. The left working arm provides additional stretch on the peritoneum that is divided accurately with the cautery hook. In a deep pelvis, the posterior dissection may not be possible all the way to the pelvic floor without dividing the right rectal attachments. In such situations, early division of the upper right lateral rectal attachments further opens up the posterior plane of dissection (Fig. 11.13B). In male patients, as the right lateral dissection is continued inferiorly the seminal vesicles come into view (Fig. 11.13C). At this point it is easier to begin the anterior dissection and define the Denonvilliers' fascia in the midline before proceeding with dissecting the rectum from the seminal vesicles and prostate. For anterior dissection, the third arm retracts the bladder anteriorly, providing the required traction and the left working arm retracts the rectum posteriorly to provide countertraction (Fig. 11.13D). This opens up the rectovesical fold that is incised with the cautery to identify the Denonvilliers' fascia (Fig. 11.14A–C) (rectovaginal septum in females). The dissection is continued

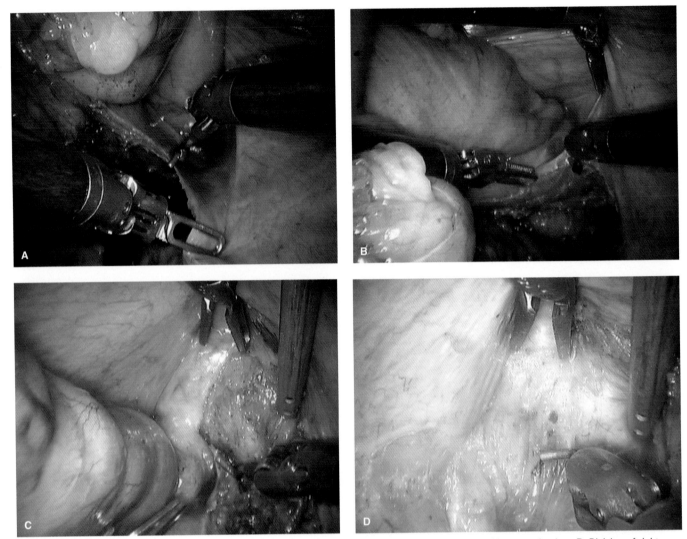

Figure 11.13 A. Transection of right pararectal peritoneum, third arm is providing macroretraction, two working arms in view. **B.** Division of right lateral rectal attachments. **C.** Right seminal vesicle exposed during division of right lateral rectal attachments. **D.** Anterior exposure: third arm is elevating the bladder, rectovesical peritoneal fold incised, right seminal vesicle exposed.

just outside the Denonvilliers' fascia. This preserves the fascia on the prostate and seminal vesicles, minimizes bleeding, and reduces the risk of sexual dysfunction (Fig. 11.14D). Similarly in the female patient an accurate dissection in the avascular rectovaginal septum reduces blood loss and reduces the risk of vaginal injury (Fig. 11.14E).

The left side of the rectum is mobilized by first incising the peritoneal fold caudal to cephalad, as a continuation of the anterior peritoneal incision (Fig. 11.15A). Conversely, this can be done by starting the lateral dissection at the level of the sigmoid fossa and proceeding distally. It is often possible to achieve a lot of the left lateral dissection as a continuation of the posterior plane around the mesorectum. This leaves just a peritoneal fold on the left side that is easily incised (Fig. 11.15B).

The final dissection at the pelvic floor is accomplished by circumferential transection of the attachments of the rectum to the levator ani muscles (Fig. 11.15C,D).

Again, a precise positioning of the Cadiere forceps in the third arm is vital for good macroretraction to get good access to the pelvic floor. The use of the bipolar forceps in the left working arm not only provides an effective microretraction but also allows for hemostasis not controlled with the cautery hook (Fig. 11.16A–C).

Distal Rectal Transection and Anastomosis

In a majority of cases, the robot is only used for rectal mobilization. Distal rectal transection can be achieved using a roticulating endoscopic stapler (Fig. 11.17), using standard

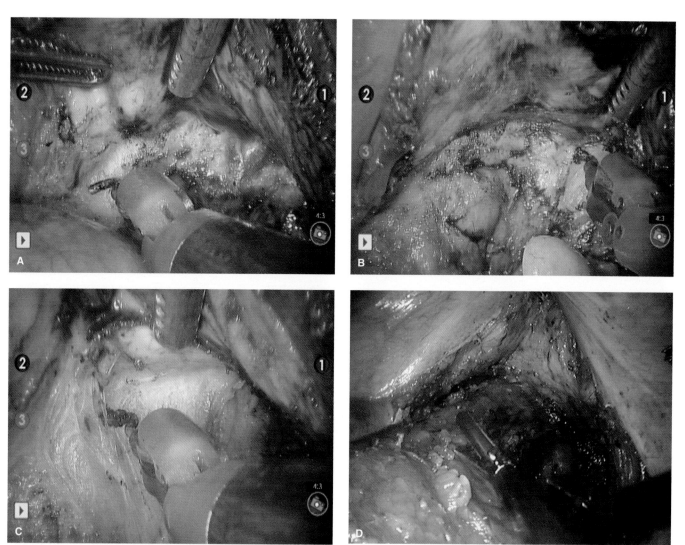

Figure 11.14 A. Both seminal vesicles exposed. **B.** Denonvilliers' fascia being incised. **C.** Dissection continued outside the Denonvilliers' fascia. **D.** Sufficient anterior mobilization in male, prostate exposed. **E.** Sufficient anterior mobilization in female, vagina exposed.

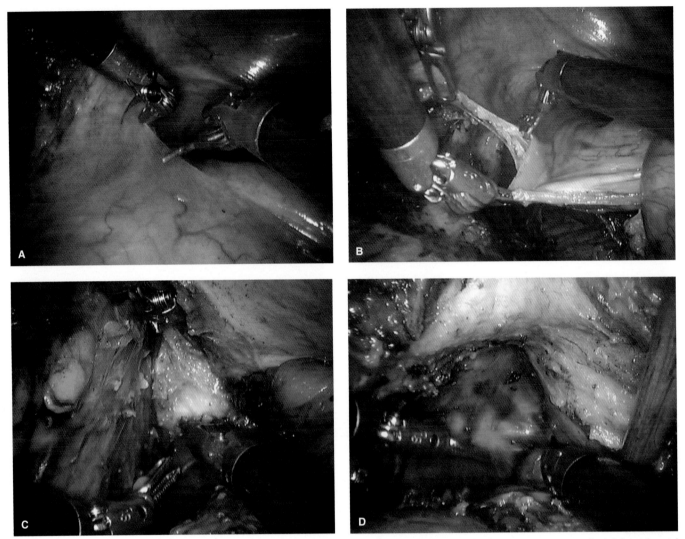

Figure 11.15 **A.** Incision of left pararectal peritoneal fold at the pelvic brim. **B.** Incision of left peritoneal fold opens an access to the left lateral rectal stalk. **C.** Transection of left lateral rectal stalk. **D.** Left lateral rectal stalk divided, prostate exposed.

laparoscopic technique. Alternatively this can also be done through the hand port with a TA stapler. In low rectal lesions and in obese male patients, distal rectal transection by the methods given in the preceding text can be a daunting task. The existing laparoscopic stapling devices, with their limited angulation, cannot achieve a right-angled rectal transection at the pelvic floor. This may compromise the distal margin.

The advanced dexterity of the robotic system can be used to achieve a controlled right-angled rectal transection and a pursestring suture placement on the distal rectal stump. This technique avoids the transecting staple lines in a doubled-stapled anastomosis and can achieve a double pursestring, single-stapled anastomosis a few centimeters from the pelvic floor (Fig. 11.18A–E). It should be mentioned, however, that this technique is under evaluation and is being tested in a large series of patients. The results of this patient series are essential to determine its safety and efficacy.

 POSTOPERATIVE MANAGEMENT

Patients undergoing robot-assisted left colon/rectal resections are managed with the routine postoperative protocol for all patients undergoing a minimally invasive colorectal resection.

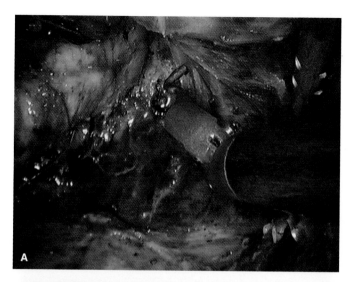

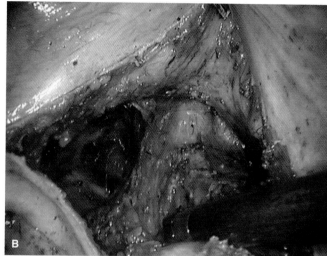

Figure 11.16 **A.** Division of low attachments at the right pelvic floor. **B,C.** Complete mobilization of the rectum.

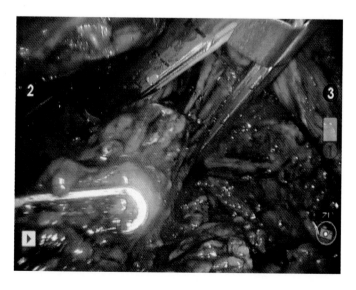

Figure 11.17 Distal rectal transection with a reticulating endoscopic stapler.

Part II: Left Colon

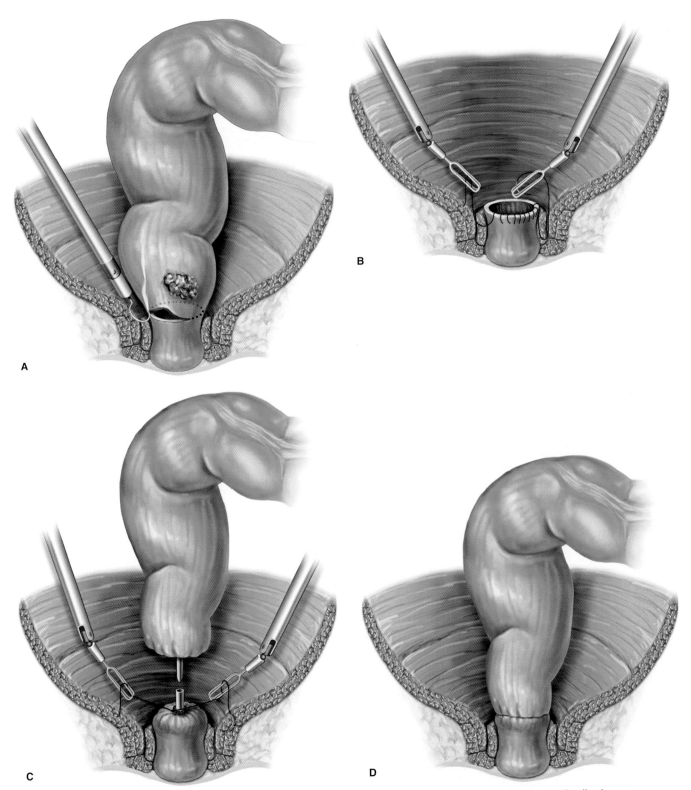

Figure 11.18 A. Transection of distal rectum with robotic hook cautery. **B.** Application of continuous pursestring suture on the distal stump. **C,D.** Single-stapled end-to-end anastomosis. (*continued*)

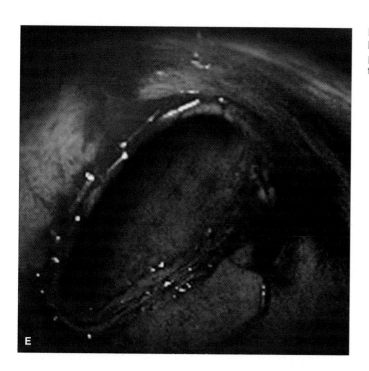

Figure 11.18 (*Continued*)
E. Endoscopic picture of double pursestring single-stapled anastomosis.

 COMPLICATIONS

There are a couple of features unique to the robot that needs to be appreciated to safely use robotic assistance without complications.

1. The absence of tactile sensation in the current version of the Da Vinci robot is one of the limitations of this system. Although this loss of tactile sensation can be more than adequately compensated by the advanced three-dimensional vision, the surgeon must learn to pay careful attention to visual cues in order to avoid trauma to the tissues. In open or laparoscopic surgery, it is possible to feel the amount of pressure being exerted on the tissues to achieve suitable retraction and exposure of the dissecting plane. In robotic surgery, this is not possible. When retracting the rectum with the robotic arms, it is possible for the surgeon to inadvertently retract too much and injure the mesorectum or the rectum. It is vitally important for the surgeon to regulate the extent of tissue retraction based on the visual cues of tissue tension. This ability to "see tissue tension" and not feel it is an important aspect of the learning curve for the robotic surgeon.

2. The imaging system of the robot enables the camera to be zoomed in very close to the line of dissection and provide a view with significant magnification. This feature is very beneficial in accurately dissecting outside the mesorectal envelop and also in visualizing and preserving the pelvic nerves. However, during the posterior dissection in the presacral space, as one goes down deep into the pelvis, it is not difficult to loose the orientation of the midline and go too much toward the lateral pelvic wall. When this happens there is a risk of injury to the internal iliac vessels. As the dissection progresses laterally, the line of dissection curves around the rectum. It is important to always know how far lateral one is to anticipate this curve in the line of dissection. This is easily done by periodically zooming out the camera to identify the sacral promontory and the midline. This also provides an opportunity to evaluate and adjust the position of the third arm on the proximal rectum to provide good "macroretraction" as one goes deeper into the pelvis.

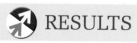 RESULTS

Published literature on robotic colorectal surgery has significantly increased in the last few years. Each group performing robotic surgery has published its own technique ranging from the use of the robot in a single cart position, to multiple cart positions, to the use of the hybrid procedure. All reports on the use of robotic assistance in colorectal procedures have confirmed its safety and efficacy.

The significant initial investment to acquire the robot together with the high recurring costs makes the issue of cost versus benefit of vital importance. Perhaps the two major concerns with the use of the robot in colorectal surgery are the increased operating time and the higher cost associated with its use. It is true that the robot provides numerous technical advantages to the operating surgeon, but is there data to show that this translates into an objective benefit?

Although it has been shown in laboratory exercises that the acquisition of robotic skills has a shorter learning curve as compared to laparoscopy, to date there is no objective evidence to claim any short-term benefit or improved long-term outcome associated with the use of the robot in colorectal procedures. Data are emerging to show that the best indication for the use of robotic technology in colorectal surgery might be for rectal dissection. Recent reports in a small number of patients show a trend toward a better mesorectal grade when the robot is used for mesorectal excision in rectal cancer. The next few years will most likely yield the necessary data for robotic surgery to either demonstrate an advantage or at least establish its equivalence as a standard of care.

✛ CONCLUSION

Robotic technology in colorectal surgery is still in its infancy. Different surgical groups, working with different patient populations, have led to the formulation of various applications and techniques for robotic-assisted left colon resections. There are no data at present to support the superiority of one technique over another, or even the superiority of robotic assistance as compared to other surgical options. At this stage it will be most appropriate to select on an individualized basis, a combination from the techniques described in the preceding text, port placements, and cart positions, which will provide the best possible clinical outcome. It should also be remembered that a structured learning protocol beginning in the laboratory and progressing to the clinical setting, all under appropriate mentoring is the safest and most effective way in acquiring the skills of robotic surgery.

Acknowledgment

The authors wish to thank Ashwin deSouza, M.S., for his help with the preparation of the manuscript and Ron Wojkovich for his contribution with the artwork.

Suggested Readings

Baik SH. Robotic colorectal surgery. *Yonsei Med J* 2008;49(6): 891–96.

Baik SH, Kang CM, Lee WJ, et al. Robotic total mesorectal excision for the treatment of rectal cancer. *J Robotic Surg* 2007;1:99–102.

Baik SH, Ko YT, Kang CM, et al. Robotic tumor-specific mesorectal excision of rectal cancer: short-term outcome of a pilot randomized trial. *Surg Endosc* 2008;22(7):1601–8.

Baik SH, Kwon HY, Kim JS, et al. Robotic versus laparoscopic low anterior resection of rectal cancer: short-term outcome of a prospective comparative study. *Ann Surg Oncol* 2009;16(6):1480–7.

Baik SH, Lee WJ, Rha KH, et al. Robotic total mesorectal excision for rectal cancer using four robotic arms. *Surg Endosc* 2008; 22(3):792–7.

Delaney CP, Lynch AC, Senagore AJ, Fazio VW. Comparison of robotically performed and traditional laparoscopic colorectal surgery. *Dis Colon Rectum* 2003;46(12):1633–9.

D'Annibale A, Morpurgo E, Fiscon V, et al. Robotic and laparoscopic surgery for treatment of colorectal disease. *Dis Colon Rectum* 2004;47(12):2162–8.

Hellan M, Anderson C, Ellenhorn JD, et al. Short-term outcomes after robotic-assisted total mesorectal excision for rectal cancer. *Ann Surg Oncol* 2007;14(11):3168–73.

Hellan M, Stein H, Pigazzi A. Totally robotic low anterior resection with total mesorectal excision and splenic flexure mobilization. *Surg Endosc* 2009;23(2):447–51.

Luca F, Cenciarelli S, Valvo M, et al. Full robotic left colon and rectal cancer resection: technique and early outcome. *Ann Surg Oncol* 2009;16(5):1274–8.

Pigazzi A, Ellenhorn JD, Ballantyne GH, Paz IB. Robotic-assisted laparoscopic low anterior resection with total mesorectal excision for rectal cancer. *Surg Endosc* 2006;20(10):1521–5.

Rawlings AL, Woodland JH, Vegunta RK, Crawford DL. Robotic versus laparoscopic colectomy. *Surg Endosc* 2007;21(10):1701–8.

Spinoglio G, Summa M, Priora F, et al. Robotic colorectal surgery: first 50 cases experience. *Dis Colon Rectum* 2008;51(11): 1627–32.

Weber PA, Merola S, Wasielewski A, Ballantyne GH. Telerobotic-assisted laparoscopic right and sigmoid colectomies for benign disease. *Dis Colon Rectum* 2002;45(12):1689–94.

12 Hand-Assisted Left Colectomy

Matthew G. Mutch

INDICATIONS/CONTRAINDICATIONS

Indications for the use of the hand-assisted approach to a laparoscopic left colectomy are the same as for an open or straight laparoscopic left colectomy. Advantages of the hand-assisted approach depend upon how it is utilized.

- Adoption—data have demonstrated faster ascension of the learning curve.
- Primary approach—data have shown shorter operative times and no difference in short-term outcomes when compared to the laparoscopic approach.
- Difficult cases—the hand-assisted approach has shown benefit in patients with complicated diverticulitis and when utilized for more complicated procedures such as total abdominal colectomy and restorative proctocolectomy.
- Alternative to conversion to laparotomy—if a surgeon needs to convert during a laparoscopic left colectomy, the hand-assisted approach offers an alternative to conversion to laparotomy.

There are no absolute contraindications to the utilization of the hand-assisted approach to a laparoscopic left colectomy. The goal is to perform a safe operation whether it is accomplished laparoscopically by hand assistance or by laparotomy. Conversions when preformed in a preemptive manner do not have a negative impact on outcomes (1,2). However, when performed reactively after a complication has occurred, the outcomes are worse than if the procedure had been performed open. There are several relative contraindications to the laparoscopic approach and they are centered on the fact of being able to progress through the operation in a safe manner (3).

- Body mass index—Patient habitus, particularly intraperitoneal fat, is one of the best predictors for successful completion of a laparoscopic case. Intraperitoneal fat present makes manipulation of the bowel, its mesentery, and the omentum much more difficult. This problem can be overcome to some extent by the use of the hand.
- Extensive adhesions—For patients with a prior history of abdominal surgery, the hand port incision is introduced to allow assessment of the adhesions before committing to

the laparoscopic approach. Extensive intraloop adhesions will require significant time to divide which may potentially lessen the benefit of the laparoscopic approach

- Large inflammatory lesions—When the inflammation prevents the safe identification of landmarks and relevant anatomy, the risk of a reactive conversion significantly increases.
- Medical issues—Disease such as COPD or cardiac disease needs special attention. The surgeon and anesthesiologist need to determine whether the patient can tolerate the pneumoperitoneum or the extremes of position. If there is evidence that cardiopulmonary function will be compromised, laparoscopy should be avoided.

The incision created for the hand port can be used to visualize the abdomen to determine the feasibility of laparoscopically completing the case.

 PREOPERATIVE PLANNING

The preoperative assessment of the patient is dependent upon the specific indication for the operation and should not alter even when an open, laparoscopic, or hand-assisted approach is utilized. The utilization of ureteral stents is left to the discretion of the surgeon and the indication for the procedure. There are two approaches to ureteral stents:

- Routinely for ureteral identification
- Selectively—utilizing them with the same criteria as used for laparotomy

SURGERY

Room Setup and Patient Position

- Mechanical bed—The patient will be put in the extremes of position to facilitate the use of gravity to retract the small bowel.
- Modified lithotomy position—The angle at the hip should be less than 10 degrees. Keeping the thigh low and knees adducted will minimize the interference of the patient's thigh with the instruments during the procedure.
- Bean bag—It is helpful to secure the patient to the operating room table. The most effective manner is with the use of a bean bag, which can be attached to the operating table with velcro. This step will allow both of the patient's arms to be tucked to their side. The patient is them cocooned it the bean bag to prevent them from moving during the operation.
- Surgeon—The surgeon stands on the patient's right side. Typically, the surgeon will place his/her right hand through the port and will use the left hand to hold the laparoscopic instrument. Alternatively, the surgeon may stand between the patient's legs, place his/her left hand through the hand port, and utilize a left lower quadrant port.
- Camera operator—The assistant that operates the camera stands on the right side and to the head of the patient.
- First assistant—If an assistant is available, they can stand between the patient's legs and utilize the left lower quadrant port.
- Monitors—The main viewing monitor is placed at the patient's left flank. It should have the ability to move to the left shoulder when mobilizing the splenic flexure and to the left thigh when dissecting in the pelvis.

Port Placement

- Hand port—The most effective site for placement of the hand port is in the suprapubic position (Fig. 12.1). This position helps to keep the hand out of the path of the camera and it puts the extraction site directly over the rectum to facilitate its division and in performing the anastomosis. The hand port can be placed through either a midline or Pfannenstiel incision.

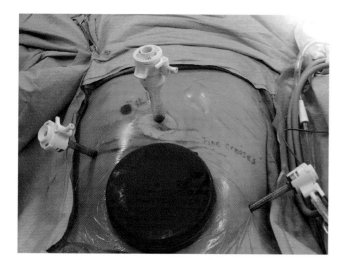

Figure 12.1   Port placement.

▤ Camera port—The camera port needs to be placed in the supraumbilical position so that it does not interfere with the skirt of the hand port.

▤ Working ports—The main working port is placed in the right lower quadrant. It should be placed half way between the hand port and the camera port and lateral to the rectus muscle. A second working port is placed in the left lower quadrant, which should be lateral to the rectus and as low as possible. This port is used for retraction and division of the lateral attachments and mobilization of the splenic flexure. The lower it is placed, the lesser time there will be for working in reverse from the camera. A third working port can be placed in the right upper quadrant based on surgeon preference.

Technique

▤ Accessing the retroperitoneum—The patient is placed in steep Trendelenburg and left side up. The small bowel is placed in the right upper quadrant. Using the medial to lateral approach, the superior rectal artery is grasped at the level of the sacral promontory with the surgeon's right hand (Fig. 12.2A and B). A long incision is made in the peritoneum medial or below the artery. With a longer incision, the exposure of the retroperitoneum will be greater (Fig. 12.3A and B). Once the retroperitoneum is accessed, the sigmoid colon mesentery is elevated and the retroperitoneum is swept down so the left ureter can be identified (Fig. 12.4). After its identification, the left

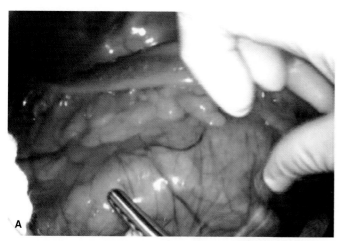
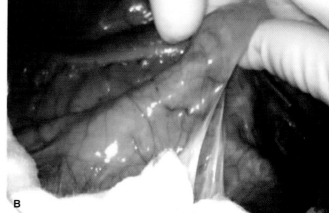

Figure 12.2   **A.** Identifying the sacral promontory. **B.** The superior rectal artery.

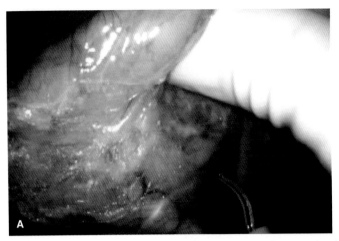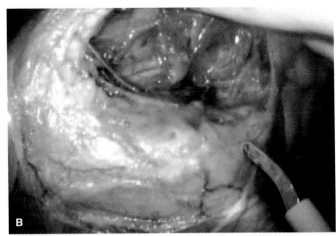

Figure 12.3 **A.** Long incision below superior rectal artery. **B.** Accessing the retroperitoneum.

ureter is then swept down and separated from the mesentery. If the ureter is not identified immediately, there are several alternative approaches. First, the retroperitoneum can be accessed at the level of the inferior mesenteric vein (IMV) (Fig. 12.5). The retroperitoneum is flat in this location. Once the proper plane is identified, it is developed in a caudad direction to connect with the space near the superior rectal artery. Second, the sigmoid colon can be mobilized in a lateral to medial direction to expose and identify the ureter. Finally, if all else fails, the top of the hand port can be removed and the ureter can be identified through the hand port in an open manner.

■ Isolation of the inferior mesenteric artery (IMA)—With the left ureter identified and safely swept out of harm's way, the IMA is then isolated at it's origin. Tension on the IMA is created by elevating the IMA with the index finger and the middle finger is used to sweep the retroperitoneum down along the course of the IMA (Fig. 12.6). A window is then created on the cephalad side of the artery and medial to the IMV (Fig. 12.7). Once isolated, the vessel can be ligated with the energy source of preference.

■ Isolation of the IMV—After the IMA has been divided, the IMV can be further elevated by incising the peritoneum and separating it from the retroperitoneum (Fig. 12.8A and B). The vein is isolated near the ligament of Treitz and the inferior border of the pancreas (Fig. 12.9).

■ Mobilization of the mesentery—At this point, the entire medial aspect of the left colon mesentery is detached and wide window of access is present. The hand is placed palm down, under the mesentery and is used as a fan retractor to elevate the left colon mesentery (Fig. 12.10). A laparoscopic instrument is used to sweep down the retroperitoneum. This dissection is carried out beyond the colon laterally from the sigmoid

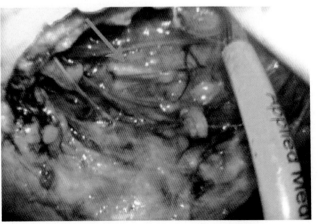

Figure 12.4 The left ureter (*blue arrow*).

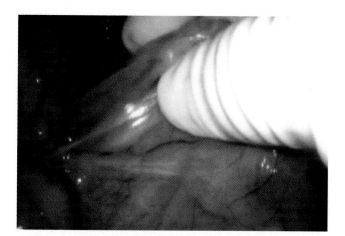

Figure 12.5 Elevation of the inferior mesenteric vein.

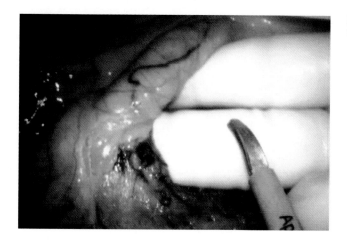

Figure 12.6 Isolating the inferior mesenteric artery.

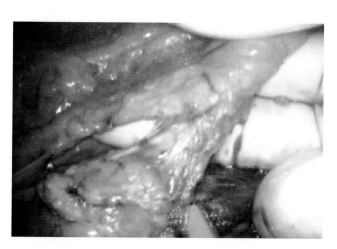

Figure 12.7 The inferior mesenteric artery at its origin.

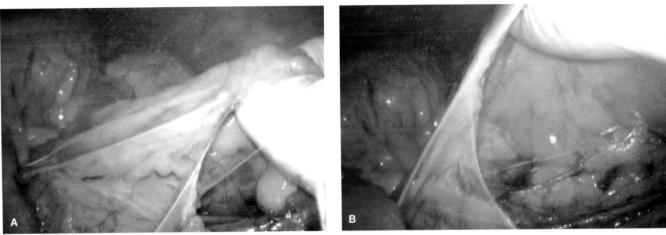

Figure 12.8 **A.** Elevating the inferior mesenteric vein off the retroperitoneum. **B.** Tracing the inferior mesenteric vein up to the ligament of Treitz.

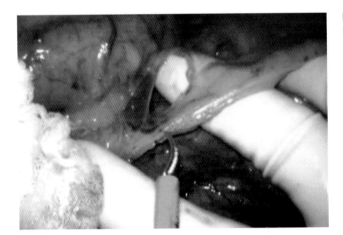

Figure 12.9 Isolating the inferior mesenteric vein at the inferior border of the pancreas.

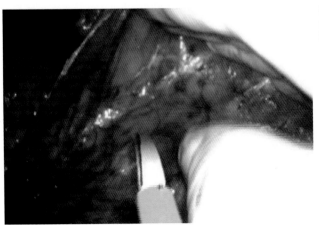

Figure 12.10 Separating the left colon mesentery from the retroperitoneum.

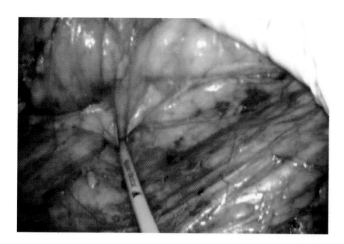

Figure 12.11 The separation is carried beyond the colon laterally.

colon up to the splenic flexure (Fig. 12.11). The more thorough this dissection is the easier the lateral and splenic flexure mobilizations will be.

- Lateral mobilization—After the colon and its mesentery have been mobilized by attaching the colon to the abdominal sidewall, from a medial approach beyond the colon laterally, all that remains is the lateral peritoneum (Fig. 12.12). This layer is incised and the hand is then placed through this defect into the medial plane of dissection (Fig. 12.13A and B). The lateral attachments are then divided along the surgeon's finger so the sigmoid colon and entire left colon are detached (Fig. 12.14).
- Splenic flexure mobilization—The splenic flexure needs to be inspected so that the relationship between the omentum and colon can be appreciated. The first step is to separate the omentum from the transverse colon all the way to or beyond the mid-transverse colon. By incising the peritoneal attachment the lesser sac is then entered (Fig. 12.15). There are varying amount of adhesions between the omentum and transverse colon mesentery (Fig. 12.16). By dividing all of these attachments the lesser sac is wide open and the peritoneal attachments between the inferior border of the pancreas and the transverse colon mesentery is exposed (Fig. 12.17). Coming from the patient's left side, the surgeon's left hand is placed behind these attachments and they are divided all the way to the midline. This allows for complete mobilization of the splenic flexure.
- Specimen extraction—The colon is then extracted through the hand port. The proximal colon and mesentery are divided and prepared for anastomosis (Fig. 12.18A and B). The rectum can be divided laparoscopically or open through the hand port (Fig. 12.19).
- Anastomosis—The circular stapled anastomosis can be performed either laparoscopically or open via the hand port (Fig. 12.20A and B). If there is an anastomotic

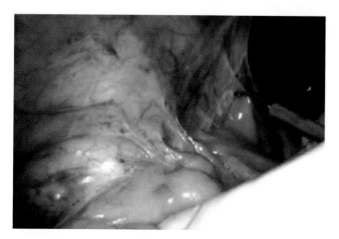

Figure 12.12 The lateral attachments of the sigmoid colon.

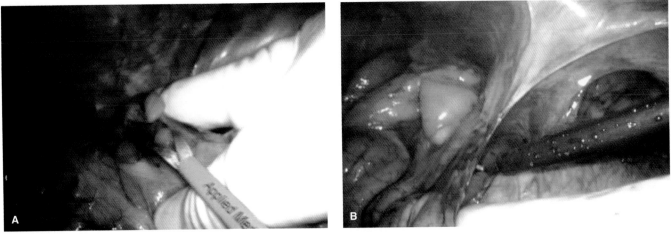

Figure 12.13 **A.** Incision of the lateral attachments. **B.** The medial plane of dissection is entered.

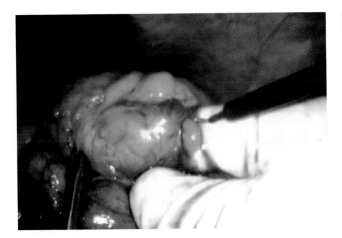

Figure 12.14 Division of lateral attachments up to the splenic flexure.

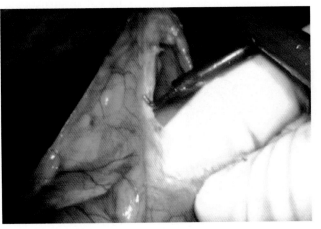

Figure 12.15 Separation of the omentum from the transverse colon.

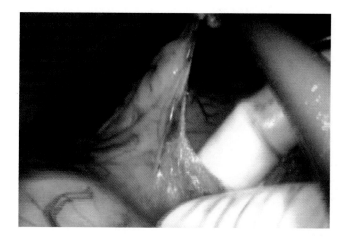

Figure 12.16 Attachments of omentum to transverse mesentery.

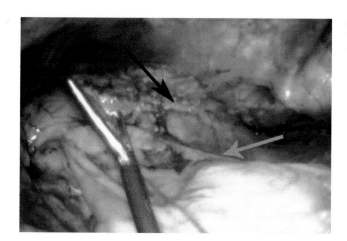

Figure 12.17 Posterior attachments of transverse mesocolon (*blue arrow*) and pancreas (*black arrow*).

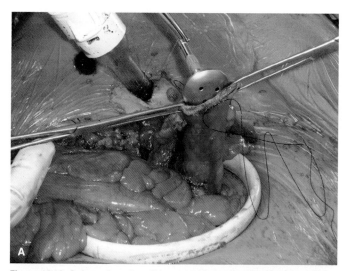
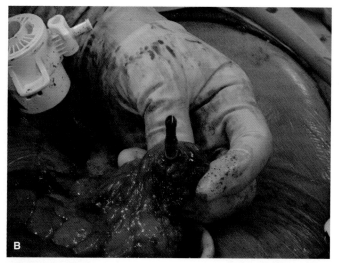

Figure 12.18 **A.** Insertion of anvil into proximal colon. **B.** Proximal colon is ready for anastomosis.

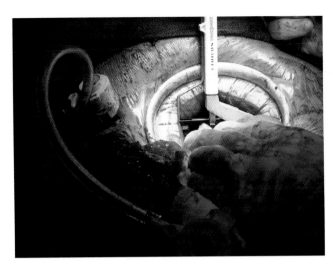

Figure 12.19 Division of rectum.

complication such as bleeding, air leak or incomplete doughnuts, it can be managed directly through the hand port.

 Closure—All 10-mm port sites should be closed. The hand port can be closed in the standard fashion with a heavy running suture or with interrupted sutures.

 # POSTOPERATIVE MANAGEMENT

Whether a left colectomy is performed open, laparoscopically, or hand assisted, there are no special alterations in postoperative care. Data have shown that accelerated pathways that consist of early ambulation and early oral feeding are beneficial and can lead to shorter hospital stays. There is no clear consensus regarding the optimal management of postoperative intravenous fluids or postoperative ileus.

COMPLICATIONS

The potential complications associated with a left colectomy include bleeding, infection, anastomotic leak, left ureteral injury, injury to other abdominal organs, thromboembolic events, and a myriad of medical complications related to cardiopulmonary or renal

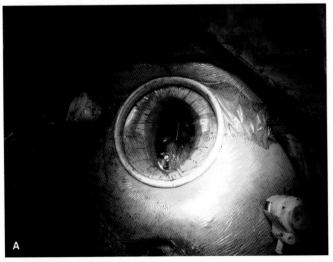

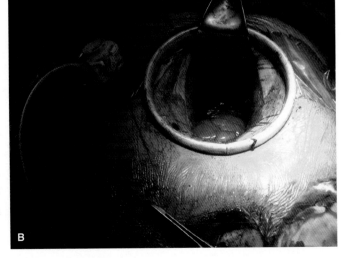

Figure 12.20 **A** and **B.** Anastomosis.

disease. The most devastating complication is a missed injury to a hollow viscus caused either by electrocautery or by instrument trauma. Thermal injuries can occur by several mechanisms; conduction by touching instruments, conduction through an instrument that has a break in its insulation, inadvertent contact with tissue, or conduction through a hollow structure such as a blood vessel. The management of any postoperative complication should not be altered just because a laparoscopic approach was used.

RESULTS

There are many short-term benefits such as faster return of bowel function, shorter hospital stay, and less narcotic use associated with the laparoscopic approach when compared to the open approach for a colectomy. There also appear to be some long-term benefits such as decreased incisional hernia rate, decreased incidence of adhesive small-bowel obstruction rate, and better preservation of fertility in women after pelvic operations (4).

The hand-assisted approach does hold selected advantages over the straight laparoscopic approach depending on how the tool of the hand port is utilized. When used as a tool to allow a surgeon to adopt laparoscopic colectomy into their practice, it has been shown to increase the amount of the case completed by the trainee and lead to more consistent and reproducible operative times (5). When used as the primary technique for left colectomy, the hand-assisted approach leads to shorter operative times with no difference in short-term outcomes when compared to the straight laparoscopic approach. A multicenter prospective randomized trial comparing laparoscopic to hand-assisted laparoscopic colectomy found the hand-assisted approach lead to 33 minutes reduction in operative times (6). There was no difference in length of stay, return of bowel function, narcotic use, or visual pain scores. For difficult cases such as left colectomy for complicated diverticulitis or restorative proctocolectomy, the hand-assisted approach can lead to faster operative times and decreased chances for conversion to open colectomy. A retrospective review comparing laparoscopic sigmoid resection for complicated diverticulitis reported a conversion rate of 5% with hand-assisted versus 14% for laparoscopy (7). This trend was also demonstrated in a European prospective randomized trial of hand-assisted versus straight laparoscopic colectomy (8). In the straight laparoscopic arm, two-thirds of the conversions utilized a hand-port to complete the case. Surgeons were also queried about the usefulness of the hand-assisted approach and the response was that 33% of the cases would not have been completed without the use of the hand.

CONCLUSIONS

The hand-assisted approach to laparoscopic left colectomy is another tool in the surgeon's armamentarium. The surgeon may implement this approach in many different situations without any difference in short-term outcomes when compared the straight laparoscopic approach.

Recommended References and Readings

1. Shawki S, Bashankaev B, Denoya P, et al. What is the definition of "conversion" in laparoscopic colorectal surgery? *Surg Endosc* 2009;23:2321–26.
2. Casillas S, Delaney CP, Senagore AJ, et al. Does conversion of a laparoscopic colectomy adversely affect patient outcome? *Dis Colon Rectum* 2004;47:1680–85.
3. Tekkis PP, Senagore AJ, Delaney CP. Conversion rates in laparoscopic colorectal surgery: a predictive model with, 1253 patients. *Surg Endosc* 2005;19(1):47–54.
4. Duepree HJ, Senagore AJ, Delaney CP, et al. Does means of access affect the incidence of small bowel obstruction and ventral hernia after bowel resection?: Laparoscopy versus laparotomy. *J Am Coll Surg* 2003;197(2):177–81.
5. Chang YJ, Marcello PW, Rusin LC, et al. Hand-assisted laparoscopic sigmoid colectomy: helping hand or hindrance? *Surg Endosc* 2005;19(5):656–61.
6. Marcello PW, Fleshman JW, Milsom JW, et al. Hand-assisted laparoscopic vs. laparoscopic colorectal surgery: a multicenter, prospective, randomized trial. *Dis Colon Rectum* 2008;51(6):818–26.
7. Lee SW, Yoo J, Dujovny N, et al. Laparoscopic vs. hand-assisted laparoscopic sigmoidectomy for diverticulitis. *Dis Colon Rectum* 2006;49(4):464–9.
8. Targarona EM, Gracia E, Garriga J, et al. Prospective randomized trial comparing conventional laparoscopic colectomy with hand-assisted laparoscopic colectomy: applicability, immediate clinical outcome, inflammatory response, and cost. *Surg Endosc* 2002;16(2):234–9.

13 Open

Juan J. Nogueras

INDICATIONS/CONTRAINDICATIONS

For the greater part of the early to mid-20th century, abdominoperineal resection with permanent colostomy was the mainstay surgical option for patients with rectal cancer. With the advent of surgical staplers and anastomotic techniques for low pelvic anastomoses, sphincter preservation surgery became the preferred option for the majority of rectal tumors. The dual objectives of modern rectal cancer surgery are to achieve excellent oncologic outcomes with adequate functional results. Low anterior resection with restorative intent is possible for tumors in the distal third of the rectum that do not invade the sphincter musculature. Anterior resection with curative intent is indicated for tumors of the mid to lower third of the rectum located below the peritoneal reflection without evidence of adjacent bony, pelvic sidewall, or sphincter musculature invasion. Palliative resection is indicated for patients without significant comorbidities and minimal metastatic disease in order to provide improved quality of life. In patients with significant comorbidities and advanced metastatic disease, nonoperative therapy is the preferred option.

The choice of operative approach today involves open, laparoscopic, and robotic techniques for anterior resection. As more surgeons become increasingly experienced with minimally invasive techniques, there is a tendency to favor these techniques over the open approach. Cheung et al. (1) published the results of a questionnaire among 386 surgeons in which they demonstrated that 77% of the study participants performed 1-20 laparoscopic resections per year (low volume), whereas a smaller percentage performed more than 20 laparoscopic resections per year (high volume). These authors demonstrated that more low volume surgeons had a preference for open anterior resection depending on specific factors, such as the age and gender of the patient, the presence of comorbidities, previous laparotomy, and locally advanced tumors.

Among experienced laparoscopic surgeons, there is a conversion rate to open surgery. In a retrospective study of 1,073 patients with carcinoma of the rectum and anus who underwent laparoscopic surgery, Yamamoto et al. (2) discovered that the conversion rate to open surgery was 7.3%. The patients who required conversion were heavier (BMI 24.6 vs. 22.7) and had a substantially higher rate of low anterior resection. Therefore, expertise in open technique for anterior resection is necessary for all surgeons who embark on minimally invasive surgery for rectal cancer.

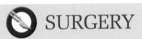

PREOPERATIVE PLANNING

Adequate preoperative staging of the patient with rectal cancer involves determination of tumor level from the dentate line, depth of penetration, lymph node involvement, and distant metastases. Based on a number of criteria, selected patients will undergo neoadjuvant therapy. After completion of neoadjuvant therapy, patients are recommended to undergo resection surgery. The timing of surgery after neoadjuvant therapy has changed over recent years, and recent data by De Campos-Lobato et al. (3) suggest that a period of at least 8 weeks is associated with a higher rate of complete pathologic response and decreased local recurrence.

Patients who undergo anterior resection should be informed of specific risks involved with the surgery, especially potential injuries to the pelvic autonomic nerves resulting in sexual and bladder dysfunction (4). Moreover, patients should have some understanding of function after restorative proctectomy, with an expectation for increased frequency and urgency in the early postoperative period.

Patients are seen preoperatively by the enterostomal nurse for stoma education and optimal stoma site marking.

SURGERY

Preparation and Positioning

All patients receive a preoperative full mechanical bowel preparation. Perioperative antibiotics are administered for 24 hours.

In anticipation of surgery in the deep pelvic space, the surgeon must ensure optimum visualization of tissue planes. In order to achieve this, preoperative procurement of adequate assistance, retraction, and illumination is important. Deep pelvic retractors, such as the St Mark's retractors, are important for adequate exposure. For patients with a narrow pelvis, the illuminated, narrow blade St Mark's retractors are especially helpful. The use of a headlight can also facilitate adequate visualization in the deep pelvis.

As was demonstrated by Pokala et al. (5), selective use of ureteral stents for adequate localization of the ureters can also be beneficial.

The patient is placed in the modified lithotomy position with careful attention to adequate padding to avoid injury to the peroneal nerve that may result in postoperative foot drop.

Technique

The surgery is approached via a midline incision. Upon entering the abdomen, a thorough exploration is performed to exclude metastatic disease. The sigmoid and descending colon are mobilized medially and the left ureter is identified. An assessment is made about the length of the descending and sigmoid colon, and the need for splenic flexure mobilization. Brennan et al. (6) reported on their experience with selective mobilization of the splenic flexure during anterior resection for rectal cancer. The ability to create a tension free and well-vascularized anastomosis determines the need for splenic flexure mobilization. The splenic flexure mobilization is facilitated with the operating surgeon standing between the legs of the patient in the modified lithotomy position. A recent study from Cleveland Clinic Florida evaluated patients referred for redo colorectal anastomosis for anastomotic stricture. In virtually every instance the splenic flexure had not been mobilized and neither the inferior mesenteric artery nor vein had been proximally divided (CCF Ref).

The peritoneum on both sides of the rectum is incised at the level of the sacral promontory, with care to avoid injury to the ureters and to the sympathetic nerves. Various means of identification of the nerves have been dissected but are rarely needed (Silva et al.). The dissection is carried underneath the superior rectal artery, and the superior rectal artery is dissected to the level of the left colic artery and inferior mesenteric artery. The decision of the location of vessel ligation is based on the need for adequate length for a tension free and well-vascularized anastomosis (7). Division at a level just inferior to the left colic artery, with preservation of the left colic artery will result in more predictable blood supply to the anastomosis, but may not give sufficient length, especially in cases where the majority of the sigmoid is resected. Division at the level of the inferior mesenteric artery, at its takeoff from the aorta, along with proximal division of the inferior mesenteric vein, will typically ensure sufficient length for the anastomosis. The anastomosis will then rely on blood supply from the marginal artery of Drummond, based on the middle colic artery. The level of vessel division has not been demonstrated to have an effect on the oncological outcome of the operation (8).

Total Mesorectal Excision

The purpose of an anterior resection for cancers of the mid and low rectum is complete removal of the lymph node bearing mesorectum along with its intact enveloping fascia, a technique referred to as total mesorectal excision (TME). The impetus for this technique dates to a paper by Heald et al. (9) in which five cases of minute microfoci of adenocarcinoma were demonstrated in the mesorectum several centimeters distal to the edge of the intraluminal rectal cancer. In 1992, Heald (10) demonstrated a 4% local recurrence rate with the technique of TME, and since then, many have adopted this technique as the standard for rectal cancer surgery.

The mesorectum is enveloped by the fascia propria (11). The proper plane of dissection is initiated by following the posterior aspect of the superior rectal artery until a shiny, filmy membrane is encountered at the pelvic brim. This plane lies between the fascia propria of the rectum containing the mesorectum and its vessels and lymph nodes, and the endopelvic fascia, which covers the hypogastric nerves and pelvic plexuses. The dissection proceeds posteriorly along this plane, keeping in mind that the fascia propria may be tethered to the presacral fascia at the level of the fourth sacral vertebra, sometimes referred to as the rectosacral fascia or ligament. At this point, it is important to avoid entering the presacral fascia for fear of injuring the presacral veins, which may result in significant bleeding. The dissection is carried posteriorly as far as can be accomplished safely under direct vision. The surgeon should avoid the technique of blind blunt dissection as this technique may result in breach of the fascia propria and an incomplete mesorectal excision. The anterolateral dissection is initiated by incising the peritoneum in the pouch of Douglas and dividing the remaining peritoneum laterally, avoiding injury to the pelvic sidewall and its vessels. The anterior dissection is carried out in front of Denonvillier's fascia, which lies posterior to the prostate and seminal vesicles in males and the vault of the vagina in females, and anterior to the extraperitoneal rectum, anterior mesorectum, and fascia propria (12). It is important to recognize that immediately anterior to Denonvillier's fascia lie the parasympathetic nerves that supply the corpora and erectile function in males. These small nerves are in very close proximity during this anterior dissection and are in jeopardy of injury (13).

The posterior dissection is carried out below the rectosacral fascia down to the level of the retrorectal space, whose inferior portion corresponds to Waldeyer's fascia (14). The entire mesorectum is thereby contained within the specimen. The location of the point of transection is determined in part by the location of the tumor. A distal resection margin of 1 cm is now considered adequate for oncological outcome (15). Ensuring accurate localization of the distal edge of the tumor, or postradiation ulcer, may require intraoperative visualization with flexible or rigid endoscopy. Once the inferior level of the tumor is identified, and the level of transection determined, the rectum is transected with a 30-mm linear stapler. For very distal tumors, a transanal mucosectomy or an intersphincteric dissection may be indicated.

Colorectal Anastomosis

The traditional end-to-end coloanal anastomosis was the default technique for many years. However, a constellation of symptoms attributed to the loss of reservoir, including urgency, clustering of evacuations, and incontinence, has prompted surgeons to seek alternative anastomotic techniques. Hallbook et al. (16) demonstrated improved function over straight anastomosis with the creation of a colonic J pouch. Numerous subsequent studies including several randomized controlled trials and meta-analysis confirmed these findings. Benefits of the colonic J pouch as compared to the straight coloanal anastomosis persist for at least 2 years (Luo et al., CCF). Huber et al. (17) demonstrated similar functional results between the colonic pouch and the Baker side-to-end anastomosis, further corroborated in a prospective randomized trial by Machado et al. (18). The Baker technique is particularly useful in situations where the pelvis is narrow and the mesentery is thick, precluding the creation of a pouch. Either technique is acceptable, keeping in mind that the size of the pouch or the length of the defunctionalized limb should not exceed 6 cm. The author prefers the use of the side-to-end anastomosis because of the ease of construction without demonstrable long-term detriment in functional results over the more technically challenging colonic J pouch. The editors, however, favor the colonic J pouch. A randomized controlled trial is currently underway to compare the two techniques.

The anastomosis is created with the circular stapler, using the double-stapled technique. For cases that involved a mucosectomy, a hand-sewn anastomosis is preferred. The anastomotic integrity is tested with air by filling the pelvis with saline, occluding the lumen proximal to the anastomosis, and insufflating air transanally. If an air leak is present, direct transanal visualization of the anastomosis with the use of an anoscope can often locate the anastomotic defect and facilitate direct repair. Routine intraoperative endoscopy rather than simple blind air insufflation has clear benefits (Li et al., CCF, 2009). A rectal washout before the creation of the anastomosis has not been shown to have any oncologic benefits over avoidance of the maneuver (19).

After completion of the anastomosis, a location is selected in the terminal ileum for exteriorization as a diverting loop ileostomy. The site of the stoma in the abdominal wall has been selected preoperatively and marked for easy intraoperative identification. Recent data demonstrate the benefits of the use of a temporary diverting loop ileostomy in reducing the incidence of anastomotic leakage when compared to no diversion (20–22).

The use of a drain in the pelvis is left to the discretion of the surgeon.

 ## POSTOPERATIVE MANAGEMENT

Immediate postoperative management is similar to any other major abdominal surgery. Perioperative antibiotics are stopped after 24 hours. Early ambulation and pulmonary toilet are strongly encouraged. Nasogastric tube decompression is not routinely administered. The urinary catheter is removed once the patient is ambulatory. The output from the ileostomy is monitored, and optimized to remain at a volume less than 1,200 cc per day. The management for high stoma output includes antidiarrheal medication, fiber supplementation, cholestyramine, and tincture of opium.

Prior to takedown of the loop ileostomy for re-establishment of intestinal continuity, a contrast enema is administered transanally in order to document anastomotic integrity. An endoscopic evaluation may also be performed at this time to visualize the anastomosis and the neoreservoir. The timing of the closure of the ileostomy will depend on whether the patient undergoes adjuvant chemotherapy. In these cases, the stoma is closed at least 4 weeks after cessation of the chemotherapy. In case of no adjuvant therapy, the stoma is closed no sooner than 8 weeks after surgery.

 ## COMPLICATIONS

Intraoperative complications can occur at any step of the operation, and the surgeon must be aware of specific potential injuries during each phase of the operation. Splenic flexure mobilization may result in inadvertent tear of the splenic capsule or laceration of the spleen. During the lateral rectal mobilization, injury to the ureters and iliac vessels may occur. At the level of the sacral promontory, injury to the sympathetic nerves may result in sexual dysfunction. Dissection of the anterior rectum at the level of Denonvillier's fascia may result in damage to the parasympathetic autonomic nerves, resulting in subsequent bladder and sexual dysfunction. Posterior mobilization of the rectum places the presacral venous plexus at risk, especially at the level of the rectosacral fascia.

A significant postoperative anastomotic complication is anastomotic leak. The overall anastomotic leak rate in a large randomized multicenter trial was 19.2%, with a rate of 10.3% in patients with defunctioning stoma compared to 28% in patients without a defunctioning stoma (21). Defunctioning proximal loop stoma decreased the rate of symptomatic anastomotic leakage. The long-term risk for a permanent stoma in patients who undergo a low anterior resection of the rectum for cancer is 19% (23). Among the reasons for a permanent stoma, the most common were unsatisfactory anorectal function and sequelae of anastomotic leakage.

CONCLUSION

Restorative proctectomy with low colorectal anastomosis is possible for the majority of patients with rectal cancer. Dissection along anatomic planes ensures complete removal of lymph node-bearing tissue in the mesorectum and preservation of vital nerves for bladder and sexual function. Creation of a reservoir in the neorectum by end-to-side anastomosis or colonic J pouch improves function. Proximal diversion with a loop ileostomy decreases the incidence of complications from anastomotic leakage.

Recommended References and Readings

1. Cheung YM, Lange MM, Buunen M, et al. Current technique of laparoscopic total mesorectal excision (TME: An international questionnaire among 368 surgeons. *Surg Endosc* 2009;23:2796–801.
2. Yamamoto S, Fukunaga M, Miyajima N, et al. Impact of conversion on surgical outcomes after laparoscopic operation for rectal carcinoma: a retrospective study of 1,073 patients. *J Am Coll Surg* 2009;208:383–9.
3. De Campos-Lobato LF, Geisler DP, da Luz Moreira A, Stocchi L, Dietz D, Kalady MF. Neoadjuvant therapy for rectal cancer: the impact of longer interval between chemoradiation and surgery. *J Gastrointest Surg* 2011;15(3):444–50.
4. Nesbakken A, Nygaard K, Bull-Njaa T, et al. Bladder and sexual dysfunction after mesorectal excision for rectal cancer. *Br J Surg* 2000;87(2):206–10.
5. Pokala N, Delaney CP, Kiran RP, et al. A randomized controlled trial comparing simultaneous intra-operative vs sequential prophylactic ureteric catheter insertion in re-operative and complicated colorectal surgery. *Int J Colorectal Dis* 2007;22(6):683–7.
6. Brennan DJ, Moynagh M, Brannigan AE, et al. Routine mobilization of the splenic flexure is not necessary during anterior resection for rectal cancer. *Dis Colon Rectum* 2007;50:302–7.
7. Buunen M, Lange MM, Ditzel M, et al. Level of arterial ligation in total mesorectal excision (TME): an anatomical study. *Int J Colorectal Dis* 2009;24:1317–20.
8. Lange MM, Buunen M, van de Velde CJH, et al. Level of arterial ligation in rectal cancer surgery: low tie preferred over high tie. A review. *Dis Colon Rectum* 2008;51:1139–45.
9. Heald RJ, Husband EM, Ryall RD. The mesorectum in rectal cancer surgery: the clue to pelvic recurrence? *Br J Surg* 1982;69:613–6.
10. MacFarlane JK, Ryall RD, Heald RJ. Mesorectal excision for rectal cancer. *Lancet* 1993;341:457–60.
11. Bisset IP, Chau KY, Hill GL. Extrafascial excision of the rectum: surgical; anatomy of the fascia propria. *Dis Colon Rectum* 2000;43:903–10.
12. Lindsey I, Warren BF, Mortensen NJ. Denonvillier's fascia lies anterior to the fascia propria and rectal dissection plane in total mesorectal excision. *Dis Colon Rectum* 2005;48:37–42.
13. Clausen N, Wolloscheck T, Konerding MA. How to optimize autonomic nerve preservation in total mesorectal excision: clinical topography and morphology of pelvic nerves and fascia. *World J Surg* 2008;32:1768–75.
14. Garcia-Armengol J, Garcia-Botello J, Martinez-Soriano F, et al. Review of the anatomic concepts in relation to the retrorectal space and endopelvic fascia: Waldeyer's fascia and the retrorectal fascia. *Colorectal Dis* 2008;10:298–302.
15. Park IJ, Kim JC. Adequate length of the distal resection margin in rectal cancer: from the oncological point of view. *J Gastrointest Surg* 2010;14(8):1331–7.
16. Hallbook O, Pahlman L, Krog M, et al. Randomized comparison of straight and colonic J pouch anastomosis after low anterior resection. *Ann Surg* 1996;224:58–65.
17. Huber FT, Herter B, Siewert JR. Colonic pouch vs side-to-end anastomosis in low anterior resection. *Dis Colon Rectum* 1999;42:896–902.
18. Machado M, Nygren J, Goldman S, et al. Similar outcome after colonic pouch and side-to-end anastomosis in low anterior resection for rectal cancer: A prospective randomized trial. *Ann Surg* 2003;238:214–20.
19. Constantinides VA, Cheetham D, Nicholls RJ, et al. Is rectal washout effective for preventing localized recurrence after anterior resection for rectal cancer? *Dis Colon Rectum* 2008;51:1339–44.
20. Huser N, Michalski CW, Erkan M, et al. Systematic review and meta-analysis of the role of defunctioning stoma in low rectal cancer surgery. *Ann Surg* 2008;248(1):52–60.
21. Matthiessen P, Hallbook O, Rutegard J, et al. Defunctioning stoma reduces symptomatic anastomotic leakage after low anterior resection of the rectum for cancer: a randomized multicenter trial. *Ann Surg* 2007;246(2):207–14.
22. Tan WS, Tang CL, Shi L, et al. Meta-analysis of defunctioning stomas in low anterior resection for rectal cancer. *Br J Surg* 2009;96(5):462–72.
23. Lindgren R, Hallbook O, Rutegard J, et al. What is the risk for a permanent stoma after low anterior resection of the rectum for cancer? A six-year follow-up of a multicenter trial. *Dis Colon Rectum* 2011;54:41–7.

Part III: Low Anterior Resection

14 Laparoscopic

Badma Bashankaev and Christina Seo

 ## INDICATIONS/CONTRAINDICATIONS

The indications for a laparoscopic low anterior resection with stapled coloanal or color-ectal anastomosis (hereafter referred to as stapled low anterior resection [LAR]) are as follow:

- Middle rectal tumors (5–10 cm from anal verge)
- Lower rectal tumors (0–5 cm from anal verge), with a distal margin of ≥1 cm, with an extra 1 cm of rectum required to perform stapled anastomosis

This procedure is absolutely contraindicated only in patients with unstable hemody-namics such as acute myocardial infarction or severe sepsis such as fecal peritonitis.

The relative contraindications depend largely upon the experience of the surgical team. They include the following:

- Morbid obesity
- Advanced age
- Severe cardiovascular or pulmonary disease
- Liver cirrhosis
- Large or enlarging abdominal aneurysm
- Severe acute inflammatory bowel disease
- Large abscess or phlegmon
- Pregnancy
- Presence of scars from multiple laparotomies
- Coagulopathy or bleeding disorders

In cases where establishing pneumoperitoneum is contraindicated due to hemody-namic or pulmonary compromise, the laparolift (gasless laparoscopy) option may be considered.

 ## PREOPERATIVE PLANNING

Informed consent is an obligatory part of every preoperative plan. A discussion with the patient regarding the risks, benefits, potential complications, and alternatives to the pro-cedure provides a realistic gauge of the patient's expectations. Specific to the laparoscopic approach, the possibility of conversion to open surgery in cases of technical difficulties or intraoperative complications ought to be discussed. Intraoperative colonoscopy may be used for precise verification of the position of the lesion, the height of the rectal stump, and final evaluation of the anastomosis. If used routinely, this procedure should be added to the informed consent.

Preoperative evaluation of patients scheduled for stapled LAR consists of standard tests, rectal cancer staging, and any further assessments needed specifically for low rectal procedures. The steps needed to stage the rectal cancer and determine the appropriate surgical procedure(s) include:

- Digital rectal examination
  - Assessment of size and degree of fixation of mid to low rectal tumors
- Flexible sigmoidoscopy/rigid proctoscopy
  - Measurement of the level of lesion from the anal verge or dentate line
  - Biopsy of the lesion
- Biopsy for pathologic examination
  - Diagnosis confirmation
  - Preliminary prognosis of disease
- Colonoscopy
  - Exclusion of synchronous colonic lesions
- Endorectal ultrasound with two-dimensional (2D) or three-dimensional (3D) sensors
  - Rectal wall penetration (T-stage)
  - Nodal involvement (N-stage)
    - Local lymph node involvement
- Magnetic resonance imaging (MRI) of the abdomen and pelvis
  - Rectal wall penetration (T-stage) and evaluation of involvement of adjacent structures
    - Determination of resectability or need for en bloc resection
  - Lymph nodes involvement (N-stage)
    - Local and regional lymph node involvement
- Computed tomography (CT) scan of the abdomen and chest
  - Detection of distant metastasis (M-stage)
- Positron emission tomography (PET) scan
  - Verification of local and distant metastasis
- Chest x-ray
  - Detection of distant metastasis

Evaluation of the patient's overall physical fitness and determination of the patient's operative risk are done with the following:

- Internal medicine evaluation
  - Cardiology, renal, hepatology, pulmonology consults if required
- Anesthesiology consult
  - Ideally before day of surgery
- Complete blood count (CBC), complete metabolic panel (CMP) blood tests
  - Carcinoembryonic antigen (CEA) level for postoperative surveillance
- ECG
- Considerations specific to stapled LAR:
  - Preoperative counseling for stoma care with ileostomy/colostomy marking
    - Obtain the optimal position of the stoma
      - Permanent tattoo with India ink or henna of stoma site if seen ≥1 week before surgery
      - Skin marker with transparent medical dressing (Tegaderm™, 3M, St. Paul, MN) if seen less than a week before surgery
    - Provide initial education about ostomy maintenance
  - Preoperative surgical nurse visit
    - Explanation of surgical procedure, including bowel preparation, and postoperative fast track protocol

- Scheduling of patient's admission to the hospital
- First step in establishing patient awareness of fast-track care protocol
- Anal manometry in patients older than 65 years
  - Diagnosis of latent fecal incontinence and impaired sphincter mechanism

Current recommendations suggest offering patients with stage II (node-negative disease with transmural invasion) and stage III rectal cancer (node-positive disease) neoadjuvant chemoradiotherapy (nCRT). It is widely accepted that nCRT results in downstaging and downsizing of the tumor with a better likelihood for successful sphincter preservation by providing a safe distal margin of 2 cm. In the USA, nCRT therapy lasts for 5–6 weeks and consists of median radiation dose of 50.4 Gy (45–65 Gy), with 45 Gy to the pelvis and 5.4 Gy boost to the tumor over 28 fractions with fluorouracil (5-FU)-based infusions. The optimal interval after completion of nCRT to surgery is around 6 weeks; this is related to the progression of acute postchemoradiation inflammation to fibrosis while maintaining a safe period to allow tumor regression.

Patients are asked to stop taking medication containing aspirin and aspirin-like products 10 days prior to the surgery. The day before surgery, patient undergoes mechanical bowel preparation. *Nil per os* (NPO) status after midnight the night prior to surgery is requested to decrease the potential risk of pulmonary aspiration with resultant chemical pneumonia. The patient is admitted on the morning of surgery. Cross-typing of blood can be done either during preoperative evaluation or on the day of surgery.

Both perioperative antibiotic prophylaxis for the first 24 hours and DVT prophylaxis with subcutaneous injection of 5,000 units of heparin and/or pneumatic sequential pressure devices for the lower extremities are standard precautions.

SURGERY

The operating room (OR) team consists of the operating surgeon, first assistant, camera assistant, scrub technician/nurse, and a circulating nurse. It is crucial that the OR team has a common understanding of the procedure and a firm knowledge of laparoscopic instruments and their handling. The surgeon and first assistant may share the camera driving throughout the case. In addition to having a solid familiarity with the surgical procedure, reverse camera driving and advanced laparoscopic skills are very important skills.

Typically, the surgeon and camera driver stand on the right side of the patient (opposite to the site of dissection), with the first assistant on the left side. During the operation, the position of surgeon may need to change in order to increase range of motion; for example, during the splenic flexure mobilization, the surgeon may need to stand between the legs of the patient.

At least two monitors are required for the laparoscopic LAR. One should be on the left side of the patient for the surgeon and camera driver, and another over the patient's head or right shoulder for the first assistant.

A laparoscopic tray with a traumatic bowel or Babcock graspers is required. Two 30 degree 10-mm cameras and one 30 degree 5-mm camera should be placed in a thermos with warm sterile water, or in a special camera warmer.

Positioning

After the patient is brought into the OR, he or she is carefully transferred to the OR table. The anesthesiologist then intubates the patient and inserts a naso-/orogastric tube. The patient is placed in modified lithotomy using Allen® (Allen Medical Systems, Acton, MA) stirrups with legs oriented so that the toes, knees, and shoulders are in line. The knees should be slightly flexed and the thighs flattened parallel to the bed so that the surgeon can maintain the greatest range of motion of his hands and laparoscopic instruments.

The use of a Bean Bag placed directly on the table with both arms tucked can prevent sliding of the patient while using steep Trendelenburg and reverse-Trendelenburg positions. The patient's extremities should be well padded to avoid any trauma at bony prominences.

It is important to provide 3–4 cm of exposure of the perineal area off the edge of the operating table before commencing the surgery to allow easy passage of the circular stapler. Additional care should be taken to regulate the temperature of the patient with the use of heating devices such as Bair Hugger®, Arizant Inc., Eden Prairie, MN.

If patient had a stoma site marked preoperatively, the site is marked with a needle tip to prevent losing the mark during the preparatory wash.

We routinely use ureteral stents for deep pelvic surgery. A urologist places these stents to facilitate safe laparoscopic pelvic dissection by providing tactile and visual confirmation of the safety of the ureter.

Rectal irrigation is undertaken with Betadine® Solution (aqueous solution of 10% povidone-iodine) (Purdue Products L.P., Stamford, CT). The abdomen is prepped and draped in the usual sterile manner, taking care to position the sterile towels along the anterior axillary line for proper trocar placement and across the xiphoid and pubis for possible laparotomy.

It is preferable to use laparoscopic draping with built-in pockets to attach the insufflation tubing, camera cord, light cable, and cautery cord around the perimeter of the patient's abdomen. The Steri-Drape™ (3M™ Medical, St. Paul, MN) plastic pouches or other holsters are useful for organizing and securing the laparoscopic instruments onto the sterile field.

Technique

The laparoscopic-stapled LAR consists of several steps (Fig. 14.1). This procedure can be performed totally laparoscopically (port site wounds only) and laparoscopic-assisted (port sites and specimen extraction site). Both approaches start by establishing pneumoperitoneum. There are two common techniques of laparoscopic entry into abdominal cavity to maintain pneumoperitoneum—closed (Veress) and open (Hasson), based on surgeon preference.

The open Hasson technique is preferable due to its ease and minimal risk of injury to peritoneal structures. The incision is made above or below the umbilicus depending upon the height of the patient and the distance of the umbilicus from the pubis. An extension of this incision may be used for specimen extraction, thereby providing somewhat better cosmesis. The Hasson technique starts with a vertical 1.5-cm long skin incision with #15 blade scalpel or diathermy, dissecting the subcutaneous tissues to the level of fascia. The fascia is grasped with Kocher clamps or similar instrument to better visualize and incise that layer. Anchoring sutures are placed on the edges of the fascial incision with 2-0 Vicryl™ (Ethicon Inc., Summerville, NJ) or silk to form handles for the Hasson trocar. The preperitoneal fat is gently spread to expose the peritoneum, which is grasped with smaller clamps and divided, taking care to ensure that there is no intervening bowel. The 12-mm Hasson trocar is then introduced into the abdominal cavity and secured with the previously placed anchor sutures. The insufflation tube is attached and carbon dioxide pneumoperitoneum with a pressure of up to 15 mm Hg is established.

A 30-degree 10-mm camera is obtained from out of the warmer or thermos and attached to the light and video processor cables. White balance of the camera is done on a laparotomy gauze or any other uniformly white surface.

The camera is then introduced into the abdominal cavity. A careful survey of the entire abdominal cavity is performed to note any adhesions and any relevant disease of the liver or peritoneal surfaces (to exclude tumor metastasis).

Placement of the ports should be done judiciously to allow for adequate triangulation of the instruments and freedom of motion unobstructed by the costal margins and iliac spines. The right lower quadrant port should be about 2–3 cm medial and superior to anterior superior iliac spine, while the right upper quadrant port should be a handsbreadth above this, allowing a centimeter or two margin from the lower ribs. Some adjustment must be made for the patient's overall body habitus and abdominal contour. There should also be some flexibility in considering the previously marked stoma site, which should be either avoided entirely or used as a port site, though it is rarely an ideal site for laparoscopic instruments. A left lower quadrant or suprapubic trocar may be useful for some cases.

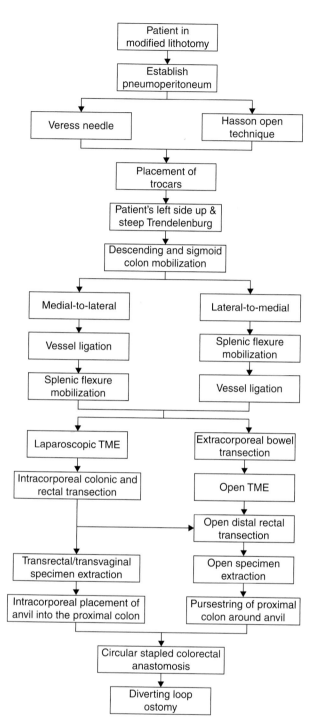

Figure 14.1 Laparoscopic stapled low anterior resection.

Using 10–12 mm ports for all port sites provides flexibility for the angle of the camera and stapler. Alternatively, one can use one 5-mm umbilical port for a 5-mm camera, two 5-mm right sided ports, and one 10–12 mm left lower quadrant or suprapubic port (4–5 cm above the pubic bone) for the endoscopic stapler.

A skin incision with a #15 blade scalpel or diathermy is made in the right lower quadrant. The 30-degree laparoscopic camera is turned 180 degrees for direct visualization of the trocar insertion. The trocar is placed in the dominant hand and slowly introduced through the skin incision with tip oriented toward pelvis. Transillumination by laparoscopic camera through abdominal wall in nonobese patients can help avoid injuring the hypogastric vessels. The right upper quadrant trocar is placed in a similar fashion.

The surgeon may require an extra lower left quadrant port for additional retraction and exposure. This port should be placed in an almost mirror image of the port on the right or suprapubically. Addition of this trocar can be done at the beginning of the case or later in the case when needed.

After the introduction of the ports, the patient is turned to right-side-down position with steep Trendelenburg. This facilitates displacement of the omentum and small-bowel loops toward the right side of the abdominal cavity. Once the left colon can be adequately visualized, the surgeon can change the grasper in the lower right port to laparoscopic shears with diathermy or any other energy source such as the laparoscopic ultrasonic Harmonic Scalpel® (Ethicon Endo-Surgery, Cincinnati, OH).

Lateral-to-Medial Dissection

Exposure for a lateral-to-medial dissection begins with gentle retraction of the left colon cranially and medially with an atraumatic nonlocking bowel grasper. The white line of Toldt in the left paracolic gutter is incised and the dissection begun in the avascular plane between the mesocolon and retroperitoneum (including Gerota's fascia). It is extremely helpful to the surgeon to have good quality monitors or HD-monitors to be able to distinguish with confidence between the subtle color and texture differences between the embryologic tissues. Mobilization should be continued to the level of the root of the mesentery and the duodenum while identifying and protecting the left ureter. In obese patients, ureteral stents facilitate this task by providing tactile feedback.

After the ureter is identified, the dissection is continued medially until the mesocolon is separated from the splenic attachments and Gerota's fascia. In thin patients, planes may be more fused. Care must be taken to stay in the plane that is above the left ureter in order to avoid entering through the sigmoid mesentery and potentially endangering the small bowel on the other side.

Once the dissection is extended toward the splenic flexure as far as can be comfortably done in the right lateral-Trendelenburg position, the patient is positioned heads-up while maintaining the patient's right side down. The surgeon can now stand between patient's legs and complete the splenic flexure mobilization with the energy source in the lower left port. This increases the right hand's range of motion in a difficult flexure. To facilitate the dissection, the omentum can be divided over the middle colic vessels to mobilize the transverse colon toward the splenic flexure. This may require a larger bipolar coagulation device such as the LigaSure Atlas (Valleylab, Boulder, CO). Once the lesser sac is opened, the first assistant standing on the left side of the patient can retract the transverse colon, while the surgeon uses the left hand grasper for countertraction on the omentum, and with energy source in the right hand finish the mobilization of the splenic flexure. Care must be taken to avoid damage to the pancreatic tail, splenic vessels, and the spleen itself.

Once the left colon and splenic flexure have been mobilized, the mesocolon is dissected off the aorta until the inferior mesenteric artery (IMA) is identified. The parietal peritoneum should be scored and the IMA should be skeletonized of mesenteric fat to do an oncologic resection of the lymph node basin. Either a high ligation of IMA or a selective left colic artery-sparing vessel ligation can be performed using an energy source such as the LigaSure Atlas (Valleylab, Boulder, CO) or an endoscopic vascular stapler load (with 2.5 mm staples, white or grey cartridges). It is imperative that the left ureter be well visualized before closing the stapler or coagulator jaws. The grasper should be used to stabilize the proximal vessel trunk while firing the stapler to maintain adequate control of the vessel stump in case of a stapler misfire or staple line bleed. If bleeding occurs, endoscopic staples or clips may be used, as energy sources are not effective when applied to staples.

Further proximal mobilization in the same plane will provide exposure of the fourth portion of the duodenum and the ligament of Treitz. The inferior mesenteric vein (IMV) can be found just lateral to the duodenum at this level. The IMV is often divided here to provide length as the proximal colon will need to reach down to the pelvis.

Medial-to-Lateral Dissection

In this approach, the patient is turned with the left side up so that the small bowel can be swept away from the root of the mesentery. The IMA is identified and skeletonized, then divided with vascular staples or an energy source such as the LigaSure device. The bare area of the mesentery is divided caudally, which brings the plane of dissection directly to the IMV as it is exposed just lateral to the duodenum. The IMV is divided in a similar manner to the IMA. The colonic mesentery is dissected bluntly away from the retroperitoneum, using the ureter as a guide for the intervening plane. This dissection is continued proximally and distally until the only remaining attachments are the lateral-most attachments to the abdominal sidewall, spleen and omentum.

Rectal Dissection

The patient is brought back to a steep Trendelenburg position to allow the small bowel and omentum to fall away from the operative field. The camera is oriented toward the pelvis and dissection is continued posteriorly while preserving the hypogastric nerves. Mobilization of that plane ultimately leads to the avascular plane between the mesorectum and the presacral fascia. The first assistant should provide adequate traction of the proximal rectum superiorly and laterally. The posterior dissection is continued distally and on either side to include the division of the lateral rectal stalks. Lastly, the anterior dissection is performed to complete the total mesorectal excision (TEM). Denonvillier's fascia in male patients is swept anteriorly, separating the seminal vesicles from the mesorectum. In female patients, uterus might obstruct the view to the deep pelvis; retraction may require either an additional port for a laparoscopic retractor or suspension to the anterior abdominal wall using extracorporeal suture a with straight Keith needle. Alternatively, the use of any curved needle can be introduced through the trocar and used to suture either through the uterine corpus or around the round ligaments in the avascular windows just lateral to the uterus. After the needle is cut and extracted through the trocar, the sutures are brought out through the skin using a Berci fascial closure device (Karl Storz GmbH & Co, KG, Tuttlingen, Germany) and tied.

The principles of a total mesorectal excision should be followed down to 1–2 cm distal to the tumor, but the mesorectal envelope should be mobilized to 5 cm below the tumor. The rectum is clamped at the level of desired transaction and an intraoperative flexible sigmoidoscopy or rigid proctoscopy can be performed to confirm the distance from the dentate line.

The alternative methods for completing the rest of the resection are as follow:

- **Open approach.** This involves a continuation of the procedure extracorporeally through a lower midline incision. The colon is transected extracorporeally with a GIA™ stapler (Covidien Autosuture, Mansfield, MA) and the mesocolon is cleared off the bowel wall for an automatic purse string clamp. The purse-string is closed around the anvil of circular stapler placed in the lumen of the proximal colon and returned to the abdominal cavity. Long purse string suture ends (like horse reins) will facilitate proper colon and anvil orientation through small abdominal incision when the ends of colon and rectum area approximated. An open rectal transection is done using a linear stapling device (TA™ stapler from Covidien Autosuture, Mansfield, MA) or curved cutting stapler (Contour®, Ethicon Endo-Surgery, Inc., Cincinnati, OH), with an open specimen extraction.
- **Laparoscopic-assisted approach.** Endoscopic stapled transection of the rectum is performed with the use of articulating endoscopic stapler (Endo GIA™ Roticulator™, Covidien Autosuture, Mansfield, MA). The proximal colon is brought down to the pelvis, and the level of transection is selected. The colon should be tension-free while in the pelvis. The selected level is marked with laparoscopic suture or several endoscopic clips for future identification. The midline/suprapubic port is extended >5 cm or a lower left quadrant incision for specimen extraction is created. An Alexis® wound protector (Applied Medical, CA) is helpful in flattening the abdominal wall and provides full circumferential retraction of the wound edges. After specimen extraction, a purse string is closed around the anvil of circular stapler in the proximal

colon similarly to the open fashion and returned to the abdominal cavity. Pneumoperitoneum is reestablished by twisting the upper ring of Alexis® wound retractor around its axis or mounting a surgical glove onto it.

■ **Totally laparoscopic approach.** Laparoscopic transection of proximal colon can be done with an endoscopic stapler (Endo GIA™, Covidien Autosuture, Mansfield, MA). Additional rectal irrigation with Betadine® Solution (Purdue Products L.P., Stamford, CT) is done. The rectum is clamped below the tumor with a laparoscopic grasper. In cases of a transrectal specimen extraction, the rectum is transected with laparoscopic shears. If a vaginal route of extraction is selected, rectum is stapled with laparoscopic articulating stapler (Endo GIA™ Roticulator™, Covidien Autosuture, Mansfield, MA). A plastic bag for specimen extraction is introduced through the open lumen of the rectum or the newly created incision of the posterior wall of vagina. The specimen is placed in the bag and brought out. Care must be taken to ensure gentle force application. The anvil head with its white plastic spike is introduced into the abdominal cavity through the same route. A diathermy colotomy of the proximal colon is performed 2 cm proximal to the transected staple line. The anvil head is introduced and milked up into the proximal colon. If the surgeon is proficient in laparoscopic suturing, the colotomy can be oversewn and the rectal stump pursestringed around the stapler central spike. Otherwise, the colotomy site is stapled off with one firing of endoscopic articulating stapler and rectal stump is closed with another one. In order to prepare a straight colorectal anastomosis, the spike of the anvil head should penetrate the colon in the center of the staple line. If a Baker type of colorectal anastomosis is selected, an site on the antimesenteric side of the colon 2–4 cm proximal to the staple line should be penetrated with diathermy assistance.

Colon and rectal transection in any of these approaches is usually performed with staplers with 3.5 mm staple height loads (blue cartridges), and more than one firing of the stapler may be needed to get across the rectum. In all cases, a perpendicular transection of the mesorectum to the rectal tube axis is required to provide adequate oncologic margins, and coning of the distal fascial fat envelope specimen must be avoided. There are obvious obstacles in endoscopic stapler angulation, especially in a narrow and deep male pelvis. Providing adequate angulation for straight rectum transection can be challenging. Most of the current reticulating endoscopic staplers are limited to 45 degrees of motion, which is not always sufficient. The articulating endoscopic linear cutter I-60 from Power Medical Interventions (Langhorne, PA) is the only 12 mm laparoscopic articulating linear stapler with a 90-degree range of angulation. Both laparoscopic approaches and open rectal transections benefit from additional help by the assistant. The assistant's fisted hand can push on the perineum to lift the pelvic floor and therefore the distal rectum, thus facilitating the placement of a straight stapler line.

It is up to the surgeon whether to form a neorectal reservoir, a coloplasty, or a straight anastomosis from the proximal colon. The relative functional inferiority of a straight anastomosis to a colonic pouch is negated after the first year after surgery. In cases of colon redundancy, the formation of a 5 cm colonic J-pouch with an end-to-side anastomosis is preferable. In a narrow male pelvis, forming a coloplasty pouch by repairing a longitudinal 10 cm incision of an antimesenteric colotomy in a transverse manner is a reasonable option.

After completion of the rectal dissection, specimen extraction, and anvil placement, a proximal colon is prepared for the anastomosis on the distal 1.5–2 cm by clearing the mesentery and the appendices epiploicae off the anvil. A circular stapler is introduced into the rectum, gently dilating the sphincter muscles. The surgeon and assistant need to coordinate the movement of the stapler relative to the pelvic anatomy with instructions from both sides of the perineum ("Angulate the stapler to the patient's right," "Lift the stapler's end up," etc.). The spike of the stapler is slowly advanced through the desired site of the rectal stump, generally near the center of the staple line. In laparoscopic approaches, the anvil grasper is helpful in steady stapler assembly in combination with an atraumatic grasper for the creation of a properly oriented colorectal anastomosis. The stapler is slowly closed under direct vision. Digital examination of vagina in females is recommended to ensure noninvolvement of the posterior wall in the stapler line. If the posterior vagina is involved, the stapler is opened, the anvil might be detached and additional rectal mobilization is performed. Visualization of the cut edge of colon mesentery and tinea is done in order to prevent anastomotic rotation. If the stapler ring is free and no colon rotation is found, the stapler is fired. The stapler is gently withdrawn out of the rectum with rotational movements and the distal and proximal "donuts" inspected for completeness, and sent to pathology.

The pelvis is filled with saline and a repeat intraoperative sigmoidoscopy/proctoscopy is recommended, both for inspection and for insufflation of the anastomosis. Gentle clamping of a proximal to the anastomosis colon is performed and an "air leak test" for anastomotic leak and staple line competency.

The abdomen and pelvis are then irrigated and suctioned out. Hemostasis is ascertained and the bowel is inspected for injuries. Routine pelvic drainage is not required and is done according to surgeon preference. A drain can be placed through the lower quadrant port or new stub wound.

The creation of a diverting ostomy is also done according to surgeon preference. In our institution, all patients who have undergone nCRT receive a diverting ileostomy. If the procedure was finished in an extracorporeal fashion, a loop of small bowel 50–60 cm proximal to the ileocecal valve that easily reaches the abdominal wall at the previously selected stoma site marking is selected. Bowel orientation is color marked with a distally placed 3-0 chromic catgut (brown) and proximal 3-0 polydioxane (blue) loose ties. A circular skin incision is made in the previously marked stoma site. The subcutaneous fat is separated, the fascia is divided with diathermy, and the muscles are gently spread along the fibers. Thus, peritoneum is then identified and divided, and the loop of bowel is extracted through the wound.

The procedure is laparoscopically performed; a loop of small bowel is selected in about 50–60 cm proximal to the ileocecal valve and secured below the stoma site with a locking bowel grasper. The stoma site incision is made in a similar way to the open technique and the loop of bowel is grasped from outside with a Babcock clamp and extracted. It is important to visually confirm that the small-bowel mesentery is properly orientated to prevent possible 180 or 360 degrees rotations.

A loop ileostomy is created routinely for diversion of low anastomosis.

- A loop of bowel oriented with the efferent (distal) limb placed inferior to the afferent (proximal) limb
- A window is created in the mesentery at the apex of the loop of bowel and a small Kelly clamp is passed through
- Stoma rod is grasped with the clamp and passed through the mesenteric defect
- 2-0 silk stitches are placed to fix the stoma rod on both sides in opposite directions to prevent rotation and slippage of the rod

The fascia of the wound extraction site and port sites are closed with PDS or Vicryl, and the skin is closed using absorbable subcuticular intradermal sutures (4-0 Monocryl™, Ethicon Inc., Somerville, NJ). A Berci fascial closure device (Karl Storz GmbH & Co, KG, Tuttlingen, Germany) can be used to close the fascia of the port sites.

After the wounds are covered with sterile towels and ostomy is maturation is finalized:

- A transverse enterotomy is made with electrocautery on the efferent side of the limb.
- The bowel wall of the afferent limb is everted and Brooked into place with Vicryl or chromic sutures.
- The mucosa of the efferent limb if approximated to the skin without eversion.

This technique provides an ostomy with low risk of skin damage and comfort ostomy appliance use.

It is important to understand that keeping a laparoscopic approach should not be a goal of surgery, and that if no progress occurs after 45–70 minutes at each step of the surgery, one has to consider a conversion to an open approach. Patient safety should

Part III: Low Anterior Resection

be the priority of the surgical team. Conversion should be proactive (before a complication occur), rather than retroactive (to a problem after it occurs).

 # POSTOPERATIVE MANAGEMENT

Patients undergoing laparoscopic stapled LAR should be enrolled in a fast track recovery protocol (enhanced recovery protocol). It starts at the preoperative level during the initial office visit and includes 12–17 steps throughout the whole perioperative period. The usual elements include:

- Preoperative care
  - Preoperative counseling
  - Preoperative feeding
  - Administration of synbiotics
  - No bowel preparation
  - No premedication
  - Fluid restriction
- Perioperative measures
  - Perioperative high O_2 concentrations
  - Active prevention of hypothermia
  - Epidural analgesia
  - Minimally invasive surgery/transverse incisions
- Postoperative
  - Avoidance of NG tubes
  - Avoidance of drains
  - Enforced postoperative mobilization
  - Enforced early postoperative oral feeding
  - Avoidance of systemic opioids
  - Standard laxatives
  - Early removal of urinary catheter

This protocol is geared toward the physiologic recovery of the patient after surgical procedures with a minimization of postoperative ileus and pain levels, as well as a reduction of cardiopulmonary, thromboembolic, infectious, and cerebral/cognitive complications.

We utilize the Cleveland Clinic Florida Enhanced Recovery Protocol in every patient after abdominal surgery (Table 14.1). It includes preoperative steps emphasizing the educational role of the surgeon and dedicated preoperative colorectal nurse, intraoperative measures and modified postoperative management. After a laparoscopic stapled LAR surgery is finished, the nasogastric tube is removed in the OR. The patient is awakened by the anesthesiologist and transferred to the postoperative recovery area. When the patient is alert and fully awake, he or she is transferred to a regular floor ward. Diet started with clear liquids and ice chips, and the medication list should include antiemetic drugs (ondansetron 4 mg intravenously every 6 hours), pain medication (patient controlled analgesia with morphine 1.5 mg every 10 minutes, no basal rate, lockout at 10 mg/hour or hydromorphone 0.1 mg every 6 minutes lockout at 1 mg/hour and ketorolac first dose 30 mg IV with then 15 mg every 6 × 48 hours for pain). Antibiotic prophylaxis is continued for 24 hours after surgery, duodenal and gastric ulcer prophylaxis is started with pantoprazole 40 mg IV daily or famotidine 20 mg IV BID change to oral medication when tolerating full liquid diet. DVT prophylaxis is continued with 5,000 U subcutaneous heparin injections every 8 hours and use of pneumatic pressure stockings when patient is in a bed rest. Vitals, status, inputs and outputs are checked and calculated every 4 hours; next morning blood tests (CBC and CMP) are ordered.

The nurse is informed to notify doctor if one of the following occurs:

- Body temperature >38.6°C (101.5°F)
- Systolic blood pressure >160 or <90 mm Hg

TABLE 14.1	Enhanced Recovery Protocol at Cleveland Clinic Florida		
	Perioperative day	**Activity**	**Comments**
Preoperative	Initial office visit	Discuss aspects of surgery, potential risks, complications, and alternatives. Defining the range of required preoperative tests (internal medicine or cardiology clearance, blood work, etc.) Handouts given to patients defining expectations of early ambulation, return of bowel function, projected discharge criteria Handouts listing medications to avoid prior to surgery for prophylaxis of intra- or postoperative bleeding	Performed by surgeon and preoperative colorectal nurse/physician assistant Performed by surgeon and preoperative colorectal nurse/physician assistant Performed by surgeon
Perioperative	0	If a stoma is considered a possibility, education by dedicated stoma nurses regarding care and management; also preoperative marking Subcutaneous heparin and pneumatic stockings Active prevention of hypothermia May receive spinal anesthesia Oro/nasogastric tube removed at extubation	
Postoperative	1	Clear liquid diet, ice chips Enforced early postoperative mobilization Incentive spirometry exercises Subcutaneous heparin, pneumatic pressure stockings	5 laps in the hallway (~100 m) 5,000 units subcutaneous every 8 hr during hospital stay Prevention of respiratory problems
	2	Awaiting flatus or bowel movement Removal of dressing Removal of bladder catheter	
	3	If flatus or BM present advance diet to full liquid Heplock IV fluids Discontinue patient controlled analgesia pump Oral pain medication If ostomy present—ostomy nurse education visit	
	4	Advance diet to low res diet unless distended Anticipate discharge home	

- Pulse >110, sustained, or <50 beats/minute
- Respirations greater than 24/minute or respiratory distress, or O_2 saturation <90%
- Change in mental status
- Urine output less than 30 ml/hour or greater than 240 ml/hour

On the morning after surgery, the patient is seen by the surgical team and his or her status is evaluated. If no negative progress is found, patient is ambulated and its importance in prophylaxis of postoperative complications is explained again. The use of incentive spirometry exercises plays a significant role in pneumonia prophylaxis. The patient is continued on clear liquids and ice chips diet until flatus or bowel movement are present. The urinary catheter and dressings are discharged on the second postoperative day. Intravenous volume can be decreased to 75–100 ml/hour. At any day when patient has a bowel movement of flatus diet should be advanced to low residue diet, intravenous hydration should be stopped with a heplock, oral pain medication administered. When patient is tolerating full liquid diet IV pain medication is switched to oxycodone 5 mg/325 mg acetaminophen, 1–2 tabs PO q 4 hours for pain. It is most important to explain to the nurse and to write an order that pain medication should be given one tablet for visual pain score of 5 or less, two tablets for pain score above 5 with total dose of acetaminophen from all sources should be less than 4 g in 24 hours from all sources.

Usually, patients in our institutions are ready for discharge at postoperative day 4–5. In some cases absence of bowel function progress at each step or the development of nausea and/or vomiting leads to the cessation of enteral feeding by a NPO diet, adequate IV hydration, correction of electrolyte imbalances, and nasogastric tube placement if needed. In case of NPO is maintained for more than 8 days, a total parenteral nutrition should considered.

COMPLICATIONS

Complications can be classified as intraoperative and early and late postoperative. Intraoperative complications include the following:

- Bleeding at any point of surgery when vessels are ligated or coagulated
  - Use of diathermy
  - Stable grasping of proximal vessel trunk when coagulated or stapled
    - If bleeding occurs, clamping the proximal vessel stump will decrease/stop bleeding and provide time for linear restapling, or applying laparoscopic clips, or use of an energy sources
- Ureteric trauma while dissecting in pelvis and mesentery mobilization
  - Visualization of the ureter at any step of surgery with cutting, diathermy use
    - Ureteral trauma The type of repair, is dependent on the laparoscopic expertise of the urologist
  - Vaginal trauma during low rectal dissection
- Vaginal assistance and retraction toward abdominal wall
  - If vaginal wall damage is diagnosed—primary laparoscopic or transperineal repair or perhaps by the gynecology is dependent on laparoscopic expertise of urologist
- Duodenal and small-bowel trauma while grasping, relocating and using diathermy
  - Gentle tissue handling with atraumatic bowel graspers
    - If a seromyotomy is diagnosed—primary intracorporeal repair with laparoscopic sutures is possible
  - Careful energy application with centered field laparoscopic view of the tips of the instrument
    - If a thermal bowel injury is seen—primary intracorporeal repair with laparoscopic sutures is undertaken

Early postoperative complications are as follow:

- Bleeding
  - Initial relaparoscopy; if it fails to identify the source, then a laparotomy should be performed

Late postoperative complications include the following:

- Anastomotic leak and pelvic sepsis
  - NPO and interventional radiology consult for drainage
  - Consider diverting ileostomy if not already diverted before
- Hypogastric nerve damage with bladder dysfunction, sexual dysfunction
  - Sharp and precise pelvic dissection, good sense in use of energy sources

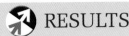 RESULTS

This procedure is a minimally invasive method of sphincter-preserving surgery. Laparoscopic-stapled low anterior resection has similar short-term functional and oncological results when compared to laparotomy.

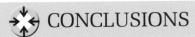 CONCLUSIONS

Laparoscopic-stapled low anterior resection is a valuable tool in the colorectal surgeons' armamentarium. It provides magnified visualization in a lower pelvis with precise rectal mobilization and nerve sparing. The procedure is associated 10–20% conversion rate, which is related to surgical team expertise and patient selection.

15 Laparoscopic Low Anterior Resection with Transanal Anastomosis or Colonic J Pouch Creation

Sharon L. Stein and Conor P. Delaney

INDICATIONS/CONTRAINDICATIONS

Laparoscopic low anterior resection with transanal anastomosis is performed primarily for oncologic indications. Patients with tumors invading beyond the muscularis mucosa or lymph node involvement should undergo enbloc resection of the rectum and mesorectum. Oncologic resections mandate negative margins: ideally 2 cm of uninvolved distal tissue in the rectum and anus although 1 cm may be acceptable in tumors with favorable pathology to preserve sphincter function. When patients present with low rectal cancers, it may be impossible to achieve appropriate margins while using a double-stapled technique. Some low lying early rectal cancers, circumferential lesions, or tumors with unfavorable pathologic findings may be inappropriate for local excision and a transanal approach should be considered. Transanal or coloanal hand-sewn anastomosis allows for removal of mucosa or internal sphincter providing greater distal margins, while preserving bowel continuity.

Occasionally, during surgical operations for benign disease, technical problems such as stapling misfiring, ischemia, or benign pathology such as low rectovaginal fistula, may call for a coloanal technique. Ability to perform a hand-sewn transanal anastomosis will allow the surgeon to reestablish bowel continuity when the patient might otherwise require a permanent colostomy.

Transanal techniques, while preserving intestinal continuity, have a greater incidence of frequent bowel movements and mild-to-moderate incontinence. Patients with poor preoperative candidates are poor candidates for this technique and should undergo creation of permanent colostomy. Patients with tumors invading the sphincters or into the lateral pelvic sidewalls should undergo abdominal perineal resection or pelvic exenteration and should not be considered for transanal anastomosis.

Laparoscopic surgery may be safely performed in experienced hands in a wide variety of patients. While laparoscopic surgery and small incisions are convenient in thin fit patients, morbidly obese patients and elderly patients are also candidates for laparoscopic proctectomy and may benefit from decreased incision lengths, earlier mobility, and decreased respiratory compromise. With appropriate retraction and preservation of appropriate oncologic margins, laparoscopic surgery can be performed on most operative candidates. Several preliminary studies on laparoscopic proctectomy have demonstrated functional and oncologic results equivalent to open surgery and a randomized trial is underway to assess the outcomes of laparoscopic proctectomy for cancer. Patients with extensive adhesions and scarring from past surgery may not be good candidates for laparoscopic surgery. In addition, laparoscopic proctectomy is an advanced laparoscopic procedure and should not be performed for oncologic indications by inexperienced laparoscopic surgeons.

PREOPERATIVE PLANNING

Prior to surgery, all patients should undergo appropriate preoperative staging for the rectal neoplasia. Local, nodal, and metastatic evaluation of the tumor should be performed. Prior to surgery, a tumor biopsy and pathologic diagnosis should be established. A rigid proctoscopy and digital exam should be performed by the operating surgeon to evaluate tumor location, fixation, and appropriate surgical approach.

In addition, depth of invasion and nodal status should be established using either endorectal ultrasound or magnetic resonance imaging. Choice of exam should be based on local expertise and tumor staging. For T1 and T2 tumors, endorectal ultrasound is more accurate for staging, while in more advance T staging MRI has been shown to be more sensitive.

Advanced tumors should be evaluated for neoadjuvant therapy prior to surgical resection. T2 tumor with unfavorable histology, any T3 or T4 tumor, and any tumor with nodal involvement are candidates for preoperative chemoradiation. Assessment of appropriate oncologic margins should be performed preoperatively, as posttreatment regression of tumor does not necessarily equate with resolution of microscopic disease.

Metastatic evaluation includes computed tomography of the abdomen and pelvis and baseline CEA level, which may be useful for postoperative monitoring. In addition, there is an 8–10% rate of synchronous polyps or neoplasia and patients without obstructing lesions should have preoperative assessment of the entire colon and rectum.

All patients should have a preoperative evaluation of baseline continence. Personal history of fecal incontinence including nighttime soilage, incontinence to liquid, solid or flatulence should be addressed. Physical exam should include digital evaluation of sphincter tone and strength of contraction. Although anal manometry may be performed, digital rectal exam has been shown to be a better predictor of postoperative continence.

Patients should be consented for temporary ileostomy and should be aware of the possibility of a permanent colostomy. Temporary ileostomy is used in very low rectal anastomosis to protect the anastomosis during immediate postoperative period secondary anastomotic leak rates of up to 17%. Permanent colostomy may be necessary if the tumor is found to invade the sphincter muscles intraoperatively. Patients should have the opportunity to meet with an enterostomal therapist for preoperative counseling and should be marked for left- and right-sided stomas prior to surgical positioning.

Appropriate preoperative evaluation of medical comorbidities should be performed as indicated by patient history. All patients receive preoperative laboratory assessment including standard metabolic, coagulation, and blood count studies. Patients should also have type and cross match of blood for possible transfusion.

Preoperative bowel preparation is controversial. Although data demonstrate that bowel cleansing may not be necessary in all colon surgery, bowel preparation avoids leaving a column of stool in the diverted colon. In addition, bowel cleansing provides the ability to perform colonoscopy intraoperatively if not completed preoperatively. The authors routinely perform preoperative bowel preparation.

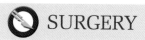 SURGERY

Essential equipments for successful laparoscopic low anterior resection include 5 or 10 mm 30-degree camera for adequate visualization especially vital in the pelvis for deep dissection, nontraumatic laparoscopic bowel graspers, laparoscopic scissors with electrocautery capability, and an energy device or staplers for vessel transection. A Lonestar retractor and lighted Hill Ferguson anal retractors facilitate perineal dissection.

Prophylaxis

Prior to incision, antibiotics with appropriate anaerobic and aerobic coverage should be given and redosed every 4 hours throughout the operation. Subcutaneous low-dose molecular heparin is given prior to induction. Sequential compression devices are used for all patients intraoperatively. Skin preparation of perineum and perianal region is performed per standard protocol.

Positioning

The authors position patients in modified lithotomy position in yellow-fin or padded stirrups. Care should be made to ensure that the lower leg is well protected to prevent injury to the perineal nerve. An electric operating table is lined with either a gel pad or bean bag to reduce the risk of pressure injury and facilitate varied positioning throughout the operation. An orogastric tube, placed after induction of anesthesia, allows for decompression of the stomach intraoperatively and is removed prior to extubation.

Steps in Laparoscopic Low Anterior Resection with Coloanal Anastomosis

1. Abdominal exploration
2. High ligation of inferior mesenteric artery and vein
3. Splenic flexure takedown and left colon mobilization
4. Protectomy with total mesorectal dissection
5. Perineal dissection
6. Removal of specimen
7. Creation of a neorectum
8. Anastomosis
9. Creation of diverting ileostomy

Abdominal Exploration

The abdomen is entered using an open technique and Hasson port. Additional ports are placed under laparoscopic guidance. Our typical port placement is shown in Figure 15.1.

Initial evaluation occurs to determine laparoscopic feasibility of the operation. If significant adhesions from prior surgery exist, the decision is made to convert to open surgery. The abdomen is evaluated for metastatic disease. The peritoneum is inspected for signs of tumor implantation. Attention is drawn to the liver, which may be elevated to examine the inferior aspect. The ovaries are inspected in female patients, as there is a 3–8% incidence of ovarian metastasis in colorectal cancer patients. The pelvis is assessed to evaluate for lateral extension of the tumor. In the case of large bulky tumor, it may be difficult to assess invasion of sphincter muscles preoperatively, and decision to convert to abdominal perineal resection may occur intraoperatively.

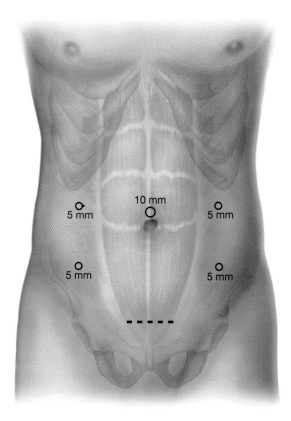

Figure 15.1 Placement of laparoscopic ports. Typically, the abdomen is opened through a supraumbilical port, which will allow for placement of a 10-mm camera. Five-millimeter ports are placed in the right upper and lower quadrant. The right lower quadrant port should be placed at the premarked ileostomy site. On the left side, an upper and lower quadrant 5-mm ports are placed. The left lower quadrant port site or a pfannenstiel incision will be used for specimen retraction sites. Port site placement may be modified for body habitus.

High Ligation of Inferior Mesenteric Artery and Vein (Fig. 15.2)

The patient is placed in Trendelenburg, left side up to isolate the left colon from the small bowel. The superior hemorrhoidal vessels are elevated at the sacral promontory and dissected in the open space caudal to the vessels. Branches of the hypogastric nerves lying between the aorta and the inferior mesenteric artery are preserved and

Figure 15.2 Dissection of the inferior mesenteric artery. At the level of the sacral promontory, the inferior mesenteric artery is tented anteriorly toward the abdominal wall, allowing for dissection parallel and deep to the artery. Note the left colic artery is preserved. Nerve fibers from the sympathetic plexus lay below the artery, and are swept down and preserved. Prior to transection, identification of the left ureter is vital to ensure it is not inadvertently transected with the vascular bundle.

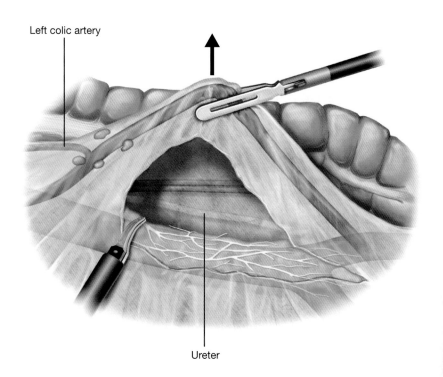

Left colic artery

Ureter

swept caudally toward the aorta. The left colic artery is conserved to maintain blood flow to the left colon. The left ureter must be definitively identified and preserved prior to transection of the inferior mesenteric artery. The artery is transected using a stapler, clips, or an energy device. A stapler is placed through the colon extraction site, most commonly the left lower quadrant incision. If an energy device is used, three firings (two proximal and one distal) are used prior to transection. The inferior mesenteric vein is located proximal to the pancreas and ligated. High ligation of the inferior mesenteric artery and vein are essential for adequate colonic length. In situations where the left colon does not reach the anus comfortably, the left colic artery may be sacrificed, but care must be taken to ensure that this does not compromise anastomotic blood supply.

Splenic Flexure Takedown and Left Colon Mobilization (Figs. 15.3 and 15.4)

Dissection proceeds in a medial-to-lateral direction, under the transected inferior mesenteric artery. The retroperitoneum can be maintained intact and swept caudally, preserving the left ureter, gonadal vessels, and psoas muscle. This dissection continues inferiorly to the pelvic brim and superiorly to the inferior border of the pancreas. Posterior and lateral attachments should be completely dissected; any posterior adhesions may compromise reach of the left colon into the pelvis.

The dissection to the splenic may begin from the iliac fossa and proceed superiorly to the splenic flexure, or from the mid-transverse colon laterally. In a superior approach, reverse Trendelenburg will help isolate the transverse colon. The plane between the omentum and colonic mesenteric is identified by triangulation of the colon and the mesentery. An avascular plane exists that allows for sharp dissection. The omentum is typically fused medially and is easiest to enter toward the midline and is confirmed by visualization of the posterior wall of the stomach. While approaching the spleen, care should be taken to avoid excessive tension that may cause capsular tearing resulting in bleeding.

The lateral dissection should stay just inside the line of Toldt, which represents the retroperitoneum. In the iliac fossa, reidentification of the ureter is vital, as this is a

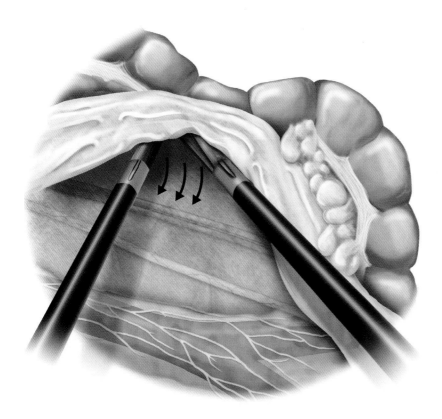

Figure 15.3 Assistant is located between the patient's legs to enable him/her to work with the camera. The medial-to-lateral dissection is facilitated by reverse Trendelenburg with left side elevated. Retractors are placed under the mesentery to keep tension on the line of Toldt and retroperitoneum. Open bowel graspers elevate the mesentery in anterior direction allowing for a wider line of traction during the dissection. The surgeon can then dissect above the retroperitoneum to the lateral sidewall, superiorly to the splenic flexure and inferiorly toward the iliac fossa. Care must be taken to ensure that the ureter and retroperitoneal structures remain with the retroperitoneum, and the plane of dissection does not veer under the distal edge of the pancreas.

Part III: Low Anterior Resection

Figure 15.4 Mobilization of the splenic flexure. An avascular plane is present between the omentum and the epiploicae of the colon. Entry is facilitated in the midline, where the omental planes are fused and proceed toward the splenic flexure.

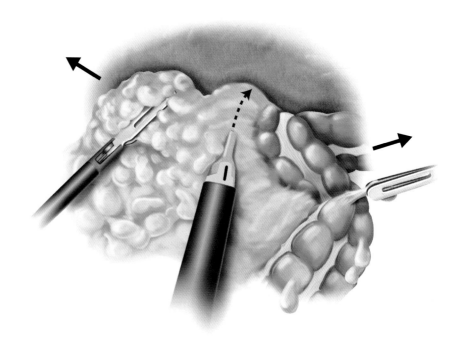

common location for ureteric injury. Often the sigmoid colon is tethered to the lateral wall in this location, hindering the view of the ureter. Superiorly, the avascular dissection plane may come close to the colon laterally, and care must be taken to ensure that there is no injury to the colon. If dissecting too far from the colon, it is easy to enter the retroperitoneal plane, resulting in increased bleeding and potential damage to retroperitoneal structures.

Protectomy with Total Mesorectal Dissection (Fig. 15.5)

The mesorectal plane is entered by elevating the rectosigmoid junction in a superior and anterior direction. The right gutter can be entered through the avascular plane at the base of the mesentry. The mesorectal dissection should be performed sharply to prevent injury to the hypogastric and parasympathetic nerves. The hypogastric nerves are visualized and preserved at the sacral promontory, coursing laterally into the pelvis. Dissection is performed posteriorly, then laterally. Posterior dissection continues through the avascular plane outside the fascia propria to Waldeyer's fascia and then to the levator muscles. The lateral stalks are a site of potential injury to the nerves of the pelvic plexus. Staying just lateral to the fascia propria helps to protect vital structures.

Obese patients may present a challenge in dissection. A fan retractor can be used to increase counter tension to allow for dissection. In a male with a thin pelvis, upward traction may be critical to allow for adequate lateral access for dissection. If using an energy device, a suction/irrigator can be used intermittently to evacuate smoke and allow for better visualization.

After posterior dissection is complete, the anterior dissection is performed (Fig. 15.6). Pulling the rectum superiorly and caudally will place tension on the anterior planes. A second retractor can be used to place tension on the anterior pelvic structures. Care must be taken to avoid injury to the seminal vesicles laterally. A very thin avascular plane exists, and must be carefully dissected using sharp dissection. Both the seminal vesicles and vagina will bleed if the dissection is not precise. If the patient has had a prior hysterectomy, the vagina can be fused to the anterior rectum. In addition, a large uterus can obstruct visualization and the ability to appropriately retract the rectum.

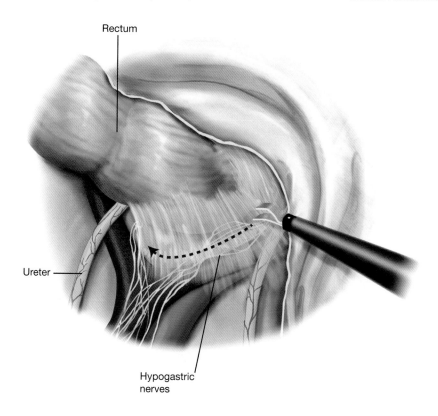

Rectum

Ureter

Hypogastric
nerves

Figure 15.5 Entering the appropriate plane for mesorectal dissection is critical to oncologic resection. By elevating the rectosigmoid junction anteriorly and superiorly, a plane may be visualized on the right side of the mesorectum. Sharp dissection should be performed in this avascular plane.

A Keith needle can be used to fix the uterus to the anterior abdominal wall to alleviate this situation.

Depending on the location of the tumor, wider margins may be required. As the dissection proceeds into the lower pelvis, a finger may be placed into the rectum to create counter traction and assess appropriate dissection planes. A uterine sound may also be placed into the vagina to prevent injury and create tension to elucidate dissection planes.

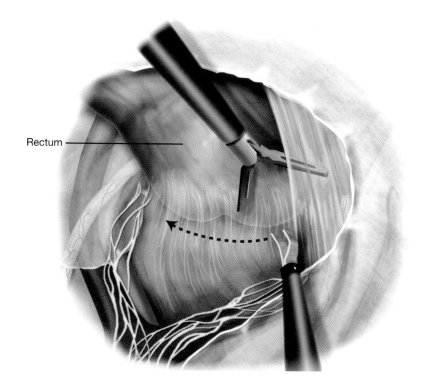

Rectum

Figure 15.6 Lateral stalks. Continued tension on the rectum by lifting the rectum anteriorly and superiorly allows for visualization of the mesorectal plane. At the lateral stalks, neurovascular bundles travel close to the dissection plane. Unless there is tumor infiltration preservation of the lateral stalks should be performed by staying close to the fascia propria of the rectum.

Part III: Low Anterior Resection

Figure 15.7 Anterior view of laparoscopic dissection. An open retractor pulls the anterior structures away from the dissection plane to allow for visualization of the appropriate plane. Care must be taken to preserve the seminal vesicles lateral to the prostate while dissecting Denonvillier's fascia.

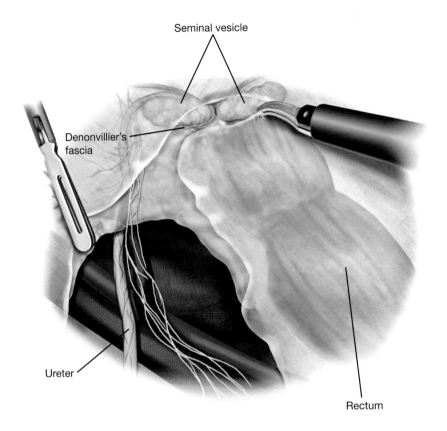

Seminal vesicle

Denonvillier's fascia

Ureter

Rectum

Perineal Dissection (Fig. 15.7)

The patient's legs are lifted and spread in lithotomy stirrups to allow the operating surgeon and assistant to access the perineum. A separate set of operative instruments should be used to prevent contamination from the perineum to the abdomen. Lonestar retractor is placed to expose the anus.

Dissection begins with a circular incision at the dentate line. This is typically performed using electric cautery to minimize bleeding. Operating in the posterior plane initially may decrease run off from the superior/lateral aspect and maximize visualization. The incision is carried down into the intersphincteric plane for a transphincteric resection or through the submucosal for mucosectomy. A solution of dilute (1/200,000) epinephrine may help to elucidate the operative plane and minimize bleeding. This can be injected into the submucosal. The external sphincter is preserved to maintain continence. The external sphincter may be distinguished from the internal sphincter by twitching of skeletal muscle fibers in response to electrocautery.

After dissection of the anal ring, superior to the puborectalis, the dissection plane widens to incorporate the full thickness of the rectal wall and enters the pelvis to connect with the abdominal dissection. The plane is entered posteriorly most safely initially and then continued laterally. Anteriorly, care must be taken to avoid entry into the vagina in females, the prostate and urethra in males. A finger placed transvaginally can help elucidate the appropriate plane. Excessive vascularity is usually associated with dissection within the vaginal or prostate wall and the appropriate avascular plane should be reestablished.

Removal of Specimen

Extraction of the colon and rectum may be done through a left lower quadrant incision, pfannenstiel incision, or transanally. A 4-cm left lower quadrant incision can be made at an existing port site and is adequate for most specimens with minimal morbidity from the incision site. A transverse or oblique incision is used; small right-angle retractors can be useful in visualization of the anterior fascia. In a thin patient, the muscles may be spared as in an open appendectomy; heavier patients and larger specimens may require transection of rectus sheath muscles.

Alternatively, a small pfannenstiel incision can be made 2 cm above the pubis symphysis. The incision is carried out to the anterior fascia, which is angled slightly superiorly. The rectus sheath is separated from the anterior sheath using upward retraction from Allis clamps. Small penetrating vessels may be cauterized with a Debakey forceps prior to retraction into the muscle. The anterior fascia is mobilized superiorly to just below the umbilicus, and inferiorly to the pubis. The abdomen is then entered through the linea alba by separating the two rectus sheath muscles.

Maintaining pneumoperitoneum while entering the abdomen can help to isolate the anterior abdominal wall from viscera and prevents inadvertent injury. A wound protector is mandatory to prevent fecal and tumor contamination of the extraction site. The specimen is exteriorized with laparoscopic guidance.

The proximal resection margin is selected on the left colon after evaluation of appropriate oncologic margins and evaluation of adequate blood supply. The sigmoid colon is not typically used secondary to potential ischemia after high ligation of the inferior mesenteric artery. Adequate blood supply can usually be verified by sharp transection of the colon and visualization of pulsatile blood flow. Transection of the colon is performed using a noncrushing bowel clamp or GIA stapler.

The specimen may also be resected through the anal canal except in the case of a large bulky tumor, which could cause damage to the sphincter muscles and should be removed transabdominally. Prior to resecting the specimen, adequate length to control the distal colon should be drawn through the anus. Stay sutures should be placed on the colon prior to transection, as the colon will otherwise have a tendency to retract into the pelvis, creating difficulty with fashioning of the anastomosis and rectal reservoir.

Creation of a Neorectum

Creation of a colonic reservoir has been shown to improve defecatory function in the first 6 months of function postoperatively by decreasing frequency of bowel movements. Colonic J pouch, coloplasty, end-to-side anastomosis each provide advantages over straight anastomosis and the authors prefer to perform a colonic J pouch if reach is adequate; a coloplasty may be performed in patients without additional reach. End-to-side anastomosis provides some of the benefits of J pouch. In males with narrow pelvis, a straight coloanal may be necessary.

A colonic J pouch is created extracorporeally with the distal 6 cm of sigmoid or descending colon folded upon itself (Fig. 15.8). A crotch stitch is placed to approximate the antimesenteric borders of the colon and to prevent twisting during manipulation. Pouches lengths greater than 6 cm have been correlated with increased difficulty with evacuation postoperatively. A 60-mm GIA stapler is inserted into enterotomies created at the proximal and distal folds of the colon. Care should be taken to staple along the antimesenteric border of the J pouch to avoid bleeding from the staple line and preserve blood supply. The efferent end of the colon is either oversewn or stapled, per surgeon preference.

Coloplasty is constructed with a longitudinal incision approximately 4–6 cm from the distal resection margin, along the antimesenteric border. The incision is extended 8–10 cm proximally (Fig. 15.9). The longitudinal incision is closed transversely to enlarge the colonic reservoir in a manner similar to a Heineke-Mikulicz pyloroplasty. Single layer of 3-0 vicryl sutures is typically used.

If the side of the colon reaches more distally into the pelvis, a side-to-end anastomosis can be created. The end of the colon is stapled or oversewn. The anastomosis will be constructed on the antimesentery border of the colon, approximately 3 cm proximal to the staple line. Blood supply may be superior at the antimesenteric border when compared to the end of the colon.

Anastomosis

After extracorporeal abdominal preparation of the proximal anastomosis and colonic reservoir, the colon is returned to the abdomen. If a wound protector is used, this incision

Figure 15.8 Perineal dissection: Dissection plane is begun at the dentate line using a lighted Hill-Ferguson retractor and carried proximally in a posterior, lateral, and then anterior manner. Mucosectomy may be facilitated with infiltration of dilute epinephrine to isolate the submucosal. Intersphincteric plane is used to achieve appropriate oncologic margins in appropriate patients. Entry into the pelvis occurs above the puborectalis.

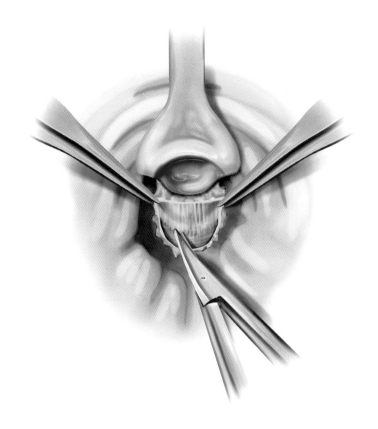

Figure 15.9 Colonic J pouch: Colonic J pouch is created on the antimesenteric side of the colon with a single firing of a GIA 60-mm stapler. Pouch length should be limited to 60 mm to prevent difficulty with pouch emptying.

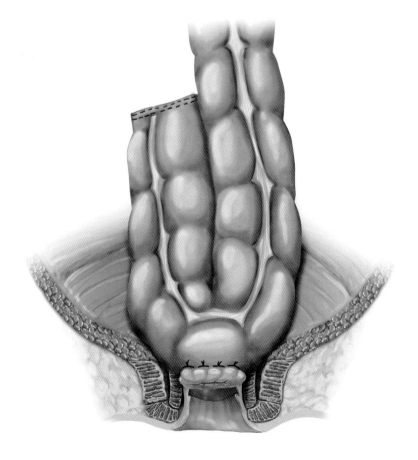

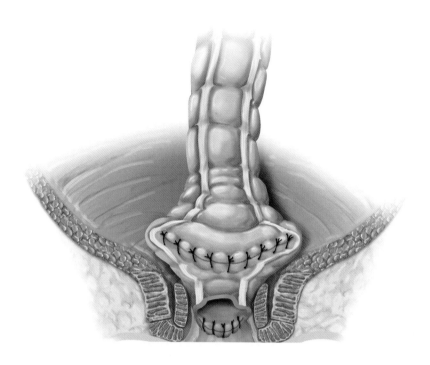

Figure 15.10 Coloplasty: A longitudinal colotomy approximately 8–10 in length starting 4–6 cm from the distal colon resection margin is closed with a single layer of polyglycolic acid sutures in an interrupted fashion.

should be occluded to reestablish pneumoperitoneum. When using a firm wound protector (Alexis Wound Retractor System, Applied Medical, Rancho Santo Margarita, CA), the incision can be closed by twisting the wound protector on itself and placing a large Kelly clamp to occlude the hole. A moist sponge may be wrapped around the protector to prevent leakage of gas.

Upon returning to the abdomen, the operative field is checked for hemostasis, mesenteric alignment, and small bowel crossing deep the colon prior to construction of anastomosis. Fixation of the colon can obscure the view of the left side of the abdomen. The colon is checked for appropriate reach into the pelvis. The colon is guided into the pelvis and operator at the pelvis may assist with guidance by placing a ring forceps or Babcock into the abdomen and guiding the colon gently to the anus.

Sutures are placed to secure the colon to the anus prior to creation of a colotomy. This ensures the colon does not retract and no soilage will occur in the pelvis. A colotomy is made in the apex of the J pouch or distal staple line and 2-0 vicryl are used to secure the colon to the dentate line, with sutures incorporating the sphincter muscles for more secure placement. Generally 6–8 sutures are necessary to ensure appropriate approximation of the colon to the dentate line.

Diverting Ileostomy

For anastomosis below 5 cm from the anal verge, the authors typically place a diverting ileostomy to minimize complications of anastomotic leak that may occur. The ileum is run laparoscopically proximally from the ileocecal valve and reach is checked to the anterior abdominal wall. Ideally, the ileostomy is created between 10 and 20 cm from the ileocecal valve. Proximal and distal orientation are checked to ensure maturation of the afferent ileum.

A trocar site on the right side is typically the premarked ileostomy site. The skin incision is enlarged to allow two fingers to reach into the abdomen. Generally the subcutaneous and anterior fascia are sharply dissected using electrocautery. The muscle will be spread using two large Kelly clamps at right angles, and the posterior sheath is opened. Care must be taken to ensure the inferior epigastrics were not injured during dissection. The ileostomy is lifted laparoscopically to the anterior abdominal wall and pulled through the abdominal wall using a Babcock clamp. A supporting rod is placed

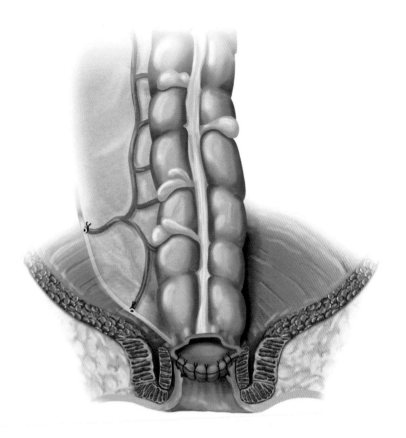

under the ileum to prevent slippage of the posterior ileal wall into the abdomen allowing for passage of fecal stream prior to maturation. The ostomy is matured in a Brooke fashion after closure of all port and specimen extraction sites.

The authors use a Jackson-Pratt drain selectively in cases below the peritoneal reflection. If the patient is not diverted, a Mallencott drain may be left in place in early postoperative period to facilitate neorectal drainage.

POSTOPERATIVE MANAGEMENT

Patients are placed on standard postoperative accelerated recovery program after surgery. Soft foods and oral analgesia are started on postoperative day number 1, and patients are encouraged to ambulate on postoperative day 0 or 1. The Foley catheter is typically removed at 24 hours. Patients should undergo postoperative enterostomal teaching for care of ostomy and ostomy bars are removed after approximately 2–3 days in most patients.

COMPLICATIONS

Complications are similar to other abdominal surgeries and include bleeding, infection, and postoperative ileus. In addition, low anterior resection with coloanal anastomosis increases risks of anastomotic leak, sexual and bladder dysfunction when compared to other colon surgeries.

Anastomotic leak rates for anastomoses below 5 cm from the anal verge are up to 18%. History of radiation, low anastomosis, immunosuppression, and technical difficulty have been associated with increased anastomotic leak rates. Creation of a diverting ileostomy helps to moderate the complications of leak but does not decrease the anastomotic leak rate. Postoperative morbidity rates are comparable between diverted and not diverted patients, but reoperative rates are lower when an ileostomy is used. In general, the authors employ the use of a diverting ileostomy for patients with low rectal cancer. However, patients with ileostomies have morbidity associated with a second hospitalization and operative intervention; a small percentage of patients may never undergo ileostomy closure.

Sexual and erectile dysfunction is increased in patients undergoing proctectomy with total mesorectal excision. Approximately 30% of males experience difficulty with erection or ejaculation following low anterior resection secondary to intraoperative injury to the sympathetic or parasympathetic nerves. Dysfunction may improve with time and studies demonstrate some improvement with the use of sidafenil postoperatively. The rate of dysfunction increases with age, preoperative radiation, and poorer preoperative ejaculatory function. Rate of female sexual dysfunction is less well described but women may have difficulty with pain, sensation, and orgasm postoperatively.

Bladder dysfunction is a less common complication. Up to 15% of patients experience some temporary bladder dysfunction postoperatively, secondary to dissection in the pelvis or injury to parasympathetic nerves. Less than 5% suffer from permanent dysfunction when employing total mesorectal dissection techniques. Some patients may require replacement of the foley catheter postoperatively.

RESULTS

The greatest risk to patients with low rectal cancers is the risk of cancer recurrence. Local or pelvic recurrence is noted to occur in 2–25% of patients within 5 years after low anterior resections, with most studies reporting recurrence rates of approximately 10%. Overall 5-year survival is stage dependent with rates ranging from 70% to 85% for resections performed for curative intent. Although results of large randomized trials are pending preliminary results on laparoscopic rectal resections for colon cancer do not appear to increase rates of local recurrence.

Postoperatively patients may experience increased frequency, bowel movements, and soilage. Most studies describe 2–4 bowel movements per day on average, with up to 25% of patients suffering from some degree of incontinence. Anterior resection syndrome, characterized by urgency, frequency, and soilage occurs in up to 10% of patients following total mesorectal excision.

Coloplasty and colonic J pouch have been proposed to decrease frequency and urgency in patients undergoing coloanal and low rectal anastomosis. Recent studies have demonstrated comparable outcomes using the two techniques, with significant reduction in number of bowel movements over straight coloanal anastomoses. Patients with reservoir creation were found to have fewer nighttime bowel movements, less incontinence to solid stool.

Alternative for coloanal anastomosis is generally abdominal perineal resection. Many patients prefer to attempt to preserve continence despite risks of functional disability. In appropriately selected patients, total mesorectal resection with coloanal anastomosis offers oncologic resection with intestinal continuity.

CONCLUSIONS

Low anterior resection with transanal anastomosis provides restoration of intestinal continuity in patients who might otherwise be left with a permanent colostomy. Preoperative staging including proctoscopy, ultrasound or MRI to evaluate depth of invasion and lymph node involvement, and full colonoscopy is essential to creation of appropriate operative plan. In addition, total mesorectal resection and attention to margins are essential to maintaining oncologic standards and low recurrence rates.

Most patients are candidates for laparoscopic low anterior resections in experienced hands. Patients with prior surgery, obese patients, and males with narrow pelvis may be assessed for laparoscopic approach and may benefit from minimally invasive techniques.

Defecatory function may be worsened in patients following low anterior resection with transanal anastomosis, with large series demonstrating 2–4 bowel movements per day and up to 25% of patients having some degree of incontinence postoperatively. Creation of a neorectum by use of a J pouch or coloplasty may improve function, especially in the early postoperative period.

Recommended References and Readings

Bretagnol F, Lelong B, Laurent C, et al. The oncological safety of laparoscopic total mesorectal excisio with sphincter preservation for rectal carcinoma. *Surg Endosc* 2005;19(7):892–6.

Chude GG, Rayate NV, Patris V, et al. Defunctioning loop ileostomy with low anterior resection for distal rectal cancer: should we make an ileostomy as a routine practice? A prospective randomized study. *Hepatogastroenterology* 2008;55(86–87):1562–7.

Delaney CP, Zutsi M, Senagor AJ, et al. Prospective, randomized controlled trial between a pathway of controlled rehabilitation with early ambulation and diet and traditional postoperative care after laparotomy and intestinal resection. *Dis Colon Rectum* 2003;46(7):851–9.

Herlot AG, Tekkis PP, Constantinides V, et al. Metaanalysis of colonic reservoirs versus straight coloanal anastomosis after anterior resection. *Br J Surg* 2006;93(1):19–32.

Orsenigo E, Di Palo S, Vignali A, et al. Laparoscopic intersphincteric resection for low rectal cancer. *Surg Oncol* 2007;12(1):S117–S120.

Ng SSM, Leung KL, Lee JFY et al. Laparoscopic-assisted versus open abdominal perineal resection for low rectal cancer: a prospective randomized trial. *Ann Surg Oncol* 2008;15(9):2418–25.

Sideris L, Zenasni F, Vernerey D, et al. Quality of life of patients operated on for low rectal cancer: impact of the type of surgery and patients' characteristics. *Dis Colon Rectum* 2005;48(12):2180–91.

Tsikitis VL, Larson DW, Poola VP, et al. Postoperative morbidity with diversion after low anterior resection in the era of neoadjuvant therapy: a single institutional experience. *J Am Coll Surg* 2009;209(1):114–8.

Wibe A, Syse A, Andersen E, et al. Onoclogical outcomes after total mesorectal excision for cure for cancer of the lower rectum: anterior vs abdominal perineal resection. *Dis Colon Rectum* 2004;47(1):48–58.

16 End-to-End, Side-to-End Anastomosis

Marylise Boutros and Anthony M. Vernava III

INDICATIONS/CONTRAINDICATIONS

Sphincter-saving resections for rectal cancer and other benign conditions of the rectum have become standard over the last 20 years, having replaced abdominoperineal resection for many patients. Our experience with low colorectal anastomosis is vast and our understanding of long-term outcomes is increasingly clear. The stapled straight end-to-end anastomosis (EEA) is the standard low colorectal anastomotic technique (1). Although this low anastomosis frees the patient from a colostomy, unfortunately, it has a high rate of anastomotic leak and bowel dysfunction.

- Anastomotic leaks after colon resection occur at a rate less than 3%, whereas rectal anastomoses have a reported leak rate of 10–20% (2). This increase in the risk of anastomotic leak is thought to be due to the devascularization ensued by a total mesorectal excision, the technical difficulty of a low pelvic anastomosis, and the impact of neoadjuvant radiation on bowel healing (3,4). The mortality (2–7%) associated with this complication is significant (5).
- Bowel dysfunction after rectal resection is common (up to 60%) (6). Patients may suffer from incontinence, increased frequency of defecation, urgency, and incomplete evacuation. The degree of symptoms correlates with the level of anastomosis (4).

Several alternate anastomotic approaches have been developed in an attempt to diminish these complications. There are restorative reconstructions, including the colonic J-pouch and transverse coloplasty, which may be used for coloanal anastomoses (discussed elsewhere in this chapter) as well as a low colorectal side-to-end anastomosis. This is a variation on the standard EEA anastomosis.

Contraindications

- In order to perform a low colorectal anastomosis, an oncologically sound resection that spares the sphincters must be possible.
- Furthermore, any patient undergoing a low colorectal anastomosis must have adequate preoperative continence and sphincter function, as increased stool frequency and diminished continence can result even in the best circumstances.

- Similarly all preexisting patient risk factors for anastomotic complications such as anemia, malnutrition, smoking, or cigarette should be corrected and the need for a proximal protective loop ileostomy be considered in all the cases.

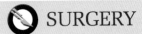 PREOPERATIVE PLANNING

- Prior to a low colorectal resection, consent should be obtained for a possible permanent colostomy or a temporary diverting ileostomy. The location of both of these stomas should be marked preoperatively while the patient is sitting and standing.
- Preoperative mechanical preparation of the bowel is undertaken before resection of the rectum.
- General anesthesia is induced. Broad-spectrum antibiotic coverage (7) for prevention of surgical site infections and prophylaxis (8) for deep vein thrombosis (with subcutaneous unfractunated heparin injection and sequential compression devices) is initiated at this time.
- A bladder catheter is placed after induction of anesthesia.

SURGERY

Patient Positioning

The patient is placed in the appropriate positioning specific to the operative approach (open, laparoscopic, or robotic). However, despite the approach a few key principles will facilitate fashioning the anastomosis:

- The patient is placed in the modified lithotomy (with appropriate stirrups) or split-leg position in Trendelenburg.
- After exploratory laparotomy, the small bowel is packed away in the upper abdomen. This positioning gives the surgeon the best access to the pelvis.

Mobilization

The splenic flexure and the distal large bowel are fully mobilized along with the rectum as described elsewhere in this chapter. For there to be enough proximal colon to fashion a tension-free anastomosis, a high ligation of the inferior mesenteric artery and inferior mesenteric vein is usually necessary. Rectal resection with total or partial mesorectal excision, as indicated by the location of the tumor, is performed. The posterior dissection plane is developed in an avascular areolar tissue plane all the way to the pelvic floor. The dissection plane can be followed around the pelvis to the lateral peritoneal attachments. The attachments are incised to release the rectum. For mid to low rectal tumors, the anterior lateral ligaments containing the middle hemorrhoid vessel are divided with electrocautery at the sidewall of the pelvis to remove all of the mesenteric fat.

Bowel Preparation for Anastomosis

The distal resection margin is chosen and the mesorectal fat is circumferentially cleared off. A linear stapler is fired across the rectum; this can be laparoscopically done using an Echelon® (Ethicon, Cincinnati, OH, USA) or Endo GIA® (Ethicon, Cincinnati, OH, USA) or in an open procedure using a number of stapling devices including the Contour curved cutter® (Ethicon, Cincinnati, OH, USA) or TA stapler. It is imperative to ensure that the rectum has been completely stapled and closed (Fig. 16.1).

Operative Technique for the EEA Anastomosis

This technique is the standard method to construct low colorectal anastomoses. Since the advent of the circular end-to-end stapler and the description of the EEA anastomosis

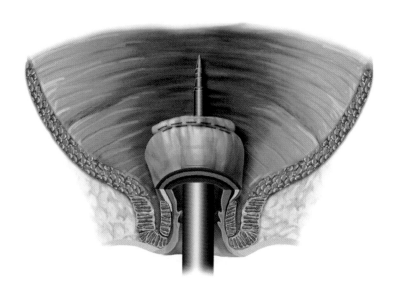

Figure 16.1 Schematic representation of the distal rectal stump with EEA stapler introduced. This is used for both the end-to-end and end-to-side anastomoses.

in 1979, this technique has evolved from a double purse-string EEA anastomosis to a double-stapled EEA anastomosis (9,10).

- The proximal resection margin is chosen in an area that is non-inflamed and free of diverticula. It is imperative at this point to confirm that the proposed proximal resection margin can easily reach the stapled rectal stump without any tension. Then, the remaining mesocolon is divided.

- A purse-string clamp is placed at the transection line and the colon is divided just distal to the clamp using a long-handled knife. Next a nonabsorbable, monofilament suture such as 2.0 nylon on a straight needle is threaded through the purse-string clamp and the clamp is removed. Alternatively, the colon is divided at the proximal transection line using a long-handled knife and a hand-sewn purse-string suture using 2.0 prolene is placed on the cut edge of the bowel. The specimen is removed.

- The circular stapler anvil (typically size 28, 29, or 33) is gently introduced into the proximal bowel and secured in place using the purse-string suture.

- It is important to ensure that there are no diverticula or mesocolonic tissue on the surface of the bowel where the EEA stapler will be fired.

- The proximal colon is gently placed into the pelvis ensuring that it is correctly oriented and that the mesentery is not twisted (Fig. 16.2).

- The stapler is then gently transanally introduced up to the stapled end of the rectal remnant. Under direct vision the stapler is opened such that the trocar pierces through the rectal remnant at or adjacent to the linear staple line. The anvil and the trocar of the stapler are then correctly mated orienting the proximal colon. Once closed, the stapler is fired, opened, and gently removed.

Operative Technique for the Side-to-End Anastomosis

Anastomotic techniques have evolved to improve the quality and function of low colorectal anastomosis. The side-to-end low colorectal anastomotic technique was initially employed to overcome large discrepancies in proximal colon and distal rectal size, as well as situations in which the operating room set-up was not prepared to allow access to the perineum for a traditional straight EEA anastomosis (11). However, more recently, it appears that this technique may confer improved functional results, and possibly, fewer complications (12,13). The technique is as follows:

- The proximal resection margin is chosen in an area that is non-inflamed and free of diverticula. It is imperative at this point to confirm that the proposed proximal

Part III: Low Anterior Resection

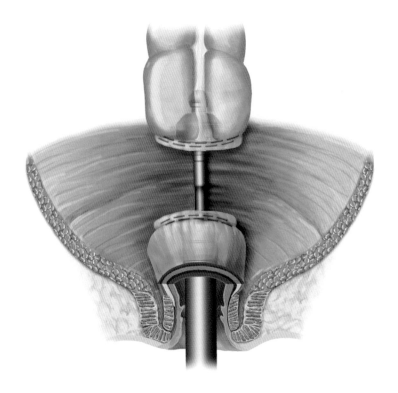

margin can easily reach the stapled rectal stump without any tension. Then, the remaining mesocolon is divided and the colon is transected using a linear cutting stapler.

- The specimen is removed.
- A 3 cm colotomy is made 3 cm from the proximal staple line. The circular stapler anvil (typically size 28, 29, or 33) is lubricated and inserted through the colotomy such that the head of the anvil is pushed cephalad and the spear is brought out through the colotomy. A purse-string suture may be placed around the anvil using 2.0 polypropylene.
- It is important to ensure that there are no diverticula or mesocolonic tissue on the surface of the bowel where the circular stapler will be fired.
- The proximal colon is gently placed into the pelvis ensuring that it is correctly oriented and that the mesentery is not rotated (Fig. 16.3).
- The circular stapler is then gently transanally introduced up to the stapled end of the rectal remnant. Under direct vision the circular stapler is opened such that the trocar pierces through the rectal remnant at the linear staple line. The anvil and the trocar of the circular stapler are then correctly mated orienting the proximal colon. Once closed, the stapler is fired, opened, and gently removed. (Fig. 16.3b)

Testing the Anastomosis

Regardless of which technique is used to perform the low colorectal anastomosis, it is important to test for anastomotic integrity.

- Once the circular stapler is removed, the stapler is opened and both tissue donuts are retrieved and inspected to ensure that they are circumferentially complete and intact. The muscular layer of the colonic wall must be intact.
- The pelvis is then filled with saline and the proximal colon is occluded with an atraumatic bowel clamp.
- A flexible sigmoidoscopy is performed, distending the rectum and the anastomosis with air, demonstrating that it is air tight by the lack of bubbling in the saline-filled pelvis. Direct visualization of the staple lines also ensures completeness, viable proximal and distal mucosa, and adequate hemostasis.

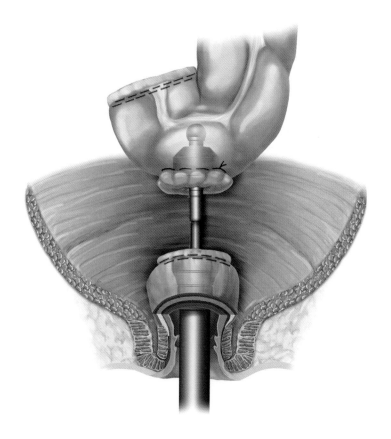

Figure 16.3 Schematic of the ends of bowel when the end-to-end anastomosis stapler is mated in fashioning an end-to-side anastomosis. Note the side limb should be about 3 cm.

Placement of Pelvic Drains

 The use of pelvic drains is controversial.

 Although previously believed to minimize the risk of anastomotic complications by preventing the collection of fluid or hematoma in the pelvis, the use of drains has not shown to be of any benefit or harm in large randomized controlled trials (RCTs) and meta-analyses (14).

 The authors and the editors selectively drain low colorectal anastomosis.

POSTOPERATIVE MANAGEMENT

Postoperative management in colorectal surgery has evolved in the last decade resulting in shorter hospital stays and decreased morbidity. This fact is partly due to the implementation of fast-tracking programs based on evidence-based management practices (15). The elements of fast-track colorectal postoperative management include:

 Use of non-narcotic analgesia and minimized use of narcotic analgesia.

 Avoidance of excess intravenous fluid and the use of goal-directed fluid administration.

 Preoperative carbohydrate administration and early postoperative feeding (clear fluid diet on postoperative day 0, advancing to low residue diet on postoperative day 1 if tolerated).

 No use of routine nasogastric tubes.

 Removal of the bladder catheter on postoperative day 1.

 Early aggressive ambulation.

 Well-defined daily care maps and discharge criteria.

These efforts have significantly reduced the standard hospital stay (14). In addition, there is evidence that the perioperative use of alvimopan, a peripherally acting μ-opioid

Part III: Low Anterior Resection

receptor antagonist, may shorten the return of bowel function and time to discharge by approximately one day without compromising analgesia (16).

COMPLICATIONS

Anastomotic complications have significant morbidity. In the acute postoperative period, there are two anastomotic complications that may present with varying severity:

Anastomotic Leak

- Low colorectal anastomoses have the highest reported leak rate compared to small bowel and colonic anastomosis; and are reported to be 10–20% (2,3).
- The incidence of leak is strongly associated with the distance of the anastomosis from the anal verge (4), with coloanal anastomoses having the highest leak rate.
- Anastomotic leaks are managed based on the patient's symptoms; a small contained leak in an asymptomatic patient may be managed solely with antibiotics, whereas a large contained leak may require radiological percutaneous drainage and a free leak presenting with peritonitis and sepsis requires operative lavage and diverting loop ileostomy if not already present or takedown of the anastomosis and creation of an end-colostomy and Hartmann's stump.
- The long-term sequelae of an anastomotic leak may be insignificant or may result in a stricture or a fistula.

Anastomotic Bleed

- Anastomotic bleeding also varies in severity, with most instances being minor and self-limited. They usually occur with passage of the patient's first stool.
- Rarely, bleeding can be massive and require transfusion, endoscopic or transanal examination with 1:10, 000 epinephrine injection, cautery, clip, or suture application.

Anastomotic complications are usually related to technical factors or to preexisting patient factors. Thus, every effort must be made to assess and optimize these factors preoperatively and intraoperatively.

Technical Factors (2–4)

- It is essential to create a tension-free anastomosis (splenic flexure mobilization recommended, high ligation of the inferior mesenteric artery and the inferior mesenteric vein are all necessary).
- Ensure good blood supply at the anastomoses. This can be done by evidence of pulsatile bleeding from the marginal artery at the level of the anastomosis or by the presence of an audible pulse with a handheld Doppler. In addition, the color of the bowel confirms viability.

Preexisting Patient Factors (2–4)

- Poor nutrition
- Radiation exposure
- Immunosuppression
- Smoking
- Anemia

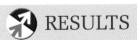 RESULTS

Multiple RCTs have addressed the question of which anastomosis confers the best functional long-term outcome. A meta-analysis of these RCTs reported that the colonic J-pouch was superior to the straight EEA anastomosis in bowel frequency, urgency, fecal incontinence, and the use of antidiarrheal medication. However, the colonic J-pouch did not confer significantly different functional outcomes in RCTs that compared it to transverse coloplasty or the side-to-end anastomosis (6). In addition, the rate of anastomotic leak is significantly higher after both end-to-end coloanal anastomosis and coloplasty compared to colonic J-pouch anal anastomosis.

A more recent RCT compared low colorectal end-to-end with side-to-end anastomoses and reported an overall clinically significant anastomotic leak rate of 16.8% with significantly less leaks in the side-to-end group as compared to the end-to-end group (5% vs. 29.2%, $P < 0.005$). This benefit was found for mid- and low-rectal resections and thus the authors postulated that this significant benefit may be due to an improved blood supply in the end-to-side anastomosis. (12)

A recent RCT examined the optimal size of the side limb in the side-to-end anastomosis. They randomly assigned patients at the time of surgery to either a short (3 cm) or long (6 cm) side limb. They found that anastomotic leaks, bowel frequency, Wexner incontinence score, urgency, and use of antidiarrheal medications and laxatives were not significantly different between the two groups. However, they did find that incomplete evacuation, as demonstrated by defecography, was significantly higher in the long limb as compared to the short limb group (59% vs. 25%, $P < 0.039$). (13) These findings mirror prior reports of colonic J-pouch limb length.

CONCLUSIONS

When a restorative rectal resection is being performed, patient and technical factors need to be optimized to minimize the risks of complications and improve long-term functional outcomes. A side-to-end low colorectal anastomosis is a technically simple alternative technique to a straight EEA anastomosis that may be used preferentially; or it may be utilized when a colonic J-pouch is not feasible because of a narrow pelvis or inadequate bowel length. However, whenever technically feasible the colonic J-pouch is the preferred method of anastomosis.

Recommended References and Readings

1. Enker W, Picon A, Martz J. Anterior and low anterior resection of the rectum. In: Fischer J, Bland K, eds. *Mastery of Surgery.* 5th ed. Philadelphia: Lippincott Williams & Wilkins, 2001: 1556–65.
2. Dietz D, Bailey H. Postoperative complications. In: Bruce W, Fleshman J, Beck D, Pemberton J, Wexner S, eds. *The ASCRS Textbook of Colon and Rectal Surgery.* New York: Springer, 2007:141–55.
3. Rullier E, Laurent C, Garrelon J, et al. Risk factors for anastomotic leakage after resection of rectal cancer. *Br J Surg* 1998;85: 355–58.
4. Ho Y, Wong J, Goh S, et al. Level of anastomosis and anorectal manometry in predicting function following anterior resection for adenocarcinoma. *Int J Colorectal Dis* 1993;8:170–74.
5. Nivatvongs S. Complications of anorectal and colorectal operations. In: Gordon PH, Nivatvongs S, eds. *Surgery of the Colon, Rectum, and Anus.* 3rd ed. New York: Informa Healthcare, 2007:1165–87.
6. Brown CJ, Fenech D, McLeod RS. Reconstructive techniques after rectal resection for rectal cancer. *Cochrane Database Syst Rev* 2008;2:CD006040.
7. Nelson RL, Glenny AM, Song F. Antimicrobial prophylaxis for colorectal surgery. *Cochrane Database Syst Rev* 2009;1: CD001181.
8. Hirsh J, Guyatt G, Albers G, et al. Executive summary: American College of Chest Physicians evidence-based clinical practice guidelines (8th Edition). *Chest* 2008;71S–109S.
9. Goligher J, Lee P, Macfie J, et al. Experience with the Russian model 219 suture gun for anastomosis of the rectum. *Surg Gynecol Obstet* 1979;118:517–24.
10. Cohen Z, Myers E, Langer B, et al. Double stapling technique for low anterior resection. *Dis Colon Rectum* 1983;26:231–35.
11. Adloff M, Arnaud J, Beeharry S, et al. Side-to-end anastomosis in low anterior resection with EEA stapler. *Dis Colon Rectum* 1980;23:456–58.
12. Brisinda G, Vanella S, Cadeddu F, et al. End-to-end versus end-to-side stapled anastomoses after anterior resection for rectal cancer. *J Surg Oncol* 2009;99:75–79.
13. Tsunoda A, Kamiyama G, Narita K, et al. Prospective randomized trial for determination of optimum size of side limb in low anterior resection with side-to-end anastomosis for rectal carcinoma. *Dis Colon Rectum* 2009;52:1572–77.
14. Urbach D, Kennedy E, Cohen M. Colon and rectal anastomosis do not require routine drainage: a systematic review and meta-analysis. *Ann Surg* 1999;229:174–80.
15. Kehlet H, Wilmore D. Evidence-based surgical care and the evolution of fast-track surgery. *Ann Surg* 2008;248:189–98.
16. Bream-Rouwenhorst HR, Cantrell MA. Alvimopan for postoperative ileus. *Am J Health Syst Pharm* 2009;66:1267–77.

17 Hybrid Robotic and Fully Robotic Procedures

Susan M. Cera

 ## INDICATIONS/CONTRAINDICATIONS

Rectal cancer surgery is technically challenging because of the limited confines of the pelvis and the close proximity of the presacral veins, autonomic nerves, and reproductive organs. In 1979, the procedure that is known as total mesorectal excision (TME) was introduced by Dr Heald (1) and is now universally accepted as the gold standard for treatment of rectal cancer. The technique involves precise dissection of the avascular plane between the presacral fascia and the fascia propria of the rectum. The goal for optimal oncologic outcome is total excision of the mesorectum including an intact mesorectal envelope without defects and microscopically tumor-free radial and distal margins. The secondary goal is autonomic nerve preservation relating to quality of life.

Rectal cancer surgery has gone through an evolution of change in the era of minimally invasive surgery. Since the first laparoscopic colectomy in 1991, the use of laparoscopic surgery for colorectal cancer has been increasing. Appropriate oncologic outcomes for colon cancer have been validated in randomized trials studies such as the COST trial (2). Likewise, laparoscopic low anterior resection (LAR) with TME has several advantages when compared with open LAR, including reduced postoperative pain, faster recovery of bowel function, improved quality of life, and decreased hospital stay and disability. However, the laparoscopic approach to LAR has inherent technical limitations, such as a two-dimensional view, limited dexterity of the long, straight instruments, and fixed instrument tips. Consequently, this technique has been proven to have a steep learning curve with a high rate of conversions. The British CLASSIC trial, a large prospective randomized study comparing laparoscopic to open colorectal surgery, reported a 34% conversion rate for laparoscopic approach to rectal resection (3).

The Intuitive Surgical® Da Vinci surgical™ system (Intuitive Surgical®, Sunnyvale, CA), FDA-approved in 2000, was specifically developed to compensate for the technical limitations of the laparoscopic approach. The magnified vision is 10 times that of the human eye and, when the image visualized through the view finder on the surgeon's console, is three-dimensional. Motion scaling is a feature that translates small hand movements outside the patient's body into precise movements inside the body. As the movements are transferred from the handle to the tip of the instrument, tremors and small movements are filtered for enhanced dexterity and smoother motion especially during fine dissections and suturing under microscopic magnification. Motion scaling is designed to allow greater precision than is normally achievable in open and laparoscopic surgery. Finally, the tips of the robotic instruments encompass endowrist technology demonstrating the same full range of motion as a human wrist and can therefore rotate 360 degrees and bend with 90 degrees of angulation.

Robotic LAR with TME for rectal cancer has been described in two ways. The first is a hybrid of laparoscopy and robotics. Vessel division and mobilization of the splenic flexure are accomplished laparoscopically followed by positioning of the robot between the patient's legs for the robotic TME. This approach was the mainstay procedure using the original design of the Da Vinci system with three arms. The second robotic approach, developed by Dr Seon-Hahn Kim of Seoul, Korea, involves robotic use for all portions of the procedure including vessel division, mobilization of the splenic flexure, and the TME. Fully robotic LAR has only been possible since the release of the Da Vinci S model that has four arms, each of which has a wider range of motion. The advantage of the fully robotic approach is that the robot is positioned over the patient's left knee allowing access to the anorectal area should digital exam, vaginal retraction, or flexible sigmoidoscopy be required during the dissection.

Indications for robotic LAR include T1 through T3 tumors. Tumor location at any level of the rectum is possible, although strategy for intestinal reconstruction may differ. For tumors of the rectum 2 cm above the anorectal ring a double-stapled anastomosis is the preferred option. Tumors less than 2 cm from the anorectal ring that demonstrate no sphincter invasion are amenable to an intersphincteric resection. For this technique, the transanal intersphincteric dissection is performed first followed by the robotic transabdominal steps of the procedure. The specimen may be retrieved transanally or through a minilaparotomy incision followed by either a hand-sewn anastomosis or a double-stapled anastomosis. Rectal carcinomas invading the anal sphincter are surgically treated with abdominoperineal resection and permanent colostomy.

Contraindications to robotic LAR are the same as for laparoscopy. Body mass index (BMI) is not a restriction and those patients undergoing preoperative chemoradiation therapy are potentially appropriate candidates. A significant history of multiple previous operations may be a relative contraindication. If significant adhesions are encountered, lysis of adhesions may be laparoscopically completed prior to docking the robot. The robot is not as adept at moving to multiple quadrants of the abdomen because of vertical limitations on range of motion of the robotic arms.

Surgeon experience plays an important role in the success of robotic LAR and in ensuring both patient safety and good oncologic outcome. The surgeon should have experience with rectal cancer surgery and good knowledge of the open techniques. He/she should demonstrate advanced laparoscopic skills and be proficient in basic robotic skills that have a learning curve. These skills include the following:

1. Docking and undocking using the various arm and port clutches to move the arms
2. Maximizing space between the robotic arms and strategic planning to avoid arm collisions
3. Learning the console controls associated with the robotic system
4. Learning the various robotic instruments that differ from the laparoscopic instruments
5. Learning to use visual cues when manipulating the bowel and mesentery without haptic feedback and with forces that are motion scaled and electronically enhanced

Contraindications to robotic LAR procedures are the same as for the laparoscopic approach. Application of all minimally invasive procedures should be tailored to the level of the surgeon experience. Minimally invasive approaches to rectal cancers are technically challenging and require advanced skills for good technique and troubleshooting. For robotic surgery, technical confidence can be overestimated during the training period since those surgeons without minimally invasive experience may find it easier to navigate the pelvis with the more stabilized system, accommodating instruments, smoother dissections, and magnified views that the robot offers.

PREOPERATIVE PLANNING

Routine preoperative staging should be performed for all rectal cancers including colonoscopy, biopsy, CT scan, and either endorectal ultrasound or pelvic MRI. Oncology consultation may be appropriate for initiation of neoadjuvant chemoradiation therapy.

 # SURGERY

The robotic hybrid procedure involves three steps:

1. Laparoscopic mobilization of the left colon and splenic flexure, ligation of the mesenteric vessels (This mobilization can be performed medial to lateral or lateral to medial based on surgeon preference)
2. Robotic TME (The robot is positioned between the patient's legs)
3. Specimen retrieval and anastomosis

The fully robotic procedure involves four steps. The robot is not moved during the procedure but the arms are undocked and redocked during the different phases.

1. Robotic vessel division and retroperitoneal dissection medial to lateral (The robot positioned over the patient's left leg to reach from the pelvis to the left upper quadrant)
2. Mobilization of the splenic flexure
3. Robotic TME
4. Specimen retrieval and anastomosis

For both approaches, the robotic TME is followed by specimen retrieval, possible anastomosis, possible diverting loop ileostomy depending on the surgical plan.

Operating Room Set Up

For the Hybrid Procedure (Fig. 17.1)
Assistant and scrub tech are positioned to the patient's right.

The robot is positioned at the patient's feet during the laparoscopic portion and then brought between the patient's leg during the robotic TME.

The video cart and additional monitors are placed to the patient's left.

For the Fully Robotic Procedure (Fig. 17.2)
The assistant and scrub tech are to the patient's right.

The video cart is at the foot of the bed.

The robot is positioned over the patient's left leg.

Patient Positioning (Fig. 17.3)
The patient is placed supine in a modified lithotomy position with the legs in padded adjustable stirrups. Both arms are tucked at the patient's sides and the patient should be secured to the bed to avoid shifting in the Trendelenburg position. Towels are placed in an x-shaped fashion across the patient's chest and tape is placed over the towels to secure the patient to the bed. For the hybrid procedure, both patient's legs should be padded anteriorly to prevent injury from the robotic arms. For the fully robotic procedure, additional padding should be placed on the left leg. Placement of ureteric stents (optional) followed by foley catheter is performed prior to initiation of the robotic procedure. During the robotic portion of the procedure, the patient is placed in steep Trendelenburg with a 30-degree right lateral rotation to keep the small bowel out of the pelvis and in the right upper quadrant.

Figure 17.1 OR setup for hybrid robotic low anterior resection (LAR).

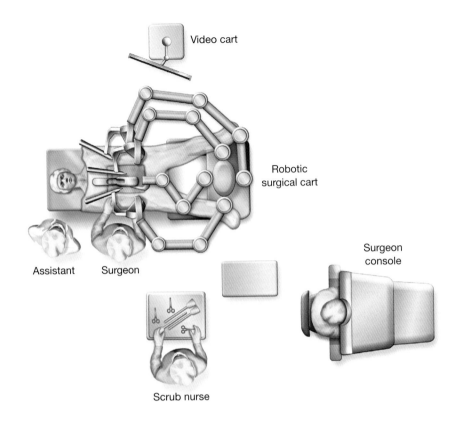

Port Placement and Docking

Hybrid Procedure Ports (Fig. 17.4)

- The 12-mm camera port is placed 3 cm either above or below umbilicus midway between the xiphoid and the symphysis pubis.

Figure 17.2 OR setup for fully robotic LAR.

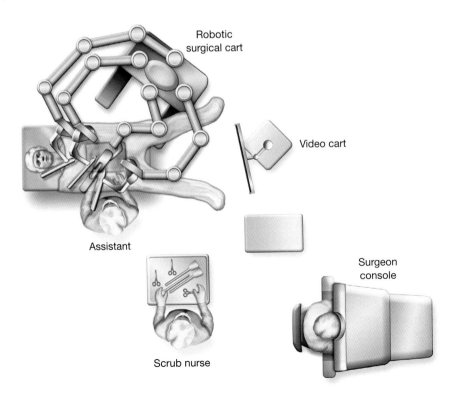

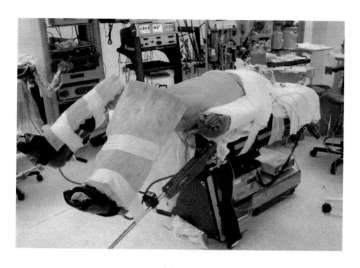

Figure 17.3 Patient positioning for robotic LAR: both hybrid and fully robotic.

- The right lower quadrant port is both L_1 (laparoscopic port 1) and R_1 (robotic port 1). This should be a disposable 12-mm port (to accommodate a stapler) through which is telescoped an 8-mm nondisposable metal robotic port (for the robotic portion of the procedure).
- The right upper quadrant port is L_2. This port is a disposable 5-mm port.
- The left lower quadrant port is R_2, with additional port R_3 placed left lower quadrant lateral to R_2 if a Da Vinci S system (four arms) is used. Both of these ports are the robotic metal nondiposable ports.

Fully Robotic Procedure Ports: Starting with Camera Port and Then Clockwise (Fig. 17.5)

- Camera port 12 mm placed 3 cm to the right and 3 cm above umbilicus.
- R_1: 12-mm port right lower quadrant (midclavicular line) through which is telescoped an 8-mm robotic port. The 8-mm port can be removed to place an endostapler.

Figure 17.4 Port placement for hybrid robotic LAR.

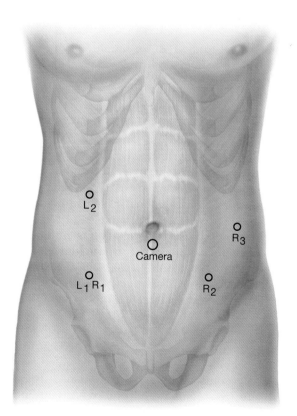

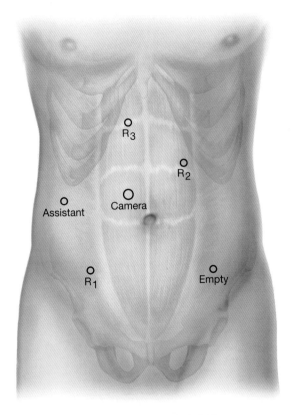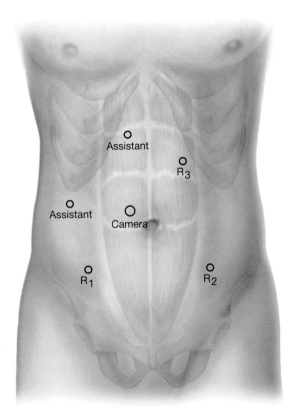

Figure 17.5 Port placement for fully robotic LAR.

- Assistant port right lateral midabdomen: 5-mm port for retracting and suctioning by assistant.
- R₃: 8-mm port right upper quadrant should be medial to midclavicular line but to the right of the falciform ligament.
- R₂: 8-mm port left upper quadrant placed just to the right of the midclavicular line midway between umbilicus and left subcostal region.
- Left lower quadrant 8-mm robotic port placed at the same height and positioned as the right lower quadrant port.

*Note: All of the 12-mm ports are disposable while the 8-mm ports are robotic metal nondisposable ports.

All of the robotic ports described in the preceding text are the 8-mm ports. The 5-mm ports are available but the 5-mm graspers have less grip and, as of this publication, there are no 5-mm shears that accommodate electrocautery. Alternatively, the 5-mm Harmonic can be used but the robotic version does not have the endowrist technology minimizing key advantages of the robotic instrument technology.

For both techniques, the camera port is inserted first using an open technique. The camera trocar used should be an extra-long standard disposable trocar (the Hasson is too short to accommodate the docking grips of the robotic arms). Stay sutures are placed to hold this trocar in place. The abdomen is insufflated, and, once pneumoperitoneum is achieved, the remainder of the ports is inserted through the abdominal wall using the 30-degree robotic scope facing upwards. The camera is held by the surgeon or the assistant while the ports are placed. The ports should be inserted to the thick black line on the port to ensure optimal port depth. At this point, inspection of the abdomen should be undertaken. Adhesions should be laparoscopically divided and, if performing the hybrid procedure, the laparoscopic portion is accomplished. Prior to docking the robot, the table is placed in the Trendelenburg position with right lateral

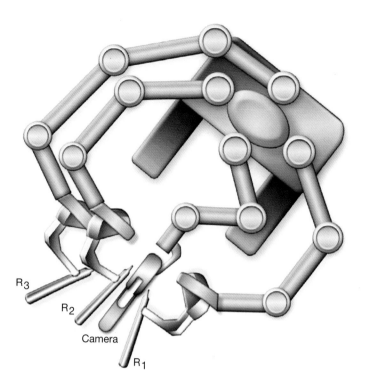

Figure 17.6 Arm configuration for robot with four arms.

R₃

R₂

Camera

R₁

rotation to ensure that the small bowel is out of the pelvis. It is imperative to ensure that all the bowels are in the right upper quadrant and the patient and the table positioned before docking the robot. *Once the robot is docked the position of the table cannot be changed.*

The camera is now removed and the robot cart is advanced to the OR table until the camera arm is directly over the camera port. If using a four-arm robotic system, the camera arm should be bent to the robot's left away from the side with arms 2 and 3 (Fig. 17.6). All ports, which are empty at this point, are docked using the various port and arm clutch maneuvers. Once docked, the arms are positioned to maximize distance between to avoid collisions and are elevated to maximize space in the abdominal cavity. *Once all ports are docked, the 30-degree scope is exchanged for a zero-degree scope which is used for the remainder of the case.* Because of the magnification of the robotic system, the zero-degree scope maximizes the view of the pelvis. The camera is inserted into the camera port and, by manually moving the robot arm of the camera, the other instruments are inserted under direct vision. *The tips of the instruments should remain in the visual fields at all times to avoid inadvertent injury to intra-abdominal contents.* This administration is more important with the robotic technique than the laparoscopic because the field of vision is much smaller and more magnified with the robotic system and there is no haptic sensation which in a laparoscopic procedure might alert the surgeon to a problem.

The surgeon should be familiar with the various instruments available. Electrocautery shears and the bipolar Maryland forceps are commonly used for sharp dissection. The Graptor™ and the double fenestrated grasper are long grasping instruments for grasping and retracting the bowel. Shorter instruments such as the fenestrated, Cadiere, and ProGrasp™ forceps are advantageous for grasping small amounts of tissue during dissection but may cause injury if used to retract the bowel. Cautery can be connected to many of the instruments and the Harmonic is available with use of a separate foot pedal not attached to the console.

A qualified assistant, such as a resident, secondary surgeon, or well-trained first-assist, is needed for the procedure and remains scrubbed at the patient bedside. This assistant should be experienced in laparoscopic maneuvers, ligating vessels, and stapling division of bowel if the attending surgeon does not wish to scrub back into the case each time for these portions of the procedure.

Technique

Hybrid Procedure

Phase 1: Laparoscopic Mobilization of the Left Colon and Splenic Flexure with Ligation of the Mesenteric Vessels

Using the camera, L_1 and L_2 ports, the laparoscopic instruments are used to perform either a medial-to-lateral or lateral-to-medial mobilization of the left colon and splenic flexure with ligation of the mesenteric vessels (the inferior mesenteric artery [IMA] and the inferior mesenteric vein [IMV]). The surgeon and the assistant are standing to the right of the patient, and the table can be repositioned to optimize the use of gravity. Upon completion of the mobilization, the patient is placed back into the Trendelenburg position with the right side down until all bowel remains out of the pelvis.

Phase 2: Robotic TME

The robotic cart is brought between the patient's legs until the camera arm is directly over the umbilical camera port. The camera scope is a zero degree scope. Port and arm clutch maneuvers are used to dock the arms to the camera and other three (R_1, R_2, and R_3) instrument ports. Typically, two graspers are placed through the left ports and the monopolar cautery shears are placed into the right. The assistant stands to the patient's right and uses L_2 for retraction and suctioning. The surgeon now sits at the console in the operating room and controls the robotic camera and the arms. The rectosigmoid junction is elevated superiorly and anteriorly using the R_3 with a bowel grasper and is then locked into place. Using the electrocautery shears in R_1 and the short grasper (such as the Cadiere forceps) in R_3, the plane between the fascia propria of the rectum and the parietal fascia is identified and entered. The hypogastric nerves are identified and preserved, as are the ureters. The dissection is carried out posteriorly first and then laterally along the pelvic sidewalls. The peritoneal reflection is incised anteriorly, and the plane between the rectum and the vagina/prostate is developed. The dissection is circumferentially undertaken to the level of the levators.

Phase 3: Specimen Retrieval and Anastomosis

Before dividing the rectum, one member of the team performs a digital rectal examination under direct visualization, and the distal margin is carefully assessed. The 8-mm robotic port is removed from its telescoped position in the 12-mm right lower quadrant port to accommodate the stapler. The distal rectum is divided by the assistant or the surgeon, if he/she chooses to scrub at this point, with a reticulating 30-mm linear stapler. The robot is now dedocked and pushed back from the table. The specimen is extracted by creating a 4-cm suprapubic or left lower quadrant (at the port site) mini-laparotomy covered with a plastic wound protector. The proximal bowel is divided and an anvil is introduced into the proximal stump. A standard circular stapled anastomosis is created under laparoscopic visualization.

The specimen may also be transanally retrieved after which either a hand-sewn or stapled anastomosis is created. After incising the distal rectum or performing an intersphincteric dissection connecting to the previously accomplished pelvic dissection, a wound protector is placed in the anus. The specimen is delivered and the bowel transected. If an intersphincteric dissection is performed, a hand-sewn colonanal anastomosis is accomplished with or without colonic J pouch. If an intersphincteric dissection is not performed and a margin of rectum remains, a stapled anastomosis is possible. The anvil is placed in the proximal bowel and returned to the pelvis. A pursestring suture is created in the distal resection margin. A circular stapler is inserted with the trocar advanced and a stapled anastomosis created. Following any of these anastomotic techniques, the anastomosis is tested for air tightness.

FULLY ROBOTIC PROCEDURE

Phase 1: Vessel Division and Retroperitoneal Dissection

The ports are placed as described in the preceding text. Before the robot is brought to the table, the camera is used to ensure that the bowel is out of the pelvis. Laparoscopic evaluation, lysis of adhesions (if needed), and division of the proximal jejunal ligament are performed. The robot is brought to the table. To ensure optimal positioning of the robot, the camera, target anatomy (left lower quadrant), and robot are aligned in a straight line over the patient's left leg. The robot arms are docked to the ports and the space between the arms is maximized to avoid collisions. The camera is inserted and the instruments are placed under direct vision. R_1 is the right lower quadrant port through which is telescoped an 8-mm robotic port. R_3 is right upper quadrant and R_2 is the left upper quadrant port (Fig. 17.5). R_2 is used to grasp and lift the sigmoid mesentery/vascular pedicle in an upward direction. It is locked in this position for the vessel transection. R_3 is a grasping instrument (Maryland or Cadiere forceps) while the R_1 port contains the electrocautery shears. The IMA is identified. The presacral space is entered and the dissection is performed underneath the IMA to its origin taking care to identify and avoid the retroperitoneal structures and ureter. The IMA is isolated and ligated with robotic hemostatic clips. After which the vessel is transected with the shears. The retroperitoneal dissection is continued more proximally until the IMV is identified and isolated. It is also ligated with clips and transected with the shears. If a coloanal anastomosis is planned, the left colic is divided to allow reach of the bowel into the pelvis (Fig. 17.7). The remainder of the retroperitoneal dissection is performed in a medial-to-lateral fashion with the extent of dissection superior to the inferior border of the pancreas separating the tail of the pancreas from the mesocolon. The gastrocolic ligament is divided from medial to lateral keeping the distal transverse colon omentum on the specimen (facilitates next portion of the procedure). The dissection is also carried laterally to expose gerota's fascia, and inferiorly to the psoas muscle.

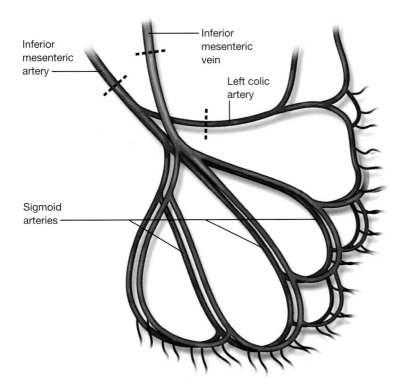

Figure 17.7 Vessel division for coloanal anastomosis.

Inferior mesenteric artery

Inferior mesenteric vein

Left colic artery

Sigmoid arteries

Phase 2: Mobilization of the Splenic Flexure

The instrument is removed from R_2 and the R_2 arm is undocked and pushed backwards to allow this phase of the procedure. R_1 and R_3 are used to incise the white line of Toldt and mobilize the splenic flexure.

Phase 3: Robotic TME

The R_3 robotic arm is undocked from its position in the right upper quadrant and moved to the left upper quadrant port. The R_2 arm is now docked to the left lower quadrant port (Fig. 17.5). Grasping instruments are placed in both of these ports. The two right upper quadrant ports are both used by the assistant for retracting and suctioning of blood and fumes. R_3 grasper retracts the rectosigmoid and uterus anteriorly while R_2 and R_1 instruments perform the TME as described in the hybrid procedure. Upon completion of the TME, the R_1 arm is dedocked and the 8-mm port removed from the 12-mm port. The stapler can then be placed through this port without having to move the robot.

Phase 4: Specimen Retrieval and Anastomosis

Specimen retrieval and anastomosis, if planned, is accomplished as outlined in the hybrid procedure.

POSTOPERATIVE MANAGEMENT

Postoperative management is similar to laparoscopic procedures for rectal cancer. The patient is kept on 24 hours of antibiotics, deep venous thrombosis prophylaxis, and encouraged to ambulate and use an incentive spirometer. With onset of flatus, the diet is advanced and patient is discharged in stable condition. If a stoma is created, stoma teaching and appropriate stoma output are ensured prior to discharge.

COMPLICATIONS

The advanced technology offered by the robotic system predisposes to complications that are specific to the robot. The increased magnification and the consequent narrower field of vision may lead to thermal or traumatic injuries that can occur outside the field of vision, particularly if moving from one quadrant to another. It is especially important to keep the tips of the instruments in the field of vision at all times.

The loss of haptic feedback may lead to unintentional tissue injury. The force exerted by the finger movements at the surgeon console is electronically magnified. The resulting force must be assessed by visual cues. Tearing of bowel and mesentery is possible either by the force exerted in closing the grasping instrument or by the torque placed on the tissue. These conditions are more common in inexperienced hands and when attention is not paid to the visual cues of the retracting instruments.

Because of the high level of technology, there are disadvantages with the system that may contribute to complications. Troubleshooting the robotic equipment often requires outside resources from the company and may cause delay or prolonging of the surgical procedure. Working in two or more quadrants (as is frequent in colorectal surgery) yields to large excursions of the arms that may lead to collisions of the arms both outside and inside the patient. Frequent collisions may be a sign of suboptimal port placement or robotic arm position and may lead to limitations in the vertical movement of the instruments. Dedocking and redocking is required for changing the decubitus of the table and it can add approximately 20 minutes or more to the length of the procedure.

With regard to anastomotic leak rate, although one study suggested that the leak rate that was statistically significantly lower using the robotic technique when compared to laparoscopic methods (4), all other comparative studies revealed similar anastomotic leak rate (5–7).

Two other disadvantages are noted with the robotic system though they may not contribute to complications. The setup time for a robotic procedure may be longer, though this time is shortened with an experienced team. A second physician or resident is required that can perform advanced laparoscopic skills such as retracting, suctioning of blood, and stapling across bowel.

RESULTS—HYBRID PROCEDURE

The hybrid procedure has been deemed safe and feasible in both case series and case-controlled studies. Pigazzi et al. (6) published a case-controlled series of six patients who underwent hybrid robotic TME in comparison to six undergoing laparoscopic TME. Although this was a small series, no differences were detected in short-term operative, pathological, or clinical outcomes. The robotic operation was not more time-consuming than laparoscopy despite the additional setup time required that was included in the operative time reported. Additional study assessed surgeon's fatigue-following robotic versus laparoscopic surgery. Their findings demonstrated much less physical and psychological strain following robotic procedures. Potential explanations include a more ergonomically sound position for the surgeon sitting at the console, a decreased need to direct the assistant holding the camera, and less eye strain because of increased visualization of pelvic structures with the robotic three-dimensional telescope. In a second publication by this same group, 39 consecutive patients underwent hybrid robotic LAR for rectal cancers of all levels of the rectum (8). Patient and oncologic outcomes are similar to rates previously reported in the literature for the laparoscopic approach; however, the conversion rate was low at 3%. These data suggest an advantage of robotics leading to less conversion to an open procedure.

A larger case-controlled study by Patriti et al. (7) included 29 patients undergoing hybrid robotic procedure matched with 37 undergoing laparoscopic procedure. Results included statistically significant shorter operative time and less conversion to open in the robotic group. Clinical, pathological, and short-term oncologic outcomes were otherwise the same between the two groups.

The group with the most widely published hybrid robotic TME data is Baik et al. They claim the first formal description of the hybrid technique of robotic TME with autonomic nerve preservation (9). A subsequent study evaluating hybrid technique with the use of four robotic arms instead of three led the authors to conclude that better exposure could be obtained with use of the fourth arm (10). This group evaluates pathologic outcomes by describing the completeness of the mesorectal envelope as a function of the precision of the robotic dissection. In an evaluation of 18 robotically performed TMEs, complete dissection was accomplished more often than the 16 laparoscopically performed TMEs (94% vs. 81%), though this was not statistically significant (11). Mean operating room time and conversion rates were the same. In a second and larger publication by this group, 56 patients who underwent hybrid robotic LAR were matched with 56 patients in whom the procedure was performed laparoscopically (4). Originally, this was a prospective randomized trial but was changed to prospective comparative study because patient preference resulted in several crossovers to the alternative method. In this study, there was statistically significant lower conversion to open, shorter length of stay, and less major complications (anastomotic leak) with the robotic technique. While not statistically significant, the number of macroscopically complete TME versus nearly complete or incomplete occurred more often in the robotic group than in the laparoscopic group. These data suggest that since robotic TME leads to pathologic results where macroscopic grading is excellent, the pathologic results may theoretically lead to improved oncologic outcomes survival. However, there are no long-term data following in robotic rectal cancer surgery. In addition, these authors suggest that the microscopic visualization using the robotic system leads to improved preservation of

Part III: Low Anterior Resection

the pelvic nerves preventing sexual and bladder dysfunction. Ongoing investigation is being undertaken and the data will be published in the future.

RESULTS—FULLY ROBOTIC PROCEDURE

Currently only a single case series has been published with regard to fully robotic procedure. Luca et al. reported on 55 consecutive patients undergoing fully robotic LAR. Their data revealed no positive margins in the surgical specimens, appropriate short-term clinical and pathologic results, and no conversions to open procedure. Their findings suggest that fully robotic LAR can be accomplished without need for robotic hybrid techniques (12).

CONCLUSIONS

Robotic surgery devices have been developed beyond investigational devices and are becoming increasingly disseminated in all fields of surgery. Robotic surgery addresses the challenges of laparoscopic surgery for rectal cancer by embodying a steady surgical field (motion scaling), a magnified and three-dimensional view, and by allowing the surgeon's wrist action to be reflected in the tips of the instrument. While the learning curve is steep, the rewards include the benefits of minimally invasive approach with potentially less conversion, less surgeon fatigue, better oncologic outcome (decreased positive margin rate and improved completeness of TEM), and less impairment in quality of life (sexual and bladder dysfunction). It should be emphasized that the studies presented in this chapter involved the experience of individual surgeons with significant skill and experience in robotic pelvic surgery. Several disadvantages with the system including the high cost of acquisition and of maintenance of the platform are still prohibiting factors in widespread use.

Costs of the surgical robot include capital acquisition, limited use instruments, team training expenses, equipment maintenance, equipment repair, and operating room setup time. The cost of Da Vinci robot is approximately 1.5-2 million dollars. The cost of a single robotic instrument (e.g., a bowel grasper) is $2,200. These instruments can be used 10 times and then must be disposed. Service for a robot is comprehensive. Software is continually added as it becomes available to the technicians employed by the Intuitive Surgical company (Sunnyvale, CA). Upkeep and maintenance can be included in extended warranties. Surgeon reimbursement for a robotic procedure is the same as the laparoscopic form. In addition, surgeon time for training is at the expense of the surgeon. Setup time for the robot can also be prohibitive in a busy surgical arena where block time can be a limited and sought-after commodity. Yet while surgical outcomes, such as cure rates of prostate cancer, may be improved with the robot, the reimbursement is not increased. Ultimately the cost of the technology is absorbed by individual hospitals/surgeons if they so choose. These decisions are often based on the size of the hospital and the types of populations treated. Hospitals located in more affluent areas are more likely to acquire the most cutting edge technology. A robot may not be possible for an urban hospital with few resources.

Other limitations of the system include the lack of haptic feedback (potential physical risk to the patient), increased operative times, inability to access all four quadrants of the abdomen, and the need for an assistant (second physician or well-trained PA for suctioning of liquids/fumes and assisting in retraction). Currently, the benefits of robotics have not yet been shown to translate into long-term improved oncologic outcome and survival. In addition, studies are needed to assess for potential advantages in quality of life such as reduced risk of sexual and voiding dysfunction. If proven, these advantages could possibly offset the significantly increased cost of health care resources.

Recommended References and Readings

1. Heald RJ. A new approach to rectal cancer. *Br J Hosp Med* 1979; 22:277–81.
2. Clinical Outcomes of Surgical Therapy Study Group. A comparison of laparoscopically assisted and open colectomy for colon cancer. *N Engl J Med* 2004;350:2050–59.
3. Guillou PJ, Quirke P, Thorpe H, et al; MRC CLASICC Trial Group. Short-term end points of conventional vs laparoscopic-assisted surgery in patients with colorectal cancer (MRC CLASICC trial): multicenter, randomized controlled trial. *Lancet* 2005;365:1718–26.
4. Baik SH, Kwon HY, Kim JS, et al. Robotic versus laparoscopic low anterior resection of rectal cancer: short term outcome of a prospective comparative study. *Ann Surg Oncol* 2009;16:1480–87.
5. Baik SH, Ko YT, Kang CM, et al. Robotic tumor-specific mesorectal excision of rectal cancer: short-term outcome of a pilot randomized trial. *Surg Endosc* 2008;22:1601–8.
6. Pigazzi A, Ellenhorn JD, Ballantyne GH, Paz IB. Robotic-assisted laparoscopic low anterior resection with total mesorectal excision for rectal cancer. *Surg Endosc* 2006;20:1521–5.
7. Patriti A, Ceccarelli G, Bartoli A, Spaziani A, Biancafarina A, Casciola L. Short- and medium-term outcome of robot-assisted and traditional laparoscopic rectal resection. *JSLS* 2009;13:176–83.
8. Hellan M, Anderson C, Ellenhorn JD, Paz B, Pigazzi A. Short-term outcomes after robotic-assisted total mesorectal excision for rectal cancer. *Ann Surg Oncol* 2007;14(11):3168–73.
9. Baik et al. Robotic total mesorectal excision for the treatment of rectal cancer. *J Robotic Surg* 2007;1:99–102.
10. Baik SH, Lee WJ, Rha KH, et al. Robotic total mesorectal excision for rectal cancer using 4 robotic arms. *Surg Endosc* 2008; 22:792–7.
11. Luca F, Cenciarelli S, Valvo M, et al. Full robotic left colon and rectal cancer resection: technique and early outcome. *Ann Surg Oncol* 2009;16:1274–8.
12. Wexner et al. The current status of robotic pelvic surgery: results of a multinational interdisciplinary consensus conference. *Surg Endosc* Published online Nov. 27, 2008.

List of Additional Recommended Readings

Baik SH, et al. Robotic total mesorectal excision for rectal cancer: it may improve survival as well as quality of life. *Surg Endosc* 2008;22:1556.

D'Annibale A, Morpurgo E, Fiscon V, et al. Robotic and laparoscopic surgery for treatment of colorectal diseases. *Dis Colon Rectum* 2004;47:2162–68.

Spinoglio G, Summa M, Priora F, Quarati R, Testa S. Robotic colorectal surgery: first 50 cases experience. *Dis Colon Rect* 2008; 51:1627–32.

Ziogas D, Roukos D. Robotic surgery for rectal cancer: may it improve also survival? *Surg Endosc* 2008;22:1405–6.

18 Hand-Assisted

Sang W. Lee and Jeffrey W. Milsom

INDICATIONS/CONTRAINDICATIONS

There are many potential benefits to the laparoscopically of performing rectal surgery. Recent meta-analysis of studies of nonrandomized trials comparing laparoscopic versus open surgery showed the usual benefits associated with laparoscopy after laparoscopic rectal surgery for cancer: shorter time to bowel function and shorter length of stay (1). In addition, compared to open surgery, laparoscopy can provide unprecedented, unobstructed views of the rectal dissection planes even in a patient with narrow pelvis, not only for the surgeon but also to the entire surgical team. Despite these potential advantages, application of laparoscopic techniques during rectal dissection has been limited partially because of technical challenges in providing adequate exposure, retraction of the bulky rectal specimen, and laparoscopic distal rectal stapling.

In order to retain some of the benefits of laparoscopic surgery while not compromising oncologic rectal dissection, some surgeons have advocated performing hybrid procedures in which colonic portion of the surgery is performed using the "pure" laparoscopic technique and rectal dissection is performed open through a limited low midline or Pfannenstiel incision (2). Alternatively, hand-assisted laparoscopic techniques can be used for rectal cancer surgery. In comparison to hybrid procedure where the incision is not created until the end of the procedure, the hand-assisted technique utilizes the incision from the very beginning of the procedure by placing the hand into the abdomen by using an access device. As shown in several studies, hand-assisted compared to "straight" technique may result in shorter operative time based on colonic portion of the operation alone (3,4).

In hand-assisted laparoscopic rectal surgery, rectal exposure and dissection can be either directly performed through the incision using the open techniques or laparoscopically undertaken. Because open rectal dissection technique has been well described in other sections, it will not be reviewed in detail in this chapter. During hand-assisted laparoscopic rectal dissection, the surgeon's hand can be utilized to retract and expose the rectal tissue planes during laparoscopic dissection. However, in patients with narrow pelvis, the hand can sometimes get in the way of dissection by obscuring laparoscopic view. Ergonomically it can be extremely awkward to use the hand to retract the rectum for long periods of time.

We previously described a novel method of laparoscopically exposing the rectal dissection planes by using a Gelport® device and exteriorizing the colorectal stump (5).

In this technique, the end of divided sigmoid colon stump is exteriorized through a Gelport® device. The property of the device maintains pneumoperitoneum during the procedure. A gentle traction on the rectal stump creates tension and exposure for posterior and lateral rectal dissection. This simple traction maneuver can be easily accomplished by even a less experienced member of the surgical team. In addition, by using this technique, distal rectal stapling can be performed using an open approach directly through the incision. This may allow us to take advantage of unmatched laparoscopic view while performing oncologically equivalent exposure and dissection techniques as in the open surgery. By performing distal rectal division directly through the incision using the open surgical staplers, hand-assisted laparoscopic rectal surgery may result in lower anastomotic leakage rate. In this section, laparoscopic rectal dissection using this technique will be described in detail.

SURGERY

Patients are placed in the modified lithotomy position with both arms tucked to the sides. We do not use a sand bag or tapes to secure the patients to the table. Gel pads, which are commonly available in operating rooms, provide excellent traction without need for physical restraint measures. A bladder catheter and orogastric tubes are placed and preoperative antibiotics and subcutaneous heparin are given prior to incision.

A standard Pfannenstiel incision is made approximately two fingerbreadths above the pubis. Alternatively, a low midline incision can be used in patients who already have a low midline incision from previous surgery or in cases where conversion to open surgery is likely. Incision length varies according to surgeon's hand size. Approximate incision length corresponds to surgeon's glove size in centimeters (7½ glove size requires 8 cm incision). The anterior abdominal fascia is divided transversely and the abdomen is entered in the midline between the rectus sheaths. A hand-access device, Gelport® (Applied Medical, Rancho Santa Margarita, CA, USA) is placed through the incision. A 10-mm supraumbilical port for the camera can be inserted either using manual assistance or under direct vision using a camera inserted via the hand-access device. Three to four additional 5-mm working ports are placed lateral to the rectus sheath as shown (Fig. 18.1).

Hand-assisted technique is used for the initial extrapelvic portion of the operation. The patient is placed in the steep Trendelenburg position with left side up. The surgeon stands between the legs of the patient and places the left hand into the abdomen. The greater omentum is placed over the liver in the cephalad direction. The small intestines are gently packed to the right upper quadrant of the abdomen. In difficult cases, a moist laparotomy pad placed through the hand port incision can be used to pack the small intestines out of the way. The mesentery of the sigmoid colon is retracted with the surgeon's hand ventrally, tenting up the inferior mesenteric artery (IMA) and inferior mesenteric vein (IMV). The assistant uses the right-sided ports to perform the dissection. A 5-mm bipolar energy device is typically used to perform the entire case. The dissection is started dorsal to the IMA pedicle starting at the level of the sacral promontory. The plane behind the IMA is relatively avascular and dissection can be carried out to the origin of the IMA with minimal bleeding. As the dissection proceeds proximally toward the origin of the IMA, the inferior hypogastric nerves need to be identified and sharply dissected away from the IMA pedicle. Creation of a wide window behind the IMA is critical in gaining an adequate access to the retroperitoneum and identifying the left ureter and gonadal vessels.

The surgeon places his other fingers behind the cut edge of the peritoneum and gently sweeps the retroperitoneum away from the mesentery of the sigmoid colon. The left ureter at this level is located medial to the left gonadal vessels. Once the left ureter and gonadal vessels were dissected away from the harm's way, the peritoneum over the IMA pedicle is scored at the planned transecton line. High ligation of vessels can be performed either proximal or just distal to the take off of the left colic vessels using a bipolar energy device. Ligation of the IMA and IMV opens up retroperitoneal spaces further. Medial-to-lateral blunt dissection is further carried out over the Gerota's fascia and laterally to the Toldt's fascia.

Figure 18.1 Trocar placements.

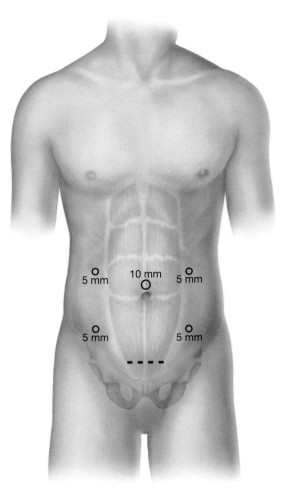

The patient is then placed in the reverse Trendelenburg position. The surgeon grasps the transverse colon and gently pulls it caudally while the assistant grasps the greater omentum and retracts it anteriorly and in the cephalad direction. The greater omentum is separated starting close to the midtransverse colon where the two leaves of the omentum are fused together. Once a window is created into the lesser sac, the index finger of the surgeon's left hand hooks the transverse colon and retracts the colon caudally and ventrally. While maintaining tissue triangulation, the greater omentum is separated from the transverse colon toward the splenic flexure. The patient is placed back in the Trendelenburg position and the surgeon's left hand is placed behind the mesentery of the sigmoid colon and the lateral attachments are exposed. The lateral attachments are sharply taken down using an energy device placed through the left lower quadrant port. It is easiest to start the detachment distally and to proceed proximally. At this point, the lienocolic ligament is sharply taken down. The best exposure is achieved when the colon is retracted caudally.

Once the colon is dissected down to the level of sacral promontory, the sigmoid colon is exteriorized through the Pfannenstiel incision and the colon is divided at the proximal margin of resection. Staple line is transected from the left colon and a purse-string suture is placed around the end of the left colon and tied around the center rod of a circular stapler anvil. The left colon is packed away in the upper abdomen with a tagged suture placed through the center rod of the anvil.

The proximal end of the rectosigmoid stump (the specimen) is drawn out through the Gelport® central opening (Gelport® left in place) and a laparotomy pad is wrapped around the colon and secured using #2 silk ties. Pneumoperitoneum is re-established. Even with colon stump drawn out through the Gelport®, pneumoperitoneum is well

Figure 18.2 Gentle cephalad traction of the externalized bowel creates excellent tension and exposure for posterior and lateral rectal dissection.

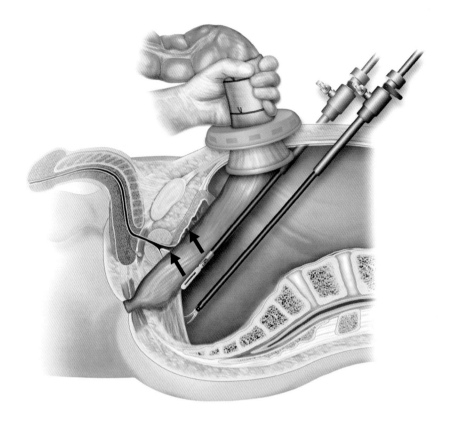

maintained. Using the laparotomy pad covering the bowel as a handle for gripping it, continuous and gentle ventral traction of the externalized bowel creates excellent tension and exposure for posterior and lateral rectal dissection (Fig. 18.2). As laparoscopic rectal dissection proceeds, constant tension is maintained by applying continuous traction on the exteriorized colon. Simultaneous additional anterior and side-to-side retraction of the rectum inside the pelvis, using laparoscopic bowel grasping instruments, provides additional exposure and tension (Fig. 18.3). This additional retraction avoids undue tension required by pulling of the rectum using the laparotomy pad, with potential inadvertent injury to the mesorectum. It also permits counter traction of the adjacent soft tissues from which the rectum is being dissected. As the rectum is dissected laterally, tension on the rectal stump should be eased, allowing lateral retraction of the rectum using a laparoscopic instrument (Fig. 18.4).

Once the rectum is fully mobilized posteriorly and laterally, the rectosigmoid stump is placed gently back through the Gelport® into the abdomen and the anterior dissection

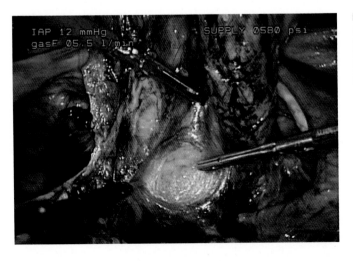

Figure 18.3 Simultaneous anterior and side-to-side retraction of the rectum inside the pelvis, using laparoscopic bowel grasping instruments, provides additional exposure and tension.

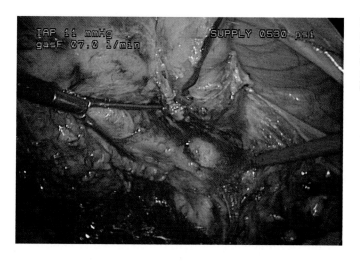

Figure 18.4 As the rectum is dissected laterally, tension on the rectal stump should be eased, allowing lateral retraction of the rectum using a laparoscopic instrument.

is performed (Fig. 18.5). Stapling of the distal rectum can be accomplished as required, either laparoscopically or directly through the hand port incision using an open method. Once the anastomosis is created, we typically perform a flexible sigmoidoscopy to examine the tissues proximal and distal to the anastomosis for adequate tissue perfusion and the staple line for hemostasis and possible defect. Air leak test is routinely performed. In case of air leak, defect in the anastomosis can be easily recognized and repaired through the incision. The incisions are closed in the usual fashion.

 ## POSTOPERATIVE MANAGEMENT

Oral gastric tubes are removed at the end of the procedure. Patients are offered liquids on the first postoperative day. Diet is advanced as tolerated. Patients are transitioned over to oral analgesics when tolerating substantial diet. Foley catheter is usually removed on postoperative day 4.

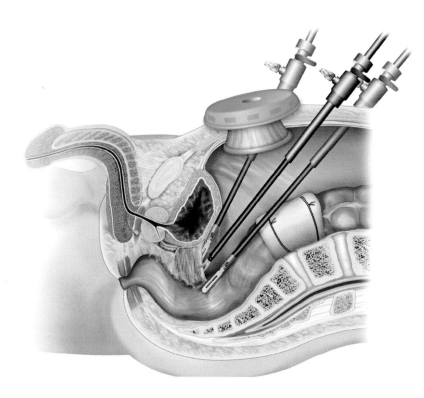

Figure 18.5 Once the rectum is fully mobilized posteriorly and laterally, the rectosigmoid stump is placed gently back through the Gelport® into the abdomen and the anterior dissection is performed.

RESULTS/CONCLUSIONS

We recently published our data of 103 patients who underwent laparoscopic and hand-assisted laparoscopic surgery for mid and low rectal cancer (6). Fifty-eight of these patients underwent hand-assisted and 45 patients underwent "straight" laparoscopic proctectomy and our overall conversion rate was 2.9%. With mean follow-up time of 42 months, local recurrence rate was 5% at 5 years. Overall survival was 91% and disease-free survival was 73.1% at 5 years.

Subgroup analysis comparing laparoscopic versus hand-assisted laparoscopic surgery revealed no significant difference between the two groups in regards to operative time and the number of lymph nodes harvested. Complication rates were similar between the two groups.

Although these results are encouraging, we cannot make any conclusion about long-term outcomes until we have results from adequately powered multicenter controlled trials. Currently, there are several ongoing multicenter trials that will hopefully provide with the answers in the near future: ACOSOG Z6051 trial from the U.S., COLOR II trial from Europe, Canada, and Asia, and Japanese JCOG 0040 trial.

Recommended References and Readings

1. Aziz O, Constantinides V, Tekkis PP, et al. Laparoscopic versus open surgery for rectal cancer: a meta-analysis. *Ann Surg Oncol* 2006;13:413–24.
2. Vithiananthan S, Cooper Z, Betton K, et al. Hybrid laparoscopic (lap) flexure takedown and open procedure for rectal resection is associated with significantly shorter length of stay than equivalent open resection. *Dis Colon Rectum* 2001;44(7):927–35.
3. Lee SW, Yoo J, Dujovny N, et al. Laparoscopic vs. hand-assisted laparoscopic sigmoidectomy for diverticulitis. *Dis Colon Rectum* 2006;49(4):464–9.
4. Marcello PW, Fleshman JW, Milsom JW, et al. Hand-assisted laparoscopic vs. laparoscopic colorectal surgery: a multicenter, prospective, randomized trial. *Dis Colon Rectum* 2009;51(6):818–26.
5. Lee SW, Sonoda T, Milsom JW. Expediting of laparoscopic rectal dissection using a hand-access device. *Dis Colon Rectum* 2007;50(6):927–9.
6. Milsom JW, de Oliveira O Jr, Trencheva KI, et al. Long-term outcomes of patients undergoing curative laparoscopic surgery for mid and low rectal cancer. *Dis Colon Rectum* 2009;52(7):1215–22.

19 Hybrid Laparoscopic/ Open Low Anterior Resection

Makram Gedeon, Richard L. Whelan, and Eric J. Dozois

Introduction

The hybrid low anterior resection (LAR), as originally described, is an operation in which the first part of the procedure (left colon mobilization) is performed laparoscopically and the second part (pelvic dissection) is accomplished using open methods via a Pfannenstiel or lower midline incision. The hybrid approach to sphincter-saving rectal resections was first introduced a decade ago when limited data existed concerning the oncologic efficacy of laparoscopic total mesorectal excision (TME) (1). In addition, concerns about the oncologic outcomes of minimally invasive methods for colon cancer existed due to early reports of port site wound recurrences. Data from the large randomized controlled trials (COST, CLASSIC, and COLOR) were not yet available. Moreover, hand-assist devices (second generation) were expensive, cumbersome, difficult to use, and therefore not very popular.

In this environment, the originators of the hybrid method, convinced of the benefits of laparoscopy, sought means of utilizing closed methods to significantly decrease overall incision length and physiologic impact, while permitting an open rectal mobilization and resection for cancer patients. The hybrid approach, as described in the following text, was the result. The hybrid method will significantly decrease incision length only if the splenic flexure would have been mobilized for an open operation. In the authors' view, flexure mobilization is indicated in the great majority of patients with rectal cancer undergoing LAR and thus most patients will benefit from this hybrid method.

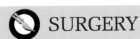 SURGERY

Order of Operation and Division of Tasks

The laparoscopic portion of the operation is performed first, followed by the open method to complete the procedure. The steps of the LAR undertaken through the laparoscopic approach include: (a) splenic flexure mobilization, (b) proximal vessel ligation, (c) division of the colon and mesentery, and (d) the initial mobilization of the rectum. After completion of the above steps, the abdomen is desufflated and a low midline or a Pfannenstiel incision is made and the case is completed using open methods.

LAPAROSCOPIC PORTION

The patient is placed in the modified lithotomy position with both arms tucked to the side with a foley catheter. Standard anesthesia monitoring, perioperative antibiotics, and subcutaneous heparin are administered. A 5-port arrangement is utilized by the authors so that both the surgeon and the first assistant have 2 ports available to them. A 5 or 10 mm camera port is placed just caudad to the umbilicus. In the lower part of the right lower quadrant a 12 mm port (to allow for intracorporeal stapling) is placed. A 5 mm port is placed more cephalad, also on the right side, at the site chosen for the diverting ileostomy, at the level of the umbilicus or to the right of the upper midline. Two 5 mm ports are placed on the left side, one low in the left lower quadrant and the second approximately at the level of the umbilicus.

The splenic flexure is mobilized first because if this portion is not amenable to laparoscopic methods, early conversion can be initiated and the subsequent incision can be limited. There are four basic approaches to flexure takedown: (a) lateral to medial, (b) medial to lateral, starting just caudal to the sacral promontory on the right side of sigmoid mesentery, (c) medial to lateral, starting at the level of the inferior mesenteric vein (IMV), and (d) starting with the omental "peel" at the level of the distal transverse colon (seldom used). Regardless of the approach that is utilized, the flexure, the descending and distal transverse colon as well as the mesentery must be fully mobilized.

Medial to Lateral Starting at the IMV

The patient is placed in the reverse Trendelenburg position with the right side down. The surgeon and cameraperson stand on the patient's right side, the latter at the level of the patient's thighs, and the former just cephalad. The second assistant stands between the patient's legs. The area to be exposed is the base of the distal transverse and descending colon mesentery adjacent to the ligament of Treitz. The distal transverse colon is gently grasped by the first assistant via the upper port on the left and retracted upwards and cephalad. The proximal descending colon is grasped, also by the first assistant via the lower left port, and retracted up and to the left. This latter move should reveal the location of the left colic vessels that appear as a bowstring. The surgeon then gently moves the small bowel to the right and caudal aspect of the abdomen that should reveal the ligament of Treitz, the proximal jejunum, and the IMV at the base of the descending mesentery. Obtaining this medial and central exposure is the most difficult part of this approach.

The peritoneum of the mesentery is then scored with a scissors parallel to and a short distance above or below the IMV depending on whether this vein is to be sacrificed or preserved. This opening is enlarged with a bipolar or ultrasonic shears (monopolar devices are avoided when working in this central location) and the plane between the posterior surface of the descending colon mesentery and the anterior aspect of Gerota's fascia is established. This is a bloodless plane that is usually more superficial than anticipated; if minor bleeding is encountered when doing this dissection it is likely that one is working dorsal to the anterior layer of Gerota's fascia. The correct plane, once found, is further developed in the lateral, caudad, and cephalad directions thus creating a pocket. The lateral limit of dissection is the white line of Toldt while the cephalad limit is the edge of the inferior border of the pancreas. Once the pocket is established, the first assistant's graspers are placed inside the pocket and used to better expose the retroperitoneal field of dissection. If the IMV is divided at this point, or earlier, then the exposure is improved.

If the inferior mesenteric artery (IMA) is to be transected early, then its location must be established and the vessel exposed by scoring the peritoneum medially and inferiorly toward the pelvis. The retroperitoneal dissection is continued caudally from the already established IMV pocket. The IMA is divided only after it is certain that the left ureter is out of harms way. If the IMA is to be divided later in the case, a second mesenteric window is made, caudal to the left colic vessels toward the base of the mesentery. The retroperitoneal avascular dissection plane between the Toldt and Gerota's fascia can then be extended beneath the distal descending colon. The left ureter and gonadal vessels are bluntly dissected away from the underside of the colon mesentery toward the left iliac fossa. After completing the medial to lateral mobilization, the descending colon is retracted medially and the remaining lateral attachments are divided sharply. The proximal left colon is released to complete this portion of the procedure.

Medial to Lateral Starting at the Sacral Promontory

The surgeon stands on the patient's right side with the camera operator while the first assistant stands on the patient's left. The patient is placed in the Trendelenburg position with the right side down so as to shift the small bowel out of the lower abdomen. The dissection is initiated at the right base of the rectosigmoid colon at the level of the sacral promontory. The first assistant grasps the sigmoid and rectosigmoid and retracts them up and to the left which places the rectosigmoid mesentery on stretch and exposes the groove between the inferior mesenteric vascular pedicle and the retroperitoneum. The surgeon then incises the peritoneum immediately beneath the IMA at the level of the sacral promontory and extends this opening into the pelvis for a distance and also cephalad toward the takeoff of the IMA. A plane is developed between the presacral structures and the colon mesentery working from the right toward the left. Care must be taken to identify and preserve the right hypogastric nerve. The left ureter and hypogastric nerve can usually be identified over the iliac artery and dissected away from the mesocolon. This posterior plane dissection is continued cephalad beneath the left colon mesentery toward the origin of the IMA. The peritoneum at the base of the left colic mesentery must be scored to expose the IMA and its branches. The left ureter and nerve in the posterior plane are dissected free of the mesentery, and the IMA is divided. If the IMA is transected at the level of the bifurcation to the left colic and superior rectal artery, the IMV can also be mobilized and divided at this point. Anteroproximal transection of the IMV requires incision of the peritoneum anterior to the aorta to the level of the ligament of Treitz to identify the vein adjacent to the duodenojejunal junction. After detaching these vessels, the medial to lateral mobilization is continued cephalad beneath the sigmoid and descending colon mesentery toward the splenic flexure.

Lateral to Medial Approach

The patient is placed in reverse Trendelenburg position with the right side down. The first assistant stands on the patient's right side with the camera operator while the surgeon stands between the legs. The first assistant, using two atraumatic graspers, retracts the distal descending and proximal sigmoid colon medially and upwards that creates tension on the lateral attachments. The surgeon initiates the dissection by dividing the white line of Toldt with a scissors or other device inserted through the lower left port. The dissection begins at the pelvic brim and continues cephalad toward the splenic flexure. As the mobilization progresses, the medial and upward traction provided by the first assistant must be increased so as to maintain traction on the attachments. The correct dissection plane between the anterior Gerota's fascia and the posterior aspect of the mesocolon must be found and developed with minimal to no bleeding. This plane is often not evident at the start, but once established, it is usually easy to maintain throughout to complete the mobilization. At the flexure it is important to make the transition from the deeper retroperitoneal plane to a more superficial plane ventral to the pancreas. As one nears the flexure, there is often a tendency to drift lateral and cephalad toward the spleen. The flexure should be pulled caudal and medial and then lifted anterior toward the abdominal wall by the assistant to expose the embryologic avascular plane that often lies well below the spleen.

Omental Peel

This step is the same regardless of the order of operation or the chosen method of descending colon mobilization. The goal is to separate the distal transverse colon from the omentum and the stomach. Most commonly the omentum is "peeled" from the colon by dividing the avascular attachments along the antimesenteric surface of the transverse colon. The omentum is reflected up and toward the head while the transverse colon is retracted caudally and dorsally. This dissection is best started just to the left of the midtransverse colon so as to facilitate entry into the lesser sac and a view of the back wall of the stomach. The surgeon must be beware of the possibility of inadvertently "overshooting" the mark and making a window in the transverse colon mesentery which is both incorrect and dangerous as the marginal artery may be inadvertently divided. Provided that the dorsal wall of the stomach can be seen through the window between the colon and the omentum the dissection plane is correct. After entering the lesser sac the remaining attachments between the omentum and the distal transverse colon are divided. The remaining splenic flexure attachments are then divided. The base of the distal transverse mesocolon, just lateral to the site of transection of the IMV anal ventral the inferior edge of the pancreas, is divided to release the final posterior attachment of the splenic flexure. Atypical mesenteric arteries in this area may require hemostatic division. Alternatively, the gastrocolic ligament can be transected outside the gastroepiploic arcade along the great curve of the stomach that detaches the stomach from the still adherent transverse colon and omentum.

Proximal Transection of the Colon and Mesentery

The proximal point of bowel transection should be chosen and the colon and mesentery intracorporeally divided prior to initiating the open portion of the LAR. Accomplishing these tasks facilitates the open part of the case. It is important to assess the mobility of the descending and distal transverse colon to determine the proximal most point that will reach into the distal pelvis without tension. The blood supply of this part of the colon should also be assessed to ensure that it is well vascularized. The mesentery is then divided starting at the base just proximal to where the IMA was transected. Great care must be taken at all times to preserve the marginal vessels close to the point of transection. Finally, the colon is divided with an intracorporeal linear stapling device completely detaching the upper and lower bowel and mesenteric segments.

Initial Rectal Mobilization

The peritoneum of the left or right pelvic gutter can be easily scored provided the rectosigmoid and distal sigmoid colon is retracted anteriorly, cephalad, and toward the opposite side. In fact, several of the descending colon mobilization methods described in the preceding text (lateral to medial and medial to lateral starting at the sacral promontory) include scoring of the iliac fossa peritoneum and partial mobilization of the rectosigmoid mesentery. A monopolar, bipolar, or ultrasonic shears can be used to score the peritoneum and to dissect beneath the rectosigmoid and proximal rectal mesentery. Traction must be maintained on the rectosigmoid to facilitate dissection posteriorly; as this plane is developed, the hypogastric nerves and the ureters need to be identified and preserved. Once started, the most caudal of the first assistant's retractors should be placed in the posterior pocket, opened wide, and then levered so as to lift the overlying mesorectum anteriorly and toward the head. Meanwhile, the first assistant's cephalad retractor is used to retract the mesorectum medially and upward at the level of the sacral promontory, thus providing more traction and improving the surgeons view of the dissection field. The peritoneum can be scored to the anterior reflection. Once completed, the peritoneal attachments on the opposite side are scored in a similar manner. It is usually a relatively simple matter to join the left and right dissection planes beneath the rectosigmoid mesentery. The anterior peritoneal reflection should be scored, if possible laparoscopically, and the dissection initiated for 1 to 2 cm.

Prior to beginning the open portion of the procedure, the proximal bowel should once again be assessed for adequate length to reach the low pelvis. Occasionally, additional mobilization will be needed and it is best done laparoscopically. In the authors' experience, retroperitoneal nonvascular attachments that have not been fully transected, can limit the downward reach of the proximal bowel. Moreover, if the ascending branch of the left colic artery has been left intact with the IMA at its origin, it may need to be transected proximally to gain additional length.

Open Portion of the Case

As originally described, after completing the closed portion of the operation, the abdomen is desufflated (through the port sites—to decrease risk of malignant cell implantation) and the laparoscopic ports removed. It is advised that prior to desufflation, the fascial suture(s) for the 12-mm right lower quadrant port be placed laparoscopically with a laparoscopic suture passer or similar device. Next, either a lower midline or a Pfannenstiel incision is made. If a midline incision is made it should start just above the pubic symphysis and extend cephalad. If a Pfannenstiel incision is made it should be placed about 2 fingerbreadths above the pubic symphysis and be centered on the midline. In both cases, the incision should be between 8 and 10 cm in length. This length will vary depending on the size of the surgeon's hand, the body habitus of the patient, and the size of the tumor. If need be, the incision can be enlarged.

The use of a wound protector of some type is advised. As mentioned, prior intracorporeal division of the proximal bowel and mesentery facilitates retraction of the proximal colon and small bowel. To start, the proximal end of the bowel specimen is identified and retracted up and out of the wound. All other bowel in the field is then retracted laterally or cephalad after placing some moist laparotomy pads. A bladder retractor is then placed and the open rectal mobilization commenced using standard open instruments and retractors (St. Mark's, wide and narrow Dever; we have found a lighted, narrow St. Mark's retractor very useful for this portion). A total mesenteric excision is then carried out and the rectum divided distally with a transverse linear stapler. If the cancer is located in the proximal rectum or proximal midrectum and the decision has been made not to divide the rectum close to the levator muscles, then the rectal mesentery will also need to be transected in addition to the rectum itself. The specimen is removed. The proximal colon is brought into the field and the proximal anvil of the circular end-to-end stapler placed into the colon and secured with a purse string. The completed anastomosis is checked for leaks and a decision made about proximal diversion. If an ileostomy is planned preoperatively, one of the right-sided ports can be placed at the site chosen for the ileostomy. The skin and fascial wounds are enlarged and the bowel exteriorized to create the stoma. The lower abdominal incision is then closed in the usual manner.

CURRENT STATUS OF LAPAROSCOPIC TME

It is possible to perform an oncologically sound rectal mobilization and TME using laparoscopic methods. A patient with a small to moderate sized tumor, and normal BMI, is appropriate for treatment with the pure laparoscopic approach (with small 3–5 cm incision made for specimen extraction and placement of stapling anvil). This should only be performed by a surgeon with significant experience in minimally invasive pelvic surgery. However, a planned hand-assisted (see in the following text) or hybrid operation is reasonable for surgeons not comfortable with laparoscopic rectal mobilization, patients with large tumors or phlegmon, and obese patients. Further, when conversion proves necessary during a straight laparoscopic operation, the hand/hybrid method is the best next approach to maintain the patient-related benefits of a minimally invasive approach.

HAND-ASSISTED LAR, DESCENDANT OF THE HYBRID

The obvious and important advantage of hand-assisted methods over hybrid methods is that it is possible to continue working laparoscopically, under pneumoperitoneum, with the hand device in place. In a planned hand-assisted LAR, the lower abdominal incision is made at the start of the case. The surgeon maintains access to all quadrants of the abdomen unlike the situation with the hybrid method. Also, if it proves difficult to complete the case under pneumoperitoneum, or if the surgeon prefers, the case can be completed using open methods via the hand-device incision. Thus, a hand device permits both closed and open surgical methods to be employed. The hybrid method alone allows only open surgery once the lower abdominal incision has been made. In the hybrid approach the lower incision is made midcase.

It is important to note that the incision needed for the hand-assisted approach is 1–2 cm smaller than that needed for the hybrid approach (1,2). One small randomized study that compared hand-assisted and straight laparoscopic left segmental or total colectomy noted that the hand method was associated with a 30-minute time savings for left segmental resection and a 56-minute reduction for total abdominal colectomy (1,2).

With several notable exceptions, it is hard to conceive of an elective situation where it would be logical or advantageous to plan preoperatively for a hybrid laparoscopic/open LAR instead of a hand-assisted procedure. Exceptions include a patient with a large bulky tumor or phlegmon or known severe pelvic adhesions. The hybrid approach also remains a reasonable approach for surgeons who do not want to undertake the pelvic dissection and distal rectal transection using closed methods. Hand-assisted methods, for the same reasons as mentioned in the preceding text, may be a choice when it becomes necessary to convert during a pure laparoscopic case. Situations where a direct conversion to open methods is logical include notable bleeding, significant bowel injury, intolerance of the pneumoperitoneum.

AUTHORS CURRENT APPROACH

Except for patients with a very large tumor, or the very obese, the case is initiated by placing a camera port periumbilically and two 5-mm working ports on the right side. A thorough exploration is then carried out. If the working conditions are reasonable, the pelvis not hostile, and the lesion not too large, an additional one or two 5-mm ports are placed on the left side and the case is carried out using straight laparoscopic methods. If, however, after exploration the attending surgeon judges that by the end of the case an incision of 8 cm or larger is likely to be needed despite the use of straight laparoscopic methods then a hand device will immediately be placed in the lower abdomen and the case carried out using hand-assisted laparoscopic methods (3). If in the course of a straight laparoscopic LAR significant problems are encountered and the judgment is made that the straight laparoscopic approach is not sufficient then the case is converted to the hand-assisted approach and then continued under pneumoperitoneum. If it proves impossible to finish the case via the hand method laparoscopically, then the case is completed using open methods through the hand incision (3). In this situation, if needed, the incision is extended to the size that would normally be used for the hybrid approach.

INCISION LENGTH

Skin incision length is one of the only objective parameters we have that can be used to assess the abdominal trauma incurred during an operation apart from operative length. It is understood by all that the fascial incision length is longer than the skin incision length. The final skin incision length should be measured at the time the dressing is being applied in the operating room and then recorded on the written and dictated operative reports. Routine measurement and reporting of largest incision length will facilitate meaningful comparison of series of operations both within and between institutions.

Recommended References and Readings

1. Vithianathan S, Cooper Z, Betten K, et al. Hybrid laparoscopic flexure takedown and open procedure for rectal resection is associated with significantly shorter length of stay than equivalent open resection. *Dis Colon Rectum* 2001;44(7):927–35.
2. Marcello PW, Fleshman JW, Milsom JW, et al. Hand-assisted laparoscopic vs. laparoscopic colorectal surgery: a multicenter, prospective, randomized trial. *Dis Colon Rectum* 2008;51(6):818–26; discussion 826–8.
3. Stein S, Whelan RL. The controversy regarding hand-assisted colorectal resection [published online ahead of print November 1, 2007]. *Surg Endosc* 2007;12:2123–6.

20 Intersphincteric Restorative Proctocolectomy for Malignant Disease

Ron G. Landmann

Intersphincteric Restorative Proctocolectomy for Malignant Disease

Background and Rationale

When addressing the issue of rectal cancer treatment, four major objectives are uniformly pursued: (a) cure—including primary local resection with negative margins and subsequent prevention of locoregional (LR) and distant recurrence, (b) decreased morbidity and mortality, (c) prevention of sexual and urinary dysfunction—as manifested by erectile dysfunction, retrograde ejaculation, vaginal dryness, dyspareunia, and difficulty voiding, and (d) maintenance of intestinal continuity/avoidance of a permanent stoma. Currently, despite the advances in chemotherapeutics, biologics, and radiation therapy, surgery is the primary modality to achieve these goals.

Current standard practice, based on preoperative staging, either with endorectal ultrasonography or magnetic resonance imaging, recommends low anterior resection (LAR) or abdominoperineal resection (APR) for most advanced (i.e., T3 or N+) distal lesions, within 0-5 cm above the dentate line. All of the advances in rectal surgery have been integral to the advent of intersphincteric restorative proctocolectomy (IRP) while continuing to meet the above primary objectives. In this procedure, the internal anal sphincter—a continuation of the rectal wall—is completely or partially excised to obtain the necessary full-thickness distal resection margin (1). Subsequent coloanal anastomosis to the remaining sphincter complex thereby restores intestinal continuity, with a goal of improved quality of life while preserving oncologic and functional outcomes. With these refinements and improvements in both neoadjuvant chemoradiation therapy and surgical techniques, patients now have another option available for sphincter preservation.

PREOPERATIVE PLANNING

Patient Selection and Preoperative Evaluation

Due to the inherent morbidity associated with a permanent stoma (2,3), a restorative proctocolectomy may be offered to all patients with tumors that are amenable to the procedure. The decision to perform a restorative procedure should be made in conjunction with the patient after discussing the likely postoperative oncologic and functional outcomes. Whereas involvement of the internal sphincter by invasive disease should not be viewed as a contraindication to intersphincteric resection (4), invasion of the external sphincter or the musculature of the pelvic floor would make the disease incurable by IRP. A digital rectal examination that shows fixation of the tumor should also be considered a contraindication as it likely means that the tumor has broken through the intersphincteric plane and has fixed the internal sphincter—an embryological derivative and continuation of the rectal wall—to the external sphincter or the pelvic floor musculature (5,6). Such disease would be better managed by APR. A preoperative pelvic magnetic resonance imaging or endoanal ultrasound is instrumental in assessing the extent of tumor spread. Indeed, any tumor that has sphincter involvement, prior to the use of neoadjuvant combined modality therapy, should be excluded from an IRP and treated by a standard APR, despite improvement after therapy. Tumors that respond with downstaging and/or down-sizing after neoadjuvant chemoradiation therapy generally would make patients candidates for LAR/IRP. A chest X-ray and a computed tomography scan of the abdomen and pelvis should be performed to rule out stage IV metastatic disease. In the case of low rectal tumors, care must be taken to examine the groins for evidence of inguinal lymphadenopathy (7). The results of these preoperative evaluations, in conjunction with those following neoadjuvant therapy, should be used to determine the distal margin of resection (8) and potential for resection with maintenance of intestinal continuity/sphincter preservation.

Body habitus also plays a significant role in operative decision making. Ideally, the patient should not be obese (body mass index [BMI] <30–32). Patients that are males, have a narrow pelvis, or a long anal canal may also make it more difficult to perform an ideal, oncologic resection. Indeed, an IRP is more likely to be performed in patients that are male, have distal tumors, or increased BMI due to difficulty introducing stapling devices (for LAR).

It is also important to determine the patient's preoperative continence. This assessment can be made by history, digital rectal examination, manometry, or a combination of these methods. In patients with good sphincter function on digital rectal examination but recent development of clinical incontinence, the dysfunction may be attributable to the neoplastic process, and it is reasonable to expect that they may benefit from an IRP. A validated incontinence score should be used. Patients with severe preoperative incontinence may be better served with a permanent stoma. However, these patients may benefit from an intersphincteric non-restorative proctocolectomy due to improved healing of the pelvic floor compared to APR, especially after undergoing neoadjuvant chemoradiation therapy. Though age *per se* is not an exclusion criterion, generally older patients have decreased sphincter tone and also less musculature needed for fecal control after undergoing radiation therapy and internal sphincter resection.

There are certain exclusion criteria that are generally accepted when evaluating ideal candidates for IRP: involvement of the external sphincter by tumor, inadequate distal margin (<1–2 cm), poor preoperative (or anticipated postoperative) sphincter function, patient preference, or an initial, pre-neoadjuvant uT3 lesion with external sphincter complex involvement (1). When looking at a nationwide database, factors that were noted to be independent predictors of sphincter preservation included younger age, proximal lesions, non-fixed lesions, and institution (9). Though not specifically addressed, individual training technique and outcomes are likely to be attributable to the success of an IRP. One cannot stress enough the importance, as with any procedure, that specialty training and experience is mandatory for selecting and then completing these procedures. There is a learning curve, which is longer when the procedure is performed laparoscopically. Furthermore, a multi- or interdisciplinary approach to evaluation and selection of these patients may help in the postoperative period.

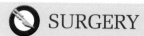 SURGERY

Surgical Technique

Various descriptions of intersphincteric restorative proctectomy have been presented in literature over the past 40 years (10–12). This extended resection for rectal malignancies is predicated on the knowledge that rectal tumor infiltration is initially limited by an embryonic plane between the visceral structures and the surrounding somatic skeletal muscles of the pelvic floor (13). An IRP attempts to rid the patient of disease while the tumor is still confined to this envelop. Throughout the dissection, particular attention is paid to minimize the damage to the sympathetic and parasympathetic fibers that are involved in bladder function and sexual potency. While damage to the sympathetic fibers leads to a decreased ability to attain orgasm, parasympathetic or combined damage results in impotence in men and vaginal dryness in women, manifesting as dyspareunia (14).

Fecal Diversion

The author's and editor's preferences are for routine temporary diversion of all patients that undergo IRP. There remains some controversy about the role of diversion in rectal surgery due to the morbidity associated with a stoma as well as a second surgery to reverse it. In our experience, as in the experience of others, the increased salvage rate, decreased rate of reoperation, and decreased clinical significance of anastomotic failures in patients with diverted stomas makes the diverting procedure justifiable (15).

Although there is one randomized prospective trial that shows decreased morbidity in terms of postoperative ileus and small bowel obstructions with a diverting transverse loop colostomy (16), our preference is to utilize a diverting loop ileostomy. As the splenic flexure is often mobilized to provide adequate length for a coloanal anastomosis during an IRP, maturing a transverse loop colostomy becomes significantly more difficult than a diverting loop ileostomy. The operation to reverse a loop ileostomy is also much easier with decreased postoperative morbidity in terms of wound infection and abdominal wall hernia formation (17).

The anastomosis is studied 6 weeks later and if the results are satisfactory, the diversion is reversed (4).

Total Mesorectal Excision

In the setting of more distal tumors requiring IRP, our preference is to perform a complete laparoscopic total mesorectal excision (TME). Based on numerous trials, and also summarized by position statements from the American Society of Colon & Rectal Surgeons and the Society of American Gastrointestinal and Endoscopic Surgeons, laparoscopic techniques for curable colon cancer have been deemed to be a safe alternative when correct oncological techniques are followed. However, it is critically important to emphasize that a laparoscopic approach to rectal cancer is not a simple procedure, and that it requires proper training and experience in advanced minimally invasive surgery (18). Most of the data presented are based upon national data evaluated laparoscopic colon surgery and extrapolated based on multicenter experience with laparoscopic rectal cancer surgery. There is currently an American College of Surgeons Oncology Group trial underway evaluating oncological outcomes of rectal cancer surgery and operative approach—open, laparoscopic, and robotic (ACOSOG Z6051).

Description of Technique

The procedure may conveniently be broken down into seven distinct steps: (a) mobilization of the sigmoid colon, left colon, and splenic flexure,(b) high intracorporeal vascular division of the inferior mesenteric artery and vein, (c) sharp TME, (d) intersphincteric distal dissection by the abdominal approach (if possible), (e) transperineal transection/intrasphincteric dissection and excision of the rectosigmoid, (f) extracorporeal transperineal creation and anastomosis of a reservoir, and (g) temporary diversion. Below is described the laparoscopic technique for an IRP.

Abdominal Phase (Steps 1–4)

The patient is placed in a modified lithotomy position and both legs are secured in Allen stirrups. Intraoperative evaluation of the rectal tumor is performed by digital rectal examination and rigid proctosigmoidoscopy to determine resectability and the site of distal resection. The rectum is then irrigated with a cytocidal solution of diluted Betadine. Both the abdomen and perineum are prepped and draped in a sterile manner. In females, the vagina is also sterilely prepped. Cystoscopy and bilateral ureteral catheter placement may be helpful in the setting of an irradiated pelvis.

Peritoneal access is obtained utilizing the open Hassan technique by a 1 cm supraumbilical incision. Upon obtaining pneumoperitoneum, a 10 mm 30-degree scope is utilized to perform a diagnostic laparoscopy. Particular attention is paid to the liver surface as well as the surface of the peritoneum to evaluate for metastatic disease. A 10/12 mm is placed in the right lower quadrant about 2 cm medial and 2 cm cephalad from the anterior superior iliac spine. An additional 5 mm port is placed in the right upper quadrant about 8 cm cephalad from the previous right lower quadrant port. A final 5 mm port may be placed in the left lower quadrant if needed for later use. This port can help with retraction of the rectum out of the pelvis, defining the anterior dissection plane, and in mobilization of the splenic flexure.

With the patient in slight Trendelenburg and airplaned to the right, the left lateral attachments of the sigmoid to the peritoneum are dissected free utilizing an ultrasonic dissector. Though some surgeons have used energized shears/electrocautery devices, the authors feel that an ultrasonic dissector may have a role in later portions of the case and maintenance of hemostasis. Care is taken to identify the left ureter and to preserve its posterolateral position. The descending colon is mobilized by freeing its lateral abdominal wall attachments along the line of Toldt. This dissection is carried proximally to the splenic flexure. The patient is then placed in slight reverse Trendelenburg and starting approximately halfway between the hepatic flexure and the falciform ligament, the gastrocolic omentum and its attachments to the transverse colon are divided. Dissection is carried out distally toward the previous dissection plane. The splenic flexure is thus completely and fully mobilized.

Placing the patient back in Trendelenburg, a high ligation of the inferior mesenteric artery (IMA) is performed. The relative anatomy of the sympathetic nerves in this region must be kept in mind while performing the next segment of the dissection. The superior hypogastric plexus and the origin of the hypogastric nerves overlie the aorta and the sacrum. They lie behind the IMA as it travels toward the rectum. These sympathetic fibers can sometimes be incorporated in the IMA pedicle if ligation of the IMA is performed too close to its origin from the aorta (14).

With the sigmoid colon on stretch and the patient airplaned to the right, mesenteric dissection is continued proximally until the vascular pedicle containing the IMA is identified. A window is created around the IMA. High ligation of the IMA is then performed just distal to its takeoff from the aorta. The author prefers to utilize a vascular stapling device for this ligation. The inferior mesenteric vein is also dissected free and divided using another firing of the vascular stapler or ultrasonic dissector. These maneuvers allow enough proximal colon length to perform reconstruction with a tension-free anastomosis.

Attention is then turned to the sacral promontory and a sharp TME is performed in the bloodless plane. The plane is maximally visualized by lateral manipulation performed with the aid of the left lower quadrant abdominal port site and cephalad-anterior retraction of the rectum performed by the right upper quadrant port site. Both hypogastric nerves are identified and preserved. Dissection is carried out initially posteriorly, followed by laterally and finally anteriorly. Care must be taken to find the correct plane of dissection, described by Heald (13) as the "holy plane of rectal surgery," just outside the fascia propria as the hypogastric nerves pass tangentially to it and medial to the ureter.

The inferior hemorrhoidal plexus (IHP) sends delicate branches to the rectum that travel in the lateral ligaments. The routine use of large clamps to ligate the lateral ligaments in an attempt to avoid hemorrhage from the middle rectal artery is unnecessary as this vessel is found in only 20% of patients. Utilization of these large clamps may increase the risk of damaging the IHP (19,20). We do not routinely include the entirety of Denonvilliers' fascia (believed to be the conglomerate of two layers of the most distal pelvic peritoneum after the space within the layers is obliterated during embryogenesis) in our surgical specimen unless there is reason to believe that it would be required to obtain an R0 resection such as with an anterior lesion.

Care must be taken not to damage the delicate cavernosal fibers while performing the anterolateral separation of the distal rectum from the prostate and the seminal vesicles during both the abdominal and perineal portions of this dissection. The fibers are highly perceptible to damage as evidenced by case reports of patients suffering from neurogenic impotence after injection of sclerosant in too deep of a plane as attempted therapy for anteriorly located hemorrhoids (21). These fibers cannot be visualized, making knowledge of their location and pathway particularly crucial. After exiting from their sacral roots, they pass from the pelvis anterolateral to the rectum on their way to pierce the urogenital diaphragm before entering the corpora (14). Damage can be avoided by performing delicate and avoiding overaggressive rectal dissection at the 2 and 10 O'clock positions, as this is where the cavernosal fibers are at greatest risk. Laparoscopy aids in this dissection by affording a high definition and magnified view of the dissection planes with minimal traction artifact. This dissection is carried down to and past the levator plate and into the intersphincteric space.

Following this step, a loop of terminal ileum approximately 25 cm proximal to the ileocecal valve is exteriorized to fashion a loop ileostomy. It is brought out through the abdominal wall at the area previously marked by the stoma nurse. A mesenteric window is created at the apex of the loop and a standard stoma bridge rod is placed within this mesenteric window and sutured into place to prevent the small bowel from reducing back into the peritoneum.

Perineal Dissection (Step 5)

Different definitions regarding the types of intersphincteric resections are abound (22,23). There is, however, uniformity in describing the total intersphincteric resection. The distal resection includes the complete internal anal sphincter complex by dissection at the level of the intersphincteric groove. The subtotal intersphincteric resection transects the internal sphincter musculature by choosing a dissection line between the dentate and the level of the more distal intersphincteric groove. A partial intersphincteric resection incorporates a distal line of dissection at or above the dentate. Occasionally, depending on the size/location of the tumor, a non-circumferential/partial internal sphincter resection may be performed.

At the beginning of the perineal dissection, a decision must be made as to the distal extent of the resection specimen. Although current literature suggests that a negative margin of less than 1 cm does not impair oncologic outcomes, these studies are able to make such claims in patients with locally advanced cancers only (24). If an attempt to perform a partial intersphincteric resection is to be made, then the author prefers to start his plane of dissection at least 1 cm distal to the furthest extent of the tumor, if not ideally 2 cm. If this is not possible or if there is preoperative evidence of internal sphincter involvement, a complete/total intersphincteric resection is advised. In such a situation, the distal plane of the resection should be started at the level of the intersphincteric groove, which may be marked by the white line of Hilton.

Once this decision has been made, a self-retaining retractor (Lone Star Retractor®, Lone Star Medical Products Inc, Houston, TX, USA) is utilized for effacement and retraction of the anal canal. Electrocautery is utilized to perform a circumferential mucosal excision at a level at least 1 cm distal to the lesion. This is extended deep past the internal sphincter muscle until the intersphincteric plane is encountered. The anal orifice (or distal resection margin) may be sutured close and the dissection is continued proximally staying in the plane within the smooth and striated muscles. We find it helpful to begin the dissection posterior and lateral before dissecting anterior as the intersphincteric plane is easier to identify in these locations. During this part of the dissection, care must be taken to avoid compromising Denonvilliers' fascia as damage to the cavernosal fibers on the other side will usually lead to sexual dysfunction. Continued dissection in these planes eventually leads to communication with the abdominal dissection. At this point, therefore, the colon and rectum are completely free and the specimen is able to be brought out per the anus. Using two bowel clamps to avoid fecal contamination, the colon is divided at an area proximal to the division of the IMA. It is sent for frozen section analysis to evaluate for distal and circumferential margins. If the margins are positive, more tissue is excised until negative margins are obtained (12,25,26). In certain cases, the procedure is converted to an APR.

A coloanal anastomosis is then performed. Techniques for the various forms of restorative anastomoses are described below. Our preference is to perform a Baker-type side-to-end anastomosis (27) when a colonic J-pouch (CJP) cannot fit or be constructed. The Lone Star retractor is removed. To reduce the risk of tumor implantation and subsequent local recurrence, cytocidal washout is performed. The puncture sites of the Lone Star retractor are also irrigated as there have been reports of local recurrence at its puncture sites (28). A rolled up hemostatic foam is placed within the neorectum.

We then return to the abdomen and perform a diagnostic laparoscopy noting the tension free anastomosis. A drain is guided behind the neorectum and brought out through the left lower quadrant laparoscopic port site. All laparoscopic port sites are removed under direct visualization and the pneumoperitoneum is released. Fascia and skin incisions are closed and the diverting loop ileostomy (step 7) is matured in the standard manner. The diverting stoma is reversed with reestablishment of intestinal continuity performed after completion of postoperative adjuvant therapy. Generally, clinical, endoscopic, and radiological examination of the anastomosis is performed prior to reversal.

Techniques of Coloanal Anastomoses (Step 6)

End-to-End Coloanal Anastomosis

Generally, cases requiring IRP necessitate a hand-sewn anastomosis as using standard end-to-end stapling devices may not be appropriate. However, stapled techniques for restorative coloanal anastomosis (CAA) after subtotal intersphincteric proctectomy have been described. In this technique, the remnant internal sphincter is first prepared for anastomosis by eversion and placement of a purse-string suture. An end-to-end stapler is then utilized to perform the anastomosis (29). Our preference is to perform a hand-sewn anastomosis with a single layer of interrupted absorbable sutures. Each suture incorporates full thickness of the wall of the colon, a portion of the internal sphincter (or external sphincter in the case of a complete intersphincteric proctectomy), and anoderm. A straight end-to-end CAA is generally performed when none of the following reconstructive modalities are feasible. Careful attention to maintain orientation of the bowel and its mesentery is assured.

Transverse Coloplasty Pouch

Another modification of the coloanal anastomosis that results in a volume effect is the transverse coloplasty pouch (TCP) (30). Much like a stricturoplasty or a pyloroplasty, the coloplasty is performed by making a longitudinal incision on the antimesenteric side of the colon and by closing it in a horizontal manner. Our preference is to make a 10–12 cm longitudinal incision starting 4 cm proximal from the most distal stapled end of the colon to be anastomosed to the anus. This incision is then closed in a horizontal manner with a single layer of interrupted 3-0 polydioxanone sutures. Alternatively, this closure can be performed with a running inner layer of absorbable suture and an outer interrupted layer of nonabsorbable imbricating sutures. The stapled end is then introduced into the pelvis. The staple line is removed by electrocautery and a hand-sewn anastomosis is performed to the anal canal with interrupted sutures by a transanal approach as previously described above for straight end-to-end anastomoses.

A TCP or straight end-to-end CAA are utilized when the pelvis is restrictively narrowed, there may be insufficient intestinal length, an excessively bulky descending colonic mesentery exists, or surgeon preference.

Colonic J-Pouch Anal Anastomosis

The CJP was originally constructed to create a stool reservoir to nullify the increased frequency of bowel movements following a CAA. The author prefers to construct a 5–6 cm J-pouch as recommended by a prospective study evaluating its optimal size (31). The distal/efferent end of the colon is stapled. The pouch consists of a 10-12 cm segment of colon, with the distal half of this segment brought alongside the proximal half in an antiperistaltic/antimesenteric manner. The colon is held in this configuration with the aid of one or two stay sutures. A colotomy is performed with electrocautery at the side wall of the colon approximately 5–6 cm proximal from the distal efferent stapled end. A gastrointestinal anastomosis stapler is introduced through the colostomy and fired to create a side-to-side anastomosis of the colon resulting in a 5–6 cm CJP. The pouch is then introduced into the pelvis and a hand-sewn anastomosis is performed to the anal canal with interrupted sutures by a transanal approach as previously described in this chapter.

Though not reviewed, in select patients a complete proctocolectomy with intersphincteric dissection may be necessary. In these cases, an ileal pouch anal anastomosis may be utilized as the neorectum and completed in a similar fashion as the CJP. The technique of proctocolectomy and formation of an ileal reservoir with an ileoanal anastomosis is well described in this textbook. However, the ileal J-pouch should be constructed utilizing a total of 40 cm with a 20 cm pouch length rather than 5–6 cm as with the CJP.

Side-to-End/Baker-Type Coloanal Anastomosis

Baker described the successful use of a colorectal side-to-end anastomosis (27). More recently, surgeons are utilizing a Baker type side-to-end coloanal anastomosis following intersphincteric proctectomy. This method, which has also been referred to as an L-pouch, appears to provide decreased frequency of bowel movements. Furthermore, the L-pouch is less bulky than a CJP, allowing it to reach the anal canal with less difficulty. The technique requires the provision of a colotomy on the antimesenteric surface of the colon, measured 5-6 cm proximal to the stapled end. This colotomy is then anastomosed to the anal canal with interrupted sutures by a transanal approach as previously described in this chapter.

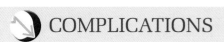

COMPLICATIONS

Complications and Anastomotic Problems

IRP suffers from an anastomotic stricture rate of 5.8% and an anastomotic leak rate between of 3–11% (32,33–35). Rates are seen to rise significantly for more distally situated anastomoses. Morbid sequelae of anastomotic leaks include anastomotic strictures, cancer recurrence, and poor postoperative anorectal function (32). These anastomotic problems, especially the leaks, lead to significant morbidity in the form of sepsis and delayed or non-closure of stoma. Also, strictures due to septic pelvic complications greatly limit continence after any of the above restorative coloanal anastomoses (6). Intra-abdominal sepsis also resulted in a decreased ability to achieve arousal (36). In an attempt to minimize these complications, authors have studied the various manners

Part III: Low Anterior Resection

of gastrointestinal restoration in these patients in an attempt to uncover the method that is most likely to heal without anastomotic problems.

There was some thought that due to a better blood supply in patients undergoing pouch procedures, their anastomosis may heal better with a resultant decrease in the rate of clinically significant anastomotic leaks. This theory seemed to be supported by initial reports indicating that there was a clinically significant lower incidence of anastomotic leaks following colonic pouch anastomosis (2%) compared to non-pouch CAA (15%) (37).

Studies evaluating the microcirculation at the anastomosis did not reveal the expected results. One group, utilizing laser fluorescence videography, evaluated the microcirculation around anastomosis after rectal resection in dogs. They compared end-to-end, side-to-end, and J-pouch coloanal anastomosis. Bowel perfusion was evaluated using IC-View laser fluorescence videography. Interestingly, it was discovered that straight coloanal anastomoses provides better anastomotic microcirculation after rectal resections than colonic-J-pouch anal anastomoses (CPA) or side-to-end anastomoses (38).

Later studies revealed the difference in leak rates between CPA and CAA to be due to a confounding variable. In this study, fecal diversion was performed in only 59% of patients with CAA and in 71% with CPA. A follow-up study by the same group with a protective ileostomy in all patients showed no significant differences. These results have since then been confirmed by other studies (6). Later, randomized studies looking at leak rates between TCP and CJP and a side-to-end anastomosis also revealed no clinically significant difference (6,34).

Reviewing the latest single and multicenter reports, anastomotic leaks and fistulae are noted to be the primary morbidity associated with IRP. Mortality is very low (Table 20.1) (1,4,22,23,32,40,39).

Quality Indicators and Pathological Comparisons

When evaluating patients undergoing IRP for rectal cancer, certain pathological results have been realized. Patients undergoing IRP generally had lower stage, (y)pT1–2, greater response to neoadjuvant chemoradiation therapy, increased rate of T downstaging, and lower grade differentiation than those patients undergoing APR (Table 20.2). Most of these reports also demonstrated an acceptable distal resection margin (DRM) as well as a generous/acceptable negative circumferential resection margin (CRM) with acceptable stage-for-stage LR recurrence rates. In the most recent data published from Memorial Sloan-Kettering Cancer Center, patients undergoing IRP and stapled anastomoses (for

TABLE 20.1	Complications After Intersphincteric Proctectomy								
	N	Anastomotic leak	Fistula	Stricture	Abdominal wound infection	Cardiac event	Pneumonia	PE/DVT	Other (ileus, UTI, bleeding, sepsis, UGIB, etc.)
Weiser, 2009 (1)	44	2	2	7	3	1	2	0	
Han, 2009 (39)	40	1			2				
Yamada, 2009 (23)	107	5		9	4		1		5
Ito, 2009 (22)	96	1						1	NR
Chamlou, 2007 (40)	90	8	1/8	1	1			1	6
Schiessel, 2005 (4)	121	6	2	11 (late, cons. Tx)				1 (fatal)	2
Tilney, 2007 & 2008 (meta-analysis) (32,41)	612	49 (10.5)		12 (5.8)					5 (3.1) Bleed

PE/DVT, pulmonary embolism/deep vein thrombosis; UTI, urinary tract infection; UGIB, upper gastrointestinal bleed.

TABLE 20.2	**Pathological Results of Intersphincteric Proctectomy**										
	Stage/(y)pTNM					**Response to CMT**				**Histology**	
	0	**I**	**II**	**III**	**IV**	**100%/pCR**	**86–99%**	**<86%**	**T dowstaging**	**Low**	**High**
Weiser, 2009 (1)	11 (25)	16 (36)	12 (27)	5(11)		11 (27)*	10 (24)*	20 (49)*	29 (66)*	42 (95)*	2 (5)*
Han, 2009 (39)		18 (45)	6 (15)	16 (40)					1/40		
Yamada, 2009 (23)		48 (45)	24 (22)	35 (33)						106 (99)	1 (1)
Chamlou, 2007 (42)	6 (8)	37 (41)	16 (18)	25 (28)	5 (6)						
Schiessel, 2005 (4)		49 (41)	33 (28)	37 (31)							

*P <0.05 when compared to APR. CMT, combined modality therapy/neoadjuvant chemoradiation therapy; pCR, pathological complete response.

higher lesions) had equivalent low LR rates, and were significantly lower than those patients necessitating APR (Table 20.3) (1).

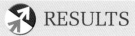# RESULTS

A meta-analysis of published cases of intersphincteric proctectomy revealed an operative mortality of 1.6%, an anastomotic stricture rate of 5.8%, and an anastomotic leak rate of 10.5% (32). Neoadjuvant chemoradiation significantly affects the patient's oncological and functional outcomes. Much effort has been spent toward finding the effects of the various modifications of this procedure on patient morbidity. The use of laparoscopy (44,45), lateral lymphadenectomy (46), and the various techniques of coloanal anastomosis have been evaluated.

Oncologic Outcomes

Some authors have wondered if the poor oncological results from APR compared with LAR are due to an unknown natural history of very low rectal cancers, with potential lymph-node metastases outside of the mesorectal envelope (7,47). An IRP is a potential intermediary that may be able to illuminate that concern as it often deals with the same tumors as an APR residing in the lowest part of the rectum.

In IRP, oncologic outcomes as measured by recurrence free survival and disease-specific survival seem not to be different, and indeed equivalent to those following LAR

TABLE 20.3	**Quality Indicators of Resection**							
	Median distal resection margin	**% + CRM ≤ 1 mm**			**LR (%)**		
		LAR/stapled	**LAR/IRP**	**APR**	**LAR/stapled**	**LAR/IRP**	**APR**
Weiser, 2009 (1)	1 cm (0.1–3.5)	0/41	2/44 (5)	8/63 (13)*	1/41 (2)	0/44 (0)	6/64 (9)*
Schiessel, 2005 (4)			3%			6/113 (5.3)	
Hohenberger, 2006 (26)			4%				
Rullier, 2005 (11)			11%			1/58 (2)	
Portier, 2007 (43)						18/173 (10.6)	
Kohler, 2000 (5)						3/31 (9.7)	
Ito, 2009 (22)	1.5 (2.2–5.5)		3/96 (3%)			12/96 (12.5)	
Chamlou, 2007 (40)	1.2 (0.5–35)		4/90 (4.4%)			8/90 (8.9, 2 pt = LR+ DR)	
Han, 2009 (39)			0/40			2/40 (5)	
Tilney, 2007 Meta-analysis (32)	0.7–2.4					51/538 (9.5)	

APR, abdominoperineal resection; CRM, circumferential resection margin; IRP, intersphincteric restorative proctocolectomy; LAR, low anterior resection.
*P <0.05
Most of these reports demonstrated an acceptable DRM as well as a generous/acceptable negative CRM with acceptable stage-for-stage LR recurrence rates. In the most recent data published from Memorial Sloan-Kettering Cancer Center, patients undergoing ISRD and stapled anastomoses (for higher lesions) had equivalent low LR rates, and significantly lower than those patients necessitating APR.

TABLE 20.4	One Year Functional Results After Intersphincteric Proctectomy						
	>5 BM/24 h	Nocturnal defecation	Urgency	Pad wearing	Flatus/feces discrimination	Stool fragmentation	Diet limitation
Chamlou, 2007 (40)	3 (4)	24 (29)	16 (19)	38 (46)	21 (25.3)	40 (41)	30 (36)
Ito, 2009 (22)	27 (36)	13 (18)	9 (12)	42 (57)	8 (11)	34 (52)	
Han, 2009 (39)			11 (31)		30 (86)	15 (43)	8 (23)
Tilney, 2008 Meta-analysis (32)		20	(19–59%)				

with stapled anastomosis. In a study comparing CAA without resection of the internal sphincter to IRP for rectal cancer, the difference in the 5-year actuarial rate for local recurrence and the overall actuarial survival rate was not found to be clinically significant (43). As with other forms of rectal resection, the distant metastasis rate for cases with lymph node metastasis is noted to be significantly higher than that for cases without lymph node metastasis (48).

It appears that IRP with negative margins is no worse than LAR, and generally better than APR from the standpoint of oncologic outcomes. Weiser published a series comparing three cohorts of patients undergoing resection for rectal cancer. Patients were stratified by those able to undergo LAR with stapled anastomosis, LAR with intersphincteric restorative proctectomy and hand-sewn coloanal anastomosis, and those necessitating APR. When looking at (y)pT3+ patients, both recurrence free survival and disease specific survival were equivalent for both LAR groups and significantly better than the APR group. The 5-year recurrence free survivals were 85%, 83%, and 47%, and 5-year disease-specific survivals were 97%, 96%, and 59%, respectively, demonstrating a statistically significant difference between the APR group and the two LAR groups (1). Similar data are obtained from other trials supporting the acceptable oncological outcomes and benefits of IRP (4,11,22,32,40,39). When able to undergo intersphincteric proctectomy, patients had comparable oncological outcomes to patients undergoing LAR with conventional stapled anastomoses, and significantly improved outcomes to those requiring APR (Table 20.4) (1).

An IRP for rectal cancer was initially proposed to obtain an adequate distal margin of resection for ultra low rectal tumors while avoiding permanent colostomy. Following initial success with IRP, the envelope was pushed, whereby a distal margin of 2 cm was deemed acceptable. The impetus to avoid a permanent ostomy in our society is such that efforts were made to reconnect the bowels in continuity with distal margins of less than 1 cm in patients who had undergone neoadjuvant chemoradiation. It is through the evaluation of the data collected from these procedures that we can confidently state that following neoadjuvant therapy, IRP with a distal margins of less than 1 cm does not appear to compromise the oncologic outcome of an R0 resection (24).

All patients, whether undergoing standard LAR with stapled coloanal anastomosis, LAR with intersphincteric proctectomy and hand-sewn coloanal anastomosis, or APR should be followed for a minimum of 5–8 years based on standard published guidelines to evaluate for recurrence and metastasis.

Functional Outcomes

Following IRP, the functional components of interest include stool incontinence and frequency. It appears reasonable that resecting the internal anal sphincter will result in increased incontinence. As expected from our understanding of physiology, intersphincteric resection resulted in a statistically significant reduction in anal sphincter resting pressure. The squeeze pressures, on the other hand, were noted to be at their preoperative levels at the time of their postoperative evaluation (4,5). When comparing coloplasty and CJP, Furst was able to demonstrate the absence of any significant difference in resting and squeeze pressure and neorectal volume between both groups, but an increased neorectal sensitivity in the coloplasty group (49).

TABLE 20.5	One Year Wexner Fecal Incontinence Score and Kirwan Class Measures of Function					
		Kirwan classification				
	Wexner score	I—Perfect	II—Incontinence to flatus	III—Occas. minor soiling	IV—Freq. major soiling	V—Incontinent/ colostomy
Ito, 2009 (22)	10	18 (25)	8 (11)	27 (37)	20 (27)	0 (0)
Han, 2009 (39)		15 (43)	10 (29)	6 (17)	3 (8.5)	0 (0)

A survey to evaluate GI function in patients that underwent IRP revealed that the mean Wexner score (50) at 1 year following stoma closure was 10. Since a Wexner score of 16 correlated with patients who experienced major and frequent soiling, this score was utilized as a cutoff for poor anal function. Following IRP, patients can expect two to five bowel movements daily and approximately a 20–60% chance of experiencing urgency. Daytime and nocturnal leakage following IRP is present in 15% and 20% of patients, respectively (51). Comparison of IRP to sphincter sparing CAA found worsening of continence as measured by the Kirwan (52) and Wexner Scores following IRP. To compensate, these patients required more utilization of antidiarrheal medications (53). In univariate analysis, both neoadjuvant therapy and the extent of internal sphincter resection were associated with poor anal function, but multivariate analysis revealed that only neoadjuvant therapy is significantly contributory with an odds ratio of over 10 (22). Overall, outcomes have been generally acceptable with minimal patient dissatisfaction (Table 20.5).

Multiple studies have looked at the functional benefits of pouch procedures versus coloanal anastomosis (6,42,54–57). When comparing the short-term functional outcomes between CJP and CAA following ISR, the frequency, urgency, Wexner Score, and Fecal Incontinence Severity Index were shown to be significantly in the favor of the CJP (6,55). Long-term studies failed to reveal these benefits. It must be noted that a difference in improved functional outcomes even over the short term may be a significant benefit given the sometimes low life expectancy of these individuals.

A meta-analysis revealed that 61% of patients after CPA and 55% after CAA experienced good functional outcomes in terms of continence (Kirwan I or II) (6). CJP resulted in decreased stool frequency than CAA. At long-term follow-up, studies failed to reveal any difference in maximum pouch volume as neorectal capacity decreased equally in both groups. This finding has led some authors to propose that the advantage of pouch procedures may not be derived from the increased volume, but rather from decreased motility (31,54).

Studies comparing the various types of pouches have noted advantages of the CJP over the side-to-end-anastomosis in the early postoperative period (56). The TCP was noted to be similar in terms of functional results to CJP (49,57,58). Though no definitive reports have been published, there is a general consensus that a Baker/side-to-end anastomosis has similar outcomes to the CJP and TCP.

Sexual Morbidity

Sexual dysfunction following rectal resection has been studied by multiple authors (3,59). It is more readily noted in males where it manifests as an inability to obtain an erection or as retrograde ejaculation. In females, the manifestation is usually in terms of dyspareunia related to vaginal dryness from decreased parasympathetic stimulation of excretory glands.

When considering sexual function or dysfunction in patients following restorative proctectomy, it is necessary to compare it to the sexual morbidity related to the alternative, an APR. In one survey, findings indicated that following APR, there was no significant change in the patient's sexual activity. The only index of sexual activity that fell postoperatively was related to marital infidelity (2). An APR with a permanent stoma adds to the sexual morbidity by adding the psychosocial barriers related to the presence of a stoma, the perceived effect of a stoma on the partner, and the fear of leakage from the stoma appliance (2). This impact is more likely to be perceived by women then by men and by patients than by their partners (60).

A more recent prospective study looking at the sexual dysfunction of APR compared to restorative procedures in 295 women revealed that women who underwent APR were half as likely to be sexually active 1 year post rectal resection when compared to their counterparts. The frequency of intercourse improved over time in the next 4 years. An APR was also associated with a sixfold higher likelihood of dyspareunia and a higher frequency of urologic dysfunctions as well (36).

The later pelvic lymphadenectomy described and published by Japanese groups appears to add to the sexual morbidity related to rectal resection by damaging the IHP overlying the pelvic vessels and associated lymph nodes. This manifests as a higher rate of impotence and bladder dysfunction (46). When conventional rectal dissection is practiced and lateral pelvic sidewall lymphadenectomy is not undertaken, the rates of impotence reported by the same authors are significantly lower, and bladder dysfunction is uncommon (61).

Stoma-Free Survival

Weiser published the most recent and largest series documenting rates of stoma-free survival in patients with distal rectal cancer undergoing LAR. A subgroup analysis comparing patients undergoing LAR with either stapled coloanal anastomosis versus intersphincteric proctectomy with hand-sewn coloanal anastomosis was performed. With an even distribution between cohorts (41 and 44, respectively), there was no statistically significant difference in the number and percent of patients being stoma-free at last follow-up (98% and 86%, $P = 0.06$). Failure to restore intestinal continuity (2% and 5%, respectively) was attributed to anastomotic leakage and one death from cardiovascular causes. Stomas were recreated in four patients in the IRP group due to anastomotic leak (1), rectovaginal fistula (2), and stricture (1). No stomas were created for poor bowel function (1).

Effect of Neoadjuvant Chemoradiation

Chemoradiation in the adjuvant or neoadjuvant setting has a dramatic effect on the oncological and functional outcomes in relation to intersphincteric proctectomy. It also has a significant effect in other aspects of a patient life as revealed in a study that found women who underwent radiotherapy in addition to IRP had a fivefold increase in dyspareunia (36).

A meta-analysis revealed a local recurrence in 51 of 538 patients (9.5%) following IRP (32). Early results revealed a significantly higher rate of LR recurrence following ISR without (46.5%) compared to with (14.2%) adjuvant chemoradiotherapy (26). In a group of 39 patients that also underwent long-course neoadjuvant radiotherapy, follow-up revealed local recurrence only in three patients (8%), all of whom had lymph node positive disease (62). Other reports of results following neoadjuvant therapy have not been as impressive with Rouanet (63) reporting a local recurrence rate of 13% in a similar cohort, while another study reported a surprisingly high recurrence rate of 21% (64). Although there have been some reports of anastomotic fistulas and pelvic hematomas in these patients, no clear pattern of high rates of anastomotic complications is evident from analyzing studies with high proportions of patients receiving neoadjuvant therapy (32). Indeed, the most recent studies evaluating LR recurrence and disease-specific survival demonstrated favorable rates despite neoadjuvant chemoradiation therapy and have been described above (1).

Studies of GI function in patients following neoadjuvant therapy note a decrease in resting and squeeze pressures as well as maximum tolerable volume following IRP. Multivariate analysis revealed only maximum tolerable volume to be correlating with

TABLE 20.6	Factors Associated with Postoperative Continence/Functional Outcome									
	Age	Gender	Tumor location	Differentiation/ grade	TNM stage	Level of IRP	Preoperative radiation	Reconstruction (J/plasty)	PSWD	Anastomotic leakage
Yamada, 2009 (23)	0.008/0.013*	0.082		0.006*/0.055*	0.778	0.897	0.139	0.054	0.751	0.536
Tiret, 2007 (8)	0.2	0.82			0.63	NS	0.035/0.04*			
Ito, 2009 (22)	0.5	0.1				0.04/0.8	<0.01/<0.01*	0.6		0.7

PSWD, pelvic side wall dissection.
*P < 0.05, significant independent factors associated with postoperative continence/functional outcome.

the Wexner/Fecal Incontinence Scores. This change was decreased with a pouch anastomosis (55). Interestingly, neorectal sensitivity was increased with coloplasty.

When examining factors thought to contribute to poor bowel function, preoperative radiation therapy was most consistently noted to be the sole prognostic factor. Age, gender, type of reconstruction technique were not significant (Table 20.6) (8,22,23).

CONCLUSIONS

Intersphincteric restorative proctocolectomy, be it subtotal or total, appears to be a viable alternative to abdominal perineal resection in terms of oncologic outcomes while maximizing quality of life in carefully selected cohorts of patients with malignant disease. Indeed, patients able to undergo IRP have excellent and equivalent recurrence free survival and disease-specific survival similar to those undergoing LAR with stapled anastomosis and significantly improved compared to those requiring APR (Table 20.7). While avoiding a stoma and maintaining intestinal continuity with sphincter preservation is a principle concern, patients must be counseled as to the expected functional outcome and the real risk of incontinence following IRP. This is particularly the case if neoadjuvant therapy is utilized for malignant disease. The use of chemoradiation therapy can offer benefits in terms of oncologic results with decreased LR recurrence, improvements in resectability, and sphincter preservation. However, this may come at the cost of worse, yet acceptable, functional outcomes (32). In these patients, even the best reported results allow for 25% of patients having occasional and major incontinence, though rarely progress to requiring permanent stomas (1,11).

TABLE 20.7	Recurrence and Survival							
	Median F/U	5-year RFS			5-year DSS			5-year OS
		LAR/stapled	LAR/IRP	APR	LAR/stapled	LAR/IRP	APR	
Weiser, 2009	47	85%	83%	47%	97%	96%	59%*	
Ito, 2009 (3-yr)	96		87%			67%		81%
Tiret, 2007	56.2		77%			75%		82%
Han, 2009	43		94%			86%		97%
Rullier, 2005						70%		81%
Shiessel, 2005	94		92.5%					
Tilney, 2007 Meta-analysis								81.5%

APR, abdominoperineal resection; DSS, disease specific survival; IRP, intersphincteric restorative proctocolectomy; LAR, low anterior resection; RFS, recurrence free survival.
*P <0.05 when compared to LAR, with either stapled or IRP/hand-sewn CAA.

Recommended References and Readings

1. Weiser MR, Quah HM, Shia J, et al. Sphincter preservation in low rectal cancer is facilitated by preoperative chemoradiation and intersphincteric dissection. *Ann Surg* 2009;249(2):236–42.
2. Dlin BM, Perlman A, Ringold E. Psychosexual response to ileostomy and colostomy. *Am J Psychiatry* 1969;126(3):374–81.
3. Bernstein WC, Bernstein EF. Sexual dysfunction following radical surgery for cancer of the rectum. *Dis Colon Rectum* 1966; 9(5):328–32.
4. Schiessel R, Novi G, Holzer B, et al. Technique and long-term results of intersphincteric resection for low rectal cancer. *Dis Colon Rectum* 2005;48(10):1858–65; discussion 65–67.
5. Kohler A, Athanasiadis S, Ommer A, Psarakis E. Long-term results of low anterior resection with intersphincteric anastomosis in carcinoma of the lower one-third of the rectum: analysis of 31 patients. *Dis Colon Rectum* 2000;43(6):843–50.
6. Willis S, Kasperk R, Braun J, Schumpelick V. Comparison of colonic J-pouch reconstruction and straight coloanal anastomosis after intersphincteric rectal resection. *Langenbecks Arch Surg* 2001;386(3):193–99.
7. Ueno M, Oya M, Azekura K, et al. Incidence and prognostic significance of lateral lymph node metastasis in patients with advanced low rectal cancer. *Br J Surg* 2005;92(6):756–63.
8. Tiret E, Poupardin B, McNamara D, et al. Ultralow anterior resection with intersphincteric dissection–what is the limit of safe sphincter preservation? *Colorectal Dis* 2003;5(5):454–57.
9. Temple LK, Romanus D, Niland J, et al. Factors associated with sphincter-preserving surgery for rectal cancer at national comprehensive cancer network centers. *Ann Surg* 2009;250(2): 260–67.
10. Lyttle JA, Parks AG. Intersphincteric excision of the rectum. *Br J Surg* 1977;64(6):413–16.
11. Rullier E, Laurent C, Bretagnol F, Rullier A, Vendrely V, Zerbib F. Sphincter-saving resection for all rectal carcinomas: the end of the 2-cm distal rule. *Ann Surg* 2005;241(3):465–69.
12. Teramoto T, Watanabe M, Kitajima M. Per anum intersphincteric rectal dissection with direct coloanal anastomosis for lower rectal cancer: the ultimate sphincter-preserving operation. *Dis Colon Rectum* 1997;40(10 Suppl):S43–S47.
13. Heald RJ. The 'Holy Plane' of rectal surgery. *J R Soc Med* 1988;81(9):503–508.
14. Keating JP. Sexual function after rectal excision. *ANZ J Surg* 2004;74(4):248–59.
15. Ulrich AB, Seiler C, Rahbari N, et al. Diverting stoma after low anterior resection: more arguments in favor. *Dis Colon Rectum* 2009;52(3):412–18.
16. Law WL, Chu KW, Choi HK. Randomized clinical trial comparing loop ileostomy and loop transverse colostomy for faecal diversion following total mesorectal excision. *Br J Surg* 2002;89(6):704–708.
17. Rullier E, Le Toux N, Laurent C, et al. Loop ileostomy versus loop colostomy for defunctioning low anastomoses during rectal cancer surgery. *World J Surg* 2001;25(3):274–77; discussion 7–8.
18. Young-Fadok TM, Fanelli RD, Price RR, Earle DB. Laparoscopic resection of curable colon and rectal cancer: an evidence-based review. *Surg Endosc* 2007;21(7):1063–68.
19. Jones OM, Smeulders N, Wiseman O, Miller R. Lateral ligaments of the rectum: an anatomical study. *Br J Surg* 1999;86(4):487–89.
20. Long DM Jr, Bernstein WC. Sexual dysfunction as a complication of abdominoperineal resection of the rectum in the male: an anatomic and physiologic study. *Dis Colon Rectum* 1959 ;2:540–48.
21. Bullock N. Impotence after sclerotherapy of haemorrhoids: case reports. *BMJ* 1997;314(7078):419.
22. Ito M, Saito N, Sugito M, et al. Analysis of clinical factors associated with anal function after intersphincteric resection for very low rectal cancer. *Dis Colon Rectum* 2009;52(1):64–70.
23. Yamada K, Ogata S, Saiki Y, et al. Long-term results of intersphincteric resection for low rectal cancer. *Dis Colon Rectum* 2009;52(6):1065–71.
24. Moore HG, Riedel E, Minsky BD, et al. Adequacy of 1-cm distal margin after restorative rectal cancer resection with sharp mesorectal excision and preoperative combined-modality therapy. *Ann Surg Oncol* 2003;10(1):80–85.
25. Park JG, Lee MR, Lim SB, et al. Colonic J-pouch anal anastomosis after ultralow anterior resection with upper sphincter excision for low-lying rectal cancer. *World J Gastroenterol* 2005;11(17):2570–73.
26. Hohenberger W, Merkel S, Matzel K, et al. The influence of abdomino-peranal (intersphincteric) resection of lower third rectal carcinoma on the rates of sphincter preservation and locoregional recurrence. *Colorectal Dis* 2006;8(1):23–33.
27. Baker JW. Low end to side rectosigmoidal anastomosis; description of technic. *Arch Surg* 1950;61(1):143–57.
28. Tranchart H, Benoist S, Penna C, et al. Cutaneous perianal recurrence on the site of Lone Star Retractor after J-pouch coloanal anastomosis for rectal cancer: report of two cases. *Dis Colon Rectum* 2008;51(12):1850–52.
29. Kasperk R, Schumpelick V. Sphincter preserving techniques: from anterior resection to coloanal anastomosis. *Langenbecks Arch Surg* 1998;383(6):397–401.
30. Fazio VW, Mantyh CR, Hull TL. Colonic "coloplasty": novel technique to enhance low colorectal or coloanal anastomosis. *Dis Colon Rectum* 2000;43(10):1448–50.
31. Hida J, Yasutomi M, Fujimoto K, et al. Functional outcome after low anterior resection with low anastomosis for rectal cancer using the colonic J-pouch. Prospective randomized study for determination of optimum pouch size. *Dis Colon Rectum* 1996;39(9):986–91.
32. Tilney HS, Tekkis PP. Extending the horizons of restorative rectal surgery: intersphincteric resection for low rectal cancer. *Colorectal Dis* 2008;10(1):3–15; discussion 15–16.
33. Karanjia ND, Corder AP, Bearn P, Heald RJ. Leakage from stapled low anastomosis after total mesorectal excision for carcinoma of the rectum. *Br J Surg* 1994;81(8):1224–26.
34. Ulrich AB, Seiler CM, Z'Graggen K, et al. Early results from a randomized clinical trial of colon J pouch versus transverse coloplasty pouch after low anterior resection for rectal cancer. *Br J Surg* 2008;95(10):1257–63.
35. Rullier E, Laurent C, Garrelon JL, et al. Risk factors for anastomotic leakage after resection of rectal cancer. *Br J Surg* 1998;85(3):355–58.
36. Tekkis PP, Cornish JA, Remzi FH, et al. Measuring sexual and urinary outcomes in women after rectal cancer excision. *Dis Colon Rectum* 2009;52(1):46–54.
37. Hallbook O, Pahlman L, Krog M, et al. Randomized comparison of straight and colonic J pouch anastomosis after low anterior resection. *Ann Surg* 1996;224(1):58–65.
38. Willis S, Holzl F, Krones CJ, et al. Evaluation of anastomotic microcirculation after low anterior rectal resection: an experimental study with different reconstruction forms in dogs. *Tech Coloproctol* 2006;10(3):222–26.
39. Han JG, Wei GH, Gao ZG, et al. Intersphincteric resection with direct coloanal anastomosis for ultralow rectal cancer: the experience of People's Republic of China. *Dis Colon Rectum* 2009; 52(5):950–57.
40. Chamlou R, Parc Y, Simon T, et al. Long-term results of intersphincteric resection for low rectal cancer. *Ann Surg* 2007;246(6):916-21; discussion 21–22.
41. Cornish JA, Tilney HS, Heriot AG, et al. A meta-analysis of quality of life for abdominoperineal excision of rectum versus anterior resection for rectal cancer. *Ann Surg Oncol* 2007;14(7):2056–68.
42. Machado M, Nygren J, Goldman S, Ljungqvist O. Functional and physiologic assessment of the colonic reservoir or side-to-end anastomosis after low anterior resection for rectal cancer: a two-year follow-up. *Dis Colon Rectum* 2005;48(1):29–36.
43. Portier G, Ghouti L, Kirzin S, et al. Oncological outcome of ultra-low coloanal anastomosis with and without intersphincteric resection for low rectal adenocarcinoma. *Br J Surg* 2007; 94(3):341–45.
44. Weiser MR, Milsom JW. Laparoscopic total mesorectal excision with autonomic nerve preservation. *Semin Surg Oncol* 2000;19(4):396–403.
45. Chung CC, Ha JP, Tsang WW, Li MK. Laparoscopic-assisted total mesorectal excision and colonic J pouch reconstruction in the treatment of rectal cancer. *Surg Endosc* 2001;15(10):1098–101.

46. Hojo K, Sawada T, Moriya Y. An analysis of survival and voiding, sexual function after wide iliopelvic lymphadenectomy in patients with carcinoma of the rectum, compared with conventional lymphadenectomy. *Dis Colon Rectum* 1989;32(2):128–33.

47. Tekkis PP, Heriot AG, Smith J, et al. Comparison of circumferential margin involvement between restorative and nonrestorative resections for rectal cancer. *Colorectal Dis* 2005;7(4):369–74.

48. Yoo JH, Hasegawa H, Ishii Y, et al. Long-term outcome of per anum intersphincteric rectal dissection with direct coloanal anastomosis for lower rectal cancer. *Colorectal Dis* 2005;7(5):434–40.

49. Furst A, Suttner S, Agha A, et al. Colonic J-pouch vs. coloplasty following resection of distal rectal cancer: early results of a prospective, randomized, pilot study. *Dis Colon Rectum* 2003;46(9):1161–66.

50. Jorge JM, Wexner SD. Etiology and management of fecal incontinence. *Dis Colon Rectum* 1993;36(1):77–97.

51. Braun J, Treutner KH, Winkeltau G, et al. Results of intersphincteric resection of the rectum with direct coloanal anastomosis for rectal carcinoma. *Am J Surg* 1992;163(4):407–12.

52. Kirwan WO, Turnbull RB Jr, Fazio VW, Weakley FL. Pullthrough operation with delayed anastomosis for rectal cancer. *Br J Surg* 1978;65(10):695–98.

53. Bretagnol F, Rullier E, Laurent C, et al. Comparison of functional results and quality of life between intersphincteric resection and conventional coloanal anastomosis for low rectal cancer. *Dis Colon Rectum* 2004;47(6):832–38.

54. Furst A, Burghofer K, Hutzel L, Jauch KW. Neorectal reservoir is not the functional principle of the colonic J-pouch: the volume of a short colonic J-pouch does not differ from a straight coloanal anastomosis. *Dis Colon Rectum* 2002;45(5):660–67.

55. Bittorf B, Stadelmaier U, Gohl J, et al. Functional outcome after intersphincteric resection of the rectum with coloanal anastomosis in low rectal cancer. *Eur J Surg Oncol* 2004;30(3):260–65.

56. Huber FT, Herter B, Siewert JR. Colonic pouch vs. side-to-end anastomosis in low anterior resection. *Dis Colon Rectum* 1999;42(7):896–902.

57. Z'Graggen K, Maurer CA, Mettler D, et al. A novel colon pouch and its comparison with a straight coloanal and colon J-pouch–anal anastomosis: preliminary results in pigs. *Surgery* 1999;125(1):105–12.

58. Heriot AG, Tekkis PP, Constantinides V, et al. Meta-analysis of colonic reservoirs versus straight coloanal anastomosis after anterior resection. *Br J Surg* 2006;93(1):19–32.

59. Lindsey I, George BD, Kettlewell MG, Mortensen NJ. Impotence after mesorectal and close rectal dissection for inflammatory bowel disease. *Dis Colon Rectum* 2001;44(6):831–35.

60. Leicester RJ, Ritchie JK, Wadsworth J, et al. Sexual function and perineal wound healing after intersphincteric excision of the rectum for inflammatory bowel disease. *Dis Colon Rectum* 1984;27(4):244–48.

61. Maas CP, Moriya Y, Steup WH, et al. Radical and nerve-preserving surgery for rectal cancer in The Netherlands: a prospective study on morbidity and functional outcome. *Br J Surg* 1998;85(1):92–97.

62. Mohiuddin M, Regine WF, Marks GJ, Marks JW. High-dose preoperative radiation and the challenge of sphincter-preservation surgery for cancer of the distal 2 cm of the rectum. *Int J Radiat Oncol Biol Phys* 1998;40(3):569–74.

63. Rouanet P, Saint-Aubert B, Lemanski C, et al. Restorative and nonrestorative surgery for low rectal cancer after high-dose radiation: long-term oncologic and functional results. *Dis Colon Rectum* 2002;45(3):305–13; discussion 13–15.

64. Wagman R, Minsky BD, Cohen AM, et al. Sphincter preservation in rectal cancer with preoperative radiation therapy and coloanal anastomosis: long term follow-up. *Int J Radiat Oncol Biol Phys* 1998;42(1):51–57.

21 Open

Eric Weiss

 INDICATIONS/CONTRAINDICATIONS

Total abdominal colectomy with ileorectal anastomosis is the surgical procedure of choice for multiple conditions requiring removal of the entire colon with preservation of the rectum. This operation typically allows for adequate bowel function in most cases with 2–4 bowel movements per 24-hour period in most patients; however, the stools are looser than normal due to lack of reabsorption of water that usually occurs in the colon. This operation is usually performed in an elective setting but can be performed in a more urgent setting when indicated. Conditions and situations requiring removal of the entire colon are multiple and are listed below:

- Familial adenomatous polyposis (>100 polyps in the colon with <20 polyps in the rectum and/or rectum "cleared" of polyps prior to surgery)
- Crohn's colitis and mucosal ulcerative colitis with relative rectal sparing and with adequate length and compliance of the remaining rectum to allow for adequate function
- Indeterminate colitis relative rectal sparing with adequate length and compliance of the remaining rectum to allow for adequate function
- Lower gastrointestinal (GI) bleeding without specific localization of a colonic segment (requires endoscopic clearance of the upper GI tract and anorectum)
- Slow transit constipation (requires normal rectal emptying by defacography and colonic inertia by colonic transit study)
- Hereditary nonpolyposis colon cancer (HNPCC)
- Obstructing left-sided colon cancer (allows for resection and primary anastomosis without stoma in an urgent or emergency situation)

The contraindications for this operation are mostly due to patient conditions that would not allow for the performance of a safe anastomosis due to the high risk of an anastomotic leak. The scenarios include the following:

- Poor nutrition (albumin <2.5–3.0)
- Hemodynamic instability
- Excessive preoperative blood loss (>10 units packed red blood cells [PRBCs] transfused)
- Poor quality of small bowel or rectum
- Patient comorbidities (cardiac, hepatic, renal and/or pulmonary)

Patients with contraindications can undergo a total abdominal colectomy with ileostomy and depending on the pathology and clinical outcomes of the initial surgery have the options of restoration of continuity at a later date, 3 or more months after the initial surgery.

PREOPERATIVE PLANNING

The preoperative planning for patients undergoing a total abdominal colectomy with a planned ileorectal anastomosis can be extensive depending on the indication for the procedure; some of the requisites have been mentioned above in the indications section. However, numerous other evaluations may be required in order to ensure that a total colectomy as opposed to a smaller or segmental resection should not be performed.

Given the magnitude of the operation adequate preoperative and perioperative evaluation and management should be undertaken. Based on age, comorbidites, and the underlying condition evaluation and maximization prior to surgery should be performed. This assessment includes adequate medical clearance, appropriate prophylactic measures according to surgical care and improvement project guidelines, and good informed consent. Further specific evaluation based on the specific conditions or indications should also be performed.

Patients with familial adenomatous polyposis should undergo endoscopic evaluation of both the upper and lower GI tracts. Colonoscopy should be performed with particular attention to the rectum. Ileorectal anastomosis can be performed when there are less than 20 polyps in the rectum that can be removed thus "clearing the rectum." Upper endoscopy with both forward and side viewing endoscopes is required to rule out gastric and periampullary lesions. A detailed family history should be obtained with particular attention being paid to a family history of desmoid tumors. A positive history of desmoid tumor should prompt a CT scan of the abdomen and pelvis to be done preoperatively to identify patients with intra-abdominal desmoids that may change the planned approach to surgery. Consideration for genetic testing should also be discussed with the patient.

Patients with Crohn's colitis, mucosal ulcerative colitis, or indeterminate colitis require complete GI tract evaluations with colonoscopy, upper GI radiography or endoscopy, small bowel imaging, and possibly CT scan of the abdomen and pelvis. The outcomes of total abdominal colectomy with ileorectal anastomosis will in part depend on whether there is any small bowel disease, rectal disease, and perianal disease. In addition, assurance of adequate preoperative nutritional status with an albumin of >2.5–3.0 and no active infections at the time of surgery will diminish the risk of anastomotic leak. Moreover, many patients with colitis receive high dose steroids and/or antitumor necrosis factor (TNF) medications. Depending on the doses and timing of medications an anastomosis may be contraindicated and an initial total colectomy with ileostomy rather than ileorectal anastomosis may be the preferred procedure.

Patients with lower GI bleeding are typically hospitalized due to ongoing GI bleeding when evaluation fails to identify a specific bleeding site within the colon. However, evaluation should be undertaken to exclude an upper GI source with upper endoscopy and an anorectal. Other diagnostic studies such as tagged red blood scan and/or angiography may not localize the site of bleeding. If blood loss persists, such that greater than 6 units of PRBCs are transfused or bleeding recurs, a total abdominal colectomy with ileorectal anastomosis may be indicated. Patients, who recover from a first bleed, are not operated on due to failure of localization and minimal risk of rebleeding. These patients should undergo small bowel imaging with radiography and capsule endoscopy to clearly exclude primary small bowel pathology.

Patients with severe constipation defined as less than three bowel movements per week or straining greater than 25% of the time who have failed conservative therapy including dietary manipulations, fiber and laxative therapy, and prokinetic medications may be candidates for surgical management of their constipation. Patients with the above history should undergo a series of anatomic and functional studies. First and foremost colonoscopy should be undertaken to exclude a mechanical cause for constipation.

A colonic transit study and defacography should be performed to find the rare patient with colonic intertia and normal rectal emptying who might potentially be a candidate for this operation. Any other indication or combination of test outcomes leads to poor postoperative results.

HNPCC patients are identified thorough family histories with patients meeting the requirements by Amsterdam or Bethesda to have HNPCC should be considered for total colectomy if a colon cancer is present in the colon with a normal appearing rectum. Genetic testing, microsatellite instability (MSI), and other tests may also be useful in helping to determine those patients with HNPCC as opposed to those with sporadic colorectal cancer. Evaluation for noncolorectal-associated malignancies such as thyroid and uterine should be performed.

Patients who present with colonic obstructions most commonly due to distal colonic malignancies have the option of three procedures: resection and stoma, resection and anastomosis or on-table lavage, resection and anastomosis. The outcomes are similar from the standpoint of anastomotic leaks but the functional outcomes are slightly worse when a total colectomy is performed but this avoids a stoma, even if temporary and is technically easier than on-table lavage.

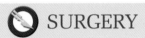

SURGERY

Positioning

Patients should be positioned in the lithotomy position so that there is access to the anus and rectum for both endoscopy and stapling techniques. Typically Allen® stirrups but Lloyd Davies or Yellowfin® stirrups may also be used. Care to pad the calfs and heals appropriately and aligning the legs in the proper orientations will decrease the risks of neuropathies and compartment syndromes. The arms can be either at the sides or out on armboards based on the surgeon's preferences. Since these operations are more complex and have the risk to be longer than segmental colectomies adequate maintenance of temperature is required.

Technique

A total abdominal colectomy with ileorectal anastomosis can be considered two segmental colectomies combined to add up to a total colectomy. The performance of a total abdominal colectomy is similar to performing a right and left colectomy on the same patient at the same time.

Adequate exposure is required which typically mandates an adequate vertical midline incision. Occasionally, the patient's body habitus and underlying condition will allow a transverse/pfannenstiel incision to be used. It is important that adequate visualization of the upper rectum and flexures is achieved. This goal often requires a generous midline incision well above and well below the umbilicus. Retraction typically using a self-retaining retractor of the surgeon's choice is employed. This retraction can include a Buchwalter, Iron Intern or Balfour type retractor and again is one of the surgeon's choice. No one retractor is necessarily better than another.

Once adequate exposure and retraction is achieved, a careful exploration for confirmation of and exclusion of other pathology is performed. This sequence should include manual palpation and visualization of the liver, gall bladder, stomach, small bowel, colon, and rectum as well as the adenexa and uterus when present in a women. Abnormalities should be documented in the operative report and intraoperative consultation with the appropriate specialists obtained when indicated.

The operation typically consists of colonic mobilization, vascular division, bowel division, and anastomosis but the specific order can vary based on the pathology, the surgeon, and the diagnosis. Typically mobilization in a lateral-to-medial fashion beginning with the right or left colon is commenced. For a lateral dissection of the right colon, one may use electrocautery or sharp dissection along the white line of Toldt. The surgeon should stand on the side of the being mobilized and the assistant retracting the colon anteriorly and medially creating tension so that the white line is easily identified. The white line is incised using either energy or sharp dissection. The colon is first mobilized from the retroperitoneal structures toward the midline. It is mandatory to identify the retroperitoneal structures of the ureter, Gerota's fascia, and duodenum on the right. One should be able to fully mobilize the cecum, ascending colon, and terminal ileal mesentery to the inferior border of the duodenum. The flexures are then liberated by dividing the hepatico colic or splenocolic ligaments. This step often requires division and ligation using clamps and ties as opposed to electrocautery alone. Advanced energy sources are excellent for this purpose and can reduce operative time and allow for a more expeditious operative procedure. Lastly, the gastrocolic omentum is divided or mobilized from the transverse colon depending on the surgeon's preference. Lifting the omentum off of the transverse colon to identify the avascular plane will allow for dissection with electrocautery which allows for preservation of the omentum and simple access to the lesser sac and transverse colon mesentery. Alternatively dividing the omentum just distal to the greater curvature of the stomach and the epiploic vessels will allow the omentum to be resected with the colon if this is one's preference. Again division and ligation using clamps and ties or the use of advanced energy sources are excellent for this purpose. At this point the entire abdominal colon is fully mobilized. Vascular division is then performed using either standard clamps and ties or a vascular sealing device of choice can be used to shorten the operative time; there is typically no need to divide the superior hemorrhoidal artery. Once the vessels are divided, division of the small bowel just proximal to the cecum and the rectum at the true rectum is performed. Identification of the "true rectum" is possible based on several anatomic landmarks including the sacral promontory, the loss of epiploica, and/or confluence of tinea. In addition, rigid or flexible endoscopy confirming a 15-cm residual rectal stump with division just above the 3rd rectal valve may be utilized. Division of the small bowel can be achieved by using linear staplers, purse-string clamps or noncrushing bowel clamps depending on the type of anastomosis one is planning. Division of the rectum is performed in a similar manner with the same choices as with the small bowel division. Once the colon is removed if an anastomosis is appropriate an ileorectal anastomosis can be performed.

Several methods of ileorectal anastomoses can be performed and include end to end or side to end. Like all anastomoses the requisite conditions include two healthy ends of bowel, excellent blood supply, no tension on the anastomosis, and a technically perfect anastomosis. These conditions can be met by all forms of anastomosis and is typically based on surgeon preference. Most commonly a circular stapled anastomosis using a double stapling technique is employed; however, double purse string or hand-sewn single or double layer anastomoses can also be performed. Most commonly the rectum is divided and closed using a linear stapler. The author's preference is to use "green" or 3.8-mm staples. Due to the relatively smaller size of the ileum typically a circular stapler of 28, 29, or 31 mm is used but 33 mm may also be used if that is the surgeon's preference. However, utilizing a 25-mm circular stapler should be avoided and if for whatever reason the small bowel is too small consider administration of glucagon or utilizing side-to-end anastomosis that will often allow for a larger diameter anvil. We typically "clear the anvil" of fat and blood vessels from the anvil post to the staple line to remove them from the planned anastomosis.

The anvil once attached should be closed under direct vision ensuring that no other structures are incorporated into the staple line. This measure is particularly important if the staple line is in close proximity to the vagina which must be clearly reflected anteriorly and inferiorly out of the staple line to prevent a rectovaginal fistula. Alternatively a compression ring or sutured anastomosis may be fashioned.

Once the anastomosis is completed some forms of testing with air either by insufflated air via the anus/rectum or endoscopic evaluation should be performed to ensure a circumferentially intact, airtight, hemostatic anastomosis. Several options are available if in an air test a leak is noted. Since the anastomosis is intraperitoneal it rarely requires diversion to protect the anastomosis in this case. Placing direct sutures at the site of the leak or redoing the anastomosis based on the size and etiology of the leak are options. Retesting after repair or revision is mandatory to ensure that no continued air leak exists.

Given that the long-term risk of small bowel obstruction is higher in patients undergoing a total abdominal colectomy compared to a segmental colectomy consideration for the placement of an anti-adhesion barrier would be recommended. Although reduction of adhesions does not necessarily decrease the long-term risk of adhesive small bowel obstruction it only makes sense that decreasing adhesions should have a positive effect. Therefore we routinely use Seprafilm® (Genzyme Biosurgery, Cambridge, Mass.) in these cases utilizing 1–4 full size sheets depending on the patients size and incision size often "sandwiching" the omentum between sheets.

POSTOPERATIVE MANAGEMENT

The postoperative management of patients following an open total abdominal colectomy is similar to that of any elective colorectal surgical procedure that was available in 2010. Regardless of whether a "fast track" protocol is formally employed many of the steps are routinely used in most practices in colorectal surgery today. These common steps include early ambulation where patients are ambulated 2–3 times per day commencing on the day of surgery or at the latest on postoperative day 1. Foley catheters used at the time of surgery can generally be removed on postoperative day 1 as long as the urine output is adequate and the hemoglobin is stable. Early oral feeding is utilized where patients are given clear liquids and their diets are advanced either as tolerated or based on passage of stool or flatus to solid food. Pain medication is usually in the form of IV PCA with additional non-narcotic pain medication such as Ketorlac for the first 3–5 days after surgery. Conversion to oral narcotic pain medication can be accomplished typically at the time patients are advanced to a solid diet. Discharge from the hospital typically 3–6 days after surgery occurs when the patient is tolerating a solid diet, having adequate pain control on oral analgesia, and moving their bowels adequately. Patients should be counseled that typically long term they will move their bowels 2–4 times per day and that the bowel movements will be looser and minimally if at all formed. This expectation is particularly true in the immediate postoperative period with improvements in function over time.

Once discharged patients may shower or bathe, ambulate up and down stairs, ride in a car and perform normal household activity for several weeks after surgery. Strenuous physical activity, weight lifting, and other physically demanding chores should be avoided for 4–6 weeks after surgery. Return to work and full activity typically occurs by 4–6 weeks after surgery but sometimes may take longer.

COMPLICATIONS

A multitude of complications can occur following a surgery of this magnitude and includes a variety of nonspecific complications that can occur regardless of the surgical procedure performed and some specific complications related to this procedure.

The nonspecific complications will be listed but not discussed, as they are common and easily managed by most surgeons.

- Cardiopulmonary (myocardial infarction, pneumonia, atelectasis, pulmonary embolus, arrhythmia)
- Wound infection
- Dehydration/acute renal failure
- Hypertension
- Impaired glucose metabolism
- Hepatic dysfunction
- Acute blood loss anemia

Specific complications to ileorectal anastomosis that require discussion include anastomotic leak, rectovaginal fistula, pelvic abscess, and prolonged postoperative ileus.

Anastomotic Leak

Anastomotic leak is the most dreaded complication of any intestinal anastomosis. An ileorectal anastomosis may have a leak rate as high as 6–8%. The time course for this complication may occur sooner than one sees with and due to the fact that the colon has been removed and there is no recovery of a colonic ileus that is required. Therefore when bowel function resumes which may be in 2–4 days, liquid stool or enteric contents may leak out of even a relatively small hole and lead to significant sepsis and contamination.

Suspicion and early identification are the two most important factors in a patient's outcome. Clinical findings of postoperative fevers, worsening abdominal pain, worsening abdominal exam, and hemodynamic compromise are all c/w an anastomotic leak but not necessarily one. If clinical findings are convincing enough no studies may be required and direct return to the OR for re-exploration may be performed. However, if the clinical scenario is not readily evident then either a water-soluble contrast enema looking for contrast extravasation or CT scan with rectal contrast may allow for identification of such a complication. If identified one still needs to decide if the leak warrants re-exploration or can be managed in a more conservative manner. Free extravasation without containment requires re-exploration. However, a small leak into a small contained cavity may be able to be conservatively managed with bowel rest, nutritional support with total parenteral nutrition (TPN), and appropriate broad spectrum antibiotics allowing for possible spontaneous healing. When free contrast extravasation occurs emergent re-exploration is required.

Re-exploration includes reopening of the prior laparotomy incision, source control of the leak, repair or takedown of the anastomosis, and fecal diversion. Prior to taking a patient back to the OR, preoperative stoma marking for an ileostomy should be performed. This precaution will allow for a better-sited stoma which will hopefully facilitate the postoperative management of the ileostomy. After the incision is reopened, immediate removal of free gastrointestinal contents should be performed. Adequate exposure should be obtained and the anastomosis examined for the site, size, and cause if possible identified. It is rare for an ileorectal anastomosis to leak due to tension and therefore further mobilization is likely unnecessary. If ischemia or necrosis is noted the anastomosis will need to be taken down and resected resulting in a Hartmann closure to the rectum and an end ileostomy. More commonly, however, a small defect for no apparent reason will be identified. In this situation either proximal diversion alone with a loop ileostomy and drainage via a closed suction drain near the anastomosis or suture repair of the defect with proximal diversion would be the options. The author tends to repair the anastomosis with interrupted absorbable suture but diversion alone has similar results. It is important to irrigate the abdomen with significant amounts of saline to dilute and thoroughly wash out the abdominal cavity. Consideration for the addition of an antifungal should be given due to the high likelihood of candida in the small bowel.

Once the patient has fully recovered and is back to his premorbid condition and assuming a minimum of 3–6 months have passed consideration for stoma closure can be given.

Rectovaginal Fistula

Rectovaginal fistulas can occur s/p ileorecal anastomosis due to one intraoperative complication and one postoperative complication. Intraoperatively incorporating a portion of the vaginal into the stapler and creating an ileorectal anastomosis with portion of the vagina in it will lead to an early rectovaginal fistula. Typically when bowel function returns the patient will experience enteric contents or stool via the vagina at the same time as moving their bowels. Due to the fact that the stool is loose as it is essentially small bowel contents this type of fistula is highly symptomatic. Due to the fact that the staples act as a foreign body these types of fistulas rarely heal spontaneously and typically require fecal diversion with a loop ileostomy and than revision/redo of the anastomosis a minimum of 3 months later. Occasionally these can be repaired at the time of fecal diversion but often there is significant inflammation at the anastomosis due to which further manipulation leads to worse outcomes.

If a postoperative pelvic abscess spontaneously erodes and drains via the vagina they can be handled like a contained leak with bowel rest, nutritional support with TPN, and appropriate broad spectrum antibiotics allowing for possible spontaneous healing. If this is not successful than similar reoperative surgery with an initial loop ileostomy for fecal diversion followed in a minimum of 3 months later with revision/redo of the anastomosis is recommended.

Pelvic Abscess

Pelvic abscesses may occur following any abdominal surgery and can occur due to intraoperative contamination or postoperative contained anastomotic leaks. Regardless these abscesses most commonly are managed by CT-guided drainage. Patients with unexplained postoperative fevers or elevated white blood cell counts should undergo CT scans of the abdomen and pelvis with PO (and/or rectal contrast) and IV contrast. If a pelvic abscess is identified either transperineal or transabdominal CT-guided drainage should suffice in controlling the abscess. Appropriate broad spectrum antibiotics and based on final cultures simplification to appropriate specific coverage should be ordered. Once the abscess is drained and there is no evidence of enterocutaneous fistula the patients may return to oral intake. The drains typically will need to stay until the outputs are minimal and reimaging reveals resolution of the collection.

Prolonged Postoperative Ileus

Prolonged postoperative ileus defined as lack of return to bowel function at 1 week following surgery may occur. This problem can occur due to partial obstruction at the ileorectal anastomosis due to swelling or structuring at the anastomosis or idiopathic. When this situation occurs it is prudent to define whether indeed this is an obstruction at the anastomosis or a nonanastomotic process. Flexible sigmoidoscopy with minimal air insufflation or water-soluble contrast enemas will allow one to determine if there is luminal patency and an ileus versus an obstruction. If an obstruction is identified than a determination needs to be made if this is edema which will resolve over time versus a stricture which will require diversion.

If an ileus is identified, then conservative treatment with supportive measures including TPN, bowel rest, naso gastric tube decompression when appropriate, and trials of prokinetics if available. One must be patient and discuss with the patient the need to be patient. There is no reason for re-exploration unless the ileus is really thought to be an obstruction. A postoperative ileus especially when the indication for the initial surgery was constipation may remain for 2–4 weeks postoperatively.

RESULTS

The "average" patient who undergoes a total abdominal colectomy with ileorectal anastomosis can anticipate a long-term functional outcome of 2–4 bowel movements per day. These bowel movements tend not to be formed and are semisolid. Continence should be satisfactory with the ability to defer the call to bowel movements for upwards of 30–60 minutes assuming that the rectum capacity is not impaired due to inflammatory bowel disease in the rectum or other cause. If more excessive numbers of bowel movements occur than the addition of fiber supplements and antidiarrheal may be required to achieve an acceptable number of bowel movements daily.

Anastomotic leak rates are 3–8% and fully described above.

✴✦ CONCLUSIONS

Total abdominal colectomy with ileorectal anastomosis can be performed for a multitude of conditions with excellent functional outcomes with acceptable bowel function and minimal complications.

Recommended References and Readings

Maeda T, Cannom RR, Beart RW, Etziona DA. Decision model of segmental compared with total abdominal colectomy for colon cancer in hereditary non-polyposis colorectal cancer. *J Clin Oncol* 2010;28(7):1175–80.

van Duijvendijk P, Slors JF, Taat CW, et al. Functional outcome after colectomy and ileorectal anastomosis compared with procto-colectomy and ileal pouch-anal anastomosis in familial adenomatous polyposis. *Ann Surg* 1999;230(5):648–54.

Gunther K, Braunrieder G, Bittorf BR, et al. Patients with familial adenomatous polyposis experience better bowel function and quality of life after ileorectal anastomosis than after ileoanal pouch. *Colorectal Dis* 2003;5(1):38–44.

Nakamura T, Pikarsky AJ, Potenti FM, et al. Are complications of subtotal colectomy with ileorectal anastomosis related to the original disease? *Am Surg* 2001;67(5):417–20.

Elton C, Makin G, Hitos K, Cohen CR. Mortality, morbidity and functional outcome after ileorectal anastomosis. *Br J Surg* 2003;90(1):59–65.

Baker R, Senagore A. Abdominal colectomy offers safe management for massive lower GI bleed. *Am Surg* 1994;60(8):578–81.

Verne GN, Hocking MP, Davis RH, et al. Long-term response to subtotal colectomy in colonic inertia. *J Gastrointest Surg* 2002;6(5):738–44.

Thaler K, Dinnewitzer A, Oberwalder M, et al. Quality of life after colectomy for colonic inertia. *Tech Coloproctol* 2005;9(2):133–7.

Pastore RL, Wolff BG, Hodge D. Total abdominal colectomy and ileorectal anastomosis for inflammatory bowel disease. *Dis Colon Rectum* 1997;40(12):1455–64.

Plummer JM, Gibson TN, Mitchell DI, et al. Emergency subtotal colectomy for lower gastrointestinal haemorrhage: over-utilised or under-estimated. *Int J Clin Pract* 2009;63(6):865–8.

Hyman N, Manchester TL, Osler T, et al. Anastomotic leaks after intestinal anastomoses: it's later than you think. *Ann Surg* 2007;245(2):254–8.

22 Laparoscopic Ileorectal Anastomosis

James W. Fleshman

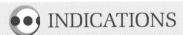 ## INDICATIONS

The more common indications for a laparoscopic total abdominal colectomy with ileorectal anastomosis are the same as for open and include synchronous colon cancers, familial cancer syndromes (HNPCC, FAP with rectal sparing, and patients with cancer under the age of 40 years), colonic inertia, Crohn's colitis with rectal sparing, and gastrointestinal bleeding.

 ## PREOPERATIVE PLANNING

The preparation of the patient is dictated by the specific indication and the appropriate evaluations should be undertaken. A mechanical bowel preparation with oral agents is not necessary but is frequently performed to reduce stool in the colon. If the patient has a history of constipation, the colon can be too heavy with retained stool to allow a safe laparoscopic approach. The left side of the colon can be adequately cleansed with several enemas prior to surgery. Routine deep vein thrombosis prophylaxis, antibiotic prophylaxis and instructions on postoperative care are required. The patients should receive education on the expected functional outcome of an ileorectal anastomosis. They can expect to have 4–5 semi-solid, pasty bowel movements a day with good bowel control after a period of accommodation (usually 6 months).

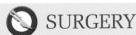 ## SURGERY

Positioning

▪ The patient is positioned in the modified lithotomy position with the legs in the Allen® stirrups with sequential compression leggings in place. A bean bag, attached

Figure 22.1

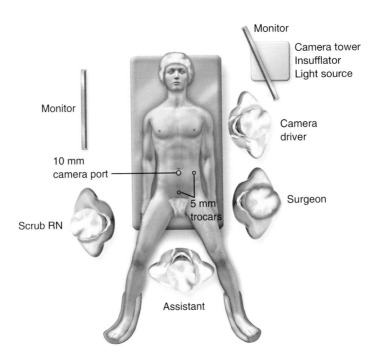

directly to the operating table with Velcro, is folded around the patient, including the shoulders, and deflated to fix the patient in position. This keeps the arms at the patient's side and allows the table to be placed in steep Trendelenburg and airplaned to the left and right during the operation. The trocar sight placement is typically at the umbilicus, right upper anterior axillary line, right lower anterior axillary line suprapubic and left flank positions. The camera operator stands to the patient's left shoulder and operates the camera through the umbilical port. The operating surgeon stands at the patient's left hip or between the legs as needed and operates instruments through the left flank and suprapubic ports (Fig. 22.1).

■ The camera cord, light cord and carbon dioxide cord are passed off of the table from the patient's left shoulder to the instrumentation tower. A monitor is placed opposite the operating surgeon and camera operator. If two monitors are available, one is at the right shoulder and one is at the right hip.

Technique

The liver should be evaluated, the omentum should be placed over the stomach to the left upper quadrant and the small bowel should be retracted from the pelvis to lie in the left upper quadrant. The 5-mm wavy grasper is a good instrument to flip the small bowel up into the left upper quadrant with a reverse "C" motion; the principle should be to avoid grasping any individual piece of bowel on the bowel itself. Using mesenteric fat or epiploic fat to move portions of intestine is appropriate. The cecum is then lifted to the anterior abdominal wall using the 5-mm grasper through the suprapubic port in the operator's left hand. An instrument with surgeon-controlled energy source can be used then to incise along the base of the peritoneum from the pelvic brim over the iliac vessels toward the duodenum at the midline of the abdominal cavity. This allows a plane to be developed in the retroperitoneum over the structures which are found posteriorly (Fig. 22.2). The right ureter is identified crossing the iliac vessels close to the bifurcation of the aorta; the gonadal vessels are further lateral and run parallel to the iliac vessels. The psoas muscle lies posteriorly and should be a boundary of dissection. The avascular plane which is encountered will be utilized as the dissection plane and can be bluntly dissected in a posterior sweeping direction to allow the mesentery and cecum to separate anteriorly from the posterior structures.

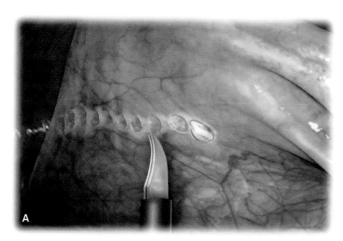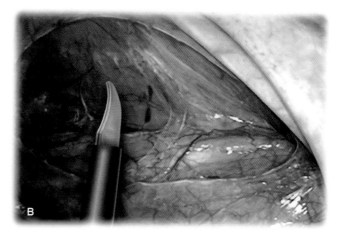

Figure 22.2

- The cecum should be completely mobilized from the retroperitoneum all the way out to the side wall of the abdomen using the left hand grasper for retraction upward and the right hand instrument to develop the plane. The dissection is carried in this posterior plane up to and around and on top of the surface of the duodenum. The duodenum should be separated from the overlying mesentery of the right colon using the left hand for anterior retraction all the way up to the hepatic flexure peritoneal attachments, thus exposing the entire sweep of the duodenum, a portion of the head of the pancreas and the lateral aspect of the middle colic vessels (Fig. 22.3). The anterior portion of the kidney will be exposed with this same maneuver with upward traction and downward counter traction. The mesentery and right colon are lifted toward the anterior abdominal wall while pulling the avascular tissue posteriorly with the blunt dissection using the instrument in the operator's right hand. Most of the retraction is accomplished with the left hand on the grasper through the suprapubic port.
- The patient is then placed in reverse Trendelenburg position and the attachments of the hepatic flexure to the retroperitoneum are lifted anteriorly and divided with an energy source along the line between the liver and the transverse colon (Fig. 22.4). This allows entry in the previously dissected plane of the right colon posteriorly in the area of purple hue in the posterior peritoneum.
- The omentum attached to the transverse colon is detached to enter the lesser sac. The transverse colon is released from the lesser sac, head of the pancreas and undersurface of the antrum of the stomach all the way out to the right side wall of the abdomen

Figure 22.3

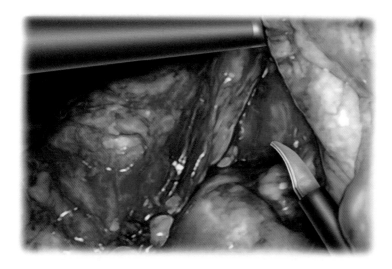

Figure 22.4

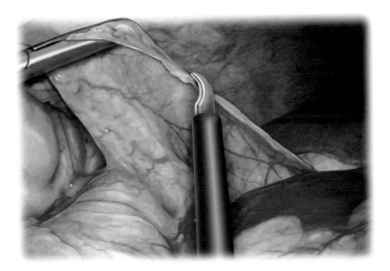

(Fig. 22.5). The hepatic flexure is completely mobilized from the under surface of the liver and the posterior dissection is connected to the right upper quadrant dissection.

- The patient is then returned to Trendelenburg position and the cecum is grasped at the ileocecal valve and lifted anteriorly to the abdominal wall. This provides the tension needed to expose the ileocolic vessel in the mesentery of the right colon.
- Dissection on either side of the ileocolic vessel will provide windows to allow transection of the ileocolic vessels at their origin along the superior mesenteric artery (Fig. 22.6).
- The right colon is then released from the lateral attachments of the colon from the right side wall of the abdomen. The cecum is grasped and lifted anteriorly. The cecum is retracted toward the midline to facilitate the division of the lateral attachments with the energy source. This maneuver allows the right colon to become a midline structure from the middle of the transverse colon all the way to the terminal ileum.

Operative Steps—Left Colon

- The patient is placed in steep Trendelenburg and airplaned to the right. The surgeon stands to the right of the patient. The small bowel is swept from the pelvis into the right upper quadrant with grasping instruments and the base of the mesentery of the left colon is exposed. The inferior mesenteric artery is identified at its origin on the aorta proximal to the sacral promontory. The space posterior to the superior hemorrhoidal artery and anterior to the sacral promontory is exposed. Anterior traction is

Figure 22.5

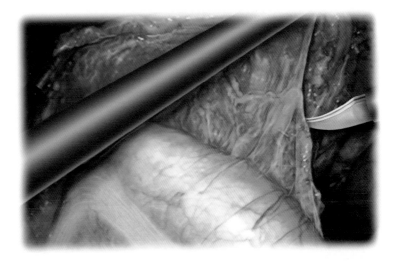

Figure 22.6

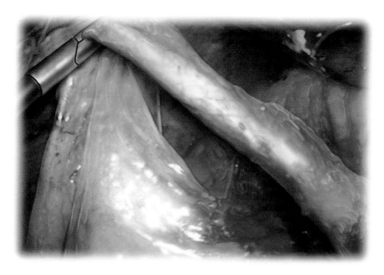

exerted on the superior hemorrhoidal artery with a clamp through the supra pubic
port. An energy source is introduced through the right lower quadrant Trocar site and
a 5 mm bowel grasper through the right upper quadrant Trocar site. The presacral
window is easily seen with this retraction plan (Fig. 22.7).

■ The peritoneum is incised along the base of the triangle to expose the areolar tissue
plane behind the superior hemorrhoidal artery, but anterior to the retroperitoneum
where the gonadal vessels and the ureter are found along the left iliac artery and vein.

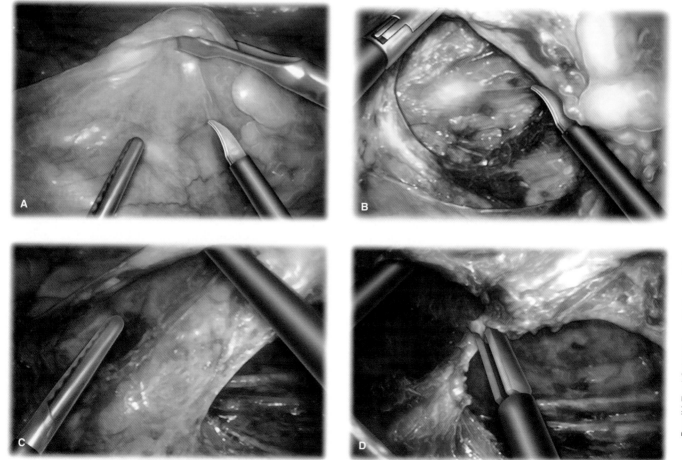

Figure 22.7

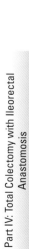

Figure 22.8

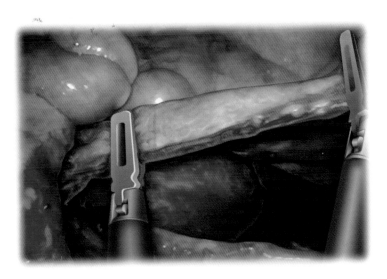

This avascular plane is bluntly developed all the way out to the left abdominal side wall behind the mesentery of the sigmoid and left colon.

■ The dissection is carried around the inferior mesenteric artery to the peritoneal window beneath the inferior mesenteric vein and anterior to the aorta. The window is incised and the opening developed cephalad to the inferior mesenteric artery. The inferior mesenteric artery is skeletonized and divided at its origin with an energy source. The artery may be divided at the bifurcation of the left colic and superior hemorrhoidal if the disease is benign to prevent all risk of injuring nerves of sexual function in the preaortic plexus.

■ Blunt dissection of the avascular plane is then carried from the pelvic brim to the tail of the pancreas and laterally to the sidewall of the abdomen beneath the left colon and its mesentery. The right upper quadrant Trocar site provides access for the retracting blunt instrument and the right lower quadrant Trocar site provides access for the energy source and/or dissecting instrument. The suprapubic site allows the second retracting grasper to lift the edge of the mesentery anteriorly to provide a tenting effect, while the camera (in the umbilical port) looks beneath and laterally.

■ The inferior mesenteric vein is then exposed at its origin at the level of the Ligament of Treitz, proximal to the first branch of the inferior mesenteric vein which travels to the splenic flexure. The vein is transected with an energy source or stapling instrument to release the base of the mesentery of the left colon (Fig. 22.8). The left colon is then released from the lateral sidewall of the abdomen from the pelvic brim to the splenic flexure, exposing the previously dissected retroperitoneum with the protected structures posteriorly.

■ The patient is placed in reverse Trendelenburg, still airplaned to the right, and the splenic flexure attachments are incised along the left sidewall of the pelvis up to the level of the spleen (Fig. 22.9). The tip of the spleen and the anterior surface of the kidney exposed as the suspensory ligaments are divided and the splenic flexure is mobilized medially. The right upper quadrant Trocar provides access for the assistant to place a 5-mm grasper and pull the splenic flexure toward the midline. The operating surgeon stands between the legs, utilizes the 10 mm grasper through the suprapubic midline and the 5-mm port in the left lower quadrant is used to place the energy source to allow the instrument to reach closer to the splenic flexure. The tail of the pancreas and tip of the spleen and anterior surface of the kidney are exposed (Fig. 22.10).

■ Finally, the omentum is released from the antimesenteric surface of the splenic flexure and transverse colon to enter the lesser sac around the corner of the splenic flexure. The right upper quadrant Trocar site provides retracting access to lift the omentum anteriorly and cephalad while the suprapubic Trocar site provides access for retracting the splenic flexure toward the feet and the left lower quadrant Trocar site provides access for the energy source to divide the attachments of the omentum to the colon.

Figure 22.9

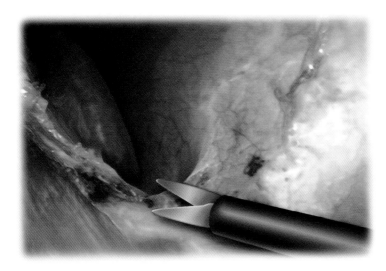

The pancreas is exposed in the base of the lesser sac and its lower edge freed from the attachments of the splenic flexure all the way to the stump of the inferior mesenteric vein at the Ligament of Treitz. The posterior wall of the stomach, the anterior surface of the pancreas, the tip of the spleen and the anterior surface of the kidney are clearly visualized with this technique (Fig. 22.11).

The Isolation of Middle Colic Vessels

- Once the left and right colon have been completely mobilized and the transverse colon completely freed from the gastrocolic ligament, the pedicle of the middle colic vessels can be identified at the inferior margin of the pancreas and the anterior surface of the third portion of the duodenum. In a hand-assisted approach, this is most easily accomplished by placing the left hand through gel port with the operator standing between the legs, and the middle colic vessels are grasped by identifying the windows of the mesentery on both sides of the vessels on either side of the midline (Fig. 22.12). This allows the middle colic vessels to be lifted anteriorly and the SMA and SMV are protected. The flexible tip camera is turned to the right upper quadrant and flexed to the right to give a transverse view of the vessels as they are stretched and lifted. An endoscopic linear cutter stapler can then be inserted through a 10-mm trocar placed in the right upper quadrant or the bipolar sealing instrument can be used through the right upper quadrant to divide the base of the middle colic vessels carefully. The time should be taken to ensure adequate hemostasis since these vessels bear the pressure of aortic flow.

Figure 22.10

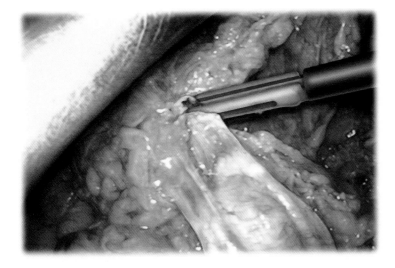

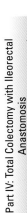

Part IV: Total Colectomy with Ileorectal Anastomosis

Figure 22.11

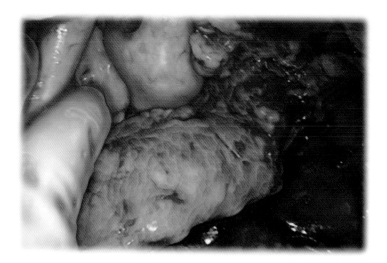

▓ The suprapubic incision is extended and a wound protector placed or in a hand-assisted case, the cap of the gel port is removed and the carbon dioxide deflated. The colon and terminal ileum are extracted. The mesentery of the sigmoid colon is identified and the mesentery divided at the level of the sacral promontory. The rectum can then be divided at the level of the sacral promontory with a transverse stapler, endoscopic stapler or linear stapler through the suprapubic incision.

▓ The terminal ileum is divided at the ileocecal valve using another firing of a gastrointestinal anastomosis (GIA) stapler. The colon and its mesentery from the right colon all the way to the top of the rectum are then passed off as specimen.

▓ The terminal ileum is returned to the abdomen. The small bowel is allowed to fall to the patient's left side, and the rectum is pulled to the right side of the pelvis. The ileum is allowed to loop down into the pelvis along the left side of the rectum and then curve back up along the antimesenteric border of the rectum to the level of the staple line. The two transverse staple lines are then aligned and the corners of the staple line are opened and a linear cutter stapler placed between the rectum and the terminal ileum to create a side to side anastomosis when fired.

▓ The transverse opening is then closed with another firing of the GIA stapler. The transverse staple line is inverted with a running monofilament absorbable suture. The apex of the GIA staple line is protected with an interrupted absorbable suture. The cut edge of the mesentery in the small bowel can usually be secured to the retroperitoneum along the side of the aorta on either side of the aorta using a running

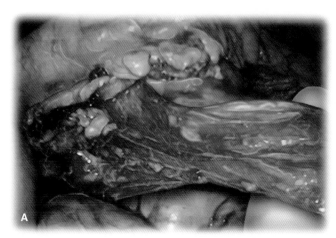

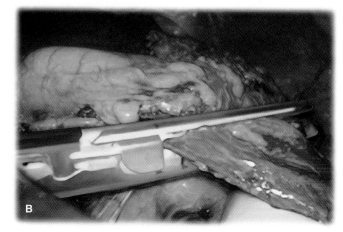

Figure 22.12

absorbable suture. This has the benefit of preventing internal herniation and guarantees that the small bowel is lying in an unrotated or twisted manner.

- The inner aspect of the umbilical trocar is closed with a figure-of-eight suture of 0 absorbable suture. The Pfannenstiel incision is closed with a running monofilament absorbable suture in the fascia. Subcutaneous tissue is irrigated with antibiotic solution at all sites, and the skin is closed with skin staples and band-aids are applied.

 # POSTOPERATIVE MANAGEMENT

Patients are ambulated early. They rely on intravenous fluid replacement to maintain a urine output of greater than 30 ml/hour. Nasogastric decompression is not required unless the patient becomes nauseated. Within 24–48 hours most patients will tolerate clear liquids and the diet can be advanced as tolerated. Patients should be given 24 hours of prophylactic antibiotic coverage, incentive spirometry, deep vein thrombosis prophylaxis, and encouraged to ambulate as much as possible during the early time period. Usual hospital stay after an open right colectomy is 4 to 5 days, or less, when placed on a fast tracking post-op regimen. Post-op analgesia is usually managed with patient controlled analgesia followed by switch to oral analgesics.

The patient will have a fairly rapid return of bowel function because of the laparoscopic approach. There will most likely be a large fluid shift because of the raw surfaces created. Adequate fluid can avoid acute renal failure, dehydration, and an ileus.

 # COMPLICATIONS

As we perform more ileorectal anastomoses for familial polyposis and Crohn's disease, the frequent development of a delayed ileus has led us to describe a syndrome known as the "ileorectal syndrome." This is possibly caused by the terminal ileum facing new high pressure intraluminally because of its attachment to the rectum with an intact sphincter only 12 cm away. The high pressure causes the ileum to interpret this as small bowel obstruction, and a high volume of intraluminal fluid is created which causes diarrhea, a bloating sensation, and even nausea and vomiting occurs. Treatment is best accomplished with a nasogastric tube, bowel rest, and total parenteral nutrition for support. This syndrome develops even when a 34 mushroom catheter is left in the rectum in the early postoperative period to decompress and equalize the pressures in the rectum. The terminal ileum responds as if it were a blocked ileostomy with high outpouring of fluid, distension, and a syndrome of nausea, vomiting, diarrhea, and all around misery. The patient should be reassured, supported, and the possibility of an anastomotic leak ruled out with a computed tomographic scan.

If the patient develops a postop obstructive picture, it is important to rule out an internal herniation, especially if the mesentery has not been secured to the retroperitoneum. The internal herniation and volvulus around the superior mesenteric artery can result in disaster, as a significant portion of the small bowel can infarct resulting in short bowel syndrome and loss of the possibility for intestinal continuity. Rapid recognition and treatment by exploration and detorsion is essential in this situation.

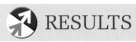 # RESULTS

Anastomotic leak occurs in less than 4% of patients who undergo total colectomy and ileorectal anastomosis. Rapid recovery as a result of utilization of the laparoscopic approach makes this a very attractive approach for those needing total colectomy. Hand-assisted approaches provide the same outcome as laparoscopic with shorter operating room (OR) times.

✦ CONCLUSION

Laparoscopic total abdominal colectomy should be considered in patients requiring removal of the entire colon.

Suggested Readings

Boushey RP, Marcello PW, Martel G, et al. Laparoscopic total colectomy: an evolutionary experience. *Dis Colon Rectum.* 2007; 50(10):1512–9.

Chung TP, Fleshman JW, Birnbaum EH, et al. Laparoscopic vs. open total abdominal colectomy for severe colitis: impact on recovery and subsequent completion restorative proctectomy. *Dis Colon Rectum.* 2009;52(1):4–10.

Marcello PW, Fleshman JW, Milsom JW, et al. Hand-assisted laparoscopic vs. laparoscopic colorectal surgery: a multicenter, prospective, randomized trial. *Dis Colon Rectum.* 2008;51(6): 818–26.

23 Hand-Assisted

David A. Margolin

 ## INDICATIONS/CONTRAINDICATIONS

Laparoscopic total abdominal colectomy is one of the more challenging laparoscopic colon procedures (LAP) as the surgeon is asked to work in all four quadrants of the abdomen. The use of hand-assisted laparoscopic (HAL) techniques has been shown not only to facilitate the technical aspects of the procedure by restoring some tactile sensation, but also to decrease the operative time. In essence, it makes laparoscopic procedures "more like open surgery." The indications for the procedure are the same whether performed open, laparoscopic, or hand assisted. However, it is up to the surgeon to determine if the patient is a candidate for minimally invasive surgery. They need to take into account the patient's overall comorbidities as well as surgical history. While multiple previous abdominal operations are not an absolute contraindication for LAP or HAL, the individual surgeon's level of comfort and experience with the planned procedure plays a large role.

 ## PREOPERATIVE PLANNING

Preoperative Preparation

Standard mechanical bowel preparation is not mandatory. However, it is the author's preference, since it is easier to handle an empty colon. Our patients use a polyethylene glycol (PEG) preparation prior to surgery and maintained on clear liquids the day before surgery. We no longer use oral antibiotics prior to surgery but ensure that standard intravenous broad-spectrum antibiotics are given within 1 hour of skin incision. Since the patients will be in a modified lithotomy position for several hours deep vein prophylaxis is mandatory. We utilize both subcutaneous heparin and sequential compression stockings commencing immediately prior to surgery and continued after surgery. All patients have an informed consent that includes the potential for conversion to an open procedure.

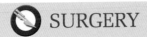

SURGERY

Patient Positioning and Preparation

The patient is placed on a gel pad to prevent slippage. After induction of general anesthesia an orogastric tube and indwelling urinary bladder catheter are placed. The patient is placed in a modified lithotomy position using Yellow Fin Stirrups™ (Allen Medical, Batesville, IN) with the thighs even with the hips and all potential pressure points appropriately padded. Care is taken to ensure that there is no pressure on the peroneal nerves and that the patient's knees are in line with contralateral shoulder. Both arms are tucked in the adducted position to facilitate securing the patients for the extremes of positioning used during laparoscopy. The patient is then secured to the table, with tape across the chest and the forehead to limit neck movement. Rectal irrigation is performed. After that the skin is prepped with a 2% chlorhexidine-based solution and draped in a standard fashion. Prior to draping the table is rotated in all directions to assure that the patient is stable.

Instrument/Monitor Positioning

Two monitors are utilized during the procedure. One is on the patient's right side at the level of the shoulder. The other monitor is placed on the patient's left side at the level of the hip. At our institution the monitors are mounted on booms from the ceiling allowing easy repositioning for optimal visualization. Because of the configuration of our operating rooms the insufflation tubing, suction tubing, cautery power cord, laparoscopy camera wiring, and a laparoscope light cord are brought off the patient's left side at the foot of the table. We routinely use a 10-mm laparoscope with a 30-degree lens. However, with the increased availability of high-definition cameras and monitors a 5-mm laparoscope may be an acceptable alternative.

Port Selection and Placement

Prior to placing any ports the outline of the hand-assist device is marked on the patient's abdomen. We use the Applied Medical GelPort® (Applied Medical, Ranch Santa Margarita, CA). By tracing the outline of the device we ensure that all of our ports are outside the outline to function throughout the procedure. We place the inferior edge of the device 2–3 cm from the pubic symphysis in the midline. Once this marking is done, we use a modified Hasson technique to enter the abdomen above the umbilicus and obtain pneumoperitoneum. A vertical skin incision is made with a scalpel followed by dissection down to the linea alba. A Kocher clamp is used to elevate the fascia in the midline at the level of the umbilical stump and the linea alba is then incised. S-shaped retractors are helpful in exposing the midline. Entry into the peritoneal cavity is accomplished sharply. Once entry into the peritoneal cavity is obtained a 10-mm blunt-tip balloon trocar is placed and inflated. A total of four additional ports are used. We use two 5-mm ports in the left and right upper quadrants and a 5-mm port in the left lower quadrant. We will often place a 12-mm port in the right lower quadrant, as this will allow placement of an endoscopic stapler if necessary; the hand port is placed later in the procedure (Fig. 23.1).

Mobilization and Transection

After establishing pneumoperitoneum and placing the necessary ports the abdominal cavity is laparoscopically explored. The patient is then placed in the Trendelenburg position and is rotated to their left. We initially begin with right colon mobilization prior to placement of the hand port. Unlike other authors, we find that placing the hand port prior to mobilizing the right colon actually slows down the operation. First, the

Figure 23.1 Laparoscopic port sites and hand port placement.

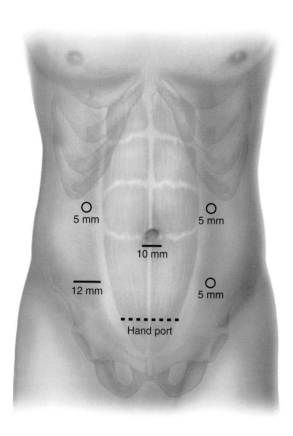

○ 5 mm   ○ 5 mm

— 10 mm

— 12 mm   ○ 5 mm

┄┄┄┄┄┄
Hand port

ileocolic artery is grasped and elevated, and the avascular plane on either side is dissected free to allow clear visualization of the duodenum. The vessels are then ligated and divided using a vessel-sealing device such as the Ethicon EnSeal® (Ethicon Endosurgery, Cincinnati, OH) although the choice of the alternate energy source is up to the surgeons' discretion. Care is taken at this point to sweep the duodenum medially. Sweeping away from the duodenum can lead to serosal tears. The lateral attachments of the right colon are laparoscopically mobilized, being careful to stay in the lateral avascular plane.

Once the colon is mobilized to the level of the hepatic flexure the patient is rotated to their right, still in the Trendelenburg position. The sigmoid colon is grasped thought the left lower quadrant port and elevated to the abdominal wall. The avascular plane inferior to the inferior mesenteric artery (IMA) is opened and the left ureter is identified. The IMA is then isolated and ligated. Superior and lateral dissection is undertaken from a medial to lateral direction behind the colon and anterior to the left ureter up to the level of the splenic flexure.

At this point in the procedure the hand port is placed. As previously mentioned, placing the hand port prior to mobilizing the right colon is more of a hindrance. A 7-cm transverse incision is made 2–3 cm superior to the pubic synthesis and dissection is continued to the fascia. The fascia is opened vertically for 7 cm, the port is placed, and pneumoperitoneum is reestablished. Standing on the patient's left side, the patient is rotated to neutral with a slight amount of reverse Trendelenburg. The surgeon places his or her left hand through the port to apply downward traction on the splenic flexure. Using his or her right hand an alternate energy source device is placed through one of the left-sided trocars and the splenic flexure is mobilized. Once free the surgeon then replaces his or her hand and with the right hand elevated the transverse colon and using one the right-sided port releases the distal transverse colon from underneath and takes the omentum off the transverse colon and subsequently divides the transverse mesocolon and the middle colic artery, completely freeing the abdominal colon. The assistant who is on the patient's left side plays a key role in the portion of the procedure. He gives countertraction through one of the left-sided ports.

An alternate approach is occasionally used, to make the hand port incision, as described above, at the beginning of the case. Using handheld retractors we then mobilize the cecum, ascending and sigmoid colon up toward their respective flexures. Once difficulty is encountered with the mobilization pneumoperitoneum is established and the trocars are placed under direct vision in the previous mentioned locations. This limited open dissection may significantly decrease operative time especially in thinner patients.

Creation of the Anastomosis

Once the colon is completely mobilized the top of the hand port is removed and the colon at the sacral promontory is divided using an open 45-mm stapler. The remainder of the colon is delivered through the hand port, the distal terminal ileum is divided, and the specimen is removed from the field. Then, using a Furness clamp a purse string is made in the distal terminal ileum and the anvil for a 29-mm circular staler is secured in the terminal ileum. A Fansler retractor is used to gently dilate the anal sphincters and allow easy transanal passage of the stapler. Once the stapler is passed into the anal canal the Fansler retractor is removed and the stapler is manipulated through the rectum to the staple line. The trocar is deployed. Care is taken to assure that the trocar does not go through the staple line but 1–2 mm anterior or posterior to the rectal staple line. After a tension-free anastomosis is created, the pelvis is filled with water, and rigid proctoscopy is performed to check for an air leak. Because of the proximal nature of the anastomosis small leaks can be repaired under direct vision through the hand port.

Closure of Port Sites

After verification of hemostasis and a sponge and instrument counts the ports are removed. The 5-and 10-mm port sites are irrigated and the skin is closed with a subcuticular monofilament absorbable suture such as 4-0 poliglecaprone (Monocryl®) suture. The fascia at the umbilical port site is closed with interrupted 0 (Vicryl®) and the hand port site is closed in layers. First the peritoneum and transversalis fascia is closed with a polyglycolic acid suture (Vicryl®) and then the anterior rectus fascia is closed with a monofilament absorbable suture polydioxanone (PDS®); the skin is closed similar to the other port sites.

 # COMPLICATIONS

HAL retains most of the potential complications associated with both the open and the laparoscopic procedures including hemorrhage, adjacent organ injury, and anastomotic dehiscence. Although still present the risk of incisional hernia and postoperative surgical site infection may be significantly decreased compared to the open procedure. One complication that is more common and fortunately preventable in HAL than open surgery is a 360-degree twist of the anastomosis. This potentially devastating complication occurs because of the decreased field of view with the laparoscope. In order to prevent this problem, it is imperative that the surgeon uses good techniques and follows the cut small-bowel mesentery proximally to verify that there are no twists and that it lays in a straight line on top of the retroperitoneum.

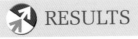 # RESULTS

Hand-assisted total abdominal colectomy has been shown to be an efficacious modality in lieu of open or strait laparoscopic surgery. Many authors have touted it as a potential hybrid procedure that maintains the advantages of laparoscopy (1–7).

Nakajima in the review of 23 patients, 12 HAL and 11 LAP, found no difference in conversion rate, blood loss perioperative complications between the two groups, and a significantly shorter operative time in the HAL group (1). Boushey in reviewing 130 nonrandomized cases again showed no difference in anything but conversion rate and a trend toward shorter operative time in the HAL group (3). Marcello et al. in a randomized prospective multicenter trial comparing HAL to straight laparoscopy for left-sided and total colostomies demonstrated a significant decrease in operative time with no loss of the benefits of laparoscopic surgery (7). Subset analysis for the patients undergoing total abdominal colostomies showed a decrease in time from 285 ± 105 to 199 ± 35 min. Although a small sample size, 14 in the HAL and in the15 straight lap group in this randomized trial there was no difference in time to flatus, diet, or length of stay. There is some concern that the long-term benefits of LAP will be lost with HAL, especially the incidence of postoperative hernias and bowel obstruction. Sonoda in reviewing 536 patients over a 5-year period, 266 Hal and 270 LAP, found no difference in either incisional hernias or the incidence of bowel obstruction with a median follow-up of 27 months (4).

 CONCLUSION

Some of the technical challenges of laparoscopic total abdominal colectomy may be overcome by the HAL approach. Most of the benefits of laparoscopy appear to be maintained while operative times may be shortened. The tactile sensation afforded by use of the hand may be beneficial to many surgeons.

References

1. Nakajima K, Lee SW, Cocilovo C, et al. Laparoscopic total colectomy: hand-assisted vs. standard technique. *Surg Endosc* 2004;18:582–86.
2. Rivadeneira DE, Marcello PW, Roberts PL, et al. Benefits of hand-assisted laparoscopic restorative proctocolectomy: a comparative study. *Dis Colon Rectum* 2004;47:1371–76.
3. Boushey RP, Marcello PW, Martel G, et al. Laparoscopic total colectomy: an evolutionary experience. *Dis Colon Rectum* 2007;50:1512–19.
4. Sonoda T, Pandey S, Trencheva K, et al. Long-term complications of hand-assisted versus laparoscopic colectomy. *J Am Coll Surg* 2009;208:62–6.
5. Aalbers AG, Biere SS, van Berge Henegouwen MI, Bemelman WA. Hand-assisted or laparoscopic-assisted approach in colorectal surgery: a systematic review and meta-analysis. *Surg Endosc* 2008;22:1769–80.
6. Martel G, Boushey RP, Marcello PW. Hand-assisted laparoscopic colorectal surgery: an evidence-based review. *Minerva Chir* 2008;63:373–83.
7. Marcello PW, Fleshman JW, Milsom JW, et al. Hand-assisted laparoscopic vs. laparoscopic colorectal surgery: a multicenter, prospective, randomized trial. *Dis Colon Rectum* 2008;51:818–26; discussion 826–28.

Suggested Readings

Agha A, Moser C, Iesalnieks I, Piso P, Schlitt HJ. Combination of hand-assisted and laparoscopic proctocolectomy (HALP): technical aspects, learning curve and early postoperative results. *Surg Endosc* 2008;22(6):1547–52.

Cima RR, Pattana-arun J, Larson DW, et al. Experience with 969 minimal access colectomies: the role of hand-assisted laparoscopy in expanding minimally invasive surgery for complex colectomies. *J Am Coll Surg* 2008;206(5):946–50; discussion 950–52.

Hassan I, You YN, Cima RR, et al. Hand-assisted versus laparoscopic-assisted colorectal surgery: Practice patterns and clinical outcomes in a minimally-invasive colorectal practice. *Surg Endosc* 2008;22(3):739–43.

Hsiao KC, Jao SW, Wu CC, et al. Hand-assisted laparoscopic total colectomy for slow transit constipation. *Int J Colorectal Dis* 2008;23(4):419–24.

Ozturk E, Kiran PR, Remzi F, Geisler D, Fazio V. Hand-assisted laparoscopic surgery may be a useful tool for surgeons early in the learning curve performing total abdominal colectomy. *Colorectal Dis* 2009 Jan 27 [Epub ahead of print].

Polle SW, Dunker MS, Slors JF, et al. Body image, cosmesis, quality of life, and functional outcome of hand-assisted laparoscopic versus open restorative proctocolectomy: long-term results of a randomized trial. *Surg Endosc* 2007;21(8):1301–07.

Roslani AC, Koh DC, Tsang CB, et al. Hand-assisted laparoscopic colectomy versus standard laparoscopic colectomy: a cost analysis. *Colorectal Dis* 2009;11(5):496–501.

Stein S, Whelan RL. The controversy regarding hand-assisted colorectal resection. *Surg Endosc* 2007;21(12):2123–26.

Watanabe K, Funayama Y, Fukushima K, Shibata C, Takahashi K, Sasaki I. Hand-assisted laparoscopic vs. open subtotal colectomy for severe ulcerative colitis. *Dis Colon Rectum* 2009;52(4):640–45.

Zhang LY. Hand-assisted laparoscopic vs. open total colectomy in treating slow transit constipation. *Tech Coloproctol* 2006;10(2):152–53. No abstract available.

Part IV: Total Colectomy with Ileorectal Anastomosis

24 Open

Ashwin deSouza and Herand Abcarian

 ## INDICATIONS/CONTRAINDICATIONS

Defining the indications for an open total proctocolectomy with ileostomy mandates the discussion of three concepts:

- the extent of surgical resection, that is, a total proctocolectomy
- the use of a permanent stoma versus an ileal pouch anal anastomosis
- the surgical approach being either laparoscopy or laparotomy.

Resection of the entire colon and rectum as a total proctocolectomy may be indicated for the following disease processes:

- Familial adenomatous polyposis
- Ulcerative colitis
- Synchronous colorectal malignancies
- Crohn's disease

Familial Adenomatous Polyposis

Patients with familial adenomatous polyposis are usually diagnosed early as a family history of this condition warrants early screening with colonoscopy. Although a total proctocolectomy is the required extent of resection, an ileal pouch anal anastomosis is the preferred surgical option in the absence of concomitant advanced rectal cancer.

Ulcerative Colitis

Surgery is indicated for ulcerative colitis in the following situations:

- Intractability despite adequate medical treatment.
- Dysplasia or malignancy in long standing ulcerative colitis.
- Acute severe ulcerative colitis with toxic megacolon.

Although a restorative proctocolectomy with ileal pouch anal anastomosis has become the preferred option for most patients with ulcerative colitis, a permanent end ileostomy is still indicated in selected individuals. Elderly patients are often unable to cope with the relatively high frequency of liquid bowel movements after an ileal pouch. These patients also have multiple medical comorbidities, putting them at high risk for complications following a lengthy operation and a difficult pouch anal anastomosis. An end ileostomy is a good option and is often well accepted in this patient population.

Documentation of good sphincter tone is a prerequisite before an ileal pouch procedure. Sphincter tone is often suboptimal in patients who have had prior obstetric injury or a fistulotomy for anorectal fistulae. Long-term quality of life is better with an ileostomy in patients with poor sphincter tone.

Restoration of intestinal continuity with an ileal pouch has the advantage of avoiding a permanent stoma but is not entirely without complications. The associated risks of anastomotic leakage, pouchitis, and pouch failure should be appreciated by the patient when consenting for the procedure. In view of the higher incidence of long-term complications, the need for pouch surveillance and an additional procedure to close the temporary diverting stoma, medically fit patients with good sphincter tone may still opt for a permanent ileostomy. The choice between a permanent stoma and a restorative procedure is therefore influenced by a number of factors with the patient having to make the final decision.

Ulcerative colitis presenting as an acute severe attack with significant colonic dilatation (toxic megacolon) and signs of impending perforation, requires urgent surgical intervention. In this setting, the patient is often hemodynamically unstable and unable to withstand a prolonged procedure. In addition, an acutely inflamed colon may also be extremely friable and can perforate with the least manipulation. A total abdominal colectomy with ileostomy is therefore the preferred option in the emergent setting. A completion proctectomy with or without an ileal pouch can be performed at a later stage after resolution of the acute attack.

Synchronous Colorectal Malignancies

The incidence of synchronous large bowel adenocarcinoma varies from 1.5–7.6%. A synchronous rectal and sigmoid lesion can most often be resected en block, with a colorectal anastomosis to restore intestinal continuity. However, for a synchronous rectal and right colon lesion, a total proctocolectomy with ileostomy is sometimes required. Although not contraindicated, an ileal pouch is best avoided in the setting of synchronous colorectal cancers and patients are usually offered an end ileostomy with a low Hartmann's procedure. Following adjuvant therapy, the option of a pouch procedure can be considered in patients showing good control of the primary malignancy.

The presence of a single malignancy in the colon or rectum puts the rest of the large bowel at a 12–62% risk of harboring polyps. If the polyps are too numerous to be removed endoscopically, or a number of polyps show malignant/premalignant changes, a total proctocolectomy with ileostomy should be considered especially in elderly patients.

Crohn's Disease

Crohn's disease with pancolitis, poorly responsive to medical management is a definite indication for a total proctocolectomy with ileostomy because an ileal pouch is an absolute contraindication in Crohn's disease. However, the procedure may have to be performed in two stages if there is severe perianal Crohn's disease. Performing a proctectomy in the presence of active perianal Crohn's with abscesses and draining fistulae significantly increases the incidence of perineal wound sepsis and nonhealing. An abdominal colectomy and ileostomy together with unroofing of the perianal fistulae is done at the first stage. Once the infection and inflammation abates, the patient may be scheduled for completion proctectomy. A number of local pedicle flaps to cover the perineum have been described but are best avoided in the presence of active infection. Fecal diversion with ileostomy together with laying open all fistulous tracts and ultimately an intersphincteric proctectomy, often results in healing in a significant number of patients, decreasing the need for flap procedures.

Although laparoscopic colorectal resections are becoming increasingly common-place, the majority of rectal resections in the United States are still accomplished by a laparotomy. Laparoscopy has its own learning curve, limitations, and technical challenges. While a limited colon or rectal resection could be completed safely and effectively within a reasonable time period, a total proctocolectomy may prove to be time consuming using a pure laparoscopic technique. Additionally inflammatory bowel disease is often associated with extensive bowel adhesions and complex fistulization, which when present add significantly to the technical difficulty of the procedure.

The benefits of laparoscopy should be prudently weighed against the technical ability of the operating surgeon, the complexity of each individual case, and the surgical risk of the patient. A decision to convert to the open approach is not a sign of failure but rather a reflection of a mature judgment and should be made early if needed.

This chapter emphasizes the surgical technique of an open total proctocolectomy with end ileostomy.

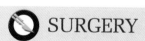 PREOPERATIVE PLANNING

A full colonic evaluation with colonoscopy is usually mandatory in all patients who require a total proctocolectomy. Additionally, a small bowel follow-through or computed tomographic (CT) enterography is necessary to rule out small bowel involvement in inflammatory bowel disease. Preoperative imaging with an abdominal and pelvic CT scan is useful to determine the presence of bowel wall thickening, adhesions, and likely sites of internal fistulization. A CT scan also helps to trace both ureters and determine the need of preoperative ureteral stenting to facilitate intraoperative identification of the ureters.

Avoiding a routine bowel prep is an evolving concept although a majority of surgeons still prescribe a full bowel prep before a total proctocolectomy.

Patients with inflammatory bowel disease requiring surgery are usually on high dose steroids or on immunosuppressive medications. Immunosuppressives can be discontinued postoperatively but steroids need to be continued through the perioperative period and gradually tapered over the next few weeks. Prophylactic antibiotics and deep venous thrombosis prophylaxis are essential because inflammatory bowel disease renders many patients in a hypercoagulable state.

Perhaps the most important aspect of preoperative planning is the marking of the stoma site as the patient will be left with a permanent ileostomy at the end of the procedure. Stoma site marking should be done preoperatively by a dedicated enterostomal therapist with appropriate patient counseling. It is important to accurately site the stoma away from incisions, bony prominences, and skin folds.

SURGERY

Patient Positioning

The patient is positioned on the operating table in the modified lithotomy position with minimal hip flexion to facilitate the abdominal part of the procedure. For the perineal dissection, the legs can be flexed to increase the exposure.

It is important to ensure that the buttocks lie outside the edge of the table after the foot portion of the table has been removed. This maneuver is to enable placing a perineal retractor such as a St. Mark's or Lone star to significantly enhance the surgical exposure during the perineal dissection.

Prolonged procedures in the lithotomy position are also known to be associated with postoperative neuropathy. Care should be taken to ensure that all pressure points are adequately padded and protected. The legs should be securely fastened in the Allen's stirrups to prevent external rotation at the hip joints. The hips may be abducted and flexed for exposure of the perineum but external rotation should be minimized to prevent undue traction on the femoral nerves. The femoral nerve at the hip and the common peroneal nerve at the neck of the fibula are the two most common nerves to be affected in the lithotomy position. As the patient is usually positioned with arms apart, the upper extremities must be adequately padded and the brachial plexus be protected from excessive abduction of the arm.

Technique

The procedure can be performed with two surgical teams working from the abdomen and perineum simultaneously.

Abdominal Dissection

Peritoneal access is achieved through a midline incision from the pubic symphysis to above the umbilicus. As is routine for every laparotomy, the abdomen is first explored to evaluate the small bowel for Crohn's disease, the liver and gall bladder for metastasis and gallstone, and the colon for a mass or a fistula.

The procedure begins with mobilization of the right colon. The cecum is retracted medially and the peritoneum is incised along the line of Toldt in the right paracolic gutter to open the retroperitoneal avascular plane. The cecum and ascending colon are then mobilized lateral to medial by developing this avascular plane till the duodenum is visualized. An accurate identification of this plane is the key to a virtually bloodless dissection that proceeds lateral to medial, exposing the Gerota's fascia, the right gonadal vessels, and the right ureter (Fig. 24.1).

Attention is then directed to the hepatic flexure. The omentum is retracted superiorly and the lesser sac is entered by incising the gastrocolic omentum in the avascular plane just above the transverse colon. This line of dissection is then carried toward the

Figure 24.1 Colon mobilization.

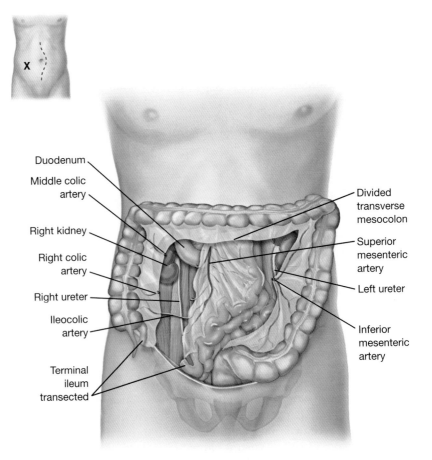

hepatic flexure to divide the hepatocolic ligament. Adhesions in the lesser sac between the omentum and the posterior wall of the lesser sac are often encountered, which should be taken down by sharp dissection. It is important to distinguish between the fat of the transverse colon mesentery and that of the omentum, as this helps in identification of the correct plane of dissection.

The hepatic flexure is then retracted medially and the final attachments to the retroperitoneum are divided to complete the mobilization of the hepatic flexure till the second portion of the duodenum is encountered. The omentum is then dissected off the transverse colon, proceeding towards the splenic flexure. At this point it is easier to begin mobilization of the descending colon before completely mobilizing the splenic flexure.

The sigmoid colon is retracted medially and the peritoneum is incised along the line of Toldt in the left paracolic gutter. This opens up the avascular retroperitoneal plane on the left side. As one proceeds to the root of the sigmoid mesocolon, the left ureter and gonadal vessels lie in close proximity to the plane of dissection and should be protected from thermal injury from the cautery. To do this, continuous traction should be applied on the sigmoid colon and dissection should proceed just outside the fat of the sigmoid mesocolon. Unlike laparoscopic dissection, the mobilization of the left colon when using the open approach is easier when performed lateral to medial.

Continuing the dissection superiorly, the descending colon is mobilized completely. Having identified the plane of dissection on either side of the splenic flexure, it becomes easy then to retract the splenic flexure medially and divide splenocolic ligament and the final attachments to the retroperitoneum to complete the mobilization (Fig. 24.2).

Having mobilized the abdominal colon completely, the vascular pedicles can then be ligated and divided. For a total proctocolectomy with ileostomy, the ileocolic pedicle need not be divided. If an ileal pouch is planned at a later stage, preserving the ileocolic pedicle is mandatory. The right colic (if present), and middle colic pedicles are then divided. When resecting for inflammatory bowel disease or familial polyposis, it is not necessary to ligate the vascular pedicles at their root. However, it is technically easier to divide the vessels at their origins before they branch.

Care should be taken when ligating the inferior mesenteric artery as a complex network of sympathetic nerves is present at the root of this vascular pedicle. These nerves are essential for ejaculation in males and bladder emptying in females and should be preserved especially when operating for benign disease. With a thick, inflamed mesentery it is sometimes easier to follow the superior hemorrhoidal artery superiorly to identify the inferior mesenteric artery, which can then be isolated on all sides and divided

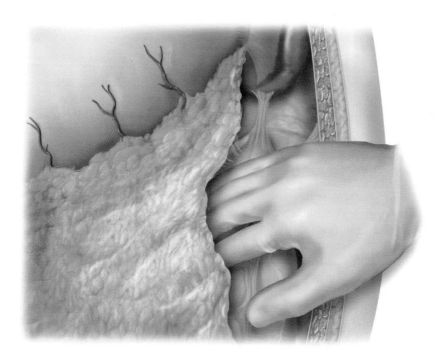

Figure 24.2 Division of the splenocolic ligament after mobilization of the transverse and ascending colon.

as proximally as needed. When operating for malignancy, however, a high ligation of the inferior mesenteric artery is mandatory to achieve an oncologically sound resection.

The terminal ileum is then transected with a linear stapler and the completely mobilized abdominal colon is then delivered out of the incision. A self-retaining retractor (e.g., Balfour or Bookwalter) is used to retract the abdominal wall, and the small bowel and omentum are packed into the upper abdomen. The patient is positioned with a slight Trendelenburg tilt to gain exposure to the pelvis.

Rectal dissection is begun posteriorly with identification of the avascular presacral plane. This plane is best identified at the level of the sacral promontory in the midline. The rectum is retracted anteriorly to stretch the rectal mesentery and the peritoneum to the right of the upper rectum is incised. This incision is then extended inferiorly on the right of the rectum while continuing to maintain anterior traction.

The presacral plane is developed just outside the mesorectal fat, keeping the mesorectal envelop intact. The pelvic hypogastric nerves run in the areolar tissue of the presacral space and must be preserved. Maintaining anterior traction on the rectum and dissecting just outside the mesorectal fat will minimize the risk of injuring these nerves.

The rectum is then retracted towards the left and the right lateral attachments of the rectum are divided. It is important to follow the curve of the rectum to avoid injury to the vascular structures on the lateral pelvic wall. The middle rectal artery, if present, will be encountered during this part of the dissection and can usually be carefully clamped, cauterized, and divided. A similar dissection is performed on the left side to divide the left lateral rectal attachments.

The anterior dissection differs slightly in both sexes. In males, the bladder is retracted anteriorly and the rectum is pushed posteriorly to expose the rectovesical fold of the peritoneum. The peritoneal incisions on the right and left of the mobilized upper rectum are then connected through this peritoneal fold. The Denonvilliers' fascia is usually adherent to the seminal vesicles and prostatic capsule and it is easier to dissect just posterior to this fascial layer. This avoids injury to the pampiniform plexus and the nervi erigentes and maintains a bloodless surgical field.

In females, the rectouterine peritoneal fold is loose and the rectovaginal septum is usually clearly defined. This makes the anterior dissection easier than in men. The uterus is retracted anteriorly to identify both uterosacral ligaments arching round the rectum from the cervix to the sacrum. The rectouterine peritoneal fold is then grasped between the uterosacral ligaments and incised to enter the areolar plane. This is then developed to mobilize the rectum from the vagina anteriorly. The abdominal dissection is complete when the rectum is circumferentially mobilized all the way to the anorectal ring.

Perineal Dissection

The patient's legs are flexed at the hip to facilitate exposure to the perineum. In the absence of rectal cancer such as when performing the procedure for familial polyposis or inflammatory bowel disease, an intersphincteric dissection is preferred as this leaves behind the substantial muscle mass of the external anal sphincter, which is well vascularized and aids in perineal wound closure. When operating for low rectal cancer, the entire sphincter complex should be excised.

For an intersphincteric dissection, a circumferential incision is made just outside the anal verge. The incision is deepened to enter the plane between the internal and external sphincters, that is, the intersphincteric plane. Dissection is continued in this plane till the anorectal ring is reached. The outer layer of the muscularis propria is then incised in the midline posteriorly to enter the dissected presacral space. The muscularis propria is then circumferentially divided at the anorectal ring and the specimen is delivered through the perineal incision.

When performing the procedure for rectal cancer, a circumferential incision is made on the perineal skin about 2 cm away from the anal verge. The incision is deepened through the ischiorectal fat to reach the levator muscles. Entry to the pelvic cavity is best achieved in the posterior midline. The coccyx is palpated, the anococcygeal raphe is incised and the levators are divided bilaterally. It often helps to have the surgeon operating from the abdomen place a finger posterior to the rectum to aid entry into the pelvic cavity from the perineum. The index finger is introduced into the pelvic cavity from below through this opening and the levators are hooked over the finger and divided with cautery. This is done on both sides to leave only the anterior attachments of the rectum to the prostate. The specimen is then brought through this posteriorly dissected space and delivered through the perineal incision. This helps in dividing the final attachments of the rectum to the prostate.

The pelvic cavity is then thoroughly irrigated with saline solution and the levators are approximated with interrupted sutures. Drainage of the pelvis is not mandatory and is a matter of surgeon preference. When opted for, drainage should be dependent, bringing the drain out through the perineum or active suction with the drains placed on the abdominal side of the pelvic floor closure.

The perineum is closed in layers and the ileostomy is matured in standard Brooke fashion after closure of the abdominal incision.

 ## POSTOPERATIVE MANAGEMENT

Oral liquids are usually tolerated by most patients on the first postoperative day. Diet can then be advanced as the stoma begins to function.

The daily stoma output should be accurately charted as a small group of patients take a few days to adjust to the end ileostomy. High ileostomy outputs can lead to dehydration without adequate fluid supplementation.

A postoperative evaluation by the enterostomal therapist is also essential to ensure a correct fit of the stoma appliance and also to counsel and educate the patient in routine stoma care.

Patients with inflammatory bowel disease are usually on steroid medications and these need to be tapered gradually over the next few weeks.

 ## COMPLICATIONS

A few common intraoperative complications deserve specific mention. These may be avoided by careful attention to a few specific surgical steps.

- The ureter and gonadal vessels may be injured while mobilizing the right and left colon. The gonadal vessels cross the ureter anteriorly as one proceeds lateral to medial. Staying anterior to the gonadal vessels helps in avoiding ureteral injury. Although both the ureters and the gonadal vessels need to be identified on either side, in obese individuals this may be difficult as there is often a significant amount of retroperitoneal fat. If one is sure that dissection has not deviated from the avascular plane, dissecting the retroperitoneal fat only to identify the ureter should be avoided. However, as a minimum, the ureter should be palpated and thus identified. In reoperations or radiated cases, placement of ureteral catheters will facilitate their intraoperative identification, even though it has been shown that it does not eliminate the risk of ureteral injury. The incidence of ureteral injury has been reported to range between 0.1–0.2%.
- While mobilizing the hepatic flexure a large vein is usually encountered, extending from the right colic or right branch of the middle colic vein. This vein is short and drains directly into the superior mesenteric vein and is at risk of a traction injury when retracting the hepatic flexure medially. Early identification and ligation of this vein will prevent this complication.
- The gastrocolic omentum is sometimes shortened and adherent to the gall bladder. In such instances, the gall bladder, stomach, and right gastroepiploic artery are at risk of injury. Careful dissection, staying close to the colon is essential for a safe dissection. An inadvertent gall bladder injury may necessitate an incidental cholecystectomy.
- A high riding splenic flexure may be a challenge to mobilize. According to the technique described above, the transverse and descending colon are first mobilized before

retracting the splenic flexure medially. This identifies the plane of dissection on either side of the splenic flexure and greatly facilitates splenic flexure mobilization. However, there may be dense adhesions between the colon and the spleen that may not be fully appreciated in a high riding splenic flexure. Undue traction while mobilizing the splenic flexure can result in a splenic tear. Therefore, gentle traction during splenic flexure mobilization is essential to avoid splenic injury.

- During rectal dissection, the outer mesorectal envelop can be clearly identified in the posterior midline as the Waldeyer's fascia posterior to it is usually well defined in this location. As the mesorectal dissection proceeds towards the lateral rectal attachments, it is vital to appreciate that the mesorectum curves anteriorly around the rectum. Failure to identify the delineation between the mesorectal fat and the fat on the lateral pelvic wall tends to take the line of dissection too lateral. The internal iliac vein is at particular risk for injury at this location and may lead to significant bleeding that may be difficult to control.

The presacral venous plexus is very rarely injured at the level of the sacral promontory as the presacral plane is very well defined at this point. However, the presacral plexus is at risk for injury at the following instances during the procedure.

- During the posterior dissection when the rectum begins to curve anteriorly, failure to curve the line of dissection anteriorly together with the rectum puts the presacral venous plexus at risk of injury, especially if the dissection is carried out bluntly.
- When the rectum is pulled forcefully out of the pelvis before division of Waldeyer's fascia, the presacral fascia is stripped and significant bleeding may occur from the venous plexus.
- During entry into the pelvic cavity from the perineal incision, one usually tends to go more posterior than necessary and may thus injure the presacral plexus. A guiding finger placed behind the rectum by the abdominal surgeon goes a long way in dentifying the correct plane.

Presacral bleeding can be significant and difficult to control. Fortunately this is a low pressure venous system and can be controlled by pressure. Repeated attempts at cauterization should be avoided as this only exaggerates the injury. A tight packing usually controls the bleeding if pressure is maintained for sufficient time. If bleeding resumes after a few minutes of pressure, argon beam coagulation, thumbtacks, and especially muscle welding is effective in the control of bleeding.

- Sexual dysfunction and infertility are probably the most important factors to consider following total proctocolectomy with ileostomy for benign disease. Autonomic nerve injury in the pelvis can be prevented in most cases by carrying the rectal dissection close to the rectum posteriorly and at the level of the seminal vesicles. Avoidance of large mass ties at the root of the inferior mesenteric artery will preserve the sympathetic nerve fibers at that location. The incidence of sexual dysfunction following proctectomy for benign disease has been reported to vary from 1–3% and the rates of infertility vary from 25–40%.

CONCLUSIONS

Complete resection of the colon and rectum is a major operative procedure and has a few definite indications. However, in most instances, a restorative procedure with an ileal pouch anal anastomosis has become the preferred option. Crohn's disease with pancolitis, unresponsive to medical treatment is probably the only unequivocal indication for a total proctocolectomy with permanent end ileostomy.

Laparoscopy has an increasing role in colorectal procedures and has been successfully used to perform a total proctocolectomy. However, the open approach offers specific advantages and is still preferred by a number of surgeons in specific patient populations. The basic surgical principles hold true both for a laparoscopic and open approach, rendering a thorough knowledge of the surgical steps of a total proctocolectomy indispensable to every colorectal surgeon.

Suggested Readings

Block GE: Total proctocolectomy for inflammatory bowel disease. In: *Mastery of Surgery* (Vol II), Nyhus LM, Baker RJ Eds, Little Brown and Company, Chapter 130, pp. 1285–1294.

Cameron JL. *Current Surgical Therapy*. 9th ed. Philadelphia, PA: Mosby/Elsevier Publishers, 2008.

Corman ML. *Colon and Rectal Surgery*. 5th ed. Philadelphia, PA: Lippincott Williams & Wilkins Publishers, 2004.

Gordon PH, Nivatvongs S. *Principles and Practice of Surgery for the Colon, Rectum, and Anus*. 3rd ed. New York, NY: Informa Healthcare Publishers, 2007.

Keighley MRB: Conventional proctocolectomy with ileostomy and protectomy alone in ulcerative colitis. In: *Surgery of the Anus, Rectum and Colon*, Keighley WMB, Williams NS Eds, 1993, WB Saunders, London, pp. 1398–1431.

Proctocolectomy and ileostomy. In Colon and Rectal Surgery (3rd ed), Corman ML Ed, 1993, JB Lippincott, Philadelphia, Chapter 17, pp. 949–952.

25 Hand-Assisted

Paul E. Wise

 ## INDICATIONS/CONTRAINDICATIONS

Hand-assisted laparoscopic surgery (HALS) for colorectal procedures allows for a hybrid-type procedure between laparoscopy and open approaches to colorectal disease. These techniques use a hand-assist device that maintains a pneumoperitoneum to perform the procedure laparoscopically while a hand is inside the abdomen or when the hand or instruments (through the hand-assist device, some devices allowing this maneuver to occur with a hand in place) are being exchanged. The bases of these devices can often be utilized as a wound protector during specimen removal or as a wound retractor during any open aspects of the procedure.

HALS can help those surgeons not yet comfortable with more complex laparoscopic colorectal procedures to gain the skills needed to perform these procedures. However, studies have shown variable results as to whether HALS actually improves the learning curve for laparoscopic colorectal procedures.

HALS advantages:

- Allows a less invasive approach when laparoscopy might not be an option, especially in a difficult situation such as fistulizing inflammatory diseases, large masses, or morbid obesity.
- Allows tactile feedback to help identify small neoplastic lesions, to find a vascular pedicle in an obese patient or to palpate ureteral stents.
- Allows the ability to provide hemostasis with the hand or to use an easily placed sponge to identify a bleeding source or clean up after a bleed.
- Allows the hand to perform blunt dissection in the setting of benign inflammatory disease.
- Allows the hand to provide retraction of heavier structures within the abdomen.
- Decreases the rate of conversion to an open procedure when compared to laparoscopy (and may allow for avoiding a conversion from laparoscopy to open by utilizing HALS).
- Shorter operative time versus laparoscopy in many comparative studies of colorectal procedures.
- Shorter hospital stays versus open colorectal procedures.
- Improved cosmesis over open colorectal procedures.

HALS disadvantages:

- Cost of the hand-assist device increases cost over open colorectal procedures and perhaps over laparoscopy.
- Operative times are longer with HALS than are with most open colorectal procedures, however, these times depend upon the underlying disease, patient, and surgeon variables.
- HALS has increased incision size (and thus increased infection and hernia rates, depending on the incision utilized for the hand-assist device) over straight laparoscopy.
- Cosmesis improvement is less than that with laparoscopy for colorectal procedures, especially in the case of total proctocolectomy, when compared to an open approach.

Indications for HALS total proctocolectomy (TPC) are the same as those described for open TPC and include the following situations:

- Ulcerative colitis when no restoration is planned due to continence issues, patient comorbidities, the presence of a very distal rectal cancer, and/or patient preference.
- Crohn's colitis when no restoration is planned due to continence issues, patient comorbidities, the presence of a low rectal cancer or proctitis, patient preference, fistulizing perianal disease, and/or the presence of ileal disease.
- Familial adenomatous polyposis (FAP) when no restoration is planned due to continence issues, patient comorbidities, the presence of a very distal rectal cancer, and/or patient preference.
- Synchronous proximal and distal colorectal malignancies including very distal rectal cancer when no restoration is planned due to continence issues, patient comorbidities, and/or patient preference.
- Hereditary nonpolyposis colorectal cancer (HNPCC, Lynch syndrome) in the presence of a very distal rectal cancer which would otherwise require abdominoperineal resection, or for a mid- to low rectal cancer that would require low pelvic rectal resection but when no restoration is planned due to continence issues, patient comorbidities, and/or patient preference.

Contraindications for HALS total proctocolectomy (TPC) are the same as those settings described for laparoscopic (or open) TPC and include the following:

- Comorbidities that preclude a general anesthetic.
- Comorbidities that preclude a laparoscopic approach due to intolerance to a pneumoperitoneum including intolerance to carbon dioxide and severe cardiovascular disease.
- Portal hypertension due to cirrhosis.
- Relative contraindications which depend upon the individual surgeon in dividing large tumors, large inflammatory masses, fistulizing Crohn's disease, adhesions due to previous operations or inflammatory disease or desmoid disease, bleeding diathesis, and/or bowel distension due to obstruction or recent endoscopic evaluation.
- Lack of surgical training and/or lack of availability of the necessary laparoscopic equipment, hand-device equipment, and/or operating room equipment.

🔊 PREOPERATIVE PLANNING

After the initial assessment for indications and contraindications to HALS TPC, a similar preoperative evaluation to open TPC is recommended and includes the following:

- Full endoscopic evaluation of the colon as well as upper endoscopy in the case of FAP and HNPCC.
- Retrograde contrast radiography when the colon cannot be completely endoscopically assessed perhaps due to malignant or inflammatory stenosis.
- Antegrade contrast radiography such as CT enterography or small bowel follow through may be preoperatively indicated.

- Appropriate staging CT scanning, endorectal ultrasound or MRI for rectal cancer and laboratory evaluation and completion, if indicated, of any neoadjuvant treatment for malignancies.

  Preoperative planning then includes the following:

- Patient education, evaluation, and marking of the proposed ileostomy site by an enterostomal therapist.
- Consideration of bowel cleansing with a mechanical (and/or antibiotic) bowel preparation. This preparation can improve the ability to manipulate the colon with the HALS and laparoscopic approaches but can increase bowel distension with any distal obstruction, so should be selectively used.
- Standard preoperative use of intravenous antibiotic and deep venous thrombosis prophylaxis as per institutional and other guidelines for all high-risk and complex operative procedures, whether open or minimally invasive.
- Ensuring that the laparoscopic instruments, hand-assisted device, operating room equipment, and appropriate assistants/personnel are available.

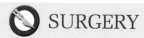 SURGERY

Positioning

As with the laparoscopic TPC, patient positioning is split-leg in the modified lithotomy position to allow perineal access and for the surgeon to stand between the legs if desired. A position-ranging operating bed is necessary to allow for steep Trendelenburg, reverse Trendelenburg, and steep side-to-side positioning as gravity is used to move the small intestines away from the point of dissection to allow for an unobstructed view. The patient must be secured to the bed. This step may be facilitated by a bean bag attached to the bed with Velcro and wrapped around the well-padded patient, who is further secured around the chest and shoulders with three-inch tape (Fig. 25.1). There should be at least two mobile monitors to allow for adequate views from either side of the table. If the monitors cannot move to the foot of the bed to facilitate the view during the pelvic dissection, a third monitor should be available (Fig. 25.2).

Instrumentation

When performing a HALS TPC, it is recommended to have a thorough understanding of the function and placement of the hand-assist device. Reusable and/or disposable

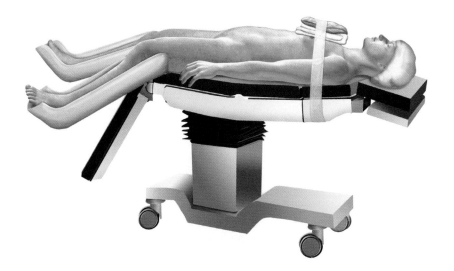

Figure 25.1 Patient positioning for hand-assisted total proctocolectomy. Arms and hands are tucked to the side and well-padded. The bean bag and tape are utilized to secure the patient to the operating table that will need to range through extreme positions. The hips are extended to keep the thighs from obstructing instrument motion when working in the upper abdomen.

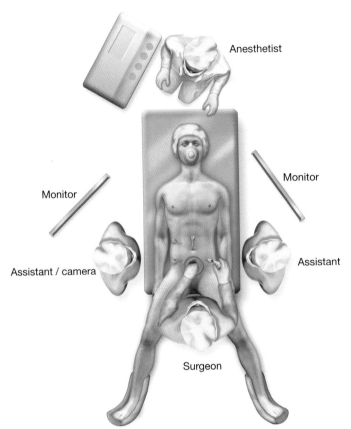

Figure 25.2 Patient, surgeon, and monitor positioning in the operating room. Monitors should be available to facilitate views into the left and right abdomen as well as the pelvis. In this example, the surgeon is performing hand-assisted takedown of the splenic flexure.

trocars of appropriate size to accommodate the available cameras, stapling devices (if needed), and any specialized energy devices to be used for dissection and/or vascular pedicle ligation should be available. Flexible-tip or angled (30° or 45°) cameras are ideal if available. Having a self-retaining retractor can facilitate the perineal dissection.

Technique

- Positioning as noted above and use of standard skin preparation
- Draping with abdominal exposure from the symphysis pubis to the xiphoid and from the bilateral anterior superior iliac spines.
- Placement of the hand-assist device can start the procedure and allow for digital inspection of the abdomen prior to the supraumbilical camera trocar placement. If there is concern for potential early conversion to an open approach based on the patient's previous operative history or preoperative radiographic assessments, a standard Hasson technique can be utilized to place a supraumbilical camera trocar first, followed by HALS device assuming the procedure can proceed.
- The hand-assist device is placed through a 5–8 cm lower midline or standard Pfannenstiel incision. It should be away from bony prominences and other trocars to allow for seating of the base of the device and to avoid the hand obstructing the instrumentation. A lower midline incision may be used if the surgeon is less comfortable with HALS or laparoscopy (and thus high concern for conversion) or high concern for the need to convert to an open approach due to the underlying pathology and/or patient factors such as obesity, adhesions, or inflammation. This lower midline incision facilitates specimen removal and lower abdominal exposure. The Pfannenstiel incision facilitates specimen removal and a better view into the pelvis as well as fewer wound complications/hernias and better aesthetics, but it can make conversion to an open procedure more problematic.

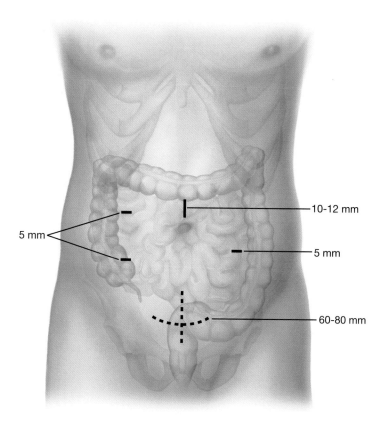

Part V: Total Proctocolectomy with Ileostomy

5 mm

10-12 mm

5 mm

60-80 mm

Figure 25.3 Trocar (solid lines) and hand-device placement (dashed lines). Incision sizes are noted but will vary depending on surgeon hand size as well as instrument/camera sizes. The hand can be placed through a lower midline or Pfannenstiel incision depending on patient factors and surgeon preference as well as the level of concern for conversion to an open approach.

- Subsequent trocar placement under direct view and after injection of local anesthetic is similar to the placement for laparoscopic TPC (Fig. 25.3). If convenient, the preoperatively marked ileostomy site can be used as a trocar site.
- The surgeon stands to the patient's left with the left hand in the abdomen and the right hand with the active instrument through a left lateral trocar. The patient is in the Trendelenburg, right side up, position. Right colectomy is initiated (as with HALS right colectomy) using a standard laparoscopic medial to lateral approach with vascular division (technique based on surgeon preference) after identification and protection of the duodenum. The hand can facilitate lateral retraction of the cecum (Fig. 25.4). The blunt dissection anterior to the retroperitoneum continues as far lateral and cephalad as possible, with further division of the ascending colon mesentery, right colic vessels, and right lateral transverse mesocolon and right branch of the middle colic vessels performed at this time or after subsequent transverse colon mobilization as described below.
- The base of the ileal mesentery along the pelvic brim is incised and the right ureter is identified and protected. The lateral ascending colon attachments and hepatocolic ligaments are divided as the patient is placed in reverse Trendelenburg. The greater omentum is elevated from the transverse colon, the lesser sac entered, and the underlying duodenum again protected. The remaining transverse mesocolon can be divided once the omentum is freed from the posterior aspect of the mesentery.
- The surgeon moves to the patient's right after the patient is again placed in Trendelenburg with the left side up. The right hand is placed in the abdomen to identify the inferior mesenteric artery (IMA) and elevate it off of the retroperitoneum (Fig. 25.5). The left hand uses the active instrument through a right lateral trocar. A standard medial to lateral approach is again undertaken (as with the HALS left colectomy or HALS sigmoid colectomy). The sigmoid mesentery inferior to the IMA is scored and blunt dissection is used to take the retroperitoneal attachments off of the posterior aspect of the sigmoid mesentery and colon with early identification and protection of the left ureter and other retroperitoneal structures prior to vascular division. The inferior mesenteric vein is then isolated and divided. Any remaining retroperitoneal

Figure 25.4 The hand can be used to laterally retract the cecum to facilitate identification and dissection of the ileocolic vessels.

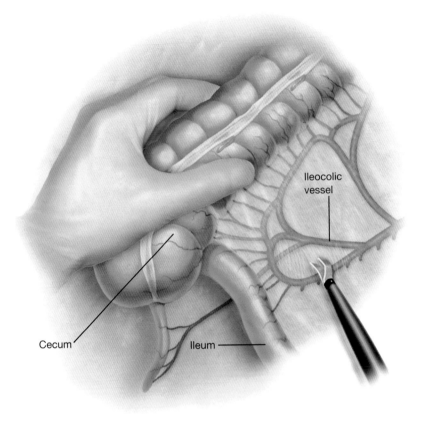

Ileocolic vessel

Cecum

Ileum

Figure 25.5 The hand can be used to identify and elevate the sigmoid mesentery to facilitate the medial to lateral approach to dissection of the inferior mesenteric artery and identification of the left ureter.

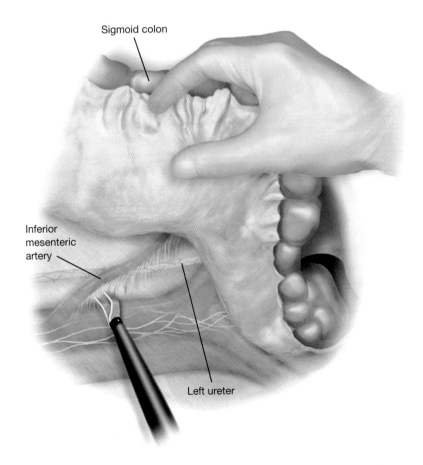

Sigmoid colon

Inferior mesenteric artery

Left ureter

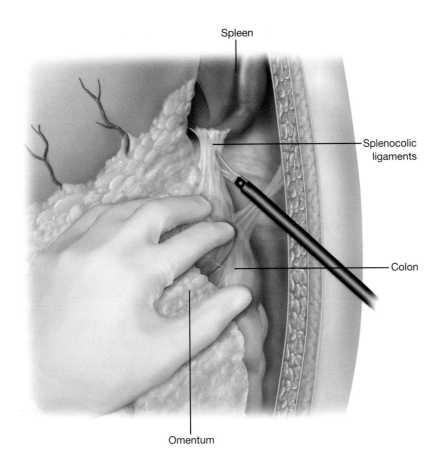

Spleen

Splenocolic
ligaments

Colon

Omentum

Figure 25.6 The hand can be used to medially retract the descending colon to facilitate division of the splenocolic ligaments and thus splenic flexure mobilization.

attachments to the descending colon and its mesentery are bluntly divided as far cephalad and lateral as possible to limit the subsequent lateral dissection.

- Lateral sigmoid attachments along the white line of Toldt are then divided from the pelvic brim to the proximal descending colon after which the patient is returned to reverse Trendelenburg. The surgeon may move to between the legs with the left hand in and the patient's left-sided trocar being used to facilitate medial retraction of the descending colon and identification and division of the splenocolic ligaments (Fig. 25.6). Any remaining greater omental and transverse mesocolic attachments are divided to completely free the colon within the abdomen.

- The patient is returned to Trendelenburg and leveled from left to right. The pelvic dissection can be performed through the hand-assist device in an open fashion after the colon is eviscerated and the ileum and its mesentery divided. Alternatively, the HALS procedure can be continued by performing a standard total mesorectal excision (TME) using the hand as a retractor of the rectum during the posterolateral dissection or the anterior peritoneum uterus/vagina or bladder/prostate during the anterior dissection. The monitors should be moved to the patient's feet with the surgeon (or assistant if preferred) using the hand standing on the patient's left with the left hand in, and the right hand maneuvering the camera or using the left lower quadrant trocar for an instrument and the surgeon or assistant on the patient's right using one or two instruments for dissection and/or retraction through the right-sided trocar(s). The dissection can be continued circumferentially to the pelvic floor in this fashion. The colon is then eviscerated through the hand-assist device and the ileum and its mesentery divided.

- The ileostomy is created in a standard fashion (see chapter on Brooke ileostomy) through the preoperatively identified site.

- The perineal dissection can be performed from between the legs while the patient remains in lithotomy and, once the dissection planes that were dissected from above are encountered, the specimen can be completely removed through the hand-assist device from the abdomen or from the perineal incision. The stoma can then be fashioned and the abdomen and perineum closed after ensuring adequate hemostasis.

■ Alternatively, after ensuring hemostasis from above, the ileostomy can be created and the abdomen closed and dressed, after which the patient can be transferred to the stretcher and returned to the re-aligned operating table in the prone jack-knife position. The perineal dissection can then be undertaken and the specimen removed from below. This prone dissection is a more ergonomic position for the surgeon and adds little to the operating time of the procedure.

■ Whether in lithotomy or prone position, the perineal dissection is performed in a standard fashion via an intersphincteric approach to preserve the external sphincter for closure and thus improve healing and decrease perineal wound complications. Complete excision of both sphincters is dictated by the underlying disease process. The pelvic floor is closed in layers, and the skin can be left open to drain and thus close by second intention or it can be closed based on surgeon preference.

POSTOPERATIVE MANAGEMENT

Postoperative management is essentially equivalent as to that following the open or laparoscopic approaches to TPC and includes consideration of the following:

■ Fast-tracking with limiting parenteral narcotic analgesics and rapid dietary advancement as tolerated.

■ Avoidance of nasogastric tubes except in the situations of bowel obstruction or prolonged postoperative ileus.

■ Enterostomal therapy education and training.

■ Appropriate postoperative medications including steroid weaning when necessary based on preoperative use, cessation of preoperative immunomodulators, and avoidance of the use of empiric antibiotics any longer than 24 hours according to institutional and other guidelines.

COMPLICATIONS

While there has never been a direct, prospective comparison between open, laparoscopic, and HALS TPC, it can be inferred from a number of studies that the rates of morbidity and mortality are similar between the three approaches.

■ Intra-operative organ and nerve injuries can occur during dissection and mobilization regardless of the approach, and, as with laparoscopy, may require conversion to an open approach. Postoperative infertility rates for women and impotence rates for men are likely similar between HALS and laparoscopy but have not been directly studied.

■ Intra-operative bleeding is a common cause for conversion during straight laparoscopy, but the ability to use the hand with HALS to control vessels, and/or the use of the hand-assist device to expose bleeding for control in an open fashion has decreased the conversion rate with HALS (from 11 to 23% with laparoscopy compared to 2–15% with HALS, depending on the diagnosis and procedure).

■ Postoperative complications with HALS TPC (as with laparoscopy and open approaches) include: wound infection (perineal and abdominal wounds), intra-abdominal abscess, incisional hernia, bleeding ileostomy complications in addition to the risks related to any major colorectal procedure.

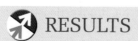 RESULTS

A few randomized as well as case-controlled trials and case series have been performed comparing HALS and straight laparoscopic approaches for colorectal procedures.

Although most studies include multiple indications and resection types, some look more specifically at TPC. There are fewer studies comparing HALS TPC to open. These studies have shown that HALS can be performed safely while, for neoplastic indications, maintaining oncologic principles of adequate lymphadenectomy and adequate margins as performed with open cancer resections equivalent to those metrics than with laparoscopy. The majority of these studies have also shown that any benefits of laparoscopy in colorectal procedures are maintained through the use of HALS including similar morbidity and mortality rates as mentioned above as well as postoperative analgesic use, time to return of bowel function, and length of hospital stay. The incision used to place the HALS device is often similar in size to the laparotomy needed to remove the specimen during a laparoscopic approach, thus equalizing the incision length between the two approaches. However, shorter incision length does favor laparoscopy when compared to HALS in most studies, but while this has some cosmetic benefit (a statistically significant 1.0–2.5 cm mean increase in incision length), the clinical significance of this appears to be minimal. HALS does significantly shorten operating times in most studies by 15–60 minutes, depending on the diagnosis and procedure. Costs are more difficult to compare but appear to be equivalent between HALS and laparoscopy. Costs also appear to be equivalent (or even lower) for HALS and laparoscopy versus open procedures due to the decreased length of stay offsetting the longer operative times.

CONCLUSIONS

The use of HALS to perform TPC, regardless of the indication, offers advantages over open and laparoscopic approaches to TPC with equivalent morbidity and mortality rates. HALS can facilitate training for, and adoption of, laparoscopic approaches while decreasing conversion rates to open approaches when compared to straight laparoscopy. HALS TPC preserves many of the advantages of laparoscopy over open TPC including excellent cosmesis with less pain and shorter hospital stays postoperatively while decreasing operative times in many cases and expanding the ability to use a minimally invasive approach to TPC.

Suggested Readings

Aalbers AG, Biere SS, van Berge Henegouwen MI, et al. Hand-assisted or laparoscopic-assisted approach in colorectal surgery: a systematic review and meta-analysis. *Surg Endosc* 2008;22(8):1769–80.

Boushey RP, Marcello PW, Martel G, et al. Laparoscopic total colectomy: an evolutionary experience. *Dis Colon Rectum* 2007;50(10):1512–9.

Cima RR, Pattana-arun J, Larson DW, et al. Experience with 969 minimal access colectomies: the role of hand-assisted laparoscopy in expanding minimally invasive surgery for complex colectomies. *J Am Coll Surg* 2008;206:946–52.

HALS Study Group. Hand-assisted laparoscopic surgery vs standard laparoscopic surgery for colorectal disease: a prospective randomized trial. *Surg Endosc* 2000;14(10):896–901.

Hassan I, You YN, Cima RR, et al. Hand-assisted versus laparoscopic-assisted colorectal surgery: Practice patterns and clinical outcomes in a minimally-invasive colorectal practice. *Surg Endosc* 2008;22(3):739–43.

Holubar SD, Privitera A, Cima RR, et al. Minimally invasive total proctocolectomy with Brooke ileostomy for ulcerative colitis. *Inflamm Bowel Dis* 2009;15(9):1337–42.

Marcello PW, Fleshman JW, Milsom JW, et al. Hand-assisted laparoscopic vs. laparoscopic colorectal surgery: a multicenter, prospective, randomized trial. *Dis Colon Rectum* 2008;51(6):818–26.

Nakajima K, Lee SW, Cocilovo C, et al. Laparoscopic total colectomy: Hand-assisted vs. standard technique. *Surg Endosc* 2004;18(4):582–6.

Ringley C, Lee YK, Iqbal A, et al. Comparison of conventional laparoscopic and hand-assisted oncologic segmental colonic resection. *Surg Endosc* 2007;21(12):2137–41.

Schadde E, Smith D, Alkoraishi AS, et al. Hand-assisted laparoscopic colorectal surgery (HALS) at a community hospital: a prospective analysis of 104 consecutive cases. *Surg Endosc* 2006;20(7):1077–82.

Targarona EM, Gracia E, Garriga J, et al. Prospective randomized trial comparing conventional laparoscopic colectomy with hand-assisted laparoscopic colectomy: applicability, immediate clinical outcome, inflammatory response, and cost. *Surg Endosc* 2002;16(2):234–9.

26 Open Restorative Proctocolectomy

Robert R. Cima

 ## INDICATIONS/CONTRAINDICATIONS

In the majority of patients with chronic ulcerative colitis (CUC), the preferred operation is the restorative proctocolectomy, also known as an ileal pouch anal anastomosis (IPAA). The advantages of the IPAA are that it removes the diseased organs, the colon and rectum, while preserving the normal route of defecation thus avoiding the need for a permanent ostomy. Since its introduction in the early 1980s, the published experience has demonstrated that IPAA is a technically challenging operation with fairly predictable functional outcomes that are durable over long-term follow-up.

The surgical approach to patients with CUC is divided into two broad categories: emergent and elective surgical intervention. Indications for emergent intervention in CUC include the following:

- Fulminant colitis
- Toxic megacolon
- Colonic perforation
- Massive hemorrhage

Fortunately, with a better understanding of the natural history of CUC and improved medical treatment options these situations arise less frequently. However, approximately 10% of newly diagnosed CUC patients present with fulminant colitis. In these emergent situations, the goal of the surgical procedure is to address a life-threatening clinical situation without precluding a future restorative procedure. In emergent situations, there is no role for proceeding to an IPAA. IPAA is time-consuming and unnecessarily increases the complexity of the surgery predisposing to significant complications.

In a patient with known CUC or indeterminate colitis who requires emergent operation, the procedure of choice is the subtotal colectomy with end ileostomy. The advantages of this approach are as follows:

- The majority of the diseased organ is removed
- Afterward the patient can improve their overall health and nutritional status

- The patient can be weaned from all immunosuppressive medications
- The rectum is left in situ allowing the patient to proceed at a later date to an IPAA without any deleterious impact on the functional outcomes

Thankfully, most IPAAs are performed under elective circumstances. In these situations the indications for surgery are as follows:

- Failure of medical therapy to control symptoms
- Relief of the deleterious side effects of medications
- The development of intestinal dysplasia
- Treatment of an intestinal malignancy

The contraindications to IPAA are steadily decreasing. Relative contraindications included the following:

- Advanced age. Traditionally, age over 55–60 was considered a contraindication to IPAA because of presumed poor functional outcomes related to incontinence. However, a number of studies have reported acceptable functional results in patients in whom IPAA was performed in their 70s and even 80s
- Planned or desired pregnancy in the near term after IPAA. IPAA has a significant negative impact on the ability to become pregnant
- History of frequent or prolonged perianal sepsis (abscesses, fistulas)
- Obesity makes the operation extremely difficult but in appropriately selected candidates it can be performed successfully
- Colonic Crohn's disease traditionally has been considered an absolute contraindication to IPAA. Recently, some authors have reported in highly selected patients without any history of small bowel or anal Crohn's disease the outcomes of IPAA are similar to CUC patients. Despite these few reports most would consider Crohn's disease an absolute contraindication to IPAA

Absolute contraindications include the following:

- Frequent incontinence episodes not associated with flares of disease activity
- Need for pelvic radiation
- Small bowel or anal Crohn's disease

⊚ PREOPERATIVE PLANNING

- Patients need to visit with an enterostomal therapist for preoperative stoma marking and to begin education regarding the care of the stoma.
- Routine use of oral antibiotics or a mechanical bowel preparation is not required. However, a patient should receive one or two tap water enemas the morning of surgery.
- If the patient is currently on steroids or has taken them within the last 6 months, a stress dose of steroids is given in the perioperative period.
- Intravenous antibiotics are administered within 60 minutes of incision.
- Ideally, a thoracic epidural catheter is placed for postoperative pain control.
- Lower extremity sequential compression devices are placed and activated prior to the induction of anesthesia.
- 5,000 units of subcutaneous heparin is administered.

INTRAOPERATIVE CONSIDERATIONS

Positioning

- All patients require a padded chest strap placed securing them to the table.
- A forced air warming device is placed over the torso and head.

- The patient is positioned in modified Lloyd-Davies lithotomy with both arms padded, protected, and tucked against the torso.
- The legs are placed in leg holder that allows the hips and thighs to be flat with respect to the abdomen but the lower leg to be positioned downward (i.e., Yellofin® Stirrups, Allen® Medical Systems).
- The use of leg holders minimize the chance of patient movement on the table during positioning changes as well as permitting access to the perineum for placement of a circular stapler or a vaginal manipulator if required.

Technique

- A lower midline incision is made and extended cephalad to gain enough exposure to safely mobilize the hepatic and splenic flexure of the colon. The lowest extent of the incision should be the top of the pubic bone. This optimizes the exposure for the pelvic dissection and performing the anastomosis. The upper extent of the incision will vary contingent upon the size of the patient and the height of the splenic flexure.
- The abdomen is thoroughly explored for any unexpected findings. Most importantly, the small bowel is inspected for any evidence of Crohn's disease.
- The entire abdominal colon is mobilized from its lateral and retroperitoneal attachments. Care is taken to identify the course of both ureters down into the pelvis.
- The mesentery of the colon is divided close to the origin of the vessels with the exception of the right colon. The mesentery of the right colon is divided close to the colon to protect the ileocolic vessel. This vessel may later need to be divided in order to achieve maximal length of the small bowel but it should be preserved initially until it is determined if the vessel must be divided.
- The small bowel mesentery is then mobilized up to the duodenum and away from the head of the pancreas. It is essential that all the small bowel mesenteric attachments to the duodenum are divided to ensure that maximal small bowel mesenteric length is achieved in order to allow the ileal pouch to reach to the upper anal canal without tension.
- The terminal ileum is divided close to the ileocecal valve by a single firing of a linear cutting stapler.
- When the abdominal colon is fully mobilized, the superior hemorrhoidal vessels are divided, and the presacral space is entered to begin mobilizing the rectum. A nerve sparing dissection is carried out to the pelvic floor. When performing the double-stapled technique, once the rectum has been dissected down to the top of the anal canal the rectum is divided with a TA-stapler approximately 1–1.5 cm above the dentate line to ensure that the pouch anal anastomosis is performed in the upper anal canal (Fig. 26.1).
- To facilitate the rectal resection, the patient is placed in steep Trendelenburg position.
- Before the ileal pouch is constructed, a check of the mesenteric length needs to be performed. Ideally, the apex of the pouch should reach 4–5 cm below the top of the pubic bone. If there is tension on the mesentery the following additional mesentery lengthening procedures can be performed:
  - The ileal colic vessel can be divided.
  - The anterior peritoneum over the course of the primary vessel supplying the pouch can be scored. This scoring is performed every 1–2 cm along the vessel's length starting near the vessel origin.
  - In the distal vessel arcade, near the pouch, small vessels can be carefully divided to construct a mesenteric window. Transient application of bulldog clamp may be helpful to verify adequacy of collateral blood supply after vascular division.
- The ileal pouch is constructed by folding the terminal ileum into a J shape. The common wall of the J-pouch is opened by firing a linear cutting stapler from the apex of the pouch with an arm of the stapler placed in each of the J limbs along the antimesenteric border of the small bowel. Ideally, the pouch should be 12–15 cm in length often requiring two firings of the 10-cm linear stapler (Fig. 26.2). Once the pouch is

Figure 26.1 Stapling across the low rectum at the top of the anal canal in preparation of performing a double stapled pouch-anal anastomosis.

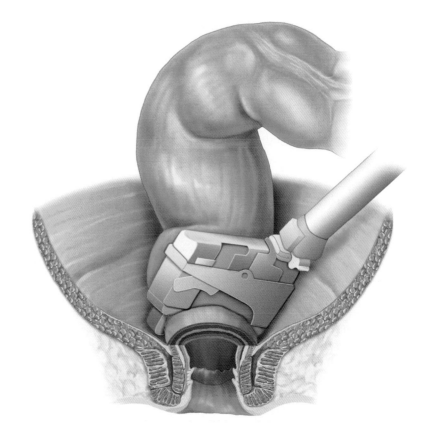

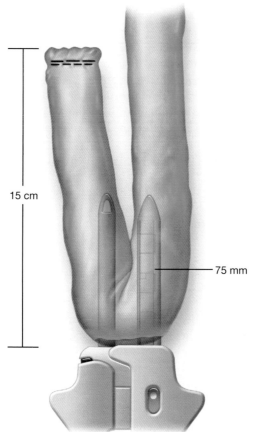

Figure 26.2 Construction of the ileal J-pouch by division of the common wall between the afferent and efferent small bowel limbs using a linear cutting stapler.

15 cm

75 mm

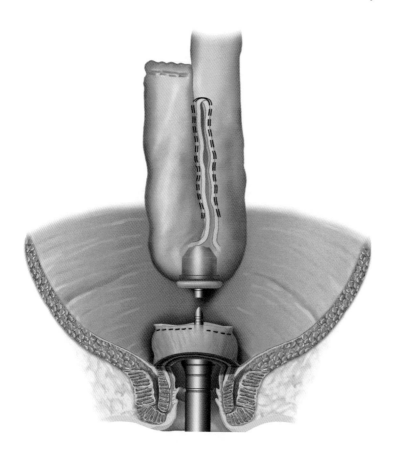

Figure 26.3 Completion of the ileal-pouch anal anastomosis using a double stapled technique.

constructed, the anvil of the EEA stapler is secured into the opening at the apex of the J pouch with a purse-string suture.

- The pouch is brought down into the pelvis and the double stapled anastomosis is fashioned ensuring there is no tension or rotation of the pouch nor any proximal small bowel trapped under the cut edge of the small bowel mesentery leading to the pouch. The cut edge of the small bowel mesentery lies along the aorta with the small bowel following to the patient's left. The pouch falls into the curve of the sacrum as the mesentery of the pouch transverses the pelvic anteriorly (Figs. 26.3 and 26.4).

- A proctoscopic exam of the pouch is performed and integrity of the pouch is tested by air insufflation.

- After the pouch anal anastomosis is completed, a diverting loop ileostomy is constructed approximately 20–35 cm proximal to the pouch.

- Two closed suction drains are placed behind the pouch and brought out of the anterior abdominal wall.

POSTOPERATIVE MANAGEMENT

Postoperative management will vary according to the unique needs of the patient. Fortunately, many CUC patients are younger and have few complicating medical problems. This permits faster mobilization of the patient. Ideally, a clinical pathway with a goal of a 3–4 day hospitalization should be utilized. Elements of such a pathway include the following:

- If a nasogastric tube remains in place at the end of surgery, it is removed the evening of surgery or the morning after surgery.

- Ambulation is started the evening of surgery. Standard venous thromboembolism prophylaxis is initiated the evening of surgery.

- Minimal postoperative intravenous fluids are provided.

Figure 26.4 Final appearance of the ileal J-pouch.

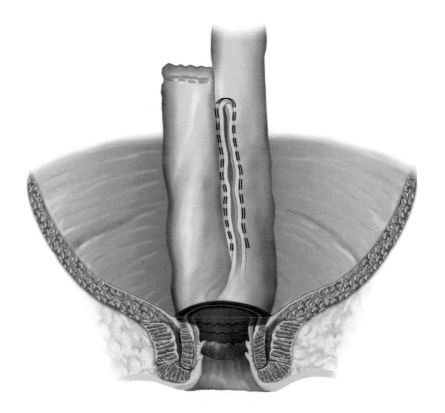

- The patient is started on a limited full liquid diet the afternoon of postoperative day 1.
- The bladder catheter is removed on postoperative day 2.
- Starting on postoperative day 2, the diet is advanced as tolerated.
- The deep abdominal drains are removed on postoperative day 3.
- Two doses of intravenous antibiotics are administered and are discontinued within 24 hours of incision closure.

The ileostomy is closed 8–12 weeks after the IPAA if there have been no major complications. Prior to closure a contrast enema is obtained through the anus to ensure that there are no visible leaks from the anastomosis or the pouch itself.

 COMPLICATIONS

IPAA is a technically challenging operation to perform and is associated with a number of early and late complications. In most reports, the 30-day morbidity of IPAA is 20–30%. The most common early complications are as follows:

- Wound infection
- Small bowel obstruction
- Diverting stoma complications
- Pouch leak and pelvic sepsis with or without an associated abscess

Pelvic sepsis occurs in 5–24% of patients after IPAA. Computed tomography (CT) is useful in demonstrating pelvic fluid collections or phlegmon. Patients with pelvic phlegmon usually respond to conservative treatment with broad-spectrum antibiotics and bowel rest, whereas patients with a pelvic abscess should ideally undergo CT-guided drainage if technically feasible, or repeat laparotomy and drainage. The most commonly cited risk factor for pelvic sepsis is chronic or high dose steroid use in the perioperative period. The pelvic sepsis may in the short-term lead to pouch excision, which is fortunately rare. However, the long-term pouch functional results are worse and there is a higher rate of pouch loss compared to patients who did not experience pelvic sepsis.

Late IPAA complications include the following:

- Anastomotic stricture
- Pouch fistulas
- Pouchitis

The most common long-term complication is an anastomotic stricture. Fortunately, this is easily treated with intermittent anal dilations. Pouch fistulas and chronic pouchitis contribute to pouch failure that may require pouch revision or excision with conversion to a permanent ileostomy. If a pelvic abscess or fistula occurs long after the operation, it raises the possibility that the patient has Crohn's disease.

The most common late IPAA complication is pouchitis, idiopathic. It is an acute inflammatory process of the pouch. In a minority of patients, it can become a chronic process. Since it rarely occurs in familial adenomatous polyposis (FAP) patients with an IPAA, pouchitis may represent an element of immune dysfunction unique to CUC patients. The exact incidence of pouchitis is difficult to measure; most series report an incidence of 12–70% depending upon the length of follow-up. No specific factors are predictive of who will develop pouchitis. An episode of pouchitis should be suspected in any patient who experiences persistent abdominal cramps, increased stool frequency, watery or bloody diarrhea, and flu-like symptoms. While many patients are treated on clinical grounds alone, accurate diagnosis requires endoscopic visualization of the pouch and histologic evaluation.

While the exact cause of pouchitis is unclear, the successful use of antibiotics, particularly metronidazole, in the treatment of acute and chronic pouchitis lends support to an interaction between pouch bacteria levels and the patient's mucosal immune system. *Probiotics may be useful in either treating or perhaps even preventing pouchitis.* Most patients with pouchitis respond to a short course of antibiotics. The primary antibiotic used is metronidazole over a 10-day course. The most commonly used alternative antibiotic is ciprofloxacin. If antibiotic treatment fails to resolve the pouchitis, then other medications, such as steroids or immunomodulators, may be used. In cases of persistent pouchitis, Crohn's disease of the pouch needs to be considered as a possible cause. Less than 8% of patients who have an IPAA will go on to develop chronic pouchitis with nearly half of those patients eventually requiring pouch excision.

RESULTS

In a review of numerous reports of outcomes for IPAA, the average stool frequency was six stools during the day, and one stool at night. Daytime and nocturnal stool frequency and the ability to discriminate flatus from stool remain stable over time, whereas the need for stool bulking and hypomotility agents declines. Major fecal incontinence (> twice per week) occurs in <5% of patients during the day and 12% during sleep. In contrast, minor episodes of nocturnal incontinence occur in up to 30% of patients at least 1 year after the operation. Pads are worn by 28% of patients for protection against seepage. Patients older than 50 years of age have a higher daytime stool frequency (eight per day) than do patients younger than 50 years (six per day). Men and women have similar stool frequencies postoperatively, but women have more episodes of fecal soilage during the day and night. Seventy-eight percent of patients report excellent continence 1 year after surgery that remains unchanged at 10 years; 20% experience minor incontinence; and 2% have poor control. Forty percent of patients with minor incontinence at 1 year remain unchanged, 40% improve, and 20% worsen by 10 years. Nocturnal fecal spotting increases during the 10-year period, but not significantly.

Postoperative quality of life is the major deciding factor for patients choosing a particular operation for CUC. Several studies have demonstrated that most patients are satisfied with the operation and lead a normal life-style regardless of the procedure. In one study of quality of life after a Brooke ileostomy or IPAA, patients were highly satisfied with either operation (Brooke ileostomy, 93%; IPAA, 95%). Daily activities (e.g., sexual life, participation in sports, social interaction, work, recreation, family relationships, travel), however, were more likely to be adversely affected with a Brooke ileostomy than by IPAA.

⬥ CONCLUSIONS

The major benefit of IPAA is that it cures the patient of the intestinal manifestations of CUC while maintaining a normal route of defecation. It is a challenging operation associated with a relatively high rate of short-term complications. The most worrisome short-term complication is a pelvic abscess that is highly correlated with a worse functional outcome and increases the most risk for pouch loss. As experience with IPAA increases, the frequency of complications decreases. Occasional incontinence appears early in almost all patients after operation, particularly at night. Fortunately, major episodes of incontinence are rare events. Although nonspecific inflammation of the pouch, or pouchitis, is the most long-term complication in most patients it is treated effectively and simply with antibiotics. When severe and recurrent, pouchitis can lead to failure of the operation; however, this is uncommon. Despite these problems, the benefits of IPAA are clear: all the intestinal disease is removed, the patient avoids a permanent stoma, and their quality of life is very good.

Recommended Readings

1. Fleshner P, Schoetz D Jr. Surgical management of ulcerative colitis. In: Wolff B, Fleshman J, Beck D, Pemberton J, Wexner S, eds. *The ASCRS Textbook of Colon and Rectal Surgery*. New York: Springer, 2007:567–83.
2. Nivatvongs S. Ulcerative colitis. In: Gordon P, Nivatvongs S, eds. *Principles and Practice of Surgery for the Colon, Rectum, and Anus*. 2nd ed. St Louis, MO: Quality Medical Publishing, 1999:831–906.
3. Pemberton JH, Kelly KA, Beart RW Jr, Dozois RR, Wolff BG, Ilstrup DM. Ileal pouch-anal anastomosis for chronic ulcerative colitis: long-term results. *Ann Surg* 1987;206:504–13.
4. Meagher AP, Farouk R, Dozois RR, Kelly KA, Pemberton JH. J ileal pouch-anal anastomosis for chronic ulcerative colitis: Complications and long-term outcome in 1310 patients. *Br J Surg* 1998;85:800–3.
5. Farouk R, Pemberton JH, Wolff BG, Dozois RR, Browning S, Larson D. Functional outcomes after ileal pouch-anal anastomosis for chronic ulcerative colitis. *Ann Surg* 2000;231: 919–26.
6. Hahnloser D, Pemberton JH, Wolff BG, Larson DR, Crownhart BS, Dozois RR. The effect of ageing on function and quality of life in ileal pouch patients: a single cohort experience of 409 patients with chronic ulcerative colitis. *Ann Surg* 2004;240:615–21.

7. Hahnloser D, Pemberton JH, Wolff BG, Larson DR, Crownhart BS, Dozois RR. Results at up to 20 years after ileal pouch-anal anastomosis for chronic ulcerative colitis. *Br J Surg* 2007;94: 333–40.
8. Fazio VW, Ziv Y, Church JM, et al. Ileal pouch-anal anastomoses complications and function in 1005. *Ann Surg* 1995;222:120–27.
9. Melton GB, Fazio VW, Kiran RP, et al. Long-term outcomes with ileal pouch-anal anastomosis and Crohn's disease pouch retention and implications of delayed diagnosis. *Ann Surg* 2008;248: 608–16.
10. Ferrante M, Declerck S, De Hertogh G, et al. Outcomes after proctocolectomy with ileal pouch-anal anastomosis for ulcerative colitis. *Inflamm Bowel Dis* 2008;14:20–28.
11. Bach SP, Mortensen NJ. Ileal pouch surgery for ulcerative colitis. *World J Gastroenterol* 2007;13:3288–3300.
12. McGuire BB, Brannigan AE, O'Connell PR. Ileal pouch-anal anastomosis. *Br J Surg* 2007;94:812–23.
13. Walijee A, Walijee J, Morris AM, Higgins PD. Threefold increased risk of infertility: a meta-analysis of infertility after ileal pouch anal anastomosis in ulcerative colitis. *Gut* 2006;55: 1575–80.
14. Hum MA, Baig MK, Wexner SD. Restorative protocolectomy ileal pouch anal anastomosis (Video). http://cine-med.com/index.php?id = ACS-2227&subnav = acs. 2003. Accessed 21 December, 2009.

27 Laparoscopic-Assisted Restorative Proctocolectomy

Joy C. Singh and Neil Mortensen

Introduction

Laparoscopic-assisted restorative proctocolectomy (LA-RP) is a hybrid colorectal procedure. It is doubtful that when Sir Alan Parks conceived the operation he originally described in 1978 (1), he saw it being performed through a small Pfannenstiel incision together with several 5–10 mm scars. This is now a viable alternative to his open technique. The first LA-RP case report was published in 1992 (2) and the first series in 1992 (3).

There is no consensus defining "a laparoscopic-assisted restorative proctocolectomy." Descriptions include procedures involving either partial or complete laparoscopic mobilization, with or without the aid of a hand-assisted port. Totally laparoscopic restorative proctocolectomy (total L-RP) combines complete laparoscopic mobilization with intracorporeal division of the rectum before conventional extracorporeal J-pouch formation (4,5). For the purposes of this article, we define a LA-RP as one in which the entire colon is laparoscopically mobilized, followed by the creation of a small Pfannenstiel incision that is used for rectal dissection. The rectum is then transected with a conventional open stapling device. Hand port techniques are associated with significantly more inflammatory response compared to laparoscopic-assisted procedures, but may be useful to reduce the need for conversion in patients with a hostile abdomen (6).

The main advantage of performing LA-RP over a totally laparoscopic procedure, particularly in males, is the ability to transect sufficiently low, just above the anorectal junction with a single staple line. The difficulties of a narrow pelvis and low rectal dissection are associated with conversion (4). Laparoscopic stapling devices are often unable to produce a satisfactory staple line in the depths of the pelvis, which may prevent construction of a safe stapled J-pouch. At present the maximum angulation obtainable by any laparoscopic stapling device is 45 degrees and multiple firings are often required. Irregular staple lines are associated with higher risks of anastomotic breakdown (7). Subsequent pelvis sepsis has devastating consequences on pouch function and can ultimately lead to pouch failure.

TABLE 27.1

Authors (Yrs)	Study type	Groups	Number of patients	Operative time (mins)	Follow up (mo)	Complication rate* (%)	Comment
Kelly 2010	Retrospective case matched	TL/open	10/10	245/208	DC	nr	50% reduction in postoperative opiate use & quicker ileostomy function in TL group
El-Gazzaz 2009	Retrospective case matched	LA/open	119 /238	272/163	60	23/21	QoL- both groups same at 1&5 yrs
Fichera 2009	Prospective	LA/open	73/106	335/321	24	63/66	Significant lower incisional hernia rate in LA group
Sylla 2009	Prospective	LA/open	50/155	198/159			Significant less blood loss in LA group
Polle 2008	Retrospective	LA/HAL/ open	35/30/30	298/214/133	3	29/20/23	QoL – equivalent at 3 months
Polle 2007	Prospective	HAL/open	26/27	nr	32	nr	Body image better in HALS group, 15% readmitted with adhesive SBO
Zhang 2007	Retrospective	TL/open	21/25	325/220	DC	38/40	Significant less blood loss, earlier return to bowel function, less postoperative stay in TL group
Larson 2006	Retrospective	LA/HAL/ open	75/25/200	320/372/230	3	36/47	Combined complication rates for LA & HAL
Larson 2005	Prospective case matched	LA/open	33/33	nr	13	45/48	Functional outcome and QoL at 1 yr was equivalent
Berdah 2004	Prospective case matched	LA/open	12/12		>36	25/25	Return to bowel function & oral intake significantly less in LA but same LOS
Maartense 2004	RCT	HAL/open	30/30	214/133	3	20 /17	QoL same for both groups at 3 months
Araki 2001	Retrospective	LA/open	21/11	215/198	DC	52/63	Significantly quicker return to bowel function in LA group, equivalent operating time and morbidity
Brown 2001	Retrospective	LA/open	12/13	150/120	DC	17/15	Equivalent findings between both groups
Dunker 2001	Retrospective case matched	LA/open	15/17	292/198	16	6/18	Body image better in LA group, but equivalent functional outcome
Hashimoto 2001	Retrospective	LA/open	11/13	483/402	DC	68/34	Less postoperative pain in LA group
Marcello 2000	Retrospective case matched	LA/open	20/20	330/225	DC	20/25	Reduced LOS and quicker return to bowel function in LA group
Schmitt 1994	Prospective case matched	LA/open	20/22	240/120	DC	68/35	Equivalent LOS

*Specific complications recorded varied between studies.
Abbreviations: DC, discharge; HAL, hand-assisted laparoscopic; LA, laparoscopic assisted; LOS, length of stay; nr, not recorded; QoL, quality of life; RCT, randomized controlled trial; SBO, small bowel obstruction; TL, total laparoscopic.

To date most surgeons favor the pragmatic approach of LA-RP over totally laparoscopic or hand-assisted procedures (Table 27.1) (8–24).

Studies examining other laparoscopic colorectal procedures have demonstrated shorter postoperative recovery, with lower analgesia requirements, fewer perioperative complications, and shorter durations in hospitals when compared with similar open procedures (25).

These short-term benefits have not been confirmed in studies comparing LA-RP with conventional open surgery. A recently published Cochrane meta-analysis compared 354 patients who underwent open RP with 253 patients who had LA-RP (including hand-assisted laparoscopic-RP) (26). There was no difference in mortality or complications. Within this analysis, no randomized controlled trial (RCT) comparing

LA-RP with open surgery was identified. There was only one RCT examining patients having either hand-assisted laparoscopic procedure or open surgery (18). In this specific study, each arm consisted of 30 patients only and there was no significant difference in complication rate, hospital stay, length of time to bowel activity, or blood loss between either group. The only significant short-term difference confirmed that laparoscopic surgery was associated with longer operative times. There are several reasons to explain the lack of overall benefit of one approach compared to another. Patient numbers in these case series examined were relatively small. The type of surgeries performed and outcomes measured demonstrated wide heterogeneity. Further, L-RP is a complex procedure composed of several distinct elements involving a total colectomy, proctectomy, followed by pouch formation and ileal anal anastomosis. Each individual procedure requires significant surgical expertise. The learning curve for segmental colonic resections is estimated at 40–50 cases to reach competency (27). Additional surgical experience is necessary to competently perform laparoscopic total colectomies (28,29). Many studies have failed to detail the previous competency of surgeons performing these cases.

Few studies have focused on long-term benefits of LA-RP. Importantly, long-term outcomes of LA-RP produce equivalent functional outcomes (9) with significantly better body image in females. Both genders preferred the cosmetic results of LA-RP compared to open procedures (13,21). This finding is in agreement with the results from other laparoscopic colorectal procedures. However, the most compelling evidence supporting a laparoscopic approach are recent studies showing that laparoscopic surgery is associated with less disruption of the anterior abdominal wall with a reduction in surgical site infection and decreased long-term wound complications including incisional hernias (30). This is especially important in patients who have poor nutrition and are receiving steroids. Further, intra-abdominal adhesions are significantly reduced (31). With respect to pouch surgery, reduction in fecundity is a major concern. Indar et al. assessed intra-abdominal adhesions in patients undergoing closure of ileostomy following total L-RP and demonstrated significantly fewer adhesions (32). In the majority of cases, adhesions both to the anterior abdominal wall and pelvic organs were absent in those undergoing laparoscopic surgery. The laparoscopic approach may potentially result in improved fecundity for females requiring surgery.

 # INDICATIONS/CONTRAINDICATIONS

Indications

Indications for LA-RP surgery are the same as for open RP surgery.

- Ulcerative colitis
  - Failed medical therapy
  - Chronic (refractory ulcerative colitis, dysplasia)
- Familial adenomatous polyposis with high rectal polyp burden
- Functional (clonic inertia)
- Indeterminate colitis
- Crohn's disease – selected cases

The diagnosis of fulminant colitis is not an absolute contraindication to laparoscopic surgery (33,34). There is evidence that this approach may result in earlier hospital discharge. LA-RP has been performed successfully in pediatric cases (35).

Contraindications

There are no absolute contraindications to an attempt at laparoscopic-assisted surgery.

Here we describe our preferred method of performing a LA-RP.

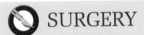

PREOPERATIVE PLANNING

Patient Positioning

The patient undergoing LA-RP is positioned lying supine with the legs in a modified Lloyd Davies position. Arms need to be tucked in closely to the sides of the trunk.

Patients are prone to injury as a result of the steep Trendelenburg and lateral tilt needed to retract the abdominal viscera by gravity.

It is important to:

- Prevent the passive movement of patients whilst on the operating table with the aid of antislip matting and a bean bag, together with additional strapping across chest and limbs.
- Prevent injuries to extremities by using extra padding to vulnerable areas around the eye, nose, face, and hands.

Due to the expected longer operative time compared to open procedures, the use of commercially available compression boots and body warmers is mandatory. The bladder is catheterized and a nasogastric tube is placed for the duration of the operation. A rectal catheter is inserted for a rectal washout.

SURGERY

Operation

Laparoscopic-assisted restorative proctocolectomy is divided into a number of key steps.

Port Placement

An open Hassan technique is the preferred method of creating the pneumoperitoneum through a periumbilical incision. A 5 mm, 30-degree laparoscope is inserted and the abdomen surveyed. Excessive adhesions and unpredicted anatomical or inflammatory conditions that prevent a laparoscopic approach should be assessed and immediate conversion initiated when appropriate.

The remaining trocars are placed under direct vision in the right iliac fossa (at the site marked for the covering loop ileostomy, if applicable) and in the right and left upper quadrants (just above the level of the umbilicus). The umbilical port acts as the position for the camera and a 12 mm port is used if a high definition camera is used. If necessary, an additional 5 mm port in placed in the epigastric region, just right of the midline, to aid mobilization of the transverse colon (Fig. 27.1).

Colectomy

Dissection of the colon begins with a medial-to-lateral mobilization of the left colon. The surgeon is positioned on the patient's right side. The left side of the colon is mobilized by placing the patient in steep Trendelenburg with left side elevated at a 30-degree angle with the lateral tilt. The inferior mesenteric artery (IMA) is exposed by the division of the peritoneum in the midline, starting at the sacral promontory and extending along a line cranially, whilst retracting the apex of the sigmoid colon toward the left pelvic sidewall. The IMA is identified but not divided. The submesenteric plane is developed, maintaining an intact Toldt's fascia below. The left ureter is identified in the retroperitoneum beneath the fascia.

The medial-to-lateral dissection is completed as far laterally and cranially as possible. At this point the sigmoid colon is retracted medially and the white line of Toldt is incised. The colon is freed from its attachments to the abdominal sidewall and mobilized medially.

Figure 27.1 Port sites and incision.

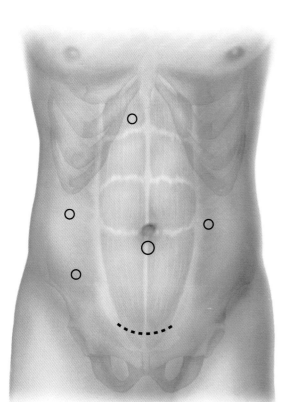

Awareness of the position of the left ureter is essential throughout dissection to prevent inadvertent damage to this structure.

The IMA pedicle is preserved if the operation is staged, in which case the left colic artery is divided and the sigmoid branches taken approximately 1 cm from the colon with a bipolar diathermy device such as LigaSure™ (Coviden, MA, USA). Vessels over 0.5 cm are secured with Hem-o-lock® clips (Tele flex Medical North Carolina, USA). In combined procedures, when proctocolectomy is planned, the IMA pedicle is not taken flush with the aorta because this technique maybe associated with hypogastric nerve injury (36). Dissection continues in a stepwise fashion heading cranially toward the splenic flexure 1 cm parallel to the mesenteric edge of the colon using a bipolar sealing and cutting device for hemostasis. It should be noted, however, if cancer is suspected or known to be present, an oncological dissection is performed and ligation of mesenteric vessels is performed as high as possible to remove all draining lymph nodes.

The patient is repositioned into reverse Trendelenburg to facilitate mobilization of the splenic flexure. The inferior mesenteric vein does not need to be divided close to the lower border of the pancreas unless indicated by the presence of malignancy. Mesenteric division continues in a retrograde fashion until the middle colic vessels are reached and divided if convenient.

The gastrocolic omentum is divided at the midline to enter the lesser sac by lifting the transverse colon toward the anterior abdominal wall. Dissection continues from medial to lateral freeing the proximal splenic flexure from the stomach and omentum. If adhesions of the omentum to the colon are dense, the omentum is sacrificed. Gentle traction of the descending colon medially and inferiorly enables the remaining lateral attachments to be divided.

The right side of the colon is mobilized by repositioning the patient into a Trende-lenburg position with the right side elevated by 30 degrees. The surgeon and camera operator stand on the patient's left side. A submesenteric window is made under the straightened ileocolic vessels by placing traction on the cecum down and out toward the right pelvic sidewall. Once again, the retroperitoneum is swept downwards separating the mesentery from the right ureter and the duodenum. Dissection continues as far laterally and superiorly as possible. The remaining gastrocolic omentum on the right hand side can be divided from medially to laterally to complete the mobilization of the hepatic flexure.

Once underlying structures have been positively identified, the ileocolic vessels can be divided after being secured with Hem-o-lock® clips. Remaining branches of the right and middle colic arteries are divided in the same fashion as the left colon, moving in an antegrade fashion.

The lateral peritoneal attachments surrounding the cecal pole are divided by retracting the cecum medially. This incision continues up toward the hepatic flexure.

The remaining peritoneum attaching the terminal ileum posteriorly may need to be incised to reveal the retroperitoneal plane and continued up to the level of the duodenum to allow maximum length of the small bowel mesentery, and as a result, the colon and small bowel should be freely mobile.

Proctectomy

We favor a Pfannenstiel incision over transverse McBurney or midline periumbilical incisions. The Pfannenstiel incision allows good access for insertion of the stapling device, specimen removal, J-pouch construction, simple regional anesthesia blockade as well as resulting in an acceptable cosmetic scar.

A small Pfannenstiel incision (5–6 cm) is made and the wound protected with an Alexis® Wound Retractor (Applied Medical, California, USA). The patient is placed in the Trendelenburg position and the colon extracted after dividing the rectosigmoid junction. The peritoneum over the right rectal wall is divided first to enter the TME plane after identifying both ureters. Our approach is aimed at reducing pelvic nerve injury associated with TME (37). Points of potential injury to nerves include the origin of the IMA, posterior dissection of the rectal tube, anterior incision of Denonvilliers' fascia or division of the lateral ligaments (36). The divided rectum is held up and the mesentery and vessels at the level of the sacral promontory are taken close to the rectum. The TME plane is then entered posteriorly after the dissection below the level of the sacral promontory. This dissection is then continued both posteriorly and laterally to the pelvic floor. Anteriorly the dissection is close to the rectal wall.

Rectal washout is performed with chlorhexidine before transection of the rectum. Accurate placement of a cross stapling device is ensured by the following.

- Assessment of the rectal stump height by placing an examining index finger in the anal canal. Transection should be performed at the tip of the finger with the proximal interphalangeal joint on the anal verge.
- Perineal pressure.
- The use of two St. Marks retractors anteriolaterally.
- An appropriately sized stapling device to transect the rectum at right angles.

After transection of the rectum at the upper anal canal, the specimen can be extracted through the Pfannenstiel incision.

Pouch Construction and Anastomosis

A standard 20 cm J-pouch with two sequential firings of a 100 mm linear stapling device is fashioned extracorporeally after identifying the point of maximal length of the terminal ileum that is able to stretch over the pubis. The anvil is secured with a purse-string suture at the apex of the J-pouch, which is returned to the abdomen. The wound protector is twisted closed and covered with a surgical glove to hold the pneumoperitoneum. The ileoanal anastomosis is performed under laparoscopic vision using an end to end anastomosis stapler. The pouch is correctly aligned without rotation by careful inspection of the small bowel mesentery and pouch along the midline. An air test is ultimately performed.

The decision to omit a diversion loop ileostomy following pouch formation is controversial. Considering the devastating sequelae of pelvic sepsis on pouch function and longevity elimination of a diverting stoma is indicated only in uncomplicated procedures in favorable patients. Care must be taken to ensure that a diverting ileostomy is not obstructed at the fascial level by creating a large enough opening in the anterior abdominal wall.

The Pfannenstiel incision and any laparoscopic port site more than 5 mm are closed at the fascial layer (Fig. 27.1). Skin incisions are closed with undyed absorbable sutures and protected with a liquid bonding agent such as Dermabond® (Ethicon, NJ , USA).

 POSTOPERATIVE MANAGEMENT

The pouch is decompressed for 48 hours postoperatively by insertion of a rectal catheter that is flushed twice daily with 20 ml of normal saline. Intra-abdominal pelvic drains are not routinely placed. Discharge is normally limited by delay of return of bowel function, the ability to care for stomas, or management of excessive pouch function resulting in electrolyte disturbance.

Following surgery, patients undergoing laparoscopic pouch surgery have less pain with lower opiate requirements as demonstrated by Kelly et al., who compared total L-RP with patients undergoing open surgery (8). Laparoscopic colorectal surgery is associated with less postoperative pain, faster mobility, and quicker return to work. Patients undergoing laparoscopic subtotal colectomies have been shown to require less opiate usage, faster return of bowel function, and shorter length of hospital stay compared to open procedure (38).

At the same time as the development of laparoscopic colorectal surgery, enhanced recovery programs have encouraged smaller incisions such as seen in LA-RP. Enhanced recovery after surgery (ERAS) programs aim to maintain normal physiology by avoiding bowel preparation, encourage the use of local anesthesia with the avoidance of opiates together with early mobilization and feeding to improve outcome measures.

Overall failure to recover in a timely manner should alert to the possibility of postoperative complications and early investigation including further laparoscopy should be considered.

 COMPLICATIONS

The following discussion will focus mainly on the impact of laparoscopic approach on complications of pouch surgery as more detailed examination of complication of pouch surgery will be discussed elsewhere.

Bleeding

Significant postoperative bleeding occurs in 3.5% of patients undergoing pouch surgery requiring re-intervention (39). However, Ahmed et al. identified no difference in postoperative blood loss comparing LA-RP with open surgery (26). However, both studies included in their analysis were published in 2001 and as such lack the benefit of modern hemostatic devices. It is thought that the newer energy source devices for vascular control have dramatically reduced intraoperative blood loss especially during closed rectal dissection.

Small Bowel Obstruction

Open RP is associated with symptomatic adhesive small bowel obstruction in 20% patients after surgery with a median follow-up of only 2–3 years (39–41). Hand assisted ports are also associated with a similar degree of adhesive small bowel complications (13). However, as discussed earlier, laparoscopic surgery may dramatically reduce this significant cause of morbidity (9).

Sexual Dysfunction

The surgical approach described here is directed to minimize injury to the nerves affecting both bladder and sexual function. The incidence of nerve injury affecting sexual function in men was 3.8% and confined to men over the age of 50 at the time of surgery (42). This study has not been repeated for patients undergoing laparoscopic RP.

Fecundity & Pregnancy

Female patient undergoing open pouch surgery have a higher rate of infertility. In a study on ulcerative colitis patients, 38% of females of childbearing age engaging in unprotected sexual intercourse failed to get pregnant within a year following open surgery compared to 13% without surgery (43). It is for this reason that the study from Indar et al. assessing adhesions in patients after total L-RP is so encouraging (32). It will be interesting if fewer adhesions translate into improved rates of fecundity.

CONCLUSIONS

At present, LA-RP is a safe and reliable approach to pouch surgery resulting in equivalent functional outcomes compared with open surgery. Although any long-term benefits of this approach are yet to be validated, at present we advocate a hybrid procedure until a laparoscopic stapling device designed to provide a single staple line at the level of the pelvic floor for all patients is available. However, in females with a deep wide pelvis we have undertaken total L-RP.

Recommended References and Readings

1. Parks AG, Nicholls RJ. Proctocolectomy without ileostomy for ulcerative colitis. *Br Med J* 1978;2:85–88.
2. Peters WR. Laparoscopic total proctocolectomy with creation of ileostomy for ulcerative colitis: report of two cases. *J Laparoendosc Surg* 1992;2(3):175–78.
3. Wexner S, Johansen OB, Nogueras JJ, Jagelman DG. Laparoscopic total abdominal colectomy. A prospective trial. *Dis Colon Rectum* 1992;35(7):651–55.
4. Rotholtz NA, Aued ML, Lencinas SM, et al. Laparoscopic-assisted proctocolectomy using complete intracorporeal dissection. *Surg Endosc* 2008;22(5):1303–08.
5. Ouaïssi M, Lefevre JH, Bretagnol F, Alves A, Valleur P, Panis Y. Laparoscopic 3-step restorative proctocolectomy: comparative study with open approach in 45 patients. *Surg Laparosc Endosc Percutan Tech* 2008;18(4):357–62.
6. Targarona EM, Gracia E, Garriga J, et al. Prospective randomized trial comparing conventional laparoscopic colectomy with hand-assisted laparoscopic colectomy: applicability, immediate clinical outcome, inflammatory response, and cost. *Surg Endosc* 2002;16(2):234–39.
7. Kienle P, Z'graggen K, Schmidt J, et al. Laparoscopic restorative proctocolectomy. *Br J Surg* 2005;92(1):88–93.
8. Kelly J, Condon ET, Redmond HP, Kirwan WO. The benefits of a laparoscopic approach in ileal pouch anal anastomosis formation: a single institutional retrospective case-matched experience. *Irish J Med Sci* 2010;179(2):197–200.
9. El-Gazzaz GS, Kiran RP, Remzi FH, Hull TL, Geisler DP. Outcomes for case-matched laparoscopically assisted versus open restorative proctocolectomy. *Br J Surg* 2009;96(5): 522–26.
10. Fichera A, Silvestri MT, Hurst RD, Rubin MA, Michelassi F. Laparoscopic restorative proctocolectomy with ileal pouch anal anastomosis: a comparative observational study on long-term functional results. *J Gastro Surg* 2009;13(3):526–32.
11. Sylla P, Chessin DB, Gorfine SR, Roth E, Bub DS, Bauer JJ. Evaluation of one-stage laparoscopic-assisted restorative proctocolectomy at a specialty center: comparison with the open approach. *Dis Col Rectum* 2009;52(3):394–99.
12. Polle SW, van Berge Henegouwen MI, Slors JF, Cuesta MA, Gouma DJ, Bemelman WA. Total laparoscopic restorative proctocolectomy: are there advantages compared with the open and hand-assisted approaches? *Dis Col Rectum* 2008;51(5):541–48.
13. Polle SW, Dunker MS, Slors JF, et al. Body image, cosmesis, quality of life, and functional outcome of hand-assisted laparoscopic

versus open restorative proctocolectomy: long-term results of a randomized trial. *Surg Endosc* 2007;21(8):1301–07.
14. Zhang H, Hu S, Zhang G, et al. Laparoscopic versus open proctocolectomy with ileal pouch-anal anastomosis. *Minim Invasive Ther Allied Technol* 2007;16(3):187–89.
15. Larson DW, Cima RR, Dozois EJ, et al. Safety, feasibility, and short-term outcomes of laparoscopic ileal-pouch-anal anastomosis: a single institutional case-matched experience. *Ann Surg* 2006;243(5):667–70.
16. Larson DW, Dozois EJ, Piotrowicz K, Cima RR, Wolff BG, Young-Fadok TM. Laparoscopic-assisted vs. open ileal pouch-anal anastomosis: functional outcome in a case-matched series. *Dis Col Rectum* 2005;48(10):1845–50.
17. Berdah SV, Barthet M, Emungania O, et al. [Two stage videoassisted restorative proctocolectomy. Early experience of 12 cases] French. *Ann Chir Gynaecol* 2004;129(6–7):332–6.
18. Maartense S, Dunker MS, Slors JF, et al. Hand-assisted laparoscopic versus open restorative proctocolectomy with ileal pouch anal anastomosis: a randomized trial. *Ann Surg* 2004;240(6): 984–91.
19. Araki Y, Ishibashi N, Ogata Y, Shirouzu K, Isomoto H. The usefulness of restorative laparoscopic-assisted total colectomy for ulcerative colitis. *Kurume Med J* 2001;48(2):99–103.
20. Brown SR, Eu KW, Seow-Choen F. Consecutive series of laparoscopic-assisted vs. minilaparotomy restorative proctocolectomies. *Dis Col Rectum* 2001;44(3):397–400.
21. Dunker MS, Bemelman WA, Slors JF, van Duijvendijk P, Gouma DJ. Functional outcome, quality of life, body image, and cosmesis in patients after laparoscopic-assisted and conventional restorative proctocolectomy: a comparative study. *Dis Col Rectum* 2001;44(12):1800–07.
22. Hashimoto A, Funayama Y, Naito H, et al. Laparoscope-assisted versus conventional restorative proctocolectomy with rectal mucosectomy. *Surgery Today* 2001;31(3):210–14.
23. Marcello PW, Milsom JW, Wong SK, et al. Laparoscopic restorative proctocolectomy: case-matched comparative study with open restorative proctocolectomy. *Dis Col Rectum* 2000;43(5):604–08.
24. Schmitt SL, Cohen SM, Wexner SD, Nogueras JJ, Jagelman DG. Does laparoscopic-assisted ileal pouch anal anastomosis reduce the length of hospitalization? *Int J Colorectal Dis* 1994;9(3): 134–37.
25. Schwenk W, Haase O, Neudecker J, Müller JM. Short term benefits for laparoscopic colorectal resection. *Cochrane Database Syst Rev* 2005;20(3):CD003145.
26. Ahmed Ali U, Keus F, Heikens JT, et al. Open versus laparoscopic (assisted) ileo pouch anal anastomosis for ulcerative

colitis and familial adenomatous polyposis. *Cochrane Database Syst Rev* 2009,(1): CD006267.

27. Tekkis PP, Senagore AJ, Delaney CP, Fazio VW. Evaluation of the learning curve in laparoscopic colorectal surgery: comparison of right-sided and left-sided resections. *Ann Surg* 2005; 242(1):83–91.

28. McNevin MS, Bax T, MacFarlane M, et al. Outcomes of a laparoscopic approach for total abdominal colectomy and proctocolectomy. *Am J Surg* 2006;191(5):673–76.

29. Antolovic D, Kienle P, Hanns-Peter Knaebel H-P, et al. Totally laparoscopic versus conventional ileoanal pouch procedure–design of a single-center, expertise based randomised controlled trial to compare the laparoscopic and conventional surgical approach in patients undergoing primary elective restorative proctocolectomy-LapConPouch-Trial. *BioMed Central Surgery* 2006;6:13.

30. Laurent C, Leblanc F, Bretagnol F, Capdepont M, Rullier E. Long-term wound advantages of the laparoscopic approach in rectal cancer. *Br J Surg* 2008;95(7):903–08.

31. Dowson HM, Bong JJ, Lovell DP, Worthington TR, Karanjia ND, Rockall TA. Reduced adhesion formation following laparoscopic versus open colorectal surgery. *Br J Surg* 2008;95(7) :909–14.

32. Indar AA, Efron JE, Young-Fadok TM. Laparoscopic ileal pouchanal anastomosis reduces abdominal and pelvic adhesions. *Surg Endosc* 2009;23(1):174–77.

33. Fowkes L, Krishna K, Menon A, Greenslade GL, Dixon AR. Laparoscopic emergency and elective surgery for ulcerative colitis. *Colorectal Dis* 2008;10(4):373–78.

34. Holubar SD, Larson DW, Dozois EJ, Pattana-Arun J, Pemberton JH, Cima RR. Minimally invasive subtotal colectomy and ileal

35. Tan WY, Jaffray B. A comparison of open and laparoscopic restorative proctocolectomy in children. *Pediatr Surg Int* 2009;25:877–79.

36. Moszkowicz D, Alsaid B, Bessede T, et al. Where does pelvic nerve injury occur during rectal surgery for cancer? *Colorectal Diseases*, 2010, Aug 16 epub in advance.

37. Quah HM, Jayne DG, Eu KW, Seow-Choen F. Bladder and sexual dysfunction following laparoscopically assisted and conventional open mesorectal resection for cancer. *Br J Surg* 2002; 89(12):1551–56.

38. Chung TP, Fleshman JW, Birnbaum EH, et al. Laparoscopic vs. open total abdominal colectomy for severe colitis: impact on recovery and subsequent completion restorative proctectomy. *Dis Col Rectum* 2009;52(1):4–10.

39. Fazio VW, Ziv Y, Church JM, et al. Ileal pouch-anal anastomoses complications and function in 1005 patients. *Ann Surg* 1995;222:120–27.

40. Francois Y, Dozois RR, Kelly KA, et al. Small intestinal obstruction complicating ileal pouch-anal anastomosis. *Ann Surg* 1989;209:46–50.

41. Marcello PW, Roberts PL, Schoetz DJ Jr, Coller JA, Murray JJ, Veidenheimer MC. Obstruction after ileal pouch-anal anastomosis: a preventable complication? *Dis Col Rectum* 1993;36:1105–11.

42. Lindsey I, George BD, Kettlewell MG, et al. Impotence after mesorectal and close rectal dissection for inflammatory bowel disease. *Dis Col Rectum* 2001;44:831–35.

43. Johnson P, Richard C, Ravid A, et al. Female infertility after ileal pouch anal anastomosis for ulcerative colitis. *Dis Col Rectum* 2004;47:1119–26.

pouch-anal anastomosis for fulminant ulcerative colitis: a reasonable approach? *Dis Col Rectum* 2009;52(2):187–92.

28 Restorative Proctocolectomy: Laparoscopic Proctocolectomy and Ileal Pouch-Anal Anastomosis

Tonia M. Young-Fadok

DEFINITIONS

Extent of Operation

To avoid confusion regarding naming conventions, this chapter will employ the following terms. *Total colectomy* describes resection of the entire colon, with either an ileorectal anastomosis (IRA) if bowel continuity is preserved, or Brooke ileostomy and retention of the rectal stump. *Proctocolectomy* refers to surgical removal of the entire colon and the rectum. The word "total" as sometimes used in "total proctocolectomy" is thus redundant and not used in this chapter.

Following proctocolectomy, the terminal ileum is either matured as a Brooke ileostomy, or, more commonly, is used for a reconstructive procedure to reestablish bowel continuity, in the form of an ileal pouch, which is anastomosed to the anal canal. Infrequently, it may be used for a continent ileostomy. Reconstruction with an ileal pouch is referred to by two common terms, *restorative proctocolectomy* (favored by the British and Cleveland Clinic) and proctocolectomy and *ileal pouch-anal anastomosis* (IPAA), a term more commonly used by Mayo Clinic. I prefer the latter description as it describes the means of restoration of bowel continuity.

Laparoscopic Procedures

Naming conventions for laparoscopic procedures, especially in the field of colorectal surgery, are somewhat open to interpretation. Most surgeons would agree on the following usages. A procedure is *laparoscopic* if the procedure is laparoscopically completed and the main incision is used only for extraction of the specimen. *Laparoscopic-assisted* usually means that a portion of the case was performed extracorporeally, such as anastomosis in a right colectomy (although if the incision is the same as used to extract the specimen, this differentiation is splitting hairs). In a *hand-assisted procedure,* a 6–8-cm incision is used to place a device that allows a hand to be inserted into the abdominal cavity to facilitate the procedure. This incision is larger than the typical 3–5-cm incision used for extraction of the specimen. In a *hybrid procedure,* a portion of the case is laparoscopically performed, such as mobilization of the abdominal colon, and then a small incision (infraumbilical midline or Pfannenstiel) is used to facilitate dissection of the rectum or deployment of a stapler. The hand-assist-incision may be used for this type of procedure, and thus many purists consider hand-assisted and hybrid cases to be similar in terms of incision length.

With regard to laparoscopic proctocolectomy and IPAA, a *laparoscopic-assisted* procedure would generally enlarge a supraumbilical port site incision, by extending it around the umbilicus to a 3-5-cm periumbilical extraction incision and then create the ileal pouch through this incision. In this chapter, a *completely laparoscopic* proctocolectomy and IPAA involves complete laparoscopic mobilization of the colon and the rectum, transection of the rectum and mesentery intracorporeally, and extraction of the specimen via the *planned ileostomy site* so that no port site is enlarged and no additional incision is employed for specimen extraction. The pouch is still constructed extracorporeally, but the ileostomy site incision is not enlarged to accomplish this goal. I prefer "completely" laparoscopic to "totally" laparoscopic given the confusion with naming conventions and the extent of procedure as noted above when the word "total" is used.

INDICATIONS/CONTRAINDICATIONS

The two most common pathologic diagnoses for which IPAA is undertaken are ulcerative colitis (UC) and familial adenomatous polyposis (FAP). Infrequently, the procedure may be appropriate in an individual with hereditary nonpolyposis colorectal cancer (HNPCC) with a rectal neoplasm, as distinct from the more common right-sided lesions that prompt a total colectomy and IRA.

The reasons for recommending IPAA in patients with UC are: disease refractory to medical therapy; complications of medications used to treat the disease; inability to wean steroids despite responsiveness of the disease; failure to thrive in pediatric patients; and patient preference in the case of those patients who prefer an operation to long-term medication. Surgeons consider IPAA to be the appropriate recommendation in patients with FAP. Others will consider total colectomy and IRA if there is relative rectal-sparing with few rectal polyps. This author's preference is for IPAA in all cases of FAP, but to consider IRA in patients with attenuated FAP with rectal sparing.

The discussion of contraindications will distinguish between contraindications to IPAA, to laparoscopic IPAA (L-IPAA), and completely laparoscopic IPAA (CL-IPAA). In the patient with UC, IPAA may not be appropriate in an emergency situation, such as perforation, toxic megacolon, and hemorrhage. This decision will depend on whether the patient is hemodynamically stable, the duration of their symptoms, and the expertise of the surgeon. Consideration must be given to stabilization of the patient and whether or not a total colectomy and Brooke ileostomy (TC&B) may be the safest and most expeditious approach. Procedures performed may range from open total colectomy and Brooke ileostomy (TC&B) in the unstable patient with perforation, to L-IPAA in the stable patient with bleeding but no evidence of malnutrition. Malnutrition (low albumin, low pre-albumin, World Health Organization definition of >10% weight loss) should prompt TC&B rather than IPAA. Emerging data suggest that recent administration of biologic medications may increase the risk of pouch complications. Thus, I will not perform IPAA in patients within 8 weeks of receiving Infliximab or 2 weeks of Adalimumab, but instead recommend a three-stage procedure. Only one additional contraindication applies to CL-IPAA—obesity. In the obese patient, the resected colorectum cannot be extracted via the ileostomy site without enlarging the incision. Although the enlarged fascial incision can be made smaller with sutures, the skin incision cannot and maturation of the stoma results in deformity that contributes to difficulty with looking after the stoma.

PREOPERATIVE PLANNING

For all patients undergoing elective surgery, a formal preoperative assessment consists of the following steps: evaluation in our preoperative clinic by a trained clinician to exclude issues pertaining to anesthesia; basic blood tests including electrolytes, complete blood count, and albumin and pre-albumin when indicated by history; chest x-ray and EKG when appropriate; type and screen within 72 hours of operation; and pregnancy test when applicable. All patients consult with our stoma nurses to mark the most appropriate site for the planned ileostomy. Some data suggest that bowel preparation is unnecessary, but these data are from open cases. Laparoscopic handling of the bowel requires a bowel preparation, and this "completely laparoscopic" approach demands it! The vast majority of patients undergoing this operation have had prior colonoscopies and can suggest which preparation has worked best for them and been tolerated. This author has no specific preference regarding bowel preparation.

On the day of operation, patients who have had a prolonged course of steroids within the preceding 6–12 months, but are now off steroids, receive a dose of methylprednisolone 20 mg intravenously on call to the operating room and then a rapid taper over 3 days. Patients who are currently taking prednisone receive a 10–20 mg higher dose of methylprednisolone (on a mg/mg basis) and then are tapered over 3 days to the preoperative dose.

NSQIP guidelines are followed; in patients who do not have a penicillin allergy, ertapenem 1 g i.v. is administered within 60 minutes of the incision with no postoperative doses required. The penicillin-allergic patient receives metronidazole 500 mg i.v. and ciprofloxacin 400 mg i.v. within 60 minutes of the incision. All patients are preoperatively given a warming blanket as this contributes to the maintenance of postoperative normothermia.

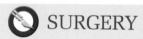 SURGERY

Positioning

Success of the operation begins with correct positioning. Three key points govern positioning: (a) steep gravity changes are used, so the patient must be safely secured to the table; (b) there must be access to the perineum for stapled or sutured anastomosis; and (c) the position must facilitate the laparoscopic approach. Thus, the patient is placed in a modified combined synchronous position (modified lithotomy). We use medical grade pink egg-crate foam to ensure that the patient does not slip or slide. This egg crate is taped to the bed *over* a drawer sheet placed beneath the foam to be used for tucking the arms. The legs are placed in padded Allen stirrups and positioned with the thighs within 5 degrees of being parallel with the abdominal wall so that instruments used in the lower trocars during dissection in the upper abdomen are not hampered by the thighs. The hands are wrapped in foam and tucked adjacent to the torso. A commercial warming device is placed over the chest, followed by a folded blanket (to prevent tearing of the Bair Hugger, so it may be used in the recovery room), and linen tape is wrapped around the patient's chest and around the table three times. A "tilt test" is then performed: the OR table is then moved into all the potential extreme positions used during the case to ensure that the patient is safely affixed to the table.

A bladder catheter is placed and an orogastric tube is inserted to be removed at the end of the procedure.

Surgical Technique

Rationale

A lateral-to-medial approach is utilized for several reasons. First, the approach is similar to the open approach and trainees more readily recognize the anatomic landmarks.

Second, a medial-to-lateral approach involves sacrificing the ileocolic pedicle. Although these vessels may ultimately be taken to obtain adequate length of the pouch, sometimes the length-limiting structure is the adjacent vessel arcade, and therefore I prefer to preserve the ileocolic pedicle until final decisions are made regarding pouch "reach" (the ability of the pouch to be anastomosed to the anal sphincter without tension). Third, in a medial-to-lateral approach, the intra-abdominal colon is devascularized early in the case prior to dissection in the pelvis; a lateral-to-medial approach avoids "dead gut" sitting in the abdomen while the pelvic dissection is completed. Finally, this approach allows for a "division of convenience" of the mesentery, avoiding dissection of the proximal vascular pedicles in a patient whose tissues may be friable from prolonged steroid use.

There are essentially three components to the laparoscopic portion of the procedure: mobilization of the left colon, mobilization of the right colon, and dissection of the rectum in the pelvis. Again, there is a rationale for this approach: the left colon is somewhat more technically challenging than is the right and once this is achieved, mobilization of the right colon is a little bit of a break before the technical challenges of the pelvic dissection! Also, even if the rectal dissection requires an open approach by those surgeons not comfortable with the laparoscopic approach, the subsequent lower midline or Pfannenstiel incision is smaller than a long midline incision required to mobilize the splenic flexure.

Laparoscopic Approach

A cutdown technique is employed for insertion of a 10/12-mm blunt port. Our population of colorectal patients is sufficiently complex that a Veress needle technique is never used. After pneumoperitoneum of 13 mmHg is achieved, the abdominal cavity is explored, and a 5-mm port is placed in the suprapubic midline and one or two additional ports (depending on BMI) are placed in the left lower quadrant. A disc of skin and subcutaneous fat are excised from the premarked ileostomy site in the right lower quadrant and a 12-mm port is placed through this site.

Left Colon Mobilization

Commencing at the left pelvic brim, the dissection commences immediately medial to the left lateral peritoneal reflection. By leaving the peritoneal reflection "with the patient," the plane of dissection identifies the left ureter, which can be gently swept laterally and protected. The sigmoid colon is mobilized to the midline and the left lateral peritoneal reflection alongside the descending colon is opened and the descending colon is mobilized medially.

The splenic flexure may be mobilized by several approaches. The easiest is in the patient with a normal BMI. Laterally, the proximal descending colon is dissected off Gerota's fascia and as the plane of dissection turns medially the lesser sac is identified, and the omentum is dissected off the distal transverse colon in a retrograde fashion. In the heavier patient, the lateral dissection is the same, but instead of proceeding in a retrograde fashion, attention turns to the mid-transverse colon. The lesser sac is identified and entered above the mid-transverse colon and the dissection is continued laterally toward the splenic flexure. The lesser sac may be entered above the omentum, thereby taking the omentum with the specimen, or between the omentum and distal transverse colon, thus preserving the omentum.

Right Colon Mobilization

The peritoneum around the base of the terminal ileal mesentery and the cecum is scored, and the correct retroperitoneal plane is entered. In a patient with normal BMI, the ureter may be identified before scoring the peritoneum; in a heavier patient, this step is easier after peritoneal incision. The right lateral peritoneal reflection alongside the ascending colon is opened and the ascending colon is mobilized medially to the midline. The medial peritoneal attachments of the terminal ileal mesentery are opened up to the level of the duodenum. Before moving the patient into reverse Trendelenburg, the dissection is checked to ensure that the right colon has been mobilized to the midline.

With the patient in reverse Trendelenburg, and the right side still inclined up, the hepatocolic attachments are divided, again taking care to identify and protect the duodenum. The management of the omentum should reflect the treatment of the splenic flexure, whether removing the omentum or leaving it with the patient. This step avoids difficulty when dividing the transverse colon and having to decide upon a point to divide the omentum when the flexures have been approached differently.

Dissection of the Rectum

The dissection of the left lateral peritoneal reflection alongside the distal sigmoid colon at the left pelvic brim is continued. The left ureter is again identified to keep it safe from the operative field. The line of dissection is continued over the level of the sacral promontory, scoring the left pararectal peritoneum. Careful inspection will reveal a line between the "white tissue" laterally that stays behind, and the "yellow tissue" medially that marks the boundary of the mesorectal fascial envelope. Scoring the left pararectal peritoneum allows entry into the presacral space at the level of the sacral promontory. This plane is developed with cautery scissors medially and distally as far as retraction and visualization permit—often to the level of the pelvic floor in a patient with normal BMI. Care should be taken to remain in the correct plane and identify the left hypogastric nerve. Attempting to remain too close to the promontory may reveal an areolar tissue plane that is actually posterior to the nerve. Therefore, it is important to identify and remain in a plane that is immediately adjacent to the mesorectum and anterior to the nerve.

Following mobilization of the left side of the rectum, the right pararectal peritoneum is scored after identifying and protecting the right ureter. The presacral plane is entered and the dissection is joined with that already performed from the left side. Again, the right presacral nerve is protected by remaining immediately posterior to the mesorectal fascia and not immediately on the presacrum. The dissection is continued to the pelvic floor.

Once the rectum is mobilized posteriorly and bilaterally, the anterior dissection proceeds. This is the most challenging portion of the rectal mobilization and is facilitated by prior mobilization of the posterior and lateral aspects of the rectum. In the male patient, care should be taken to identify and protect the seminal vesicles and prostate. In the female patient, a sponge stick is placed in the vagina to retract it anteriorly to facilitate identification and dissection in the rectovaginal septum. In this manner, the rectum is completely circumferentially dissected down to the level of the pelvic floor. This maneuver will take several position changes, as each quadrant of dissection of the rectum will allow for improved retraction of another quadrant and thus dissection circumferentially proceeds.

Once the pelvic floor is reached (the fascia and muscle are easily discerned once at the correct level), then a digital rectal examination (with an overglove on the examining hand) is performed to confirm that the correct level of dissection has been reached. In slim patients, this dissection level is often in the intersphincteric groove and care must be taken not to transect at *too* low a level.

At this point, the decision is made regarding stapled anastomosis versus mucosectomy and handsewn anastomosis. In most cases, the decision is already made. My preference is for stapled anastomosis at the top of the anal canal, with preservation of the anal transition zone as there is evidence suggesting better function in such cases. I reserve mucosectomy for ulcerative colitis with rectal cancer or dysplasia, or FAP with polyps in the rectal mucosa of the proximal anal canal, both of which are rare indications.

For a stapled transection of the rectum at the level of the pelvic floor, consideration must be given to appropriate choice of stapler. An articulated laparoscopic stapler is mandatory. I prefer to deploy the stapler via the right lower quadrant 12-mm port with a subsequent transverse staple line, but some surgeons prefer to use a suprapubic port (this preference should be considered ahead of time when the ports are placed). The length of the staple cartridge is usually dictated by the diameter of the pelvis, and thus by the gender of the patient. In female patients, a 45-mm or even a 60-mm cartridge may be used, whereas in male patients with a narrower pelvis, several applications of a 30-mm cartridge are often required.

Transection of the Mesentery

Once the rectum is transected, the colon and rectum are now a midline structure centered beneath the umbilicus, and in a patient with a normal BMI, the entire colon and rectum can be exteriorized via a 3–5-cm periumbilical incision by extending the supraumbilical port-site incision around the left side of the umbilicus (so as not to interfere with subsequent application of an appliance around the ileostomy) and the mesentery can be extracorporeally transected; this approach is the simplest.

For a "completely laparoscopic" approach, the mesentery is intracorporeally divided. In the relatively rare case when there is a cancer or dysplasia present, then the vascular pedicles should be divided at their base. In the majority of patients, the mesentery may be divided where it is most convenient. We start at the top of the sacral promontory, with the mobilized sigmoid colon and use a vessel sealing device to sequentially transect the mesentery from distal to proximal. The transverse colon is often the most technically challenging segment and is usually related to a discrepancy in how the two flexures are approached, with preservation of the omentum at the splenic flexure but mobilization of the omentum with the hepatic flexure. In such cases, a decision has to be made regarding transection of the omentum at some point, usually easiest toward the right side of the transverse colon.

As this transection of the mesentery continues toward the right colon, awareness must be maintained of landmarks. It is prudent to retain the ileocolic pedicle and, therefore, when this landmark is reached, the mesenteric transection is complete. A grasper is placed on the cut end of the rectum and the abdominal cavity is inspected to ensure that loops of small bowel do not lie over the colon as they will impede its exteriorization.

Exteriorization and Pouch Creation

The pneumoperitoneum is evacuated and the 12-mm port through the ileostomy site is removed. To create the ileostomy site, the anterior rectus fascia is incised in a cruciate fashion, the rectus muscle fibers are separated, and the posterior fascia elevated and incised similarly. The end of the rectum is then passed up through this incision and the entire specimen is exteriorized until the distal ileum is reached. The remaining small portion of mesentery is divided close to the colon to preserve the ileocolic pedicle, and the terminal ileum is transected with a linear stapler.

A point on the ileum ~15 cm from the cut end is tested to determine if it reaches to the pubis. In a slim patient, the fact that the ileum is exteriorized through a non-midline incision does not affect this test. In a heavier patient with a thicker abdominal wall, this test is less accurate and experience should determine whether pouch-lengthening techniques are required. A 15-cm J-pouch is constructed deploying two firings of a 100-mm linear stapler via an enterotomy on the antimesenteric edge of the ileum at the apex of the pouch. The small tongue of redundant tissue created at this apical enterotomy following stapling is excised, and the anvil of a circular stapler is secured within the cut edge of the pouch with a 2-0 monofilament suture. The blind end of the pouch is tacked to the adjacent afferent limb with imbricating seromuscular 3-0 silk sutures, burying the staple line. These sutures theoretically reduce leaks from this staple line and prevent elongation of the blind end.

The pouch is returned to the abdominal cavity, placing the anvil in the pelvis to facilitate finding it again. After irrigation, the fascia of the ileostomy site is closed with sutures, and the port is secured within the incision again between two of the sutures, allowing the pneumoperitoneum to be reestablished.

Creation of the Ileal J-Pouch Anal Anastomosis

After locating the anvil and pouch, the cut edge of the small bowel mesentery is traced completely along its length up to the duodenum to ensure that there is no twisting of the pouch. The anus is gently dilated and the handle of the stapler inserted. The spike is brought out *adjacent* to the staple line (rather than *through* the staple line, which can cause separation of the staples for a distance longer than that which is subsequently incorporated within the circular stapling circumference). The anvil is docked onto the handle and (after again checking the cut edge of the pouch mesentery) the stapler is reapproximated, fired, and removed. Both tissue rings in the device are examined to ensure that they are intact and the distal ring is sent to pathology as part of the specimen.

A 15-Fr round drain is placed in the pelvis adjacent to the pouch via the suprapubic port, which is removed. A loop of ileum approximately 10–12 in. proximal to the pouch is chosen for the ileostomy and brought up to the ileostomy site to check for length. The fascial sutures are removed from the ileostomy site and the loop brought up and held securely. The remaining ports are removed under direct vision. The fascia of the 12-mm supraumbilical port is secured with sutures. All skin incisions are closed with subcuticular monofilament 3-0 suture, and the ileostomy is matured in standard loop fashion with full-thickness 3-0 monofilament sutures. A 20–24-Fr red rubber catheter is transanally placed within the pouch to keep it decompressed.

 ## POSTOPERATIVE MANAGEMENT

The orogastric tube is removed at the end of the case. Patient-controlled analgesia (PCA) and scheduled ketorolac are used. Postoperative antibiotics are not required if ertapenem is used preoperatively as it has 24-hour coverage, but two more doses of ciprofloxacin and metronidazole are given if the patient is penicillin-allergic. Limited clear liquids (500 ml) are introduced on the first postoperative day and unrestricted clear liquids on the morning of the second day. If these are tolerated, an ileostomy diet (low residue diet with thickening snacks) is introduced on the evening of the second day or the morning of the third. The PCA is discontinued after tolerating solid food, and the Foley is removed after the PCA is stopped. Ileostomy care teaching is instituted on postoperative day 1, and home health services are arranged for postdischarge stoma teaching. Patients are discharged when they are tolerating adequate oral intake, and producing <1,000 ml from the ileostomy. All patients are discharged on loperamide 2–4 mg, 30 minutes prior to meals and at bedtime.

 ## COMPLICATIONS

The potential complications of this completely laparoscopic approach are similar to the standard laparoscopic and open approaches, although some complications may be reduced compared with the open procedure. The commonest immediate complications are postoperative ileus, high output from the ileostomy, partial small bowel obstruction, wound infection, and pouch leak. The wound infection rate may be less with the laparoscopic approach. In the long term, the outcomes are similar to open proctocolectomy with the exception that after a laparoscopic approach patients form fewer adhesions, and this may ultimately translate into fewer episodes of small-bowel obstruction and also maintenance of fecundity in women of child-bearing age.

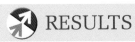 ## RESULTS

After the second stage of the operation, with closure of the ileostomy, the vast majority of patients have a pattern of bowel frequency that is acceptable to them, certainly when compared to the frequency and urgency of active colitis. In the surgical literature, the range is four to six bowel movements during the day and zero to two at night. This author's experience is that teenagers and patients in their 20s will often attain a frequency of two to four bowel movements per day depending on their dietary habits.

✦ CONCLUSIONS

A completely laparoscopic approach is feasible for proctocolectomy and IPAA, meaning that the entire colon and rectum can be mobilized, intracorporeally transected and then brought out through the ileostomy site, without the need for an additional extraction incision, or an incision for a hand-assisted device or to perform the dissection in the pelvis. This approach is an option for patients of normal to slightly overweight BMI. In heavier patients, the ileostomy extraction site can become larger than required for the ileostomy itself and it is difficult to judge the "reach" of the pouch in such patients. A lateral-to-medial approach duplicates the tissue planes used for the open approach, allows a choice regarding the level of mesenteric vessel transection, and avoids ischemic bowel sitting in the abdominal cavity while the pelvic dissection is performed. The cosmetic results are favorable, mimicking an appendectomy incision plus three port-site incisions after final closure of the ileostomy.

Suggested Readings

Ahmed Ali U, Keus F, Heikens JT, et al. Open versus laparoscopic (assisted) ileo pouch anal anastomosis for ulcerative colitis and familial adenomatous polyposis. *Cochrane Database Syst Rev* 2009;(1):CD006267.

Bemelman WA. Laparoscopic ileoanal pouch surgery. *Br J Surg* 2010; 97:2–3.

Berdah SV, Mardion RB, Grimaud JC, et al. Mid-term functional outcome of laparoscopic restorative proctocolectomy: a prospective study of 40 consecutive cases. *J Laparoendosc Adv Surg Tech A* 2009;19:485–88.

Chung TP, Fleshman JW, Birnbaum EH, et al. Laparoscopic vs. open total abdominal colectomy for severe colitis: impact on recovery and subsequent completion restorative proctectomy. *Dis Colon Rectum* 2009;52:4–10.

El-Gazzaz GS, Kiran RP, Remzi FH, et al. Outcomes for case-matched laparoscopically assisted versus open restorative proctocolectomy. *Br J Surg* 2009;96:522–26.

Fichera A, Silvestri MT, Hurst RD, et al. Laparoscopic restorative proctocolectomy with ileal pouch anal anastomosis: a comparative observational study on long-term functional results. *J Gastrointest Surg* 2009;13:526–32.

Hasegawa S, Nomura A, Kawamura J, et al. Laparoscopic restorative total proctocolectomy with mucosal resection. *Dis Colon Rectum* 2007;50:1152–56.

Indar AA, Efron JE, Young-Fadok TM. Laparoscopic ileal pouch-anal anastomosis reduces abdominal and pelvic adhesions. *Surg Endosc* 2009;23:174–77.

Larson DW, Dozois EJ, Piotrowicz K, et al. Laparoscopic-assisted vs. open ileal pouch–anal anastomosis: functional outcome in a case-matched series. *Dis Colon Rectum* 2005;48:1845–50.

Lawes DA, Young-Fadok TM. Minimally invasive proctocolectomy and ileal pouch-anal anastomosis. In: Frantzides CT, Carlson MA, eds. *Atlas of Minimally Invasive Surgery.* Philadelphia, PA: Saunders Elsevier, 2009:139–46.

McAllister I, Sagar PM, Brayshaw I, et al. Laparoscopic restorative proctocolectomy with and without previous subtotal colectomy. *Colorectal Dis* 2009;11:296–301.

Polle SW, Dunker MS, Slors JF, et al. Body image, cosmesis, quality of life, and functional outcome of hand-assisted laparoscopic versus open restorative proctocolectomy: long-term results of a randomized trial. *Surg Endosc* 2007;21:1301–07.

Rotholtz NA, Aued ML, Lencinas SM, et al. Laparoscopic-assisted proctocolectomy using complete intracorporeal dissection. *Surg Endosc* 2008;22:1303–08.

Vivas D, Khaikin M, Wexner SD. Laparoscopic proctocolectomy and Brooke ileostomy. In: Asbun HJ, Young-Fadok TM, eds. American College of Surgeons Multimedia Atlas of Surgery; Colorectal Surgery Volume. Chicago, IL: American College of Surgeons, 2008:111–16.

Young-Fadok TM, Nunoo-Mensah JW. Laparoscopic proctocolectomy and ileal pouch-anal anastomosis (IPAA). In: Asbun JH, Young-Fadok TM, eds. American College of Surgeons Multimedia Atlas of Surgery; Colorectal Surgery Volume. Chicago, IL: American College of Surgeons, 2008:117–29.

29 Hand Assisted

Peter W. Marcello

 INDICATIONS/CONTRAINDICATIONS

Restorative proctocolectomy is the procedure of choice for patients with ulcerative colitis requiring surgical intervention who wish a restorative procedure. The procedure is also indicated in patients with familial adenomatous polyposis with extensive rectal polyp formation. Unless otherwise contraindicated a laparoscopic approach is the preferred approach. Whether the procedure is performed by laparoscopy or by a hand-assisted approach is based upon the individual surgeon's experience. In the author's experience, hand-assisted approach has been associated with a reduction in operative time and conversions as compared to the laparoscopic technique, and therefore is the author's preferred approach. There are rare contraindications as follow:

- Extensive adhesion formation from prior surgery
- Inability to tolerate pneumoperitoneum

 PREOPERATIVE PLANNING

There are no specific preoperative needs for a laparoscopic or a hand-assisted approach as compared to conventional open surgery. Appropriate preoperative antibiotics, heparin administration, and marking of a site for temporary fecal diversion should be planned.

 SURGERY

Positioning

The patient is placed in a modified lithotomy position on a spilt-leg electric table.

- The arms are at the sides surrounded by a beanbag.
- Three-inch silk tape wrapped around the patient and beanbag to the table.

Figure 29.1

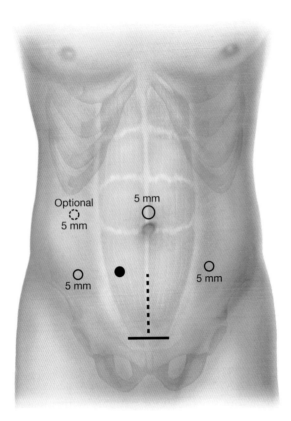

Technique

The operation begins with partial creation of the ileostomy (Fig. 29.1).

■ A core of skin and subcutaneous tissue is removed.
■ The anterior rectus sheath is incised vertically.

This maneuver is done to prevent the development of an obstruction of the loop ileostomy by the anterior rectus sheath following closure of the fascia in the Pfannenstiel incision. When a Pfannenstiel incision is created, the anterior rectus sheath is dissected from the rectus muscle and will be folded upward. If the ileostomy is made after the Pfannenstiel incision is created, it can act as a "shutter valve" when the fascia is closed, and may cause an obstruction at the ileostomy. This step is only done in cases where a temporary loop ileostomy is planned.

An 8-cm Pfannenstiel incision is made two fingerbreadths above the pubic symphysis.

■ The anterior rectus sheath is transversely incised and superior and inferior flaps are created over the rectus muscles.
■ The peritoneum is vertically opened between the rectus muscles.
■ The sleeve for the hand device is placed.
■ Five-millimeter trocars are positioned in the left lateral, supra umbilical, and right lateral positions. The right lateral trocar is placed lateral to and above the ileostomy site. Trocars are placed with the hand inside the abdomen to protect the intestine from injury (Fig. 29.1).

Right Colectomy—Medial Approach

The surgeon stands at the patient's left side with the left hand through the hand port and the right hand with a laparoscopic instrument (Fig. 29.2). The assistant stands cephalad to the surgeon, holding the camera. The patient is in slight Trendelenburg position with the right side up.

Figure 29.2

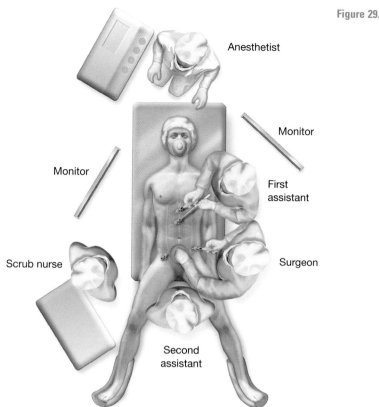

Anesthetist

Monitor

Monitor

First
assistant

Scrub nurse

Surgeon

Second
assistant

- An exploration is undertaken. The colon is examined to determine the extent and the severity of disease. The small bowel is examined to exclude Crohn's disease.
- The cecum and the terminal ileum are elevated and laterally retracted with the hand.
- A medial to lateral dissection of the right and traverse mesocolon is performed. An incision is made under the ileocolic pedicle and the duodenum is swept downward (Fig. 29.3). The ileocolic pedicle is then isolated. The fingers are quite useful for isolating the pedicles. The ileocolic vessels are then divided and ligated using a bipolar vessel sealing device (Fig. 29.4). The 5-mm bipolar sealing device is the author's preferred method of vessel ligation and division. Multiple applications of the device are used before the pedicle is divided. Although somewhat controversial, the ileocolic vessels are divided when performing a proctocolectomy and ileoanal pouch construction.

Figure 29.3

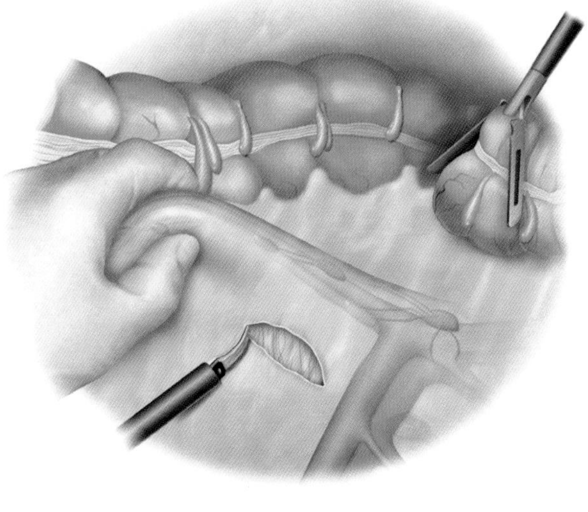

Figure 29.4

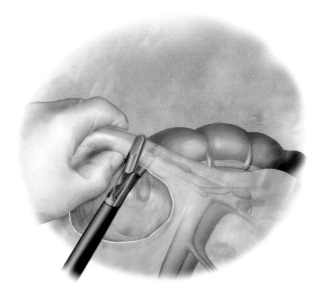

- The right-sided colon is mobilized from medial to lateral (Fig. 29.5). The colon mesentery is freed from the retroperitoneum and duodenum. A hand is used to create traction while the scissors are used to perform the dissection.
- If present, the right colic vessels are isolated and divided.

Transverse Colectomy—Medial Approach

Attention is then shifted to the transverse mesocolon. The assistant moves from the patient's left side to stand between the legs. The assistant's left hand elevates the transverse mesocolon and a laparoscopic instrument is placed through the right lateral port. The assistant's right hand controls the camera through the supra umbilical port. The surgeon remains on the patient's left side with the left hand through the hand device and the right hand with a laparoscopic instrument. The assistant elevates the transverse mesocolon with a grasper in the left hand through the right-sided trocar, while the surgeon isolates each of the individual middle colic vessels. The dissection generally begins to the left of the midline in the transverse mesocolon (Fig. 29.6). This plane often has fewer adhesions into the lesser sac. The lesser sac is entered and the distal transverse mesocolon sharply divided.

Working back toward the patient's right side, the main trunk middle colic vessel is isolated and divided (Figs. 29.7 and 29.8). The middle colic vessels may sometimes be ligated together or individually. Excessive tension on the vessels should be avoided

Figure 29.5

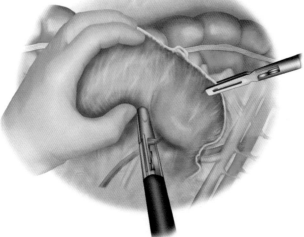

Figure 29.6

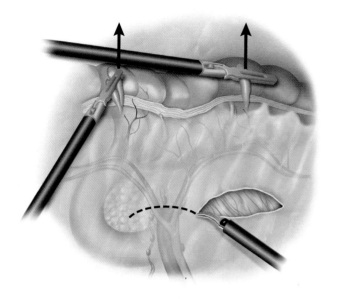

Figure 29.7

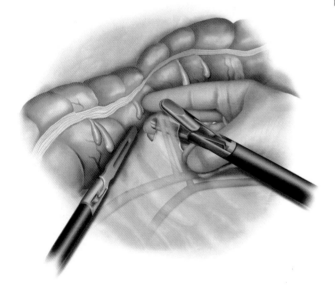

Figure 29.8

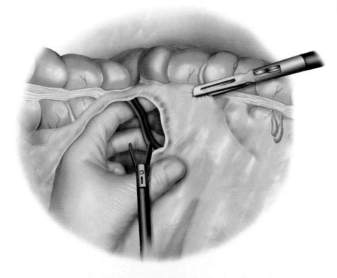

Figure 29.9

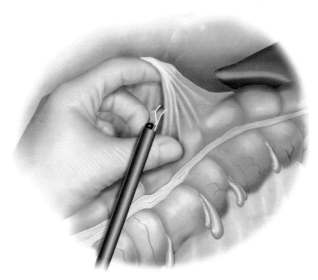

when using a bipolar vessel-sealing device. The entire proximal and mid-transverse mesocolon is thus fully divided.

Right and Transverse Colectomy—Lateral Approach

The terminal ileum and right colon are laterally mobilized. This portion begins by a laparoscopic technique.

- Scissors are placed directly through the hand device, and a grasper through the left lateral trocar. The cecum and terminal ileum are mobilized.
- The hand is then used to help mobilize the terminal ileal mesentery up to and then over the duodenum to the pancreas and superior mesenteric vessels. This lengthening maneuver is critical when performing ileoanal pouch construction.
- The remaining lateral attachments are divided with the assistant using the hook cautery through the right lateral trocar, and the surgeon remaining in the same position with the left hand in and the right hand with a laparoscopic grasper.
- The bipolar vessel sealer may also be used to help separate the omentum and control any minor bleeding (Figs. 29.9 and 29.10). With the right and transverse colon mobilized

Figure 29.10

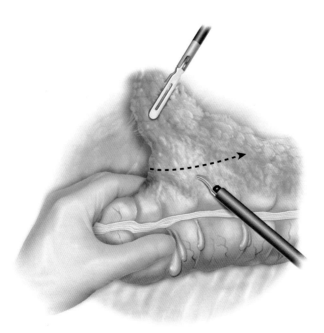

Figure 29.11

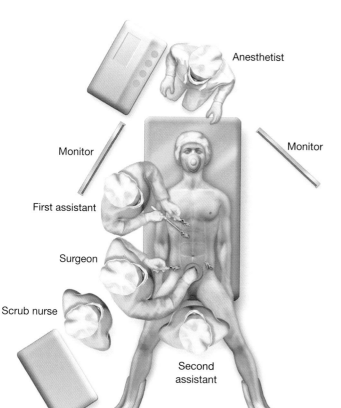

Anesthetist

Monitor

Monitor

First assistant

Surgeon

Scrub nurse

Second
assistant

and devascularized, it is placed back into anatomical position before turning to the
left colectomy.

Left Colectomy

The surgeon stands at the patients' right side with the right hand through the hand
device and the left hand with an instrument through the right lateral trocar site. The
assistant stands cephalad to the surgeon, holding the camera (Fig. 29.11). The patient
is in a mild Trendelenburg and left-side up position. The small bowel is packed out of
the pelvis to the right upper quadrant with a sponge.

■ The right hand elevates the internal mammary artery (IMA) pedicle and an incision
  is made along the right peritoneal fold of the rectosigmoid mesentery extending into
  the pelvis (Fig. 29.12). The plane beneath the inferior mesenteric pedicle is a developed heading to the left side. Care is taken to sweep down the sympathetic nerve
  fibers of the hypogastric nerves (Fig. 29.13). A plane is developed over the left ureter
  and left ovarian vessels, and the IMA pedicle is isolated and divided below the takeoff of the left colic vessels (Fig. 29.14).
■ The left-sided colon is then mobilized from medial to lateral in a plane overlying
  Gerota's fascia (Fig. 29.15). This dissection will continue to the left pelvic sidewall,
  inferiorly, into the upper retrorectal space, and superiorly, under the mesentery toward
  the splenic flexure.
■ The left colon mesentery is divided medially and the left colic vessels are isolated
  and divided. The medial dissection continues to the lateral sidewall where the line
  of Toldt can be divided.
■ The lateral attachments may now be divided. The white line of Toldt is divided
  through the left lateral trocar (Fig. 29.16).

Figure 29.12

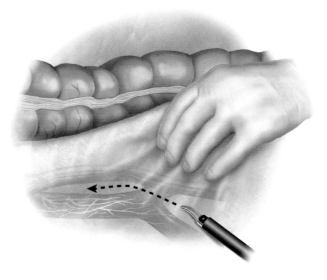

Figure 29.13

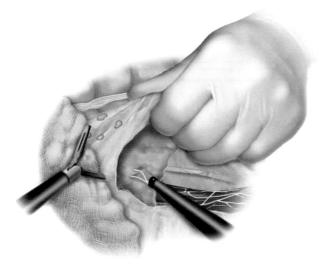

Figure 29.14

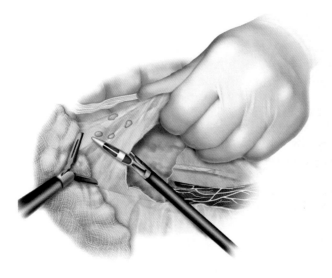

Figure 29.15

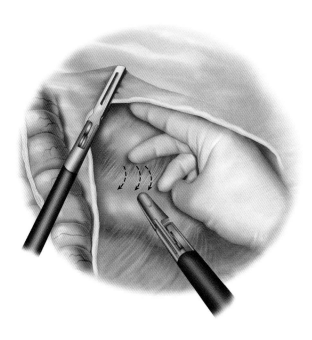

- The splenic flexure and remaining transverse mesocolon are divided. The assistant stands between the legs, holding the camera with their left hand and the hook cautery with their right hand (Fig. 29.17). This approach is similar to that used to separate the omentum from the proximal transverse colon (Figs. 29.18 and 29.19).
- With the omentum separated, the remaining portion of the distal transverse mesocolon is divided. Here, the assistant elevates the mesentery with a grasper, and the surgeon divides the mesentery with instruments, using the left hand.

With the entire mesocolon now divided, the retroperitoneum and major pedicles are examined with a sponge to ensure excellent hemostasis. The table is tilted into a Trendelenburg position with the right side up, allowing all of the small intestine to shift to the left upper quadrant. The colon is brought over the small intestine, beginning at the splenic flexure, to the right lower quadrant (Fig. 29.20). The terminal ileal mesentery can be followed up to, and then over the duodenum, with the entire small bowel to the left of the midline (Fig. 29.21). This step is critical to ensure proper orientation of the small-bowel mesentery for ileoanal pouch construction, and should be performed before moving on to the mobilization of the rectum.

Rectal Mobilization and Transection

The rectal mobilization can be done in a hand-assisted approach, a laparoscopic approach, or by an open technique through the Pfannenstiel incision depending on the

Figure 29.16

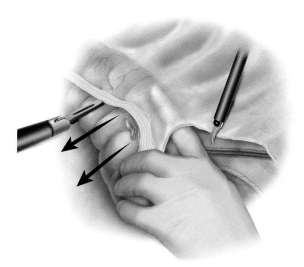

Figure 29.17

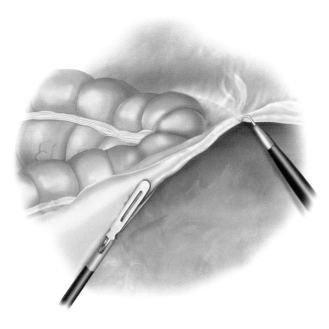

Figure 29.18

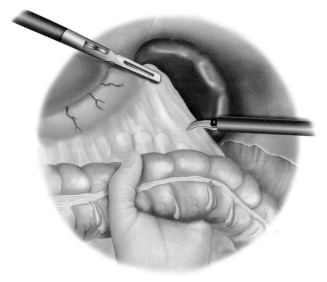

Figure 29.19

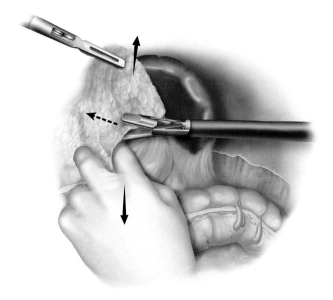

Figure 29.20

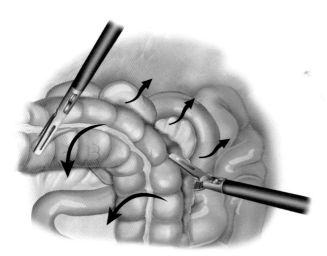

surgeon's preference, the surgeon's skill with laparoscopic proctectomy, and specific patient characteristics as it relates to the pelvic anatomy. Typically, the right hand can elevate the rectum and posterior mobilization begun with sharp electrocautery dissection (Fig. 29.22). The surgeon's right hand elevates the rectum while the left hand uses a laparoscopic grasper to provide countertraction. The assistant, standing at the patient's left side, uses the hook cautery, through the left lateral port, and holds the camera with their right hand through the supraumbilical port (Fig. 29.23). Care is taken to remain medial to the hypogastric nerve complex.

The remainder of the pelvic dissection may now be done by a laparoscopic technique, a hand-assisted technique, or through the open Pfannenstiel incision. The colon and terminal ileum are delivered through the wound (Fig. 29.24). Through the open wound, one should follow the terminal ileal mesentery up to and over the duodenum, confirming proper orientation. The terminal ileal mesentery is divided between clamps and ligated. The terminal ileum is divided with a stapler, and tagged with a suture, so that it may be packed out of the pelvis. A moist lap is used to keep the small bowel out of the pelvis. The rectal dissection continues and is completed through the open would. A full circumferential mobilization of the rectum is undertaken down to the levator floor and upper anal canal. A 30-mm stapler is used on the lower rectum. In the female patient, the vaginal cuff is visualized anteriorly. A finger is placed within the anal canal to confirm that the staple line is ~1 cm above the dentate line, and a finger is placed into the vagina to ensure that there is no entrapment before the stapler is fired.

Figure 29.21

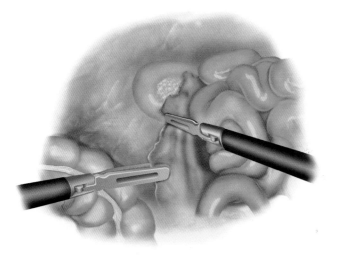

Figure 29.22

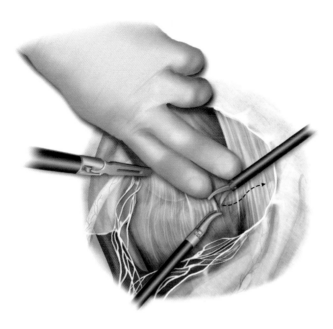

Ileoanal Pouch Construction, Anastomosis, and Abdominal Closure

The small bowel is brought back through the Pfannenstiel incision, and the ileoanal pouch is constructed through the open wound. Two to three firings of the 75-mm linear stapler are utilized. Once the orientation of the pouch is confirmed, the circular stapler is brought through the anus, the anvil is secured, and the stapler is closed. Following the anastomosis, an air leak test is performed.

The ileostomy aperture is completed by splitting the rectus muscle, and opening the posterior rectus sheath and peritoneum. The site for the ileostomy is marked on the bowel edge with chromic and polydioxanone (PDS) sutures to ensure proper orientation of the ileostomy. In the female, the peritoneum adjacent to the fallopian tube is sutured to the lateral side wall. This "oophoropexy" is performed in an attempt to prevent the development of a peritoneal inclusion cyst.

The peritoneum of the Pfannenstiel incision is vertically closed. The rectus muscle is reapproximated loosely with interrupted sutures. The anterior rectus sheath is closed transversely, and the incisions are closed with absorbable suture. Ultimately, the wounds are covered and the ileostomy is primarily matured.

Figure 29.23

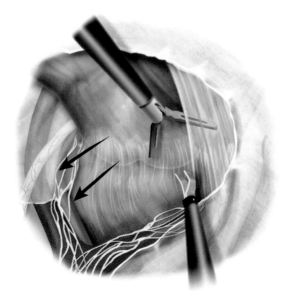

Figure 29.24

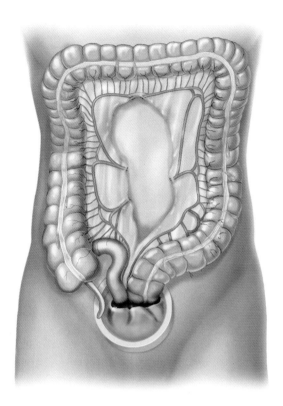

 POSTOPERATIVE MANAGEMENT

The patient is placed on a standardized accelerated postoperative care plan. Diet is slowly advanced, the patient is transitioned to oral analgesics, and the Foley catheter is removed on postoperative days 2–4 depending on the procedural details and postoperative recovery. Appropriate education of ileostomy care is initiated before, during, and after hospitalization. A water-soluble enema and flexible endoscopy is performed 6 weeks postoperatively and plans are made for ileostomy closure ~8 weeks following the original procedure.

 COMPLICATIONS

Numerous complications can occur following restorative proctocolectomy whether performed laparoscopically, by hand-assisted method, or by laparotomy. The only complication that is unique to a hand-assisted technique compared to conventional open surgery or laparoscopic pouch surgery is the risk of small-bowel obstruction at the level of the ileostomy as described above. Creation of the ileostomy aperture through the anterior rectus sheath before creation of the Pfannenstiel incision has greatly reduced the risk of this complication.

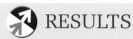 RESULTS

Extensive colorectal resections and reconstructions, including total abdominal colectomy and total proctocolectomy with ileal pouch-anal anastomosis (IPAA), are undoubtedly among the most technically challenging operations to perform laparoscopically. Hand-assisted techniques prove to be particularly relevant in allowing the adoption of minimally invasive total colorectal resections by a wider group of surgeons.

Rivadeneira and colleagues reported 23 prospectively collected cases of restorative proctocolectomy performed using hand-assisted technique or laparoscopy. The authors found that HALS was associated with shorter operative times (247 vs. 300 min, P <0.01), but with otherwise comparable postoperative variables. A similar retrospective review of 23 patients by Nakajima et al. reported comparable results, including a shorter operative time of 63 minutes favoring the HALS group. Both case series represent early experiences with HALS total colorectal resections, and, as such, were likely underpowered.

Boushey and colleagues have published the largest such prospective database series to date, in which they compared two groups of patients undergoing HALS (n = 45) or laparoscopic (n = 85), total abdominal colectomy, and total proctocolectomy. Again, the authors found a trend toward reduced operative times, in addition to significantly decreased conversion rates favoring the HALS group (2.2% vs. 7.1%, $P < 0.01$). As with segmental resections, this group also demonstrated that non-laparoscopic colorectal staff surgeons performed a much larger proportion of cases using the hand-assisted technique compared to a laparoscopic procedure (20% vs. 4.7%, $P = 0.02$).

As part of their multicenter RCT comparing HALS to straight laparoscopy, Marcello and colleagues published data pertaining to total colectomies and total proctocolectomies. Although reporting on a small number of patients (n = 29), this portion of the trial did demonstrate a significant decrease in skin-to-skin operative time associated with HALS of almost 1.5 hours (199 vs. 285 min, $P = 0.015$). This difference was also evident when the time to colectomy completion was analyzed (127 vs. 184, $p = 0.015$). Despite this significant time saving, this group did not found any significant difference between the two groups in terms of postoperative recovery.

CONCLUSIONS

Hand-assisted laparoscopic restorative proctocolectomy is the author's procedure of choice for patients requiring proctocolectomy who wish a restorative operation. The procedure as described earlier combines the advantages of laparoscopy while allowing the critical portions of the operation to be performed through the Pfannenstiel incision. For surgeons skilled in both laparoscopic segmental colectomy and open restorative proctocolectomy this approach allows for reduction in operative time and a low rate of conversion while maintaining minimally invasive benefits to the patient.

Suggested Readings

Boushey R, Marcello PW, Martel G, et al. Laparoscopic total colectomy: an evolutionary experience. *Dis Colon Rectum* 2007;50:1512–19.

Marcello PW, Fleshman JW, Milsom JW, et al. Hand assisted laparoscopic versus laparoscopic colorectal surgery: a multicenter, prospective, randomized trial. *Dis Colon Rectum* 2008;51:818–28.

Martel G, Boushey RP, Marcello PW. Hand-assisted laparoscopic colorectal surgery: an evidence-based review. *Minerva Chir* 2008; 63:373–83.

Milsom J, Bohm B, Nakajima K, eds. *Laparoscopic Colorectal Surgery*. 2nd ed. New York: Springer-Verlag, 2006.

Nakajima K, Lee SW, Cocilovo C, et al. Laparoscopic total colectomy: hand-assisted vs standard technique. *Surg Endosc* 2004; 18:582–86.

Rivadeneira DE, Marcello PW, Roberts PL, et al. Benefits of hand-assisted laparoscopic restorative proctocolectomy: a comparative study. *Dis Colon Rectum* 2004;47:1371–76.

30 Pouch Configurations

R. John Nicholls and Paris P. Tekkis

Introduction

The only reason for restorative proctocolectomy (ileal pouch-anal anastomosis [IPAA]) is to avoid a permanent ileostomy. A conventional proctocolectomy gives otherwise excellent results. Where there is no medical objection, the choice lies between a restorative and a conventional proctocolectomy and is almost entirely the patient's wish to make. This decision is possible only if the disadvantages are fully discussed. These include failure and complication rates, total treatment time, the possibility of pouchitis, and the likely functional outcome. A pouch support nurse, stomatherapist, and patient-support group can offer valuable advice, but in the end the patient must decide.

HISTORICAL BACKGROUND

The configuration of the pouch or reservoir is only part of the operation of restorative proctocolectomy. When the operation was first reported by Parks, a three-loop form of reservoir was used. This S-pouch was connected to the anal canal after a mucosectomy by an anastomosis between a point just above the dentate line and a segment of the terminal ileum projecting from the reservoir a few centimeters long. Parks said at the time that his main aim was to avoid incontinence and to do so he favored this form of reconstruction. Although this goal was achieved as reported in the first few publications (1–3), the price paid was failure of spontaneous evacuation in at least half of the patients having the procedure. This problem was radiologically shown (4) to be due to the distal ileal segment, which acted as an impedance to outflow. The two-loop reservoir described by Utsunomiya (5) did not have this feature, it being directly joined to the anal canal without any intervening ileum. Evacuation was spontaneous in almost all patients.

For this reason and also for its ease of construction by linear stapling the two-loop or "J" reservoir has become the most widely used reconstruction. Other configurations have included the "H" reservoir described by Fonkalsrud (6), the Kock, "K" design used with ileoanal anastomosis (IAA), and a four-loop reservoir, the "W" (7) (Fig. 30.1). The last was developed with the intention of achieving lower frequency of defecation, which followed the J reservoir since it was more capacious with an inverse relationship between frequency and capacitance having been demonstrated for straight ileoanal (8), ileal pouch-anal (9), and colonic pouch-anal (10,11) reconstructions.

Figure 30.1 Various pouch designs.

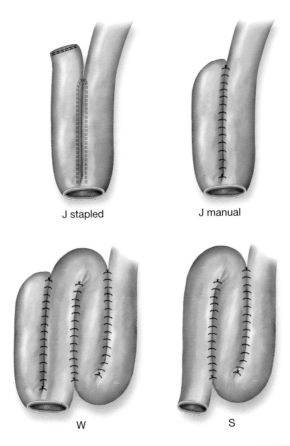

J stapled   J manual

W   S

INDICATIONS

The general indications for restorative proctocolectomy have been dealt with elsewhere. In considering the specific indication for using a reservoir as opposed to a straight segment of small intestine, there has never been a trial in adult patients comparing no reservoir (straight ileoanal) with a reservoir reconstruction. One of the few pieces of evidence for lower frequency with the latter comes from a nonrandomized comparison by Martin et al. in which 16 patients having a straight ileoanal reconstruction had a frequency of 8 defecations per 24 hours compared with 4 per 24 hours in 14 patients having an ileal reservoir (12). Other evidence comes from physiological studies of patients who have had either a straight or a pouch reconstruction (13) and from patients who have shown an inverse relationship between frequency of defecation and capacitance of the reservoir measured by balloon volumetry (8–10).

There are no particular indications other than the surgeon's preference in choosing which pouch should be used other than the "S" reservoir, which with its evacuation difficulty has almost died out. In current practice, therefore, the J pouch predominates, with a much smaller proportion of patients having a W pouch. The latter is still used in some units, however, and in recent years it may have increased its use following some evidence that long-term function is better (Table 30.2). The length of small intestine used for each is similar and the mobility of the mesentery that determines whether or not there will be some tension on the anastomosis is also similar for both "J" and "W" reservoirs.

PREOPERATIVE PLANNING

As long as an ileoanal anastomosis is possible, there is no particular preoperative planning required for the reservoir. The choice of configuration is unaffected by general factors such as the patient's condition or medication requirements. There are no local anatomical or pathological factors, which would lead to one or other type being preferred. Thus, the width of the pelvis, mobility of the mesentery, the state of the anal sphincter, and the extensiveness of any adhesions do not influence the choice of reservoir.

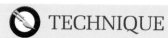 TECHNIQUE

The technique forms only a part of restorative proctocolectomy (IPAA), which has been described in detail in the foregoing sections. Briefly, it involves removal of the colon and the rectum using either an open or laparoscopic technique followed by the construction of an ileal reservoir, which is then joined to the anal canal by an IAA. The IAA can be carried out using a manual or stapled technique.

General Points

The following precautions should be observed:

- Antibiotics—Single-dose perioperative antibiotic cover should be used, but if the duration of operation exceeds 3 hours, a second dose of antibiotic is advisable, particularly if the antibiotic has a short half-life. In immunosuppressed patients receiving drugs such as cyclosporin or biological sulfonamides may still have a role in protecting against *Pneumocystis carinii* pneumonia.
- Anti-embolism prophylaxis using subcutaneous heparin, pneumatic compression, and anti-embolism stockings for prophylaxis.
- Anesthesia—Blood (usually 4 units) should be crossmatched and available if necessary. If a central venous line is needed for total parenteral nutrition, this should be inserted at the end of the operation. If the operation is carried out by an open technique, the abdominal wound will be an important cause of pain and an epidural anesthetic should be given.
- Positioning—The reversed Trendelenburg position with the legs raised (Lloyd-Davies) should be used, thereby allowing access to the anus, and the tip of the coccyx should lie over the end of the operating table to gain adequate exposure of the perineum. Whether an open or laparoscopic technique is used, this position gives excellent access to the abdomen and suitable deployment of surgeon and assistants around the patient.
- The bladder is routinely catheterized. It is helpful to insert a proctoscope before starting to drain the bowel of as much liquid feces and flatus as possible.

Surgical Technique

General Considerations of Pouch Construction

There are three principles that should be observed in constructing a reservoir:

- Minimal tension in the mesentery
- Adequate capacitance of the pouch
- Absence of distal ileal segment

To minimize tension, as full a mobilization of the mesentery as possible combined with division of selected mesenteric vessels if necessary should be performed combined with a trial descent. To achieve adequate capacity a minimum length of small bowel of 40 cm is required. Using the apex of a folded pair of loops as the point for the enterostomy to form the IAA will avoid any distal ileal segment.

Mobilization of the Mesentery

Once the colon and the rectum have been removed, an assessment of the mobility of the small bowel to descend to the pelvis is made by holding the apex of a loop of terminal ileum intended to form part of the IAA down into the pelvis. This most mobile point is around 15 cm from the ileocecal junction. If there is no evidence of tension,

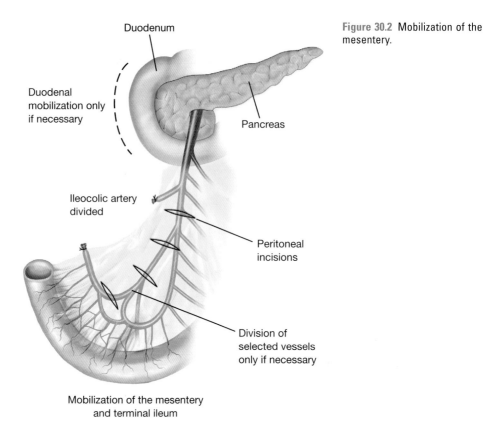

Duodenum

Duodenal
mobilization only
if necessary

Pancreas

Ileocolic artery
divided

Peritoneal
incisions

Division of
selected vessels
only if necessary

Mobilization of the mesentery
and terminal ileum

Figure 30.2 Mobilization of the mesentery.

no further mobilization of the mesentery is carried out. If, however, there is some tension, then further mobilization of the mesentery is required. This goal is achieved in three ways (Fig. 30.2):

- Mobilize the mesentery
- Perform transverse incisions of the peritoneum
- Divide selected vessels if necessary

It may be necessary to mobilize the duodenum using Kocher's maneuver. The uncinate process of the pancreas can be freed from the origin of the superior mesenteric artery and vein if necessary. Care should be taken to avoid damage to the superior mesenteric vein or its major tributaries. Usually, however, this step is not required. Four or five small transverse cuts made in the peritoneum on each side of the mesentery result in lengthening by 1 or 2 cm.

If, despite these maneuvers, there is still tension sufficient to restrict descent of the apex of the terminal ileal loop into the pelvis, then division of a selected restraining vessel in one of the vascular arcades will be necessary. This maneuver must be done with great care to avoid ischemia. The vessel restraining mobility is identified by putting gentle stretch on the mesentery and using transillumination it is then dissected from its connective tissue bed. A bulldog clamp is applied to the vessel and the end of the terminal ileum is inspected to see whether there is adequate perfusion. If vascularity is satisfactory, the vessel is then divided. This maneuver is rarely necessary if a stapled ileoanal anastomosis is used.

A trial descent of the small bowel testing its ability to descend to the level of the anal canal is recommended where the bowel has been divided to leave an open anal stump as would have been done in patients in whom a manual IAA with mucosectomy is intended. Where the anorectal stump has been closed by a transverse stapler in preparation for a stapled IAA this is not possible, but in this circumstance there is less tension on the mesentery as the IAA will be at a slightly higher level. The trial descent is undertaken by abdominal and perineal operators. A stay suture is placed on the apex of the

Stapled 'J ' Reservoir

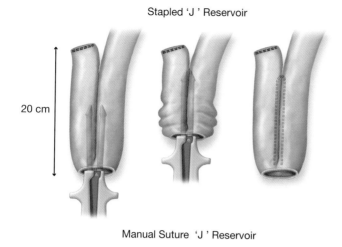

20 cm

Figure 30.3 Trial descent before making the pouch.

Manual Suture 'J ' Reservoir

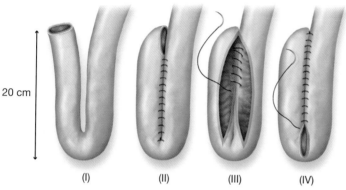

20 cm

(I)   (II)   (III)   (IV)

loop selected for the IAA and this is passed through the pelvis and anal canal to be taken by the perineal operator. Gentle traction is applied and the small bowel is drawn down to the anal canal. If it reaches the dentate line, it will do so after the pouch is formed. If it does not, then further mobilization is necessary as described earlier (Fig. 30.3).

The Pouch

In current practice, the "J" and, to a lesser extent, the "W" reservoirs are the most common types of pouches used and the technical description below will be confined to these types.

"J" Pouch

Once adequate mesenteric length is assured, the pouch is constructed by stapling or manual suture (Fig. 30.4). Most surgeons now use the former technique, but stapling may not be better since it leaves a short distal stump (the "dog ear"), which can fistulate. A "J" pouch should have a volume of at least 300 ml at the time of construction. A 20 × 20 cm loop achieves an intraoperative volume of more than 300 ml with a postoperative capacity of 380 ml.

Stapling

Three stay sutures are placed on the antimesenteric border of the ileum to ensure that the staple line is truly antimesenteric. The limbs of the pouch should each measure 20 cm in length. A transverse enterotomy not more than 3-cm long is made at the apex of the folded loops. The procedure is performed entirely through this enterotomy, concerning the limbs of the ileum over the stapler. A linear cutting stapler is introduced into the two loops of ileum and the limbs are advanced as far as possible. The stapler is closed and an inspection is made to ascertain that no mesenteric vessels are included in the shafts of the stapler. If not, the instrument is fired. A second stapler is introduced and advanced beyond the

Trial descent

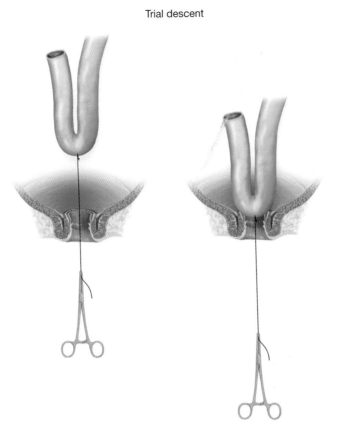

Figure 30.4 Construction of "J" pouch; stapled and manual techniques.

now open loops of ileum and closed and fired. The number of cartridges required will usually be two: a 90-mm or 100-mm stapler. The four for a 50-mm stapler and three for the 75-mm instruments; the aim should be to achieve a pouch of 17–20 cm limb length. The pouch may be everted through its mesentery to expose the posterior staple line to look for any defect and to assess hemostasis. The integrity and capacity of the pouch are tested by placing a noncrushing clamp over the afferent limb while injecting saline into the pouch through a catheter introduced through the apical enterotomy.

The terminal ileum will have been closed by a transverse stapler applied before constructing the pouch. This results in a "dog ear" at its most distal part, which is oversewn. Care should be taken to ensure that it is no more than 2 cm in length and is intact as fistulation can occur from leakage at this point.

Manual Suture

The two loops are approximated using a seromuscular continuous suture of absorbable material. The bowel is then opened and a full-thickness continuous suture is carried out from the posterior layer coming round to the anterior layer of the two loops. In this manner, the "dog ear" deformity is completely avoided since the anatomical end of the terminal ileum is incorporated end to side into the pouch. The suture is continued to the apex of the pouch and terminated at a point, which leaves the enterotomy for the IAA just able to take two fingers comfortably. If a stapled IAA is intended, however, the last few sutures up to this point should be interrupted to avoid unravelling of the continuous suture line, which might occur as it is cut by the knife of the circular stapler. It takes about 30 minutes to construct a sutured "J" pouch, but there is the advantage of maximizing volume by using all the bowel length for constructing the reservoir, avoiding the "dog ear" with its risk of fistulation and lowering the cost. It may, however, result in more contamination.

"W" Pouch

It is not practical to construct a four-loop pouch by stapling. The terminal 40 cm of the ileum is folded into four 10-cm loops. The proximal two limbs are offset from the distal two limbs by about 2 cm. The loops are united using a continuous absorbable suture. The bowel is then opened along the suture lines and a full-thickness suture is applied along the posterior layer of the pouch. As with the "J" construction, this is continued onto the anterior surface of the pouch finally to leave an aperture for the IAA, which comfortably takes two fingers.

Harms et al. (14) suggested that it is better to construct the W pouch with a slightly longer distal loop so that it fits more comfortably into the pelvis for ileoanal anastomosis, rather than using four equal lengths of ileum. These authors suggest a configuration measuring 11, 13, 10, and 10 cm. Thus, the distal enterotomy forms an apex, which is used for the ileoanal anastomosis. This detail is a modification of the description above. The integrity and capacity of the pouch should then be checked by distending it with saline as for the "J" pouch.

Ileoanal Anastomosis

In the description of pouch construction, the technique of the IAA requires some mention. This is relevant to the degree of mobilization of the mesentery required and also to the completeness of removal of the disease whether ulcerative colitis (UC) or familial adenomatous polyposis (FAP). A manual anastomosis with mucosectomy is more distal but has the advantage of being accurately placed under direct vision. The disadvantage is increased tension in a few cases, but the advantage is that there is very little remaining disease. Although it is said that function after a manual IAA with mucosectomy is less satisfactory than after a stapled anastomosis, the studies in which they have been compared have not shown any difference. In the case of a stapled IAA, although there is the advantage of less liability to tension owing to a more proximal IAA, there is the danger of making it too proximal such that a length of inflamed rectal mucosa is left in the patient. This may not matter in most cases but in some with severe inflammation and ulceration, function after closure of the ileostomy may be poor with anal burning, urgency, and blood due to the presence of the inflamed mucosa itself and the frequent passage of small-volume stool due to incomplete emptying of the pouch owing to the presence of the distal anorectal stump. A stapled IAA must therefore be sufficiently distal to avoid this complication. The relative merits of stapled and manual IAA have been reviewed in a large meta-analysis (15).

Stapled IAA

For the stapled anastomosis of a stapled "J" Pouch to the anorectal stump, a purse-string suture is placed in the distal opening of the pouch and the anvil of the circular stapler (CEEA 28 or 29 mm) is inserted into the pouch and the suture tied. The stapler is inserted into the anus and the anastomosis performed firing it in the normal way.

For the stapled anastomosis of a hand-sutured "J" pouch the technique differs in one important respect as described earlier. The last few sutures of the anterior wall of the pouch are placed in an interrupted manner to prevent cutting and unravelling of the continuous suture. Otherwise, the insertion of the purse-string suture and firing of the instrument are identical.

Manual IAA

A manual IAA requires a mucosectomy, which is undertaken through the anus after division of the bowel. If the anorectal stump is short, the entire residual mucosa is very accessible to endo-anal removal, which is effected by scissor excision facilitated by submucosal injection of saline solution containing adrenaline (1:300,000). The pouch is then brought down to the anal level by traction of two sutures (2.0 Vicryl on a 26-mm taper-cut needle—W9350, Johnson & Johnson), which have already been placed at the right and left edges of the enterotomy. The needles are not removed and having drawn the sutures through the anus, each suture is placed in turn into the anal canal at the level of the mucosectomy in the 3 and 9 o'clock position. Having placed these initial sutures the remaining sutures (12 in all; one for each hour of the clock) are inserted.

COMPLICATIONS

Morbidity occurs in 20–40% of patients. It is difficult to separate those complications due to the reservoir itself and others with the exception of fistulation directly from the reservoir as can occur in a stapled "J" pouch developing leakage from the "dog ear" stapled line at the point of distal division of the ileum. They may be divided into early and late and can be classified into those general to any surgery and those specific to restorative proctocolectomy. Any patient undergoing major surgery is at risk of developing general complications such as infections of the chest, wound and urinary track, thromboembolic disease, and hemorrhage.

The commonest complications specific to major restorative surgery and restorative proctocolectomy in particular include the following:

- Sepsis
- Poor function
- Pouchitis
- Neoplastic transformation

Failure defined by the need for a permanent or indefinite ileostomy, progressively occurs with time, being ~10% at 10 years rising to 15% or more at 20 years (16) although Hahnloser et al. (17) reported a lower rate of 6% at 20 years for patients who had not failed due to Crohn's disease. Failure is due to sepsis in 50%, poor function in 30%, and pouchitis in 10% (18). There is no evidence that failure is related to the type of pouch.

The most important complication is pelvic sepsis usually due to a degree of breakdown of the IAA in the early postoperative period. If the clinical presentation is delayed, the patient may develop fistulation into the vagina or the perineum. Such late fistulation can present months to years after the primary restorative proctocolectomy. The occurrence of pelvic sepsis is not related to the type of reservoir. When manual and stapled IAAs have been compared, there is no difference in this complication. There is no difference in the propensity of any reservoir design to pouchitis.

RESULTS

The results following different reservoir designs are essentially those relating to function. Reservoir configurations have been developed to improve frequency of defecation as the main aim. Set against this is the need to simplify the method of construction as far as possible.

Various authors have critically reviewed the results and reported a low incidence of complications, bowel frequency of 4–7 movements in 24 hours and no emptying problems (19–21). Stool frequency falls considerably in the first 12 months after ileostomy closure. Likewise, the volume of the J pouch increases with time, reaching a maximum by 2 years (3,22,23). Pouch volume is directly related to the length of ileum used for pouch construction. Volume is not, however, the only predictor of outcome: small-bowel motility, bacterial overgrowth, anal function, pouch evacuation, and villous atrophy index are also important determinants of outcome (24,25). Nevertheless, most data suggest that a large capacity and compliant pouch are probably the most important variables in achieving low bowel frequency, provided anal sphincter function is preserved (22,26–28).

The shape of the J pouch more closely resembles the normal rectum than the S or W pouches. None of the large clinical series indicate that catheterization is necessary (29,30) although frequency of defecation with the 15 × 15 cm J pouch, and particularly with the 10 × 10 cm J pouch, does seem to be greater than with the S pouch (9,26). There is, however, tremendous variation in the frequency of defecation from day to day, which is influenced a great deal by dietary intake. Furthermore, there is a long period of ileal adaptation after J-pouch construction and frequency of defecation falls substantially with time. Soiling, nocturnal defecation, discrimination, and deferment of defecation also improve. Consequently, Oresland et al. (31) showed that there was a

Part VI: Restorative Proctocolectomy

progressive improvement in the functional score over a period of at least 2 years. On account of the simple design, ease of stapling and evidence that the J pouch is from the more spherical W pouch most surgeons use the J-pouch design.

However, there is evidence that in the long term, function following "J" and "W" configurations may be different (see below for meta-analysis). Setti Carraro et al. (32) reported night evacuation in 50% of 24 patients with a "J" pouch followed for a minimum of 5 years compared with 20% of 31 patients with a "W" reservoir. The proportions of patients not having any night evacuation were 29% and 68%, respectively. In a recent article reporting 30 patients with a "J" and 19 with a "W" reconstruction, Wade et al. (33) found a significant lower frequency in the "W" group (6 vs. 4.5/24 hr) but other parameters of function and quality of life were no different. Although the "J" design is the most used owing to its ease of fashioning, some surgeons may use the "W" design owing to the chance of better function.

A meta-analysis performed identified eight comparative studies published between 1988 and 2000, of "J" pouch versus "W" pouch (34). There were four prospective randomized controlled trials (26,35–37), one prospective nonrandomized study (9), and three retrospective comparative studies (38–40). A total of 995 patients were included for analysis, comprising 689 J pouches and 306 W pouches. The characteristics of the eight included studies are summarized in Tables 30.1 and 30.2. There was no significant difference in postoperative complications between the groups. Data on function were available in 194 patients from six studies. The stool frequency was greater in the J pouch than in the "W" population, by one stool per 24 hours, $P = 0.01$ a difference which

TABLE 30.1	Adverse Outcomes by Reservoir Design			
Outcome	No. of patients	No. of studies	Odds ratio (95% CI)	*P*-value
Anastomotic leak				
J vs. W	106	3	1.04 (0.26–4.23)	0.96
S vs. W	179	3	1.70 (0.55–7.81)	0.36
S vs. J	286	5	1.21 (0.44–3.29)	0.71
Anastomotic stricture				
J vs. W	199	6	0.71 (0.24–2.06)	0.52
S vs. W	179	3	1.75 (0.64–4.83)	0.28
S vs. J	213	4	1.43 (0.50–4.05)	0.50
Wound infection				
J vs. W	199	6	0.81 (0.29–2.27)	0.68
S vs. W	179	3	1.06 (0.29–3.81)	0.93
S vs. J	158	3	1.23 (0.20–7.36)	0.82
Pelvic sepsis				
J vs. W	175	5	1.85 (0.71–4.80)	0.21
S vs. W	179	3	3.06 (0.97–9.70)	0.06
S vs. J	158	3	2.27 (0.75–6.93)	0.15
Small-bowel obstruction				
J vs. W	199	6	1.23 (0.48–3.12)	0.67
S vs. W	129	2	2.79 (0.81–9.54)	0.10
S vs. J	286	5	0.99 (0.34–2.94)	0.99
Pouchitis				
J vs. W	190	5	1.75 (0.39–7.85)	0.47
S vs. W	88	2	1.66 (0.50–5.49)	0.40
S vs. J	257	4	1.20 (0.36–4.07)	0.77
Pouch failure				
J vs. W	129	4	4.97 (0.80–30.90)	0.09
S vs. W	141	2	4.89 (0.26–90.20)	0.29
S vs. J	248	4	1.05 (0.36–3.12)	0.93

Source: Adapted from Lovegrove et al. *Colorectal Dis* 2007;9(4):310–20.
OR, odds ratio. Values <1 favor design 1; values >1 favor design 2.

TABLE 30.2	Functional Outcomes by Reservoir Design			
Outcome	No. of patients	No. of studies	OR/WMD (95% CI)	P-value
Stool frequency per 24 hr				
J vs. W	194	6	0.97 (0.20–1.74)	**0.01**
S vs. W	166	3	1.14 (−0.10–2.38)	0.07
S vs. J	433	6	−1.48 (−2.10−−0.85)	**<0.001**
Stool frequency (night)				
J vs. W	133	4	0.21 (−0.14–0.56)	0.25
S vs. W	128	3	0.13 (−0.06–0.32)	0.19
S vs. J	112	3	−0.06 (−0.28–0.15)	0.55
Seepage (daytime)				
J vs. W	129	3	2.42 (0.70–8.36)	0.16
S vs. W	88	2	3.01 (0.80–11.42)	0.10
S vs. J	148	4	0.83 (0.34–2.07)	0.69
Seepage (night)				
J vs. W	83	2	1.56 (0.46–5.30)	0.47
S vs. W	50	1	2.67 (0.60–11.76)	0.20
S vs. J	110	3	0.60 (0.16–2.20)	0.44
Daytime pad usage				
J vs. W	204	5	3.72 (1.24–11.17)	**0.02**
S vs. W	76	1	3.90 (0.81–18.71)	0.09
S vs. J	127	3	1.59 (0.59–4.30)	0.36
Nocturnal pad usage				
J vs. W	30	1	3.21 (0.12–85.20)	0.49
S vs. J	57	2	0.81 (0.26–2.56)	0.72
Urgency				
J vs. W	358	7	1.35 (0.47–3.92)	0.58
S vs. W	167	3	2.63 (0.47–14.74)	0.27
S vs. J	360	5	0.59 (0.23–1.54)	0.28
Incontinence				
J vs. W	387	7	2.31 (0.34–15.72)	0.39
S vs. W	217	4	1.02 (0.26–3.97)	0.98
S vs. J	338	4	0.95 (0.29–3.14)	0.93
Antidiarrheal medication				
J vs. W	354	6	3.55 (2.04–6.20)	**<0.001**
S vs. W	207	4	0.87 (0.29–2.65)	0.81
S vs. J	487	8	0.36 (0.16–0.81)	**0.01**
Pouch intubation				
J vs. W	300	4	0.06 (0.01–0.33)	**0.001**
S vs. W	207	4	4.23 (0.22–81.63)	0.34
S vs. J	316	5	6.19 (1.12–34.07)	**0.04**

Source: Adapted from Lovegrove et al. *Colorectal Dis* 2007;9(4):310–20.
OR, odds ratio. Values <1 favor design 1; values >1 favor design 2.
WMD, weighted mean difference. Negative values favor design 1; positive values favor design 2.
P-values in bold are of statistical significance.

reflected in a 3.55-fold increase in the likelihood of the need for antidiarrheal medication in the "J" compared with the "W" pouch group (*P* < 0.001).

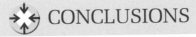 CONCLUSIONS

A reservoir is used in restorative proctocolectomy to achieve better function than follows a straight ileoanal reconstruction. The configuration used should be simple to construct with adequate capacitance and emptying characteristics. The "J" design is the most used in practice followed by the "W." There is little difference between them other than lower frequency of defecation per 24 hours and at night and less antidiarrheal medication requirement with the latter. This is offset by the greater ease of construction of the former. There is little place in current practice for the "S" and "H" designs. The "J" reservoir can be constructed by manual suture or stapling with advantages for manual suture in avoiding a "dog ear" segment, which can be a source of fistulation. Adequate mobilization of the mesentery is essential in all types of reconstructions.

Recommended References and Readings

1. Parks A, Nicholls RJ. Proctocolectomy without ileostomy for ulcerative colitis. *Br Med J* 1978;2:85–88.
2. Parks AG, Nicholls RJ, Belliveau P. Proctocolectomy with ileal reservoir and anal anastomosis. *Br J Surg* 1980;67(8):533–38.
3. Nicholls J, Pescatori M, Motson RW, Pezim ME. Restorative proctocolectomy with a three-loop ileal reservoir for ulcerative colitis and familial adenomatous polyposis. Clinical results in 66 patients followed for up to 6 years. *Ann Surg* 1984;199(4):383–88.
4. Pescatori M, Manhire A, Bartram CI. Evacuation pouchography in the evaluation of ileoanal reservoir function. *Dis Colon Rectum* 1983;26(6):365–68.
5. Utsunomiya J, Iwama T, Imago M, et al. Total colectomy, mucosal proctectomy and ileo-anal anastomosis. *Dis Colon Rectum* 1980; 23:459–66.
6. Fonkalsrud E. Endorectal ileal pullthrough with lateral ileal reservoir for benign colorectal disease. *Ann Surg* 1981;194:761–66.
7. Nicholls RJ, Lubowski DZ. Restorative proctocolectomy: the four loop W reservoir. *Br J Surg* 1987;74:564–66.
8. Heppel J, Kelly KA, Phillips SF, et al. Physiologic aspects of continence after colectomy, mucosal proctectomy and ileo-anal anastomosis. *Ann Surg* 1982;195:435–43.
9. Nicholls RJ, Pezim ME. Restorative proctocolectomy with ileal reservoir for ulcerative colitis and familial adenomatous polyposis: a comparison of three reservoir designs. *Br J Surg* 1985;72:470–74.
10. Lazorthes F, Fages P, Chiotasso P, et al. Resection of the rectum with construction of colonic reservoir and coloanal anastomosis for carcinoma of the rectum. *Br J Surg* 1986;73:136–38.
11. Parc R, Tiret E, Frileux P, Moszkowski E, Loygue J. Resection and colo-anal anastomosis with colonic reservoir for rectal carcinoma. *Br J Surg* 1986;73(2):139–41.
12. Martin L, Fischer JE. Preservation of anorectal continence following total colectomy. *Ann Surg* 1982;196:700–04.
13. Taylor BMC, Kelly B, Phillips KA, et al. A clinico-physiological comparison of ileal pouch-anal and straight ileoanal anastomoses. *Ann Surg* 1983;198(4):462–68.
14. Harms BAH, Yamamoto JW, Starling DT. Quadruple-loop (W) ileal pouch reconstruction after proctocolectomy: analysis and functional results. *Surgery* 1987;102(4):561–67.
15. Lovegrove RE, Constantinides VA, Heriot AG, et al. A comparison of hand-sewn versus stapled ileal pouch anal anastomosis (IPAA) following proctocolectomy: a meta-analysis of 4183 patients. *Ann Surg* 2006;244:18–26.
16. Tekkis PP LR, Tilney HS, Smith JJ, et al. Long-term failure and function after restorative proctocolectomy—A Multi-Centre Study of Patients from the UK National Ileal Pouch Registry. *Colorectal Dis* 2009 [Epub ahead of print].
17. Hahnloser D, Pemberton JH, Wolff BG, Larson DR, Crownhart BS, Dozois RR. Results at up to 20 years after ileal pouch-anal anastomosis for chronic ulcerative colitis. *Br J Surg* 2007;94:333–40.
18. Tulchinsky H, Hawley PR, Nicholls RJ. Long-term failure after restorative proctocolectomy for ulcerative colitis. *Ann Surg* 2003;238(2):229–34.
19. Taylor BM, Beart RW Jr, Dozois RR, et al. The endorectal ileal pouch-anal anastomosis. Current clinical results. *Dis Colon Rectum* 1984;27(6):347–50.
20. Cohen ZM, McLeod RS. Proctocolectomy and ileoanal anastomosis with J-shaped or S-shaped ileal pouch. *World J Surg* 1988; 12(2):164–68.
21. Fazio VW, Ziv Y, Church JM, et al. Ileal pouch-anal anastomoses complications and function in 1005 patients. *Ann Surg* 1995; 222(2):120–27.

22. Oresland T, Fasth S, Nordgren S, et al. Pouch size: the important functional determinant after restorative proctocolectomy. *Br J Surg* 1990;77(3):265–69.
23. Chaussade SM, Hautefeuille S, Valleur M, et al. Clinical and physiological study of anal sphincter and ileal J pouch before preileostomy closure and 6 and 12 months after closure of loop ileostomy. *Dig Dis Sci* 1991;36(2):161–67.
24. Stryker SJ, Kelly KA, Phillips SF, et al. Anal and neorectal function after ileal pouch-anal anastomosis. *Ann Surg* 1986;203(1): 55–61.
25. O'Connell PR, Pemberton JH, Brown ML, Kelly KA. Determinants of stool frequency after ileal pouch-anal anastomosis. *Am J Surg* 1987;153(2):157–64.
26. Nasmyth DG, Williams NS, Johnston D. Comparison of the function of triplicated and duplicated pelvic ileal reservoirs after mucosal proctectomy and ileo-anal anastomosis for ulcerative colitis and adenomatous polyposis. *Br J Surg* 1986;73(5):361–66.
27. Keighley MR, Yoshioka K, Kmiot W, Heyen F. Physiological parameters influencing function in restorative proctocolectomy and ileo-pouch-anal anastomosis. *Br J Surg* 1988;75(10):997–1002.
28. Lindquist K. Anal manometry with microtransducer technique before and after restorative proctocolectomy. Sphincter function and clinical correlations. *Dis Colon Rectum* 1990;33(2):91–97.
29. Metcalf AMD, Kelly RR, Beart KA, et al. Ileal "J" pouch-anal anastomosis. Clinical outcome. *Ann Surg* 1985;202(6):735–39.
30. Cohen Z, Smith D, McLeod R. Reconstructive surgery for pelvic pouches. *World J Surg* 1998;22:342–46.
31. Oresland T, Fasth S, Nordgren S, Hulten L. The clinical and functional outcome after restorative proctocolectomy. *Int J Colorectal Dis* 1989;4:50–56.
32. Setti Carraro P, Ritchie JK, Wilkinson K, Hawley PR, Nicholls RJ. The first 10 years experience of restorative proctocolectomy for ulcerative colitis. *Gut* 1994;35:1070–75.
33. Wade A, Mathiason MA, Brekke EF, Kothari SN. Quality of life after ileoanal pouch: a comparison of J and W pouches. *J Gastrointest Surg* 2009;13:1260–65.
34. Lovegrove R, Heriot AG, Constantinides V, et al. Meta-analysis of short-term and long-term outcomes of J, W and S ileal reservoirs for restorative proctocolectomy. *Colorectal Dis* 2007;9(4): 310–20.
35. de Silva HJ, de Angelis CP, Soper N, et al. Clinical and functional outcome after restorative proctocolectomy. *Br J Surg* 1991; 78(9):1039–44.
36. Keighley MR, Yoshioka K, Kmiot W. Prospective randomized trial to compare the stapled double lumen pouch and the sutured quadruple pouch for restorative proctocolectomy. *Br J Surg* 1988;75:1008–11.
37. Selvaggi F, Giuliani A, Gallo C, et al. Randomized, controlled trial to compare the J-pouch and W-pouch configurations for ulcerative colitis in the maturation period. *Dis Colon Rectum* 2000;43(5):615–20.
38. Hewett PJ, Stitz R, Hewett MK. Comparison of the functional results of restorative proctocolectomy for ulcerative colitis between the J and W configuration ileal pouches with sutured ileoanal anastomosis. *Dis Colon Rectum* 1995;38:567–72.
39. Neilly P, Neill ME, Hill GL. Restorative proctocolectomy with ileal pouch-anal anastomosis in 203 patients: the Auckland experience. *Aust N Z J Surg* 1999;69:22–27.
40. Romanos J, Samarasekera DN, Stebbing JF, Jewell DP, Kettlewell MG, Mortensen NJ. Outcome of 200 restorative proctocolectomy operations: the John Radcliffe Hospital experience. *Br J Surg* 1997;84:814–18.

31 # Open Abdominoperineal Resection

David A. Rothenberger and Genevieve B. Melton Meaux

 ## INDICATIONS/CONTRAINDICATIONS

Abdominoperineal resection (APR) is generally performed for patients who have a rectal adenocarcinoma but may also be performed for benign conditions such as inflammatory bowel diseases or incontinence and is sometimes appropriate for other low anorectal and pelvic malignancies or as a salvage procedure for anal canal cancers. The technique discussed in this chapter is intended to achieve radical clearance of anorectal malignancies; more conservative techniques of APR used for benign conditions are not discussed here in detail. Both open laparotomy and minimally invasive laparoscopic approaches are used for APR of rectal cancer. Some surgeons now use a hybrid laparoscopic approach to explore the abdomen, mobilize the left colon, and then convert to an open or hand-assisted procedure via a lower midline incision to complete the abdominal phase. A prospective trial is now being done by the American College of Surgeons Oncology Group to determine if laparoscopic technique for rectal cancer resection is a safe and effective alternative to the open technique. Other similar trials are underway in other countries. This chapter focuses on the operative technique used during an open approach for APR. The principles and techniques described here are applicable with minor modifications to extended operations for rectal cancer including *en bloc* sacrectomy, vaginectomy, or pelvic exenteration.

The decision to do an anterior resection (AR) and anastomosis versus an APR and permanent colostomy is dependent on oncologic considerations, technical considerations, the surgeon's skills and experience, anticipated functional outcomes, and patients' desires. Important oncologic and technical considerations include preoperative level of the lesion and in particular its relationship to the anal sphincters and levators, pretreatment stage of the cancer including any local organ invasion or distant spread, histology predictors of poor outcome, and threatened or involved margins and the tumor response to neoadjuvant therapy. In general, obesity and the narrow male pelvis add to the technical challenges encountered by the rectal cancer surgeon. Both open APR and open AR curative-intent radical resections for rectal cancer use the same total mesorectal excision (TME) technique to mobilize the rectum with its mesorectum and achieve proximal, lateral, and radial margin clearance. The choice of APR versus AR is primarily dependent on the surgeon's ability to achieve distal mural clearance of 2 cm and distal mesorectal clearance of 5 cm and to perform a reliable sphincter-sparing anastomosis that will preserve good anorectal function. In general, the more distal the anastomosis is located, the higher the risk of anastomotic complications and the less good the function. Pelvic irradiation generally increases the risk of anastomotic problems and worsens the functional outcome. While patients understandably may prefer a sphincter-sparing proctectomy to APR, they should be informed that sphincter preservation is not uniformly associated with better quality of life (1). It is generally counterproductive to compromise control of the cancer in a heroic attempt to avoid a permanent colostomy as recurrences often result and/or functional results are so poor that quality of life is unacceptable. The ultimate decision making with respect to selecting AR or APR may not be possible until intraoperative assessment and mobilization of the rectum is complete.

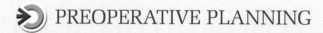

PREOPERATIVE PLANNING

Assessment and Staging

All patients with a newly diagnosed rectal cancer should undergo full clinical assessment, pretreatment staging of the primary cancer, as well as a search for metastases and synchronous colonic abnormalities. A full discussion of this topic is beyond the scope of this chapter. A history of pain with defecation may be indicative of involvement of the anal sphincters, whereas tenesmus may suggest a large or possibly fixed tumor. It is important to assess preoperative bowel function, including the presence of bowel incontinence as well as baseline sexual and urinary function. For distal rectal cancers, digital rectal examination can define tumor size, location from the anal verge, relationship to the anorectal ring, orientation within the anal canal (anterior, posterior, left, or right), and relative fixation (fixed, tethered, or mobile). Confirmation of these characteristics and biopsy for histologic confirmation of the diagnosis of rectal adenocarcinoma may be achieved by either flexible sigmoidoscopy or rigid proctoscopy. The latter is preferred by some surgeons as the most accurate method to assess precise distance and location of the lesion from the anal verge or dentate line. Complete colonoscopy is essential to exclude synchronous lesions or other colonic diseases. Pulmonary metastases are identified by chest x-ray or CT scan while hepatic metastases may be identified by abdominal CT scan. Carcinoembryonic antigen (CEA) may be useful as a baseline.

Primary tumor staging has become increasingly important to determine whether neoadjuvant chemoradiation therapy is indicated. While CT scanning is the mainstay for initial assessment of distant disease and is useful to assess gross pelvic abnormalities such as direct extension to adjacent organs, it is not adequate for primary rectal tumor staging. Endorectal ultrasonography (ERUS) appears most useful to stage early lesions and is a reliable method to assess tumor depth within the rectal wall (T1 and T2) and moderately accurate at assessing enlarged mesorectal lymph nodes (N-stage). For more extensive tumors, pelvic phased array magnetic resonance imaging (MRI) should be considered using a protocol specific for staging rectal cancer. Pelvic MRI appears to have several advantages over ERUS: (a) It is less operator dependent; (b) it provides a larger field of view beyond a few centimeters of the primary including the pelvic sidewall and other adjacent structures; (c) it is probably more accurate in assessing lymph node involvement; and (d) it provides anatomically relevant information to the surgeon. Not surprisingly, pelvic MRI has become increasingly utilized to stage rectal cancer (2). ERUS and pelvic MRI specific for rectal cancer staging may not be widely available or of adequate quality throughout the United States, so some patients may need to be referred to experienced centers to obtain these tests.

In the United States, most advanced mid or low rectal cancers with evidence of lymph node involvement and/or transmural spread of the primary are treated with neoadjuvant chemoradiotherapy followed 8–10 weeks later by radical surgical resection. Tattooing the distal edge of the tumor is sometimes useful to guide the subsequent resection and selection of a distal margin should a complete clinical response to the neoadjuvant therapy occur. The rationale for such neoadjuvant therapy is to decrease the risk of local recurrence and thus improve survival. Postoperative adjuvant chemotherapy is generally used as well to decrease the risk of distant metastases. In many parts of the world, the American approach is criticized for overtreating many patients. Many other protocols call for use of a less morbid, short-course neoadjuvant radiotherapy followed by radical surgery or for radical surgery alone if preoperative MRI suggests that TME can clear the rectal cancer adequately (3).

Role of Multidisciplinary Team

While the colorectal surgeon usually has the primary responsibility to assess and direct the treatment of a patient with rectal cancer, appropriate decision making to optimize outcomes is enhanced by a multidisciplinary team of professionals similarly focused on rectal cancer care. Preoperative consultation with other specialty colleagues to plan the optimal treatment, achieve the optimal oncologic outcome with the least morbidity, and to implement a coordinated and safe operation is essential. For many advanced stage rectal cancers, medical and radiation oncologists will oversee a course of neoadjuvant chemoradiation. If there is involvement of the genitourinary tract or sacrum, preoperative consultation with a urologist, neurosurgeon, or orthopedic surgeon is advised. Patients with distal or mid rectal cancer should be seen preoperatively by an enterostomal therapist for counseling and marking of the abdominal wall for any potential stomas. In cases where it is not clear whether the procedure will be an APR versus AR and low anastomosis with a diverting ileostomy, both sides of the abdomen should be marked. Perineal wound closure may require plastic surgical consultation to plan a rotational myocutaneous flap.

SURGERY

Special Surgical Considerations

Pelvic Floor Anatomy
APR requires that the surgeon be intimately familiar with the anatomy of the pelvis and in particular, the pelvic floor and perineum (Figs. 31.1 and 31.2). The perineum is the

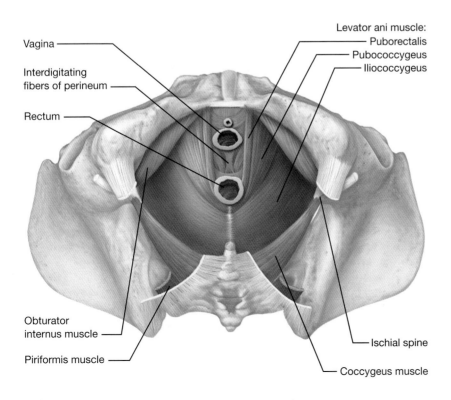

Figure 31.1 Caudal view of pelvic floor muscles.

Vagina

Interdigitating fibers of perineum

Rectum

Levator ani muscle:
Puborectalis
Pubococcygeus
Iliococcygeus

Obturator internus muscle

Piriformis muscle

Ischial spine

Coccygeus muscle

Part VII: Abdominoperineal Resection

Figure 31.2 Lateral view of pelvic floor muscles.

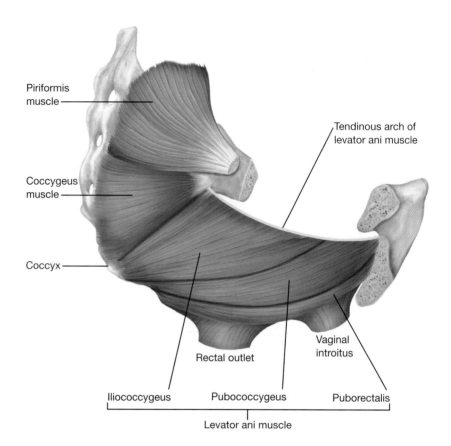

Piriformis muscle

Tendinous arch of levator ani muscle

Coccygeus muscle

Coccyx

Vaginal introitus

Rectal outlet

Iliococcygeus   Pubococcygeus   Puborectalis

Levator ani muscle

area between the thighs extending from the pubis to the coccyx. Its upper boundary is the lower surface of the levator ani. It is typically divided into an anterior urogenital region and a posterior anal region. The pelvic floor is a funnel-shaped, bilateral muscular plate that includes the three muscles of the levator ani (puborectalis, pubococcygeus, and iliococcygeus muscles) as well as the coccygeus muscle. The levator ani muscles are attached anteriorly to the pubis just lateral to the symphysis and posteriorly to the ischial spine. The puborectalis is a muscular loop without attachments to the coccyx with anterior fibers merging into the external sphincter. The pubococcygeus and iliococcygeus muscles arise from the arcus tendineus that extends from the pubis to the ischial spine. They insert on the ventral and lateral surfaces of the coccyx as well as to the anococcygeal raphe. The coccygeus muscle arises from the ischial spine and inserts into the lateral surface of the caudal part of the sacrum and the coccyx (Fig. 31.2). The pelvic floor muscles are covered by a parietal endopelvic fascial layer on their pelvic surface. The presacral Waldeyer's fascia is a thickened part of the parietal fascia that covers presacral vessels and nerves and is attached to S3 and S4 sacral segments. Anteriorly, Denonvillier's fascia separates the rectum from the seminal vesicles and prostate (Fig. 31.3).

Recent Oncologic Insight—The "Waist"

Curative intent APR is associated with higher rates of perforation, positive margins, and local recurrence than observed after AR. These poor outcomes seem independent of tumor stage or size (4). Some authors have suggested that distal rectal cancers have a different biology and routes of spread compared to proximal lesions. For instance, 25% of transmural cancers in the distal half of the rectum have lateral pelvic lymph node metastases located well beyond the dissection plane followed by TME (5). While this may explain some of the poor outcomes observed after APR, there is increasing concern that the poor results may be due in large part to anatomic and technical considerations not previously considered. Specifically, it has been suggested that the poor outcomes after APR are due to the close proximity of the cancer to the circumferential resection margin at the level of the anorectum distal to the levator muscle sling (6). As opposed

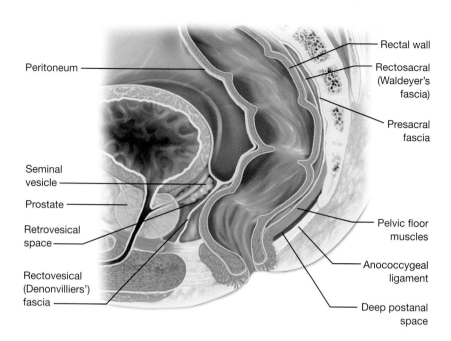

Peritoneum

Seminal vesicle

Prostate

Retrovesical space

Rectovesical (Denonvilliers') fascia

Rectal wall

Rectosacral (Waldeyer's fascia)

Presacral fascia

Pelvic floor muscles

Anococcygeal ligament

Deep postanal space

to a more proximal rectal cancer that is surrounded by the mesorectum enveloped within the endopelvic fascial plane, cancer in the distal anorectum has no comparable tissue surrounding it (Fig. 31.4). Nagtegaal et al. (4) assessed cancers <5 cm from the anal verge and found that there was little or no levator and sphincter muscles surrounding the specimen at the level of the cancer. This area has now been termed the "waist" in an APR specimen. Salerno et al. (6) found that the location of the "waist" was between 35 and 42 mm proximal to the anal verge, a site that correlates with the puborectalis.

It is possible that a well-intentioned surgeon focused on performing a low anastomosis after TME for a distal rectal cancer may follow the mesorectum distally to the point where it thins and blends with the intersphincteric plane leaving almost no surrounding tissues on the cancer-bearing anorectum where it is excised, that is, at the "waist." This is thought to result in high local recurrence rates. We agree with others that it is reasonable to modify the technique for radical APR to eliminate the "waist" and hopefully improve the poor results currently observed. The modifications described

Conventional APR with waist

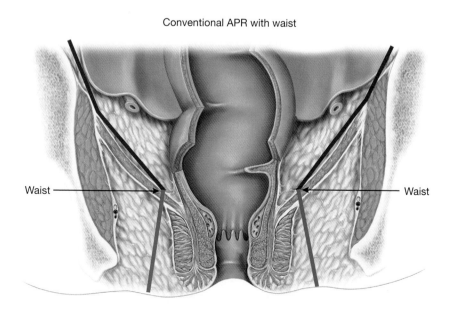

Waist

Waist

Figure 31.4 Conventional abdominoperineal resection (APR) dissection planes resulting in "waist."

Figure 31.5 Suggested oncologic dissection planes with total ischioanal excision.

APR with total ischioanal excision

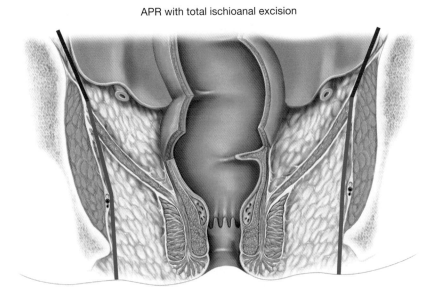

in detail include: (a) stopping the abdominal dissection at the proximal level of the levator muscles and then (b) performing a more radical perineal excision of the levators including the puborectalis in the prone jackknife position. Thus, instead of following the levators distally and inward to the anorectal ring, the surgeon can purposefully dissect through the levators laterally along the side wall and include the soft tissue around the proximal aspect of the anorectal ring as part of the intact APR specimen. When done properly, the specimen will appear as a "cylinder" rather than as an APR with a distal "waist." Holm terms this modified technique of APR for distal rectal cancers as a "total ischioanal excision" (Fig. 31.5) (7). Like Holm, we also believe that this modified technique is greatly facilitated by undertaking the perineal dissection with the patient in the prone jackknife position.

Peter McDonald and John Northover (8) recently recovered old films from the archives of St. Mark's Hospital in London, England, showing Percy Lockhart-Mummery performing a perineal excision, William Gabriel doing a perineoabdominal excision, and Oswald Lloyd-Davies undertaking a synchronous combined abdominoperineal excision of the rectum. These remarkable films were edited by Northover and shown at the American Society of Colon and Rectal Surgeons meeting in 2003 during his Ernestine Hambrick Lecture, "Rectal Cancer Surgery: The Century Since Ernest Miles." They clearly demonstrated the extensive nature of the perineal phase used by these pioneering surgeons to excise rectal cancer. In the films, after an extensive perineal incision and coccygectomy, the pelvis was cleared with lateral division of the levator muscles posterolaterally and the anterior dissection was carried up to the pouch of Douglas (Fig. 31.6).

One wonders why modern surgeons abandoned this more radical perineal phase in favor of the more conservative "conventional APR dissection" that predisposes to "the waist" of an APR specimen. We speculate that the recent emphasis to do more distal low and ultra-low anastomoses predisposed surgeons to alter what may be a key component of the deep pelvic dissection during an APR. Normally, when the dissection of a rectal cancer that is clearly amenable to resection and anastomosis reaches the level of the levators, the surgeon selects a site for division of the rectum such that there will be an adequate distal margin thus leaving the levators intact. We suggest that modern surgeons inappropriately apply the same basic technique used for low AR to the pelvic dissection for APR. Thus, when the dissection reaches the level of the levators, they follow the pelvic floor inward close to the anorectal wall before again widening the dissection plane at the level of the ischiorectal fossas. This technique unintentionally creates the "waist" in the specimen. When this method is utilized for more distal rectal cancers at or near the level of the puborectalis, surgeons may increase the likelihood of local recurrence by not adequately clearing the soft tissues from the pelvis at the

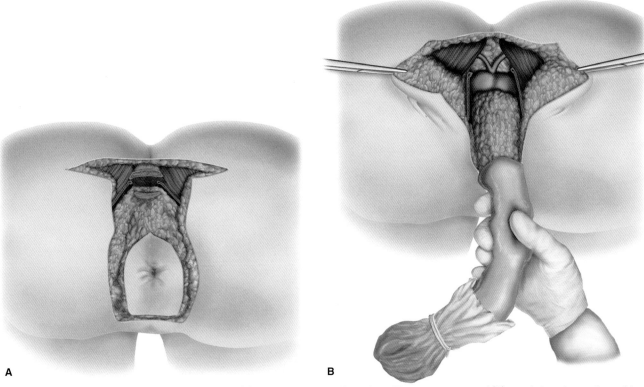

A   **B**

Figure 31.6 Drawings from St. Mark's hospital showing (**A**) extensive perineal dissection with coccygectomy and (**B**) completion of posterior and lateral dissection with delivery of specimen prior to proceeding with final anterior dissection. (Figures courtesy of Dr. John Northover, St. Mark's Hospital, East London, England.)

level of the cancer. Indeed, a less radical APR can be done using either the intersphincteric (Fig. 31.7A) or the extralevator (Fig. 31.7B) planes. Such techniques may be appropriate for APR for proximal and mid rectal cancers in patients with poor sphincter function or some other contraindication for a sphincter-preserving anastomosis and may be the preferred APR technique for benign diseases such as inflammatory bowel disease. However, for distal rectal cancers requiring APR, the surgeon is advised to consciously avoid the tendency to "cone in" on the dissection plane at the level of the levators.

Sequential Versus Synchronous APR and Patient Positioning

APR includes abdominal and perineal phases, which may be done sequentially or synchronously. The perineal phase can be done in modified lithotomy, lateral, or prone jackknife position. We prefer the sequential approach beginning with the abdominal portion of the procedure with the patient in modified lithotomy position followed by the perineal portion with the patient in the prone jackknife position. We find that this greatly improves exposure of the perineal field and improves access for an assistant surgeon. This sequential approach is particularly helpful for obese or heavily muscled patients, those with a deep anal canal, those for whom a concomitant vaginectomy or sacrectomy is planned, and those with distal tumors where anterior and anterolateral clearance may be difficult to achieve. In cases where perineal wound closure is achieved by the use of a vertical rectus abdominis muscle flap, the patient is generally repositioned in modified lithotomy following the APR. Alternatively, the flap can be developed during the initial abdominal phase of the APR and left within the abdomen for subsequent retrieval after the APR. The main disadvantages of the sequential approach are not having simultaneous access to both operative fields, the time required to change positions, and the potential dangers associated with changing position of an anesthetized patient. If we anticipate that the rectal resection will be unusually difficult because of lateral fixation, we should use the synchronous two-team technique. The patient is carefully positioned with the buttocks elevated on a pad such that the perineum extends over the edge of the operating table; retractors are used to spread the buttocks and to expose the anorectum.

APR with intersphincteric excision

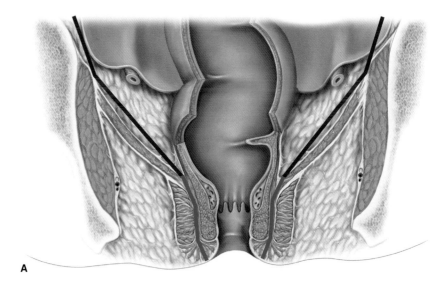

A

Extra levator APR

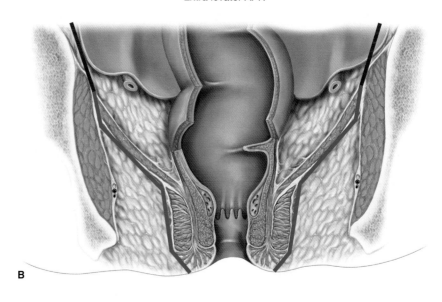

B

Perineal Wound Management

Perineal wound complications are common after APR. They range in severity from minor to serious and occur both in the immediate postoperative period and during the long-term follow-up. Radical APR results in a large pelvic "dead space" that predisposes to the development of postoperative pelvic seromas, hematomas, and abscesses, as well as to adhesive bowel obstruction as loops of intestine adhere to the presacrum deep in the pelvis. Neoadjuvant radiation and/or extended resections accompanying APR such as *en bloc* sacrectomy significantly increase the risk of perineal wound problems and make subsequent reoperation more hazardous. To minimize the risk of pelvic fluid collections, most surgeons routinely place a large suction drain in the pelvis. Many surgeons also routinely mobilize a pedicle of omentum and place it in the pelvis to fill the "dead space" and keep the small bowel from adhering to the distal sacrum. In our experience, this is rarely effective. Today, we increasingly utilize myocutaneous flaps such as the vertical rectus abdominis, gracilis, or gluteus to fill the pelvis, close large perineal defects, and simultaneously reconstruct the perineum and vagina (7,9,10). Rectus abdominis flaps have been widely reported with consistently good results. While less widely reported, the use of bilateral gracilis flaps and inferior gluteal flaps both have good results when used for the perineum. Our practice is to strongly consider the use of a myocutaneous flap in patients undergoing APR for rectal cancer in the setting of neoadjuvant radiation, extended resections, recurrent cancer, and in patients with additional comorbidities such as obesity, long-standing or poorly controlled diabetes mellitus, or smoking, which could adversely impact wound healing. The detailed use of such flaps is beyond the scope of this chapter but is addressed in chapter.

Technique

Operative Preliminaries

Generally, outpatient mechanical bowel preparation is performed the day before operation. In recent years, the need for a full bowel preparation has been questioned though most colorectal surgeons in the United States still use at least a modified preparation such as enemas prior to radical surgery for rectal cancer. APR is usually performed under general anesthesia and an epidural catheter can be considered to provide postoperative analgesia. Perioperative prophylaxis for deep venous thromboembolism is standard and an intravenous antibiotic is administered within 30 minutes of the incision.

After administration of general endotracheal anesthesia, a bladder catheter is inserted and ureteral stents may be placed to facilitate intraoperative identification and protection of the ureters. This is especially useful in the presence of a bulky primary rectal cancer invading other organs or a pelvic recurrence. An orogastric tube for decompression of the stomach is inserted. Patients are placed into modified lithotomy position with buttocks brought down to the edge of the table and legs placed into Allen™ or Yellow Fin stirrups. In general, hips should be slightly flexed and abducted with feet positioned to be flat within the stirrups. Proper alignment is maintained with an imaginary line that keeps the ankle, knee, and opposite shoulder in alignment. The risk of peroneal nerve injury can be minimized by avoiding pressure along the lateral aspect of the leg by checking that a hand can be inserted between the posterolateral portion of each leg and the stirrup.

A preoperative briefing allows the surgeon to share the plan with the entire operative team and is used to confirm the presence of appropriate instruments including self-retaining retractors such as Balfour, Bookwalter or Omni-track, the St. Mark's pelvic retractors, and the Wylie renal vein retractors, a variety of staplers and other devices including long instruments. Headlights or lighted retractors facilitate deep pelvic dissection. The assistance of an experienced second surgeon or a highly trained technician is invaluable.

The surgeon can then reassess the rectal cancer by digital rectal examination and proctosigmoidoscopy to irrigate the rectum and confirm the degree of involvement of the anal sphincter or other organs, the level of the distal edge of the tumor, and the response of the tumor to chemoradiation. The abdomen and perineum, including the vagina in females, should be prepped into the field; a midline incision is used.

Step 1: Mobilization of Colon

After abdominal exploration to identify metastatic disease or other unexpected pathology, the small bowel is packed into the upper abdomen, the patient is placed in a slight Trendelenburg position and a self-retaining retractor is placed. While some surgeons practice a medial to lateral "no-touch technique" approach and divide the inferior mesenteric vessels prior to lateral mobilization, we typically begin by laterally mobilizing the colon. The sigmoid colon is retracted to the right, and the peritoneal attachments to its left are incised along the avascular plane (white line of Toldt) distally into the pelvis and as far proximally as needed to ensure sufficient mobilization so that a tension-free end descending colostomy elevated above the skin level can be constructed. Generally, this mobilization includes a portion of the descending colon but complete takedown of the splenic flexure, as we do routinely if a low anastomosis is planned, is often unnecessary for APR. The left ureter and gonadal vessels are identified and preserved by using sharp and gentle blunt dissection to separate the retroperitoneal tissues from the left colonic mesentery.

Figure 31.8 Anatomic depiction of vascular ligation techniques. **A.** "High ligation" refers to ligation of the inferior mesenteric artery nears its origin. **B.** "Low ligation" refers most commonly to ligation of the superior rectal artery.

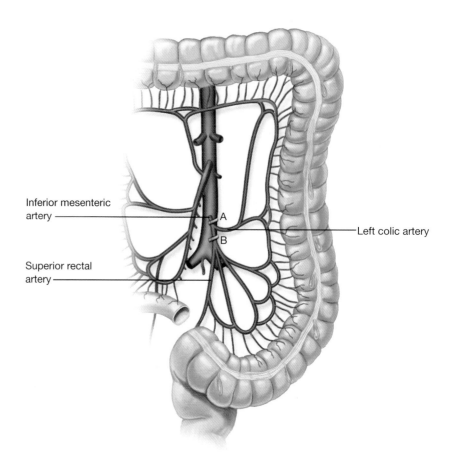

Inferior mesenteric artery

Superior rectal artery

Left colic artery

Step 2: Ligation of Inferior Mesenteric Artery

The mobilized rectosigmoid is retracted anteriorly to the left to expose the inferior mesenteric artery (IMA). Transillumination of the mesentery facilitates identification of an avascular space adjacent to the IMA at the base of the mesentery. The peritoneum overlying this space is incised on either side of the IMA and, after identifying the right ureter, the peritoneal incision is extended on the right side of the mesentery to the pelvic brim. Surgeons vary in opinion about the precise level of IMA ligation for rectal cancer resection (1,11). Some surgeons prefer a high ligation of the IMA at its origin from the aorta suggesting that this level of transection not only maximizes the mesenteric lymph node harvest, but also improves the oncologic outcomes. Other surgeons prefer a low ligation of the IMA just distal to the left colic artery, suggesting that this approach ensures better blood supply to the proximal colon and prevents nerve injury at the base of the IMA, thus minimizing functional impairment (Fig. 31.8). At present, there is not enough evidence to recommend one approach over the other. After ligation of the proximal vascular pedicle, it is convenient to clamp, divide, and ligate the mesentery to the colon at the descending-sigmoid junction where the colon is then divided with a linear stapler.

Step 3: Total Mesorectal Excision, Preservation of Autonomic Nerves, and Mobilization to Levators

TME along the areolar plane between the visceral fascia of the mesorectum and the parietal fascia of the pelvis is a standard component of APR for rectal cancer. The sigmoid with its intact and fully mobilized mesentery is retracted anteriorly and inferiorly toward the pubis to expose an avascular plane posterior to the rectum at the level of the common iliac vessels. Sharp incision of the pelvic peritoneum in this avascular plane while traction is placed on the rectosigmoid typically allows air to enter the areolar tissue posterior and lateral to the rectum in the retrorectal space. The surgeon follows the air, sharply dividing the loose areolar tissue posteriorly and laterally. Traction with the nonoperating hand and appropriate repositioning of handheld retractors is essential to keep the plane of the mesorectal dissection in view and accessible to sharp division with scissors or cautery. During the retrorectal portion of the mesorectal dissection, the hypogastric nerves are identified at the sacral promontory. These nerves descend in the presacral space in a wishbone shape and must be preserved to maintain postoperative sexual and urinary function. As the dissection proceeds posteriorly, the rectosacral (Waldeyer's) fascia located at the level of the third sacral vertebra is divided sharply, and the dissection proceeds distally. As noted above, to avoid creating a "waist" in the APR specimen, the dissection is purposefully stopped at the proximal level of the levator muscles just as the mesorectum begins to taper and thin. This transition usually occurs at the level of the fifth sacral vertebra and we find it usually corresponds to the level where the rectum changes its course from posterior to anterior. At that level, the rectum is mobilized in a posterior-to-lateral direction, with care taken to maintain the integrity of the endopelvic fascial envelope encasing the bilobed mesorectum and not to dissect further distally than the proximal levator, which will now be posterolaterally visible in the depths of the pelvis.

Exposure for the anterior dissection is facilitated by reducing the angle of the Trendelenburg position or even shifting the patient to a reverse Trendelenburg position. The anterolateral dissection is begun by incising the peritoneum of the rectovesical or rectouterine pouch in the midline and dividing soft tissue attachments anterolaterally to connect to the dissection laterally. Most often, the middle rectal artery is not present as a distinct vessel and the anterolateral dissection at the level of the proximal levator is done with electrocautery with minimal bleeding. Occasionally, however, the middle rectal artery is large enough that ligation is necessary. During this phase of the dissection, the nervi erigentes are identified and preserved on the lateral pelvic sidewalls. A conscious effort is made to avoid dissecting centrally into the pelvis along the levator or distally beyond the proximal levator.

Step 4: Sequential APR—Abdominal Closure and Colostomy Formation

In cases were a sequential approach is used, the abdominal phase is completed before positioning the patient prone. A circular incision ~2½ cm in diameter is made at the previously marked stoma site, usually in the left lower quadrant of the abdominal wall. The skin aperture, subcutaneous tissue, and fascia are kept in alignment to create a straight tract. The subcutaneous fat is cored out or separated to expose the anterior rectus fascia that is opened with a cruciate incision. The rectus muscle is split with a clamp to expose the posterior rectus sheath, which is then opened to create an aperture of adequate size (typically two finger breadths) to accommodate passage of the appropriately mobilized descending colon. A Dennis or Babcock clamp is placed through the aperture to deliver the staple-closed end of the descending colon through the abdominal wall. Care is taken to avoid twisting the colonic mesentery. Tension-free elevation of the descending colon 2 to 3 cm above the skin level is ideal to ensure that an adequate stoma can be created.

The surgeon should check the position of the ureters to be sure that they are not vulnerable to injury during the perineal dissection. If they are close to the anticipated line of resection, it may be useful to mobilize them out of the field of dissection and/or to encircle them with a vascular tape to aid their identification during the perineal dissection. The operative field is irrigated, hemostasis is secured, and correct sponge and needle counts are confirmed. We generally place a large, fluted suction drain in the pelvis through a separate abdominal stab wound placed in an area that will not interfere with the stoma or a planned rectus abdominis flap for perineal wound closure. Typically, we suture the distal end of the drain to the proximal end of the sigmoid colon that will be retrieved and resected *en bloc* during the perineal phase. If desired, a rectus abdominis myocutaneous flap can be prepared at this time. The abdomen is closed and the colostomy is then matured using an eversion (Brooke) technique with interrupted absorbable sutures (typically 3-0 Vicryl or chromic) to create a budded, everted os that will pouch more easily. The patient is then positioned prone.

Step 5: Synchronous Two-Team APR—Completion of Abdominal Dissection

If a synchronous two-team approach is used, the patient remains in the modified lithotomy position. As the pelvic surgeon initiates the perineal dissection as described below, the abdominal surgeon may proceed with additional distal posterior mobilization of the rectum to the level of the coccyx and with further anterior and anterolateral dissection of the rectum. Deep pelvic retractors are used to protect the seminal vesicles and prostate in males or the vagina in females. Heald et al. (12) considered Denonvilliers' fascia as the most anterior limit of the mesorectum and thus remove it with the specimen during the TME. We similarly excise Denonvilliers' fascia for circumferential and anterior rectal tumors to obtain a negative circumferential margin. For posterior tumors, Denonvilliers' fascia may be incised in the midline anteriorly and then the visceral fascia propria of the rectum is followed, thus sparing the parietal Denonvilliers' fascia to minimize risk of injury to the nearby pelvic nerves. The abdominal and perineal surgeons must work synchronously to develop proper dissection planes vital for curative and safe *en bloc* excision of the tumor without compromising curability. Performing the perineal phase with the patient in the lithotomy position can be very demanding technically. It is easy for the perineal surgeon to dissect slightly too posteriorly into the presacral fascia and cause venous bleeding. This can be avoided if the abdominal surgeon guides the perineal surgeon's posterior dissection into the presacral plane. It is similarly important that the abdominal surgeon protect the seminal vesicles and prostate or the vagina as the perineal surgeon performs the anterior dissection, an area difficult to visualize well in lithotomy.

The elements of the perineal dissection whether done in modified lithotomy position or in prone position are similar. As noted earlier, the major challenge during the synchronous technique is to avoid the tendency to follow the levator plate and dissect centrally, thus creating a "waist" in the specimen at the level of the puborectalis, which is associated with increased local recurrence rates. It is for this reason that we prefer the sequential approach. On occasion, the synchronous technique is necessary, but this approach demands the collaboration of two experienced surgeons.

Step 6: Perineal Dissection

After carefully positioning the patient prone over a hip roll with the table jackknifed and the buttocks spread by tape, the distal anorectum is irrigated to remove feces or tumor debris, and the perineum is prepped (including the vagina in females). The anus is then closed with a purse-string suture to minimize the risk of spillage into the operative field. In the absence of local spread beyond the anorectum, the landmarks used for dissection include the coccyx posteriorly, the perineal body anteriorly, and the ischial tuberosities laterally (Fig. 31.9). An elliptical incision is made incorporating

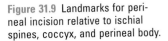

Figure 31.9 Landmarks for perineal incision relative to ischial spines, coccyx, and perineal body.

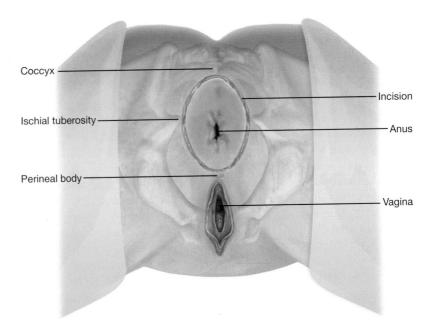

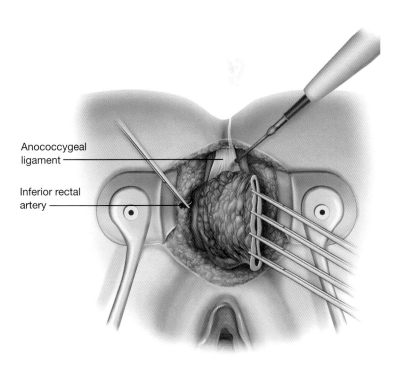

Figure 31.10 Extension of perineal dissection to pelvic floor with incision through the anococcygeal ligament to enter the true pelvis.

Anococcygeal ligament

Inferior rectal artery

Part VII: Abdominoperineal Resection

these landmarks. A Lone Star retractor is placed to separate the skin edges and the incision is deepened to the level of the ischiorectal fat bilaterally. A variety of retractors including self-retaining springs, deep Gelpi retractors, and deavers are used to maintain visualization as the dissection proceeds (Fig. 31.10). Branches of the inferior rectal vessels within the ischiorectal fossa typically can be controlled with electrocautery.

To assure adequate lateral clearance and avoid the "waist" problem described earlier, the surgeon directs the dissection in each ischiorectal fossa through the fat to the levator ani muscles laterally and the coccyx posteriorly. The posterior dissection is performed first beginning in the midline, leaving the more challenging anterior dissection until last. The anorectum is retracted anteriorly, and the postanal space is entered by sharply dividing the anococcygeal ligament at the tip of coccyx. If needed for exposure, a coccygectomy can easily be done usually with electrocautery and a heavy scissors or a periosteal elevator.

Once the true pelvis is entered posteriorly, a finger can be inserted to "hook" the levator ani muscles, which are then divided along the pelvic bone posterolaterally and then laterally (Fig. 31.11). This avoids narrowing the dissection plane and avoids the "waist" problem. While some surgeons divide the muscle with cautery, we prefer to maintain absolute hemostasis by either using the LigaSure device or by clamping, dividing, and suture ligating the coccygeus, iliococcygeus, pubococcygeus, and puborectalis. At this point in the operation, the perineal dissection has merged with the previously performed abdominal presacral dissection. The lateral resection margin is extended anterolaterally. When about two-thirds of the planned resection is complete, we generally find it convenient to retrieve the mobilized rectosigmoid with the attached drain and gently deliver it through the large posterior pelvic wound (Fig. 31.12). This maneuver provides better exposure for the remaining anterior dissection, which is often the most challenging part of the APR.

The anterior perineal incision is deepened using the posterior border of the superficial transverse perineal muscle as the guide to the rectoprostatic or rectovaginal plane. Allis clamps are used to maintain counter-traction between the perineal body anteriorly and the everted specimen posteriorly as the surgeon develops the anterior dissection plane. In a female patient, an anterior lesion may necessitate a posterior-wall vaginectomy to ensure adequate margins. If a vaginectomy is not required the rectovaginal septum is

Figure 31.11 The lateral portion of the perineal dissection is completed by dividing levator muscles from posterior to anterior on each side.

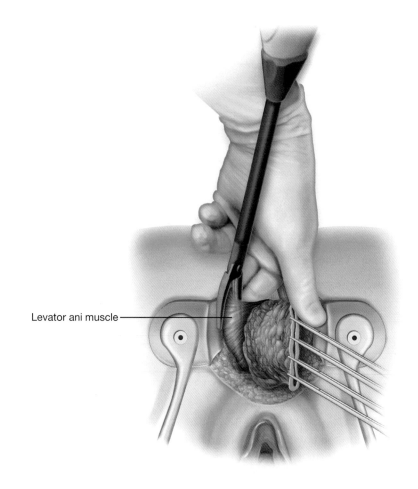

Levator ani muscle

Figure 31.12 The anterior portion of the perineal dissection is typically performed with the proximal colon and rectum delivered through the posterior/lateral pelvic defect with the attached pelvic drain. The rectourethralis muscle (or rectovaginal septum) is the remaining structure that is divided. Care should be taken not to violate the prostatic capsule in men or posterior vaginal wall in females.

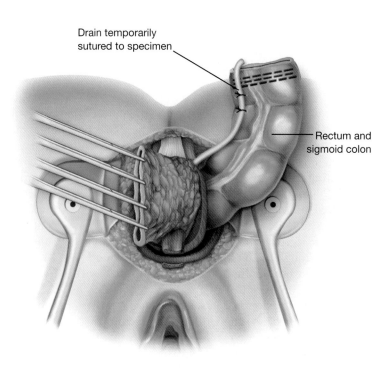

Drain temporarily sutured to specimen

Rectum and sigmoid colon

dissected proximally, often with a guiding digit in the vagina to avoid inadvertent vaginal perforation. In a male patient, anterior dissection is facilitated by palpating the Foley catheter to help avoid injury to the urethra and the prostate. The median raphe of the rectourethralis and puborectalis is divided, and the remaining attachments are divided.

Before sending the specimen for pathology examination, the surgeon should inspect it for completeness of margins and for any sign of perforation. It should appear as a "cylinder" with an intact bilobar mesorectum and overlying smooth surface. A poor-quality specimen with clefts and defects along the mesorectal fascia or a "waist" is associated with higher rates of recurrence (13,14).

Step 7: Perineal Wound Closure

The pelvis is irrigated and the hemostasis ensured. The transabdominal drain is trimmed to fit into the pelvis. Primary perineal wound closure may be undertaken in several layers with 2-0 and 3-0 absorbable sutures, but, because the levator muscles were divided laterally along the pelvic bones, it is only possible to reapproximate the subcutaneous tissues and the skin. This excision leaves a large "dead space" deep in the pelvis that predisposes to postoperative morbidity. To overcome the perineal wound morbidity, we increasingly use myocutaneous flaps as discussed earlier.

POSTOPERATIVE MANAGEMENT

The orogastric or nasogastric tube is routinely removed at the end of the procedure. If there was no extensive dissection or manipulation of the small bowel, the patient may begin clear liquids on the first postoperative day with advancement to a low-residue diet once the patient has return of bowel function. In the absence of a specific infection, postoperative antibiotics are not used. The patient should be maintained on postoperative prophylactic doses of subcutaneous heparin or low-molecular-weight heparin for prevention of thromboembolic events. Because the pelvic dissection is extensive, the Foley catheter remains until postoperative day 3. The pelvic drain is typically removed before discharge from the hospital.

Like most complex abdominal surgery done today, perioperative mortality following APR is 2–3% primarily as a result of cardiopulmonary events. Despite the major improvement in mortality in recent decades, both immediate and long-term morbidity remain high in modern series. Postoperative abdominal and perineal wound morbidity occurs in up to 50%. The majority are infections and most can be managed with local wound care and closure by secondary intention or CT drainage of pelvic collections. In some instances, abscesses necessitate through the perineum or abdominal wound to cause wound disruption, major wound fistulas, and delayed healing. Vacuum-assisted closure (VAC) dressings or reoperation may be needed to resolve the issue.

Genitourinary complications occur in up to 50% of patients. While the majority are minor including urinary tract infection, some patients suffer troublesome urinary retention and control problems following APR. In most cases, voiding dysfunction is temporary with resolution in the first 3–6 months following surgery. Ureteral or bladder injury can occur but typically can be managed readily without long-term consequences if discovered and addressed at the time of surgery. Sexual dysfunction is estimated to occur in up to 50% of men following rectal cancer resection. Women also commonly have sexual dysfunction, although the exact incidence is not known.

Other long-term morbidity specific to APR includes stoma-related problems such as stricture and paracolostomy and perineal hernias. Small-bowel obstruction from adhesions deep in the pelvis to the sacrum are common causes for reoperation on long-term follow-up. All patients experience significant body-image changes after APR and for some, this change is a major and lasting impediment to full recovery (1).

Five-year survival rates after APR by stage are reported from 78% to 100% for Stage I disease, 45–73% for Stage II disease, and 22–66% for Stage III disease. When adjusted for tumor stage, rates of overall survival, local recurrence, and disease-specific survival are better in patients with proper TME excision (14).

CONCLUSIONS

APR remains an important procedure for distal and advanced rectal cancers, particularly those cancers invading and abutting the sphincter. The importance of maintaining proper planes of dissection with the TME and careful wide perineal dissection avoiding a waist in the specimen are important considerations in performing APR. Surgeons should have candid discussions with patients with respect to expected functional and oncologic outcomes following APR.

Recommended References and Readings

1. Pachler J, Wille-Jorgensen P. Quality of life after rectal resection for cancer, with or without permanent colostomy. *Cochrane Database Syst Rev* 2005;(2):CD004323.
2. MERCURY Study Group. Diagnostic accuracy of preoperative magnetic resonance imaging in predicting curative resection of rectal cancer: prospective observational study. *BMJ* 2006; 333(7572):779.
3. Valentini V, Aristei C, Glimelius B, et al. Multidisciplinary Rectal Cancer Management: 2nd European Rectal Cancer Consensus Conference (EURECA-CC2). *Radiother Oncol* 2009;92(2):148–63.
4. Nagtegaal ID, van de Velde CJ, Marijnen CA, van Krieken JH, Quirke P. Low rectal cancer: a call for a change of approach in abdominoperineal resection. *J Clin Oncol* 2005;23(36):9257–64.
5. Hojo K, Koyama Y, Moriya Y. Lymphatic spread and its prognostic value in patients with rectal cancer. *Am J Surg* 1982; 144(3):350–4.
6. Salerno G, Chandler I, Wotherspoon A, Thomas K, Moran B, Brown G. Sites of surgical wasting in the abdominoperineal specimen. *Br J Surg* 2008;95(9):1147–54.
7. Holm T, Ljung A, Haggmark T, Jurell G, Lagergren J. Extended abdominoperineal resection with gluteus maximus flap reconstruction of the pelvic floor for rectal cancer. *Br J Surg* 2007;94(2):232–8.
8. Northover JM. Personal communication to Rothenberger, D. A., 2003.
9. Chessin DB, Hartley J, Cohen AM, et al. Rectus flap reconstruction decreases perineal wound complications after pelvic chemoradiation and surgery: a cohort study. *Ann Surg Oncol* 2005;12(2):104–10.
10. Ricciardi R, Virnig BA, Madoff RD, Rothenberger DA, Baxter NN. The status of radical proctectomy and sphincter-sparing surgery in the United States. *Dis Colon Rectum* 2007;50(8): 1119–27; discussion 1126–1117.
11. Lange MM, Buunen M, van de Velde CJ, Lange JF. Level of arterial ligation in rectal cancer surgery: low tie preferred over high tie. A review. *Dis Colon Rectum* 2008;51(7):1139–45.
12. Heald RJ, Husband EM, Ryall RD. The mesorectum in rectal cancer surgery—the clue to pelvic recurrence? *Br J Surg* 1982; 69(10):613–6.
13. den Dulk M, Marijnen CA, Putter H, et al. Risk factors for adverse outcome in patients with rectal cancer treated with an abdominoperineal resection in the total mesorectal excision trial. *Ann Surg* 2007;246(1):83–90.
14. Quirke P, Steele R, Monson J, et al. Effect of the plane of surgery achieved on local recurrence in patients with operable rectal cancer: a prospective study using data from the MRC CR07 and NCIC-CTG CO16 randomized clinical trial. *Lancet* 2009; 373(9666):821–8.

32 Laparoscopic Abdominoperineal Resection (APR)

John H. Marks and Joseph L. Frenkel

Introduction

While discussing laparoscopic abdominoperineal resection (APR) two major issues come to the forefront. One is the role of laparoscopic surgery in the treatment of rectal cancer, and the other is the indications for APR for low rectal cancer.

Since the publication of the COST Trial, few questions remain regarding the application of laparoscopic surgery in the treatment of colon cancer. However, concerns regarding the ability to perform laparoscopic total mesorectal excision (TME) still exist. To this end, the American of College Surgeons Oncology Group (ACOSOG) Z6051 trial is currently accruing patients at the time of this writing, which should definitively address this issue in a multi-institutional randomized trial. The issues of paramount importance regarding laparoscopic surgery in the treatment of a rectal cancer include proper performance of TME, as well as visualization and retraction during deep pelvic dissection. The last issue, that of transection of the distal rectum to perform an anastomosis, is a major one in laparoscopically performing sphincter-preserving surgery in the low rectum. However, this becomes a moot point in performing an APR as there is no anastomosis since the sphincter mechanism is excised.

Having performed over 350 laparoscopic TMEs with a local recurrence rate of 3% overall, we feel confident that the laparoscopic approach will be validated as a safe option for rectal cancer. This approach clearly affords a much better visualization in the pelvis and exactness of dissection. In this chapter, we highlight the methods we use to laparoscopically accomplish this operation.

●● INDICATIONS

Clearly, the issue of sphincter preservation surgery versus permanent colostomy has to do with the level of the rectal cancer, bulk of the tumor, and the patient's baseline continence. Indications for permanent colostomy include patients with incontinence, patient preference

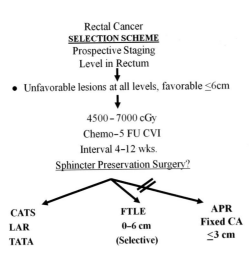

Rectal Cancer
SELECTION SCHEME
Prospective Staging
Level in Rectum

• Unfavorable lesions at all levels, favorable ≤6cm

4500 – 7000 cGy
Chemo–5 FU CVI
Interval 4–12 wks.
Sphincter Preservation Surgery?

CATS   FTLE   APR
LAR   0–6 cm   Fixed CA
TATA   (Selective)   ≤3 cm

Figure 32.1 Selection scheme for sphincter preservation employing neoadjuvant chemoradiation for low rectal cancers.

for lifestyle reasons, or direct involvement of the puborectalis. The advent of preoperative chemoradiation therapy has allowed us to alter these indications, greatly diminishing the need for APR. In a multimodal rectal cancer treatment program having treated over 800 cases, we have been able to obtain a sphincter preservation rate of 93%. In the large national trials, APR rates in the last decade have still ranged from 25% to 60%.

Our treatment algorithm for sphincter preservation employing neoadjuvant chemoradiation for low rectal cancers is shown in Figure 32.1. In the properly motivated patient with good sphincter function, the decision regarding sphincter preservation is based on tumor characteristics after completion of neoadjuvant therapy. Only patients whose cancers remained fixed in the distal third of the rectum after completion of chemoradiation therapy undergo APR. Keys to expanded sphincter preservation include (a) *basing decisions regarding sphincter preservation on the downstaged rectal cancer after completion of neoadjuvant therapy,* (b) a higher dose of radiation therapy to improve downstaging of the rectal cancer to our ideal level of 5,580 cGy, (c) allowing 8–12 weeks following radiation before making a decision regarding surgery, and (d) transanal abdominal transanal resection (TATA) technique for tumors in the distal third of the rectum, which includes an intersphincteric dissection beginning at the dentate line, assuming an adequate distal margin.

It is important to emphasize that the indications for laparoscopic APR are exactly the same as they are for an open APR. Clearly, it is poor trade for the patient to gain the benefits of laparoscopy at the expense of a permanent colostomy.

PREOPERATIVE PLANNING

Patients undergo a standard oncologic evaluation including CT scan of the abdomen and the pelvis and basic lab work, including liver function studies, complete blood cell count, metabolic profile coagulation studies, blood chemistries, and carcinoembryonic antigen (CEA) level. Endorectal ultrasound is also performed. Oftentimes this assessment is coupled with an MRI of the pelvis. In patients older than 60 years and in those individuals with coronary artery disease, hypertension, diabetes, or smokers, a full preoperative cardiac evaluation is undertaken.

Digital rectal examination and flexible sigmoidoscopic evaluation are performed in the office. Patients are then seen at 3-week intervals during their neoadjuvant treatment until the time of surgery. Final decisions regarding sphincter preservation are made based on the digital rectal and flexible endoscopic evaluation between 8 and 12 weeks following their neoadjuvant therapy. In general, patients are treated with 4,500 cGy of radiation to the entire pelvis with a boost of 1,000 cGy to the tumor in the presacral hollow. The limits of this chapter preclude us from being more expansive in this regard. All patients undergo a full bowel preparation. The patients are seen by a stoma nurse preoperatively and marked for a permanent colostomy. This is an essential point as the positioning and function of the stoma will have a major impact on the patient's quality of life.

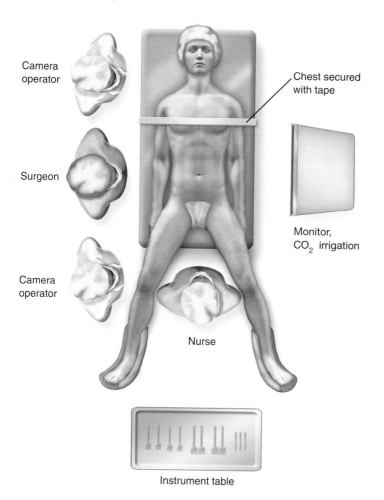

Figure 32.2 Setup of operating room to facilitate procedure.

Camera operator

Chest secured with tape

Surgeon

Monitor, CO_2 irrigation

Camera operator

Nurse

Instrument table

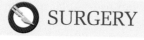 SURGERY

Positioning

Generally, patients are positioned in lithotomy. The exception to this rule is the patient with a very large bulky tumor that may require coccygectomy to obtain adequate exposure to the pelvis. In this case, the operation is started with the patient in a right Sims' position. It is essential that they are secured firmly to the table as both extreme Trendelenburg and airplaning the table to the "right side down" position will be utilized. This achieves proper retraction of the small bowel, so we can see into the pelvis clearly and position the small bowel out of the way. Shown in Figure 32.2 is our method of securing the patient to the operating room table as well as the overall setup of the operating room that facilitates the procedure.

With the patient in supine position, a strong strap of tape is used to secure the chest to the table. We feel strongly that pads on the shoulders should be avoided as this will predispose the patient to brachial plexus injury.

Technique

Perineal Dissection

It is our preference to start the operation perineally and then proceed abdominally (rendering the operation a perineal-abdominal resection rather than an APR). This is the same strategy that we use in open operations. This order dramatically facilitates the laparoscopic operation, as the most challenging portion of the laparoscopic procedure, the distal most rectal dissection, has already been done from the perineal approach.

After induction of anesthesia, the patient is placed in stirrups and digital examination is carried out to verify the location of the tumor and make the final determination regarding the need for permanent colostomy. The perineum is prepped and an O-Vicryl suture is used to place a purse string suture around the anal canal, so there is no soilage to the field at the time of surgery. The abdomen and perineum are fully prepped and draped. We find that securing the drapes around the perineum with a few interrupted 2-0 nylon sutures keeps the drapes from moving even when the patient is placed in extended lithotomy position.

As the procedure commences, the patient is put in an exaggerated lithotomy position to gain access to the perineum. A lighted suction device (Vital Vue™, Covidien, Norwalk, CT) greatly facilitates the dissection. Electrocautery is used to incise the skin with a 1-cm margin around the anal canal; the size and position of this incision can be adjusted based on tumor location. Dissection continues circumferentially into the fat of the perirectal space. The safest area for the initial approach into the pelvis is the posterior midline. The anococcygeal ligament is incised and the dissection is extended through the levators. At this point, a finger can be placed through the pelvic floor and one can excise a portion of the levators with an adequate margin. In doing this dissection, it is imperative to avoid coning in on the rectum at the levators, as it is this area where tumor margins are at greatest risk. Once one has entered into the plane above the levators, the dissection is brought around circumferentially, taking care in the male patient to avoid going into the prostate anteriorly. Special attention needs to be paid to the infraprostatic urethra in this region to avoid injury. In a straightforward case, the anterior portion of the dissection is the most challenging, and in the male is the last part to be addressed. In the event that there is tumor fixity or a large bulky cancer in another quadrant, it is better to leave this to the end of the dissection having dissected around the right or left so that the best decisions can be made in terms of where to transect. When operating for cure, any area of fixity requires that the adjacent tissue be excised *en bloc*.

It is well worth noting that in women the vagina is always prepped so that a finger can be placed here to help guide the anterior dissection. The posterior wall of the vagina does not need to be routinely excised when performing an APR in a woman unless there is an anterior fixation.

Once the perineal portion of the operation is completed, a lap pad is placed into the wound and a Tegaderm™ placed over the pad to avoid leakage of gas during insufflation for the laparoscopic portion. The legs are taken out of extended lithotomy and the thighs are placed flat with the abdomen to avoid the right thigh getting in the surgeons way when performing the laparoscopic aspect of the surgery. Gowns, gloves, and instruments are changed and the abdominal portion commences.

Laparoscopic Abdominal Portion

There are two aspects of the laparoscopic portion of the dissection: the abdominal portion and the pelvic dissection, a laparoscopic TME. Port positions are shown in Figure 32.3. The patient's body habitus will determine whether we use the #4 (5 mm) port site for the eventual stoma site. It is generally ill advised to make any compromises in the ultimate location of a stoma in an effort to accommodate a port site used for a retractor, and the relative morbidity of an additional 5-mm port in the left lower quadrant is minimal. If the port site is not going to be used as the eventual stoma site, we like to move it well away so that it will not be underneath the stoma wafer as this position would predispose it to infection.

Laparoscopic Abdominal Dissection

Once the ports are placed, the 10-mm, 30-degree camera is utilized for a full exploration of the abdominal cavity. The splenic flexure does not need to be taken down for an APR. The patient is put in steep Trendelenburg right-side-down position to get the small bowel out of the pelvis. We perform the left colon mobilization in a medial to lateral approach. The medial aspect of the retroperitoneum is incised from the sacral promontory to the duodenal-jejunal junction, the hypogastric nerves are identified inferior to the IMA and swept posteriorly (Fig. 32.4). This is the essential landmark to assure that

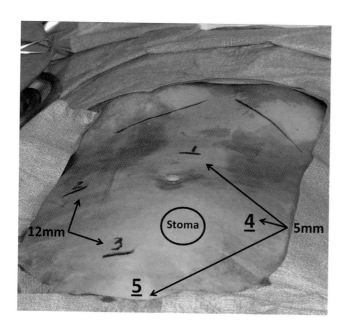

Figure 32.3 Port positions.

one is in the proper plane. There are areolar planes both posterior and anterior to the hypogastric nerves and one wants to be certain that they are anterior to avoid sexual or bladder dysfunction (Fig. 32.5). As the hypogastric nerves are swept down and the dissection is taken out laterally, the left ureter is identified. The dissection is taken up above the IMA. The IMV is dissected free from posterior retroperitoneal attachments leaving this intact. The IMV does not need to be ligated when performing an APR, but dissecting out along this plane will facilitate putting the surgeon in the proper space for the rest of the mobilization.

Once the mesentery of the left colon is mobilized fully in a medial to lateral fashion, the area of transection in the sigmoid colon is marked using a stitch placed intracorporeally for future recognition. The mesentery is transected by dividing the IMA distal to the takeoff of the left colic artery and extending the transection line to the sigmoid colon. We typically use a vessel sealing system (LigaSure™, Covidien, Norwalk, CT) to accomplish this maneuver, but it can also be done with a vascular stapling device or by dissecting out the vessel and placing clips or ties on it. Intracorporeal vascular control will facilitate the subsequent stoma creation.

The lateral attachments are incised along the white line of Toldt and in this way the colon is fully mobilized. The proximal extent of this dissection is taken to the

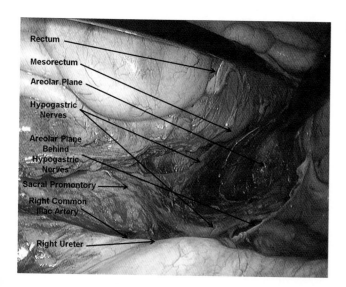

Figure 32.4 Posterior dissection.

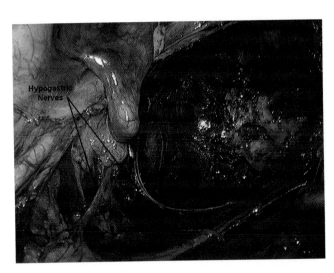

Figure 32.5 Total mesorectal excision.

splenic flexure, but the splenic flexure itself is not fully released. In some patients with a long redundant sigmoid colon, it is not necessary to do this more proximal release. Lastly, the sigmoid is transected with an Endo-GIA™ stapler. Once this is complete, attention is turned to the pelvis.

Laparoscopic Total Mesorectal Excision

The essential points to a laparoscopic TME are highlighted in Table 32.1.

A key to successful pelvic dissection has to do with minimizing blood in the field as this will both make it difficult to keep your endoscope lens clean and absorb light that significantly impairs visualization. The operation is started with the camera in the #2 port. The surgeon's left hand utilizes a laparoscopic Babcock grasper in the #1 port, while the right hand uses laparoscopic scissors in the #3 port. Through the #4 port in the left lower quadrant, a retracting grasper is placed and positioned anteriorly to hold up the pouch of Douglas and put the tissue on stretch in similar fashion as is done with a St. Marks retractor in open surgery. A suprapubic 5-mm port is placed and through this your first assistant uses a 5-mm suction device to retract the right pelvic sidewall laterally as well as aspirate at the time of activation of the energy source to clear the smoke and small amounts of blood that come onto the field. It is helpful to keep the area dry in order to facilitate a safe dissection and to minimize obscuring the view in the pelvis.

The incision along the retroperitoneum that went from the sacral promontory to the duodenum-jejunal junction is extended (Figs. 32.6 and 32.7) down along the right pararectal sulcus in the avascular crevice, which is identified. This dissection is best done with scissors or hook with electrocautery as they are thinner and thus are more precise than other instruments. A single cell layer of the retroperitoneum is incised down the right pararectal sulcus anteriorly, and then similarly down the left pararectal sulcus. Once this is opened (which we refer to as "opening the box"), a more substantial dissection can be carried out. This step entails additional retraction and duplication of steps to accomplish this.

Once the space is opened, the dissection continues posteriorly using sharp dissection with diathermy scissors or another energy device. The presacral space is dissected and opened anterior to the hypogastric nerves, which are visualized and protected. The

TABLE 32.1	Key Points to Laparoscopic TME

1. Three-dimensional retraction
2. Opening the box
3. Standardized dissection plan—posterior to anterior
4. Retraction with suction device

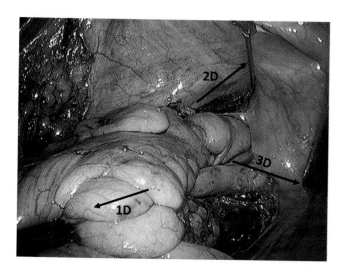

Figure 32.6 3D retraction.

grasper in the surgeon's left hand is used to anteriorly retract the rectum, with a suprapubic retractor placed, and finally by using the suction to retract the lateral rectal tissues to the side. The dissection is carried posteriorly extending to the level of the levators, after which it is brought around to the right side following the nerves for direction. By retracting as one comes along the right side with the left hand grasping the rectum and the suprapubic suction retractor of the assistant pulling out tissue laterally to the right, the areolar tissue plane is put in sharp contrast. Quite often, the perineal dissection can be entered from above posteriorly. This option is an additional advantage of starting the operation transanally, which facilitates the laparoscopic approach.

Dissection is then taken anteriorly. Oftentimes the #4 retractor needs to be repositioned to get exposure and the assistant using the suction device in the #5 port retracts anterior and laterally while the hand of the surgeon is pulling in a contralateral fashion toward the left shoulder. Once this is completed, the dissection is brought around in a similar fashion on the left side. Again following the hypogastric nerves, one stays anterior to this with the suprapubic retractor placed laterally while the #1 port retractor is in the surgeon's left hand superiorly retracting the mesorectum. The energy source is brought down along the areolar plane anterior to the nerves and the dissection is connected to the front, completing the TME.

Once this step is completed, the rectum can be brought out of the pelvis and the area inspected. If the dissection has been fully completed and the rectum brought out of the pelvis without difficulty, it is passed back down into the pelvis. Next, the previously placed proximal staple line of the sigmoid colon is brought out through the stoma

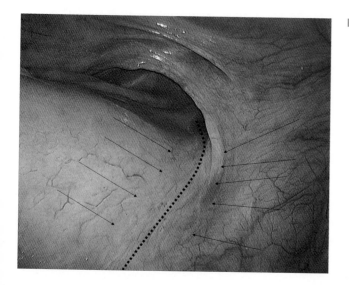

Figure 32.7 Line of incision.

Part VII: Abdominoperineal Resection

site in the left lower quadrant through a standard muscle-splitting technique. All port sites are closed and the stoma is matured. Gloves are changed and the specimen is removed through the perineal wound.

At times when the anterior portion of the dissection is particularly difficult from above, the abdomen is desufflated, the sigmoid colon is delivered posterior to the rectum through the perineal wound and brought out. In this way, the rectum is everted and leaves the last bit of adherence to be put on tension. This can then be completed from below without difficulty.

After delivery of the specimen the pelvic floor is closed using interrupted 0-Vicryl sutures. A drain is placed via a separate stab wound through the perineum. The skin is closed with 2-0 nylon suture in vertical mattress fashion. It should be noted that if there is a very large defect from extensive growth of tumor into the sidewall or vagina, consideration should always be given to muscle flap reconstruction at that time. The best flap is the right rectus abdominus muscle, in which case the entire operation would not have been done laparoscopically but through a midline laparotomy.

POSTOPERATIVE MANAGEMENT AND COMPLICATIONS

Postoperative management and complications are quite similar to these noted after open APR. We do not routinely employ nasogastric tube decompression. A bladder catheter is generally left in place until postoperative day 5 or taken out the night before discharge if they are going home sooner. Patients are generally started on clear liquid diet the day of or the day after surgery and then advanced to a GI soft diet the following day if their abdomen is nondistended, or they are not having excessive nausea or eructation. Perioperative antibiotics are used. It is important that the patient undergoes education with the stoma nurse regarding colostomy care. The perineal wound and the sutures in the perineum are generally left in place for at least 3 weeks. If there is any question about proper healing, they are taken out one at a time so that there is no problem with wound dehiscence.

RESULTS

Between January 1997 and October 2010, we have performed 370 laparoscopic TME, including laparoscopic APR, low anterior resection, proctectomy, total proctocolectomy, and TATA. Because the TATA procedure involves an intersphincteric dissection from the dentate line for tumors as low as 5 mm beneath the anorectal ring, we are able to avoid an APR in the majority of our patients with low rectal tumors. The only real distinction between APR and TATA is the perineal dissection, with the laparoscopic portion of the procedure being virtually the same. That being said, we have performed 49 true laparoscopic APRs for rectal adenocarcinoma (42), anal squamous cell carcinoma (4), anal gland carcinoma (1), radiation proctitis (1), and Crohn's disease (1). All procedures were elective and the average EBL was 320 ml; there were no significant intraoperative complications or conversion. The average number of lymph nodes harvested was 10 and the average length of stay was 6.4 days; there was no postoperative mortality. Postoperative complications included urinary retention, anemia requiring transfusion, DVT, prolonged ileus, erectile dysfunction, and perineal wound issues.

CONCLUSIONS

Laparoscopic APR and TME offer a significant secondary benefit for patients with rectal cancer. Clearly of paramount concern in the rectal cancer patient is the ability to have their cancer properly controlled, not metastasize elsewhere, and not develop a local recurrence. It is imperative that the surgeon never lose sight of these points. That said, the secondary benefits of less trauma to the abdomen, recovering more quickly from surgery as well as potential benefits of decreased bowel obstruction, less blood loss and transfusions, and the immediate diminution of pain make laparoscopic APR a real benefit to patients requiring an APR. The ACOSOG Z6051 trial and COLOR II trial reports will possibly be complete by the time of publication of this chapter and the issues regarding the safety and adequacy of laparoscopic TME and APR will likely be firmly established. Our experience, as well as that of other centers in the world, clearly shows that this procedure is safe and feasible. These trials will establish the general application of these techniques.

The major technical point we tried to highlight in this chapter is the significant benefit of opening the peritoneum, which facilitates the surgeons' staying in the proper plane laparoscopically when doing a TME. We have found that, in particular, the three-dimensional retraction technique as described earlier is essential in terms of improving our visualization and outcomes for full TME in laparoscopic surgery of the rectum.

Suggested Readings

Baker R, White E, Titu L, et al. Does laparoscopic abdominoperineal resection of the rectum compromise long-term survival? *Dis Colon Rectum* 2002;45:1481–85.

Chmielik E, Bujko K, Nasierowska-Guttmejer A, et al. Distal intramural spread of rectal cancer after preoperative radiotherapy: the results of a multicenter randomized clinical study. *Int J Radiat Oncol Biol Phys* 2006;65:182–8.

Clinical Outcomes of Surgical Therapy Study Group. A comparison of laparoscopically assisted and open colectomy for colon cancer. *N Engl J Med* 2004;350:2050–9.

Folkesson J, Birgisson H, Pahlman L, et al. Swedish rectal cancer trial: long lasting benefits from radiotherapy on survival and local recurrence rate. *J Clin Oncol* 2005;23:5644–60.

Jensen L, Altaf R, Harling H, et al. Clinical outcome in 520 consecutive Danish rectal cancer patients treated with short course preoperative radiotherapy. *Eur J Surg Oncol* 2010;36:237–43.

Leroy J, Jamali F, Forbes L, et al. Laparoscopic total mesorectal excision (TME) for rectal cancer surgery: long-term outcomes. *Surg Endosc* 2004;18:281–9.

Marks G, Bannon J, Marks J. Transanal-abdominal transanal-radical proctosigmoidectomy with coloanal anastomosis for distal rectal cancer. In: Baker R, Fischer J, Nyhus L, eds. *Mastery of Surgery*. 3rd ed. Philadelphia, PA: Lippincott Williams & Wilkins, 1996; 1524–1531.

Marks J, Mizrahi B, Dalane S, et al. Laparoscopic transanal abdominal transanal resection with sphincter preservation for rectal cancer in the distal 3 cm of the rectum after neoadjuvant therapy. *Surg Endosc* 2010;24:2700–7.

Mehigan B, Monson J. Laparoscopic rectal-abdominoperineal resection. *Surg Oncol Clin N Am* 2001;10:611–23.

Ng S, Leung K, Lee J, et al. Laparoscopic-assisted versus open abdominoperineal resection for low rectal cancer: a prospective randomized trial. *Ann Surg Oncol* 2008;15:2418–25.

Roh M, Colangelo L, O'Connell M, et al. Preoperative multimodality therapy improves disease-free survival in patients with carcinoma of the rectum: NSABP R-03. *J Clin Oncol* 2009;27::5124–30.

Swedish Rectal Cancer Trial. Improved survival with preoperative radiotherapy in resectable rectal cancer. *New Engl J Med* 1997; 336:980–87.

33 Hand-Assisted Laparoscopic Abdominoperineal Resection (HAL-APR)

Hak-Su Goh and Dean C-S Koh

INDICATIONS/CONTRAINDICATIONS

Abdominoperineal resection (APR) is not just a mutilating operation. It also profoundly alters the lifestyle of a patient. It is therefore the most dreaded of all colorectal operations, and as such it is not uncommon for a surgeon to be told, "I would rather die than to have a stoma." Fortunately, in current practice, APR is fast disappearing to become an "endangered" operation.

Diminishing requirement for APR is brought about by a combination of advances in anastomotic techniques, advent of transanal local excision, advances in chemoradiotherapy, and a better appreciation of the natural history of anorectal cancer (Table 33.1).

For over 50 years, following the description by Miles in 1908 (1), APR was the only treatment for anorectal cancer until the introduction, followed by the slow acceptance, of anterior resection by Dixon in 1948 (2). This was a high-risk operation with significant anastomotic leak rates and mortality. Circular surgical staples popularized in the 1980s, and now accepted worldwide, allow for a safer and lower anastomosis.

A seminal advance in surgical technique is total mesorectal excision (TME) as championed by Heald (3). It dramatically improves local control of rectal cancer and allows ultra-low anterior resection to be performed. APR can be further avoided by using intersphincteric dissection with coloanal anastomosis (4,5). Functional results are not necessarily compromised by such low anastomoses because of colonic pouches, end-to-side anastomosis, or coloplasty, as well as adopting very precise rectal dissection that preserves pelvic sympathetic and parasympathetic nerves (6–9). Although transanal local excision and transanal endoscopic microscopic (TEM) excision have significant recurrence rates of 20–25%, it is an important option for the very elderly and infirmed patients who are not suitable for major surgery (10).

TABLE 33.1	Reasons for Diminishing Abdominoperineal Resection	
Timeline	**Surgical progress**
1900	Abdomino-perineal resection. Mile's operation
1950	Anterior resection
1980	Surgical staples. Safer and lower anastomosis
1990	TME—total mesorectal excision. Ultra-low anastomosis
2000	Intersphincteric dissection. Coloanal anastomosis
	Advent of local excision
1980	Transanal local excision
1980	TEM—transanal endoscopic microscopic excision
	Advances in chemoradiotherapy
1970	Nonsurgical treatment of anal cancer. Nigro regime
1990	Neoadjuvant chemoradiotherapy. Downstage, shrinkage and complete response
	Better understanding of natural history of rectal cancer
2000	Rational treatment of metastatic rectal cancer

In 1974, Norman Nigro pioneered the use of chemoradiotherapy in place of APR for anal cancers (11). The results were just as good, with the bonus of avoiding a permanent stoma. It quickly became the treatment of choice for nonadenocarcinoma anal cancers. APR is therefore reserved for salvaging failed chemoradiotherapy.

At present, neoadjuvant chemoradiotherapy can achieve a response rate of up to 60% for rectal adenocarcinomas, and a complete response rate of 20% in some cases (12,13). These response rates will continue to improve with ever-improving chemotherapeutic agents. With significant shrinkage and downstaging of tumors, more sphincter-saving procedures can be performed, which otherwise would require APR. The most exciting information would be the long-term outcomes of those cancers with clinical complete response. If survival and recurrence rates are similar to those of surgical excision, the need for APR will be further reduced. With metastatic rectal cancer, the standard approach has been rectal surgery first, including an APR, before chemotherapy, followed by liver or lung resections when possible (14). The rationale is to have surgical reduction of tumor bulk as well as to prevent future complications from the primary tumor such as intestinal obstruction or bleeding. The removal of the primary tumor may also prolong survival by about 5 months (15,16). This paradigm may need to be changed.

The age-standardized relative survival ratio for metastatic colorectal cancer in the United States is 5.4% for males and 7.5% for females. In Singapore, which has similar cancer survival data as Europe, it is 3.5% and 2.8%, respectively (17). With such poor survival, surgeons must take a step back to reflect on the wisdom of rushing into a mutilating operation. There are reports suggesting that, with improved chemotherapy, the incidence of future primary tumor complications is 10% or less, much lower than what is generally assumed (18). The response rate, including complete response, to neoadjuvant chemoradiotherapy is gradually increasing. It is therefore increasingly difficult to justify APR for metastatic rectal cancer especially if there is complete response to chemoradiotherapy.

APR should be an operation of last resort when surgery is needed and sphincter salvage is not possible, such as when an adenocarcinoma has invaded the sphincter muscles or when chemoradiotherapy has failed (Fig. 33.1). Palliative APR is sometimes indicated for symptom control, but accurate preoperative assessment is critical because cutting through tumor tissues would invariably lead to local recurrence. Tumor fungating through a perineal wound is one of the most distressing problems to manage. To the purist laparoscopic colorectal surgeons, hand-assisted laparoscopic abdominoperineal resection (HAL-APR) is an oxymoron. The ultimate goal of laparoscopic surgery is to avoid having a tumor extraction abdominal scar; therefore, APR is an ideal full laparoscopic operation as the tumor is removed from the perineum. Nevertheless, the advantages of hand-assisted laparoscopic colorectal surgery over conventional open

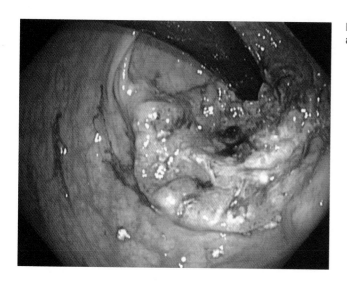

Figure 33.1 Invasive adenocarcinoma at the anorectal junction.

surgery have been shown to be similar to full laparoscopic surgery (19). The remaining problem is the incisional scar from placement of the handport. Although it can be partially hidden in the skin crease of a Pfannenstiel incision, it is best to position the scar on the planned end-colostomy site to hide the scar completely.

PREOPERATIVE PLANNING

In a case of low rectal cancer, a careful digital examination of the location, position, and fixity of the tumor is important. The critical landmark is the puborectalis muscle. It is possible to feel the distance of the tumor above the muscle as well as invasion of the muscle.

The distance between the lower margins of the tumor from the anal verge is then measured with a rigid rectoscope (sigmoidoscope) and recorded. The position of the tumor: anterior, posterior, right, or left lateral, is also determined. This orientation will influence the rectal dissection such as dissecting in front of, or behind the Denonvilliers' fascia (20); resecting a posterior cuff of the vagina; or preserving the left or right inferior hypogastric nerves (nervi erigentes). Digital examination can also differentiate mobile tumors from fixed tumors according to fixity to the underlying muscles, especially the sphincter muscles.

For a mobile tumor, it is best to evaluate with transrectal ultrasound (TRUS), which is sensitive and accurate in assessing tumor invasion of the submucosa or the muscularis propria. For a tumor with only minimal invasion of the submucosa, the best treatment option is local excision or TEM. For a fixed tumor, the examination of choice is rectal magnetic resonance imaging (MRI). The depth of muscle invasion and probable lymph node involvement (size >8 mm, irregular border or mixed signal intensity) are better demonstrated than TRUS or CT scan. Following TRUS examination, CT scan of the thorax, abdomen, and pelvis is performed to assess for distant metastasis. If rectal MRI has been performed, CT scan of the thorax and the abdomen would suffice.

Before major rectal surgery is planned, it is absolutely essential to have a positive histological diagnosis of an adenocarcinoma. Squamous or epidermoid cancers are treated by chemoradiotherapy. Tuberculous masses or atypical inflammatory masses, which may mimic rectal cancers are not to be treated by APR. If distant metastasis is present, the patient is again best treated with chemoradiotherapy first. APR is reserved for those who have failed chemoradiotherapy or palliation of distressing symptoms. When APR is inevitable, the preoperative general preparation is similar to that of any major surgery. Patients with colorectal cancer are usually elderly with significant comorbidities. Cardiac, respiratory, or renal insufficiencies need to be corrected and optimized.

Diabetes is a major problem worldwide, not just a problem of developed countries. In Singapore, 20% of colorectal cancer patients are diabetic. They are converted to insulin on a sliding scale for their surgery with close blood glucose monitoring postoperatively until regular diet is reestablished.

Specific preoperative preparation includes the following:

- Height and weight of patients to calculate their body mass index (BMI). Morbidly obese patients, BMI >35 kg/m^2, have significantly higher risks of wound infection and dehiscence, pulmonary embolism (PE), and renal failure (21). Perineal wound breakdown is already a major problem in patients who have received neoadjuvant chemoradiotherapy.
- Serum carcinoembryonic antigen (CEA) and Ca 19.9 levels. Both may be useful in patient follow-up as persistently raised or rising cancer marker levels would indicate residual disease or recurrent disease. In addition, CEA may have a prognostic value especially in Stage II disease. In colon cancer, combination of raised CEA, lymphovascular invasion, and poorly differentiated adenocarcinoma is found to carry a poorer prognosis (22).
- Deep vein thrombosis prophylaxis. For Caucasian patients, a combination of mechanical foot pumps and low-molecular-weight heparin prophylaxis is routine, but it remains a controversy in Asian patients. There is evidence that PE following surgery is less common among Asians, especially in Chinese patients (23,24). For these patients, full prophylactic measures are reserved only for high-risk patients (those with a history of DVT or PE, morbidly obese patients, and patients with a large tumor load). For average-risk patients, only mechanical foot pumps are used routinely.
- Preoperative siting of colostomy. If a stoma therapist service is available, this is most helpful. If not, the surgeon performs the siting himself or herself. Clear instruction and stoma education go a long way to reduce patient bewilderment and anxiety.
- Pain team and patient controlled anesthesia (PCA). One of the major fears of any surgical patient is pain. A pain team giving clear instruction on pain-relieving procedures such as PCA is very reassuring to patients. They can reduce not only physical pain, but also anxiety.
- Physiotherapy. Physiotherapists play a very important part in the surgical team. Preoperative breathing exercises with the aid of a spirometer is important for minimizing postoperative chest atelectasis and infection especially for smokers. Education on the benefits of early postoperative mobilization and ambulation will encourage patients to ambulate early. The basic belief in many Asian communities is that staying immobilized in bed for as long as possible is best for recuperation and wound healing.
- Bowel preparation. Traditionally, full mechanical bowel preparation is routine for APR. Recent evidence has shown that this is not necessary. Fleet enema to clear the rectosigmoid fecal loading is now considered sufficient.

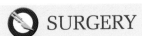

SURGERY

Conventional synchronous combined APR involves two teams of surgeons operating on the abdomen and perineum simultaneously. With the laparoscopic approach, this procedure is performed sequentially. For laparoscopic dissection, the thighs have to be positioned horizontally at the hip joints for optimal laparoscopic light, instrument, and hand access to the pelvis, while the perineal dissection requires the thighs to be fully flexed to adequately "present" the perineum; for laparoscopic surgery, the abdomen needs to be distended with carbon dioxide (CO_2) and this would be lost once the pelvis is entered from the perineum.

Positioning

Under standard general anesthesia, epidural analgesia is optional, the patient is positioned on the operating table as in a standard laparoscopic anterior resection (Fig. 33.2).

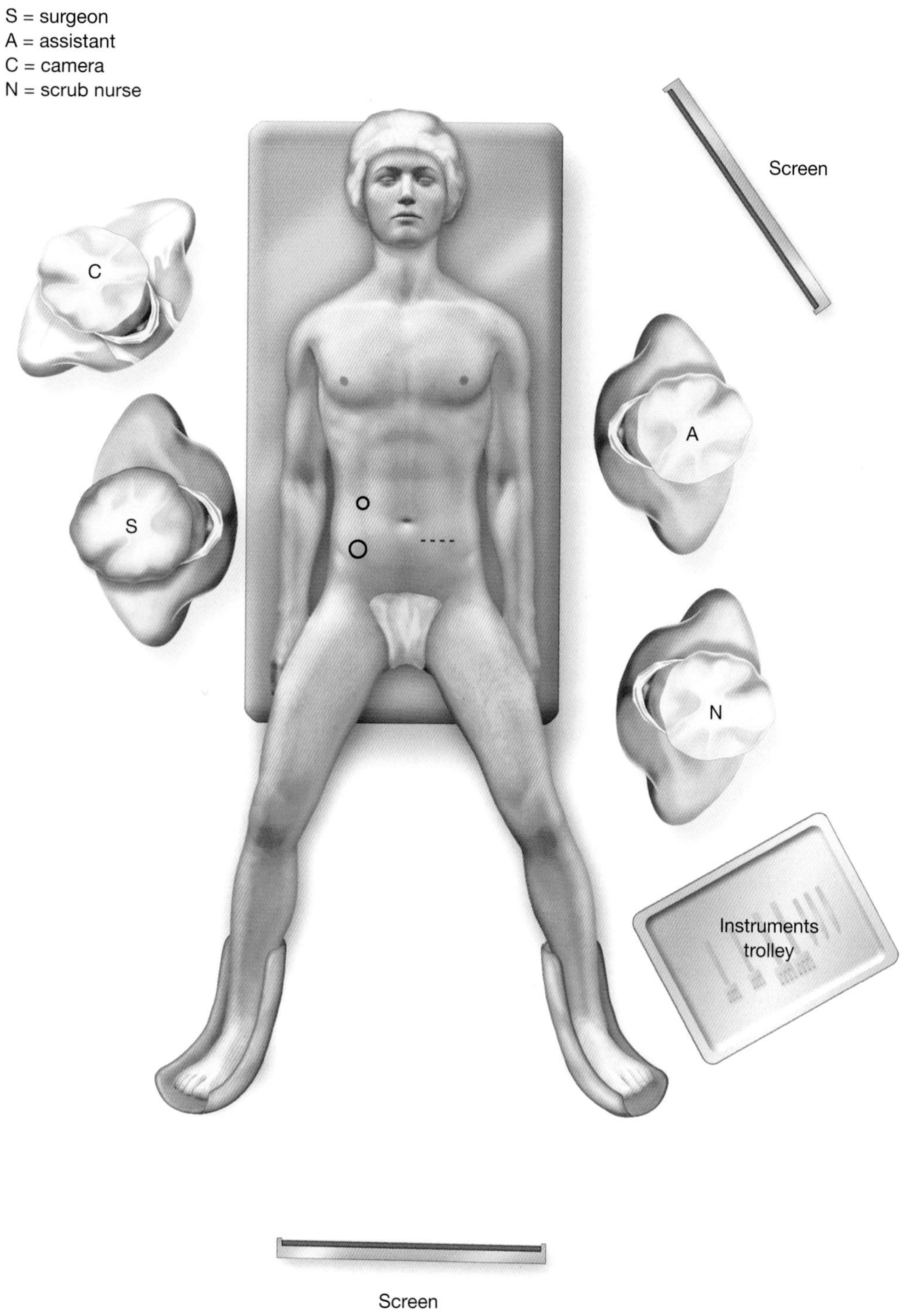

S = surgeon
A = assistant
C = camera
N = scrub nurse

Figure 33.2 Operating team
positions.

Screen

C

A

S

N

Instruments
trolley

Screen

There are two pertinent requirements, the legs need to be in adjustable stirrups like Allen or Yellowfin stirrups for easy flexing of the thighs, and the perineum needs to be lifted off the table by placing the sacrum on a sand bag, or placing the patient on a bean bag.

Both arms are tucked- in on the sides of the patient and it is important to ensure that the patient does not slide when tilted. The use of shoulder supports is necessary if the patient is not on a bean bag. A purse string is stitched round the anus to seal it off to avoid fecal spillage to the perineal wound.

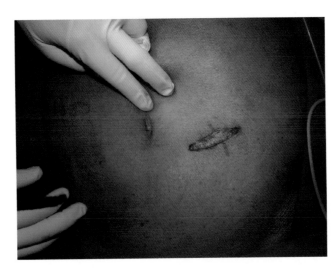

Figure 33.3 Incision for handport and colostomy.

Abdominal Part

Depending on personal preference, either the GelPort (Applied Medical, Rancho Santa Margarita, CA, USA) or Dextrus (Ethicon Endosurgery, Cincinnati, OH, USA) can be used for the handport. A horizontal line is marked on the colostomy site. Depending on the shape and size of the patient, the handport extends on both sides of the colostomy, or if possible, it extends only from the lateral side (Fig. 33.3). The length of incision should be one size, in centimeters, less than the surgeon's glove size. Once all the layers of the abdominal wall are cut through, the wound is first entered and stretched with a smaller hand of a female assistant or nurse (Fig. 33.4). Once that is done, the surgeon's hand can be inserted after lubricating with water or an aqueous based gel. This maneuver allows a smaller incision to be used.

Another technique, based on the concept that the skin is stretchable, as advocated by Dr. L. Sasaki (25) is to use a three-finger breath skin incision followed by undermining of subcutaneous and muscular layers to individual glove size. The opposing abdominal wounds are then held open by two stay-sutures (which hold together the skin, subcutaneous fat, muscles, and peritoneum) for easier insertion of the retractor ring of the handport. The well-lubricated surgeon's nondominant hand is then slowly inserted into the abdomen by progressively stretching the skin. With this technique, a median skin incision of 4-cm length can be achieved. A 10-mm port is then inserted through the GelPort cover before it is clicked into position. CO_2 insufflation can then start, the gas flow should be adequate (usually 10–20 l/min) as moving the hand in and out of

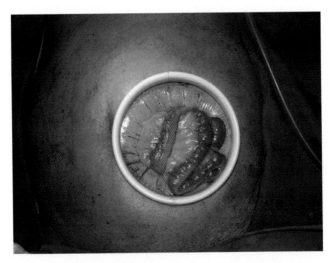

Figure 33.4 Handport retraction ring in place.

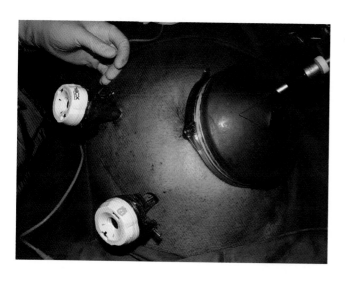

Figure 33.5 Camera through handport for initial laparoscopy and port placements.

the GelPort tends to fully deflate the abdominal insufflation. The camera is then introduced for a careful laparoscopic examination of the abdomen (Fig. 33.5).

In surgery, it is best to adopt a philosophy of "sensible expedience rather dogmatic purism." If at this early stage, adhesions are seen and easily accessible from the handport incision particularly in a patient with previous surgery, they should be quickly taken down with the diathermy or scissors. There is no need to wait for such adhesiolysis to be performed laparoscopically, which takes longer. A 10-mm port is then inserted cephalad and lateral to the umbilicus and a 12-mm working port is placed medial and cephalad to the anterior superior iliac spine. It is advisable to use the Xcel Bladeless port (Ethicon Endo-Surgery, Cincinnati, OH, USA) as it provides the flexibility for using a vascular endostapler, LigaSure (Valleylab, Boulder, CO, USA), or 10-mm Hem-o-lock clips (Weck Closure Systems, Triangle Park, NC, USA) for securing large vessels like the inferior mesenteric artery (IMA). A left lower quadrant 5-mm port is best inserted at the later stage of dissection when retraction of the anterior peritoneal reflection is required. This helps to reduce the chance of "clashing" of instruments (Fig. 33.6).

After careful laparoscopy and palpation with the hand in the abdomen, it is always worthwhile to take time to organize the abdominal content to have a good view of the operative field. With the body in a steep Trendelenburg position and with the left side tilted up, the omentum is first "placed" over the transverse colon, which is pushed as far over the liver as possible. The small bowel is then coaxed with a pair of bowel forceps to the right upper quadrant away from the pelvis and the left colon to expose the right side of the mesorectum and the root of the IMA. If the small bowel is not directed away nicely, it tends to fall into the operative field obscuring the view and getting into danger of heat injury from either an ultrasonic or a diathermy-dissecting device. The trocar through the GelPort is then removed and the left hand is inserted to lift up the mesorectum (Fig. 33.7). In a female patient, if necessary it is possible to pass a 2.0 Prolene stitch on a straight needle to secure the uterus to the abdominal wall, out of the operative field.

The Ace Harmonic Scalpel (Ethicon Endo-Surgery, Cincinnati, OH, USA) is a versatile and suitable dissecting device. With the hand-control switch, it is more convenient as it allows the surgeon to move positions easily dispensing with the need to transfer the foot pedals around with changes of the operator's position. The peritoneum at the base of the mesorectum at the level of the sacral promontory is incised (Fig. 33.8). This allows air to insinuate into the right tissue plane to aid dissection. Dissection is then carried cephalad and the left thumb can now lift up the IMA. The hypogastric nerves are identified next, the plane of dissection is between the nerves and the artery. Dissection is then extended laterally from the medical position. The thin areolar tissue enveloping the left ureter and gonadal vessels is next identified. It is dissected from its attachment to the peritoneum above and continued laterally until the white line of Toldt comes into view. With the nerves, ureter, and gonadal vessels identified, dissection can

Figure 33.6 Port positions.

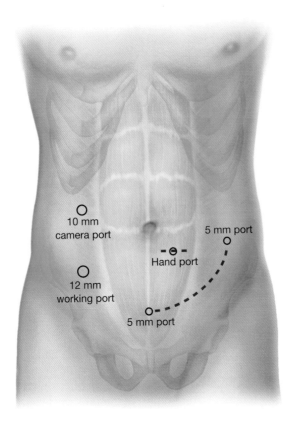

10 mm
camera port

5 mm port

Hand port

12 mm
working port

5 mm port

safely proceed proximally to the origin of the IMA (Fig. 33.9). If enlarged lymph nodes are present, they are carefully dissected off their posterior attachments and removed *en bloc*. The IMA is then skeletonized and the left colic artery identified. High or low ligation depends on whether the ligation is above or below the left colic arterial branch. The IMA is ligated and transected with LigaSure, Hem-o-lock clips, or a vascular endostapler (Fig. 33.10). Attachment of the sigmoid colon to the lateral abdominal wall are then released and the peritoneum along the white line of Toldt dissected. Attention can now turn to the pelvis. From the promontory with the rectum pulled forward, a thin areolar plane (the "Holy Plane" becomes clear) (Fig. 33.11). This plane is dissected with the harmonic scalpel in a sweeping curve following the curvature of the sacrum keeping in front of the hypogastric nerves and Waldeyer's fascia and behind the mesorectal

Figure 33.7 Rectum retracted by hand to show medical aspect of the mesorectum.

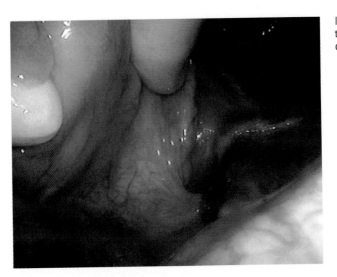

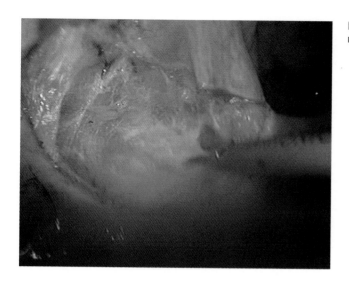

Figure 33.8 Dissection of the mesorectum.

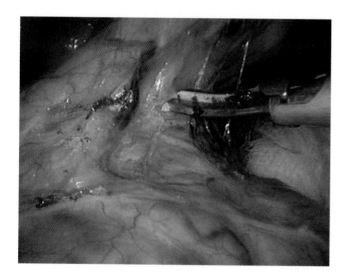

Figure 33.9 Dissecting toward origin of inferior mesenteric artery.

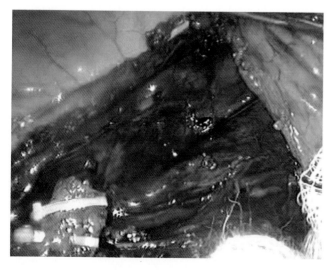

Figure 33.10 Ligated inferior mesenteric artery with view of left ureter and gonadal vessels.

Part VII: Abdominoperineal Resection

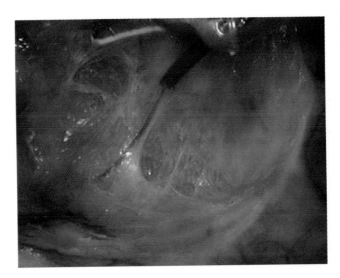

Figure 33.11 Entering the "Holy Plane" of mesorectum with sacral promontory in the foreground.

envelope, the lateral margins of the pelvis become clear and can be dissected downward, which would help dissection of the lowest posterior part of the rectum. Once the median artery is ligated, the rectum can be lifted and posterior dissection completed. With hand-assisted rectal surgery, it is easy to mobilize the posterior aspect and right lateral margin of the rectum but for the left lateral margin, the hand may sometimes gets in the way of the camera and harmonic scalpel. This is remedied by removing the hand and inserting a 5-mm port through the GelPort; the left pelvic margin can be dissected as in full laparoscopic dissection. If there is blood in the pelvis, pieces of gauze swabs can be introduced through the GelPort to keep the operating field dry and clear.

Anteriorly, the peritoneal reflection is mobilized next. At this point, an optimal position in along a line between the suprapubic region and the left anterior superior iliac spine (Fig. 33.6) the left lower quadrant is selected to insert the 5-mm port for a grasper to lift up the peritoneal reflection. When proceeding caudally, the Denonvilliers' fascia will come into view. With preoperative chemoradiotherapy, this fascia is more prominent. For a posterior tumor it is best to dissect behind the fascia, which is easier and less likely to bleed. However, with an anterior tumor, it is better oncologically, to dissect in front of the Denonvilliers' fascia, which is more vascular.

Next, the deep lateral walls are mobilized keeping close to the pelvic wall. It is important to note the position of the nervi erigentes. Up to 50% of APR can result in sexual and urinary dysfunction including impotence. If it is a laterally located cancer and one side of parasympathetic nerves needs to be sacrificed, care should then be taken to preserve the opposite set of nerves. It is important to note that these nerves are difficult to identify with the naked eye, especially when there is bleeding during the dissection. Again with conventional laparoscopic camera system, the nerves are difficult to see. But with high definition (HD) camera system, they are quite visible. With a robot, especially one from the newer generation, which has 3D vision, HD camera system and magnification, the nerves are very obvious (Fig. 33.12 and 33.13).

For an ultra-low anterior resection, dissection would converge to the center once the pelvic floor is reached. For APR, converging dissection could create "waisting" and might compromise the circumferential margin and surgical outcome. It is important to remember the tumor location and allow for 1-cm lateral clearance whenever possible. "Cylindrical APR" is another technique to maximize circumferential clearance by cutting the pelvic floor muscles at the pelvic wall.

End-Colostomy

At this stage, one is ready to prepare for the end-colostomy. As a good practice, it is best to irrigate the pelvis and to ensure complete hemostasis. A good way to locate small bleeding vessels is to instill water and to look for small "springs" of red in the clear water.

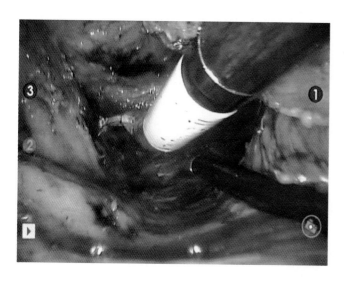

Figure 33.12 Left nervi erigentes in robotic dissection of lower mesorectum. (Courtesy of Prof. SH Kim and Dr. DN Sohn, Seoul, South Korea.)

The sigmoid colon is next delivered through the handport after detaching the GelPort cover. The laparoscope is removed, insufflation turned off and the theater operating lights switched on. A suitable section of the sigmoid is selected for fashioning a colostomy. The mesentery is divided appropriately. To be sure of a good blood supply, the marginal artery is transected without clamping to check for pulsatile blood flow. The ends of the blood vessels are then tied or sealed with the harmonic scalpel. The selected section of the colon is transected with a linear stapling device such as the TLC 75 Linear Cutter (Ethicon Endo-Surgery, Cincinnati, OH, USA) (Fig. 33.14). The divided ends of the colon are cleansed with antiseptic (chlorhexidine) soaked gauze.

Perineal Dissection

For the perineal dissection, the surgeon sits facing the perineum with a small instrument table in front. The patient's hips and knees are adequately flexed to "present" the perineum, which is cleared off the table by the sandbag supporting the sacrum. In a female patient, the vagina needs to be prepared with the perineal skin preparation. In a male patient, a "shield" incision is made with a blade with the transverse incision over the perineal body. The incision is developed further with a cutting diathermy pencil maintaining strict hemostasis when the cutaneous layer is cut through. The medial margins are folded together and held with three pairs of "tissue" clamps (Littlewoods). The lateral margins are then spread laterally outward with the Goligher's perineal retractor. This

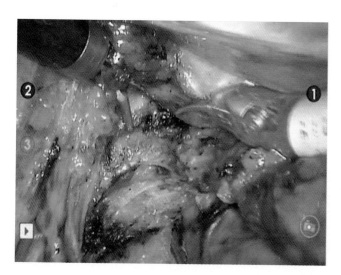

Figure 33.13 Latero-anterior course of left nervi erigentes in robotic dissection. (Courtesy of Prof. SH Kim and Dr. DN Sohn, Seoul, South Korea.)

Part VII: Abdominoperineal Resection

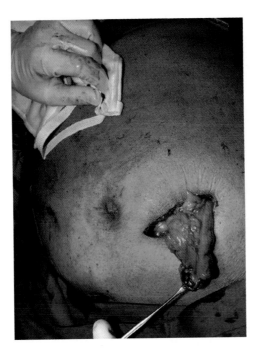

Figure 33.14 Transected colon through handport incision.

will create a bloodless plane in between the fat surrounding the anal canal and the ischiorectal fossae. This plane is developed circumferentially. Blood vessels can be identified, cauterized, and divided to create a bloodless field. This is proceeded circumferentially until the inferior aspect of the levator ani muscle is seen (Fig. 33.15).

To enter the pelvis, it is safest to approach posteriorly, dissecting anteriorly from below the tip of the coccyx. Once the Waldeyer's fascia is breached, the pelvis proper is entered. The pelvic floor can now be safely and accurately divided by placing the index finger of one hand into the pelvis and hooking down a section of the pelvic floor for division with a diathermy point set in coagulation mode to minimize bleeding. The posterior section is divided first followed by each lateral wall. Individual blood vessel can be identified and cauterized. In this manner, the whole circumference around the rectum is dissected free and the specimen is delivered perineally (Fig. 33.16).

If the anterior plane is not clearly defined, the transected rectum may be delivered out of the pelvis from the divided pelvic floor posteriorly, tension applied downward, and the anterior plane of dissection will be clearly exposed. In a female patient with an anterior rectal tumor, the perineal incision is modified to include a segment of the posterior vaginal wall to obtain optimal cancer clearance. When there are two entry points into the pelvis, anteriorly and posteriorly, resection of the pelvic floor is much easier.

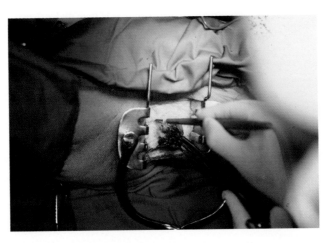

Figure 33.15 Perineal dissection of the rectum with Goligher's retractor.

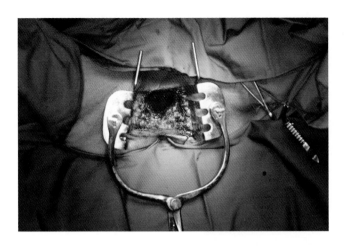

Figure 33.16 Completed resection of the rectum.

Once the rectum is removed, meticulous hemostasis is carried out, facilitated by water irrigation poured from the pelvis above. The perineal wound is closed with two layers of interrupted 2.0 Vicryl (polyglactin) sutures. It is preferable to close the vagina rather than to leave it open for drainage and this is done using 3.0 Vicryl. The perineal skin can be sutured or closed with skin staples.

Attention is now moved to the abdomen and pelvis. To prevent the small bowel from dropping into pelvic cavity, it is best to close the pelvic peritoneum with continuous or "figure-of-eight" interrupted 2.0 Vicryl accessing from the handport incision (Fig. 33.17). In a female patient, with an intact uterus, this can be used to "plug" the pelvic inlet. Before closure, a soft drain such as a Jackson-Pratt drain (Cardinal Health, McGaw Park, IL, USA) is first inserted into the perineum and brought out of the abdominal wall. It is more comfortable than having a drain sticking out of the perineum.

Closing Handport Wound and Fashioning of End-Colostomy

The rectus fascia is closed with interrupted PDS I (polydioxanone) on one side or both sides of the terminal colon, which is held snugly. The subcutaneous fat is apposed with 3.0 Vicryl. A subcuticular suture is then applied with "buried" suture ends to accurately appose the skin. The skin is finally sealed with Dermabond skin adhesive (Closure Medical Corp., Ethicon, Inc.). The colostomy is then matured with interrupted undyed absorbable 4.0 Vicryl (Figs. 33.18 and 33.19).

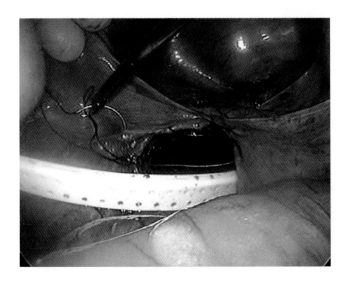

Figure 33.17 Closure of pelvic peritoneum with JP drain in the pelvic cavity.

Part VII: Abdominoperineal Resection

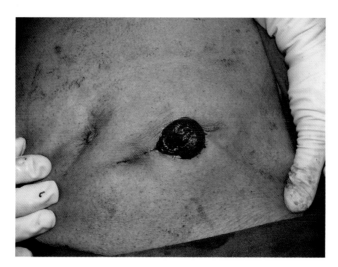

Figure 33.18 Subcuticular suture of handport incision and maturing of end-colostomy.

 POSTOPERATION MANAGEMENT

As for any patient undergoing major surgery, an HAL-APR patient is closely monitored in the first 24 hours after surgery paying particular attention to possible reactionary hemorrhage, cardiac or respiratory dysfunctions, and to ensure adequate urine output and satisfactory pain control.

Hematological investigations are performed in the first postoperative day to check for hemoglobin (Hb) level, total white cell count, urea, electrolytes, and creatinine levels, and liver enzymes, protein, and albumin. These are to be corrected if abnormal. Blood transfusion is usually not necessary if the Hb is 10 gm% or more. Clear feeds are allowed as soon as the patient is conscious. It is very difficult to talk and communicate if the mouth is dry. Full feeds are started on the first postoperative day and soft diet the following day. Oral medications, including analgesics can be started early and parenteral narcotics, including PCA, can be tailed off quickly.

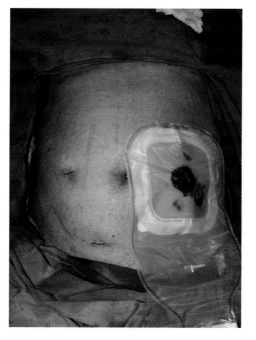

Figure 33.19 Handport incision completely hidden by colostomy bag.

The patient is started on chest physiotherapy and mobilized on the first postoperative day. As soon as the colostomy starts to function, a stomatherapy nurse begins to teach the patient and the family members on the care of the permanent stoma. Postoperative recovery and return to normal activity for HAL are similar to full laparoscopic APR.

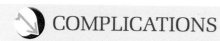

COMPLICATIONS

Complications specific to HAL-APR relate to the use of the handport incision at the end-colostomy site. The worry is that of wound infection, but this is minimized, when the incision is closed properly and perioperative antibiotic prophylaxis is given.

The other concern is parastomal hernia occurrence. This is a problem shared by all end-colostomies. In the presence of a wound dehiscence, an eventual parastomal hernia is inevitable. In addition to preventing wound dehiscence, it is possible to reduce the incidence of a parastomal hernia by prophylactically delivering the end-colostomy through a "holed" prolene mesh (26), which is placed in the extraperitoneal layer of the abdominal wound.

RESULTS

There is a paucity of publication on HAL-APR. A literature search yielded only one article, which is in Chinese from the Peking Union Medical College, Beijing, China. Six cases of HAL-APR for low rectal cancer were reported with one conversion because of pelvic adhesions. The mean operating time was 180 minutes and the mean hospital stay was 14 days. The conclusion was that HAL-APR is a "safe and simple" procedure (27). Our own experience of HAL-APR is limited to nine cases of low rectal cancer. The mean operating time was 208 minutes (150–295) and mean length of incision for the GelPort was 6.1 cm (6–6.5 cm). After a mean follow-up of 23.3 months, there were no wound infection and no local recurrence, but two patients developed parastomal hernias.

The largest experience of laparoscopic rectal cancer resection is probably from Michael Li's group from Hong Kong (28). A total of 579 patients had full laparoscopic resection, including 92 laparoscopic APRs, over a period of 15 years. The cancer-specific 5- and 10-year survival was 76% and 56%, respectively. Seventy-one of the 92 laparoscopic APRs were entered into a nonrandomized but prospective trial with 31 open APRs (29). The median operating time was similar (145 min laparoscopic vs. 156 min open), but there were significantly less blood loss, less abdominal wound and chest infection, as well as better overall survival in the laparoscopic group. The conclusion is that laparoscopic APR is safe, it confers short-term health-related benefits, and it may have long-term survival benefit.

For colonic surgery, HAL resection has been shown in a prospective randomized trial (19) as well as a systematic review and meta-analysis (30) to have the same short-term benefits as laparoscopic colon resection but carries a significant operating time advantage. For rectal surgery, a prospective nonrandomized study for ultra-low anterior resection with TME, HAL resection was found to have similar short-term benefits as laparoscopic resection and again have significantly shorter operating time (31).

With anecdotal experience of HAL-APR and with the excellent results of laparoscopic rectal cancer resection reported by premier institutions, it is tempting to extrapolate the fine results of laparoscopic APR to HAL-APR. Such extrapolation should be tempered with caution. A recent review of laparoscopic and open elective colon and rectal resections in the English National Health Service Trusts hospitals between 1996 and 2006, in which laparoscopic surgery was only 1.9% of 192,620 total number of cases, showed that patients after laparoscopic rectal resection for malignancy were more likely to be readmitted after discharge from hospital (32).

The final answer of the role of HAL for APR can only be found in a properly conducted prospective randomized trial. But such a trial would be difficult, if not impossible, to do because of the diminishing number of APR. Even a trial such as the European multicenter COLOR 11 Trial, comparing laparoscopic and open rectal cancer removal is taking a long time to complete. It started in 2003, and is estimated to be completed in 2017 (33).

A possible solution is to establish collaboration with institutions in China or India where the number of colorectal cancer is very huge and furthermore, its incidence is increasing. In parallel with their fast economic developments, their acquisition of expertise in laparoscopic surgery and uptake of surgical technology are phenomenally rapid. A case in point is the West China Hospital, Sichuan University, Chengdu, China; it sees around 1,400 cases of colorectal cancer a year and complex laparoscopic ultra-low anterior resection with TME as well as lateral lymph node dissection is widely performed (34).

✥ CONCLUSION

APR is now a rare operation. HAL-APR has the same advantages as a full laparoscopic APR of less pain, shorter hospital stay, and earlier return to normal activity. Its advantages over full laparoscopic APR include easier orientation in the abdomen and pelvis, better retraction, and a shorter operating time. To many surgeons who migrated from open to laparoscopic colorectal surgery, HAL-APR is probably less "stressful" as one can still "feel" the tissues to be divided or protected and when there is accidental hemorrhage due to injury of a blood vessel, the hand is there to "pinch" the bleeding point for corrective hemostasis, as in any open surgery. Its main disadvantage is the presence of an abdominal scar, which can be kept small and carefully camouflaged in the planned end-stoma wound.

Recommended References and Readings

1. Miles WE. A method of performing abdomino-perineal excision for carcinoma of the rectum and the terminal portion of the pelvic colon. *Lancet* 1908;2:1812–13.
2. Dixon CF. Anterior resection for malignant lesions of the upper part of the rectum and lower part of the sigmoid. *Ann Surg* 1948; 128:425–42.
3. Heald RJ, Ryall RD. Recurrence and survival after total mesorectal excision for rectal cancer. *Lancet* 1986;28:1479–82.
4. Schiessel R, Novi G, Holzer B, et al. Technique and long-term results of intersphincteric resection for low rectal cancer. *Dis Colon Rectum* 2005;48:1858–67.
5. Saito N, Sugito M, Ito M, et al. Oncologic outcome of intersphincteric resection for very low rectal cancer. *World J Surg* 2009;33:1750–56.
6. Seow C, Goh HS. Prospective randomized trial comparing J colonic pouch-anal anastomosis and straight coloanal reconstruction. *Br J Surg* 1995;82:608–10.
7. Hallbook O, Pahlman L, Krog M, et al. Randomized comparison of straight and colonic J-pouch anastomosis after low anterior resection. *Ann Surg* 1996;224:58–65.
8. Ho YH, Brown S, Heah SM, et al. Comparison of J-pouch and coloplasty pouch for low rectal cancers: a randomized, controlled trial investigating functioning results and comparative anastomotic leak rates. *Ann Surg* 2002;236:49–55.
9. Jiang JK, Yang SH, Lin JK. Transabdominal anastomosis after low anterior resection: a prospective, randomized, controlled trial comparing long-term results between side-to-end anastomosis and colonic J-pouch. *Dis Colon Rectum* 2005;48:2100–10.
10. Madbouly KM, Remzi FH, Erkek BA, et al. Recurrence after transanal excision of T₁ rectal cancer: should we be concerned? *Dis Colon Rectum* 2005;48:711–21.
11. Nigro ND, Vaitkevicuis VK, Considine B Jr. Combined therapy for cancer of the anal canal: a preliminary report. *Dis Colon Rectum* 1974;17:354–56.
12. Bosset JF, Collette L, Calais G, et al. Chemotherapy with preoperative radiotherapy on rectal cancer. *N Engl J Med* 2006;355: 1114–23.
13. Verhoef C, Van Der Pool AEM, Nuyttens JJ, et al. The "liver-first approach" for patients with locally advanced rectal cancer and synchronous liver metastases. *Dis Colon Rectum* 2009;52: 23–30.
14. Temple LK, Hsieh L, Wong WD, et al. Use of surgery among elderly patients with stage IV colorectal cancer. *J Clin Oncol* 2004;22:3475–84.
15. Bajwa A, Blunt N, Vyas S, et al. Primary tumor resection and survival in the palliative management of metastatic colorectal cancer. *Eur J Surg Oncol* 2009;35:164–67.
16. Ruo L, Gougoutas C, Paty PB, et al. Elective bowel resection for incurable stage IV colorectal cancer: prognostic variables for asymptomatic patients. *J Am Coll Surg* 2003;196:722–28.
17. Lim GH, Wong CS, Chow KY, et al. Trends in long-term cancer survival in Singapore: 1968–2002. *Ann Acad Med Singapore* 2009;38:99–105.
18. Poultsides GA, Servais EL, Saltz LB, et al. Outcome of primary tumor in patients with synchronous stage IV colorectal cancer receiving combination chemotherapy without surgery as initial treatment. *J Clin Oncol* 2009;27:3379–84.
19. Marcello PW, Fleshman JW, Milsom JW, et al. Hand-assisted laparoscopic versus laparoscopic colorectal surgery: a multicenter, prospective, randomized trial. *Dis Colon Rectum* 2008;51: 818–28.
20. Lindsey I, Warren BF, Mortensen NJ. Denonvilliers' fascia lies anterior to the fascia propria and rectal dissection plane in total mesorectal excision. *Dis Colon Rectum* 2005;48:37–42.
21. Merkow RP, Bilimoria KY, McCarter MD, Bentrem DJ. Effect of body mass index on short-term outcomes after colectomy for cancer. *J Am Coll Surg* 2009;208:53–61.
22. Quah HM, Chou JF, Gonen M, et al. Identification of patients with high-risk stage II colon cancer for adjuvant therapy. *Dis Colon Rectum* 2008;51:503–07.
23. Molina JAD, Jiang Gabriel ZW, Heng BH, Ong BKC. Venous thromboembolism at the National Healthcare Group, Singapore. *Ann Acad Med Singapore* 2009;38:470–77.
24. Cheung HYS, Chung CC, Yau KKK, et al. Risk of deep vein thrombosis following laparoscopic rectosigmoid cancer resection in Chinese patients. *Asian J Surg* 2008;31:63–8.

25. Sasaki L. Bossier City, LA, USA. Personal communication, 2009.
26. Jänes A, Cengiz Y, Israelsson LA. Preventing parastomal hernia with a prosthetic mesh: a 5-year follow-up of a randomized study. *World J Surg* 2009;33:118–21.
27. Wu J, Shao Y, Rong W, et al. Hand-assisted laparoscopic surgery in colorectal carcinoma resection: a report of 14 cases. *Zhonghua Zhong Liu Za Zhi* 2002;24:599–601.
28. Ng KH, Ng DC, Cheung HY, et al. Laparoscopic resection for rectal cancer: lessons learned from 579 cases. *Ann Surg* 2009; 249:82–6.
29. Wong DCT, Chung CC, Chan ESW, et al. Laparoscopic abdominoperineal resection revisited: are there any health-related benefits? A comparative study. *Tech Coloproctol* 2006;10:37–42.
30. Aalbers AG, Biere SS, van Berge Henegouwen MI, Bemelman WA. Hand-assisted or laparoscopic-assisted approach in colorectal surgery: a systematic review and meta-analysis. *Surg Endosc* 2008; 22:1769–80.
31. Tjandra JJ, Chang KY, Yeh CH. Laparoscopic- versus hand-assisted ultralow anterior resection: a prospective study. *Dis Colon Rectum* 2008;51:26–31.
32. Faiz O, Warusavitarne J, Bottle A, et al. Laparoscopically assisted versus open elective colonic and rectal resection: a comparison of outcomes in English National Health Service Trusts between 1996 and 2006. *Dis Colon Rectum* 2009;52: 1695–1704.
33. Aly EH. Laparoscopic colorectal surgery: summary of the current evidence. *Ann R Coll Surg Engl* 2009;91:541–4.
34. Zhou ZG. Chengdu, Sichuan, China. Personal Communication, 2008.

Part VII: Abdominoperineal Resection

34 Laparoscopic Total Mesorectal Excision

Hester Yui Shan Cheung, Michael Ka Wah Li, and Chi Chiu Chung

 ## PREOPERATIVE PLANNING

Operating Room Setup and Position of the Patient

A dedicated team consisting of at least two experienced surgeons and one camera assistant is essential in practicing advanced laparoscopic procedures like laparoscopic total mesorectal excision (TME). These operations are ideally undertaken in an integrated endo-laparoscopic operating suite, where there is a universal plug and play system for various endoscopes and laparoscopes (1). The position of the patient and the surgical team are shown in Figure 34.1. Throughout the operation the patient is predominantly put in a 20 degree Trendelenburg position with right-side-down tilt, a position that helps clear the small bowel away from the lower abdomen and pelvis.

Recommended Instruments

(1) A 30 degree telescope
(2) Two atraumatic forceps for handling of bowel and soft tissues
(3) Two grasping forceps for holding cotton tapes
(4) Laparoscopic energy devices such as an ultrasonic dissection device or bipolar sealing and cutting devices
(5) Endo-staplers of various sizes and stapler height for bowel transection and vascular division
(6) Circular stapler for transanal anastomosis
(7) A sterile plastic zip-lock bag or an Alexis® wound retractors (Applied Medical, California, USA), used as parietal protective drape during specimen retrieval

Pneumoperitoneum and Insertion of Trocars

Pneumoperitoneum is first established by a subumbilical blunt trocar using an open technique. Other trocars are inserted under direct vision (Fig. 34.2).

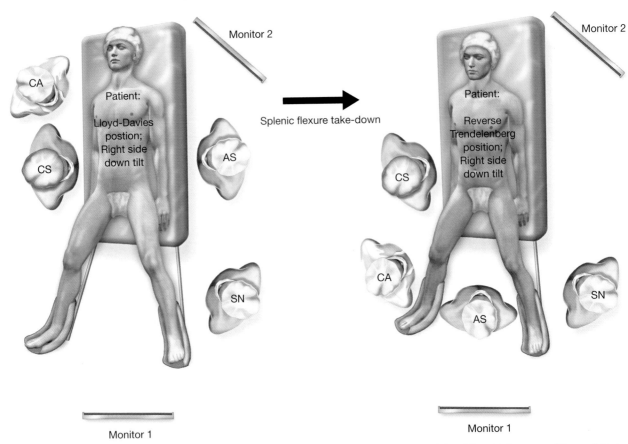

Figure 34.1 Positions of the patient and the surgical team in laparoscopic total mesorectal excision; CS = chief surgeon; AS = assistant surgeon; CA = camera assistant; SN = scrub nurse. Monitor 2 is used for splenic flexure mobilization.

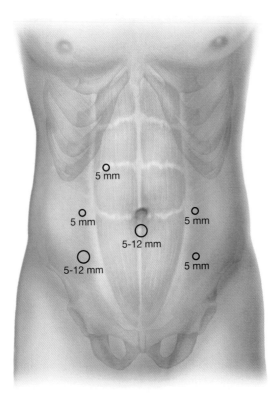

Figure 34.2 Port sites for laparoscopic total mesorectal excision or laparoscopic assisted abdominoperineal resection. An additional 5 mm port is created in the right upper quadrant if splenic flexure mobilization is necessary, as in the case of sphincter-saving resections. The chief surgeon and the camera assistant can use the subumbilical and the right iliac fossa ports interchangeably during splenic flexure mobilization.

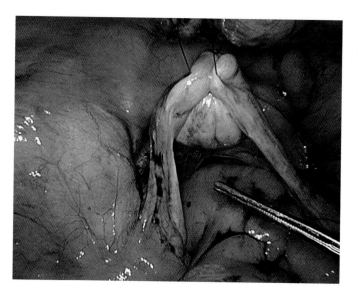

Figure 34.3 For optimal exposure of the pelvis, the uterus is hitched up to the lower anterior abdominal wall.

Exposure of the Pelvis

In female patients, for optimal exposure the uterus is first hitched up by passing sutures (00 Prolene on a straight needle) underneath the two fallopian tubes near the uterine cornua and tying them to the lower anterior abdominal wall (Fig. 34.3). The stitch should pass through the skin and be secured over a piece of gauze as a reminder to the surgeon to replace the uterus at the end of the procedure.

SURGERY

Splenic Flexure Mobilization

Splenic flexure mobilization is required, especially when colonic J-pouch construction is intended.

We favor a medial-to-lateral approach in splenic flexure mobilization. The small bowel is kept in the right side of the abdomen by tilting the operating table to the right (right-side-down position). The inferior mesenteric vein is identified lateral to the duodenojejunal flexure, and is controlled and divided. Blunt dissection is then undertaken in the avascular plane between the mesentery of descending colon and the retroperitoneal fascia (Fig. 34.4). This dissection is laterally continued toward the splenic flexure

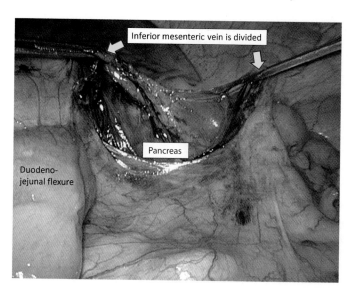

Figure 34.4 The inferior mesenteric vein is identified lateral to the duodenojejunal flexure, and is controlled and divided. Blunt dissection is then carried out in the avascular plane between the mesentery of the descending colon and the retroperitoneal fascia.

for as far as possible, until Gerota's fascia is exposed. The pancreas is identified and the dissection is maintained anterior to the pancreas. If this medial dissection is adequate, the lateral dissection is relatively simple. Starting from mid-transverse colon, the greater omentum is peeled off from the colon by incising the fascia just above the transverse colon. The posterior wall of the stomach should be clearly seen once the lesser sac is entered. By keeping close to the colon, further incision along the upper and lateral border will bring down the splenic flexure entirely. Mobilization is considered adequate if the splenic flexure can reach the midline and the descending colon can reach the anterior peritoneal reflection.

Sigmoid Mobilization

After splenic-flexure mobilization, the sigmoid is mobilized. First the lateral peritoneal attachment of the sigmoid at Toldt's fascia is divided. A 15–20 cm long cotton tape is secured around the rectosigmoid junction through a mesenteric window to facilitate counter-traction by the assistant surgeon (2) (Fig. 34.5). Laterally the left gonadal vessels and medially the left ureter are identified under the retroperitoneum (i.e., the posterior parietal peritoneum). The retroperitoneum is then incised medial to the left ureter, and the left hypogastric nerve is identified. The presacral space is entered at a plane anterior to the left hypogastric nerve, which is located approximately 1–2 cm lateral to the midline at the level of the sacral promontory. Following this step, the sigmoid colon is then rotated to the left side, the right ureter is outlined, and the retroperitoneum at the base of the sigmoid mesentery is incised, first at the level of the sacral promontory. Caution must be taken to avoid damage to the underlying right hypogastric nerve. A generous retromesenteric window is then made at the base of the mesosigmoid. Division of the retroperitoneum can be safely continued upward anterior to the aorta, until the inferior mesenteric artery is encountered. Division of the inferior mesenteric artery proximal to the origin of the left colic artery is performed with either a vascular endostapler, a bipolar sealing and cutting device or between clips. Further upward mesenteric division is then carried out until the divided inferior mesenteric vein window is met. Caution is taken to avoid injury to the left branch of the middle colic vessels.

Pelvic Dissection

The rectum is then retracted upward and forward, and the loose areolar plane between the mesorectum and the presacral fascia, with the hypogastric nerves, is identified. The right and left hypogastric nerves should be clearly visualized on the presacral fascia as two structures radiating downward and diverging outward in the pelvis. Using a

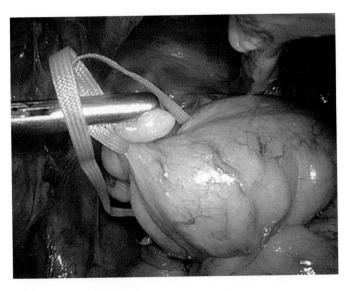

Figure 34.5 A cotton tape is tied around the rectosigmoid junction through a mesenteric window to facilitate counter-traction by the assistant surgeon.

combination of sharp and blunt dissection, wide opening of this presacral space is continued posteriorly, respecting the presacral fascia, down to a level distal to the tumor. Laterally, the left and right dissection are likewise performed by first dividing the posterior parietal peritoneum along the pelvic brim. Anteriorly, the peritoneum is incised 1–2 cm anterior to the rectouterine (female) or rectovesical (male) reflection; dissection is kept close to the vagina or seminal vesicles so that the fascia of Denonvilliers' is included in the specimen. The posterior vaginal wall or the seminal vesicles and prostate are carefully freed from the specimen after which both the lateral ligaments are divided. Further posterior dissection distally into the true pelvis is facilitated by turning the 30 degree laparoscope 180 degree upward; by doing so a much better view can be obtained, and the sacrum and presacral fascia can be seen curving downward and forward. The exposure of the pelvic floor muscles marks the end-point of pelvic dissection. The rectum is then divided with an endo-stapler just above the pelvic floor after cytocidal lavage. Endo-staplers of longer staple height such as a green cartridge may be used after pelvic radiation (3).

Specimen Retrieval and Intracorporeal Anastomosis

Specimen retrieval and intracorporeal anastomosis are the final stages of the operation. Pneumoperitoneum is abolished, and the specimen is delivered and excised by a 5–6 cm Pfannenstiel's incision. Alternatively, the pre-marked ileostomy site can be used for specimen extraction if the tumor is not bulky. A sterile plastic zip-lock bag or equivalent is used as parietal protection drape during specimen extraction. A 5 cm long colonic J-pouch is fashioned with a 60 mm linear cutter using either the descending or the proximal sigmoid colon. The detachable anvil of a circular stapler is then inserted into the apex of the pouch and secured with a 00 Prolene purse-string suture. The pouch is returned into the peritoneal cavity, and after the pneumoperitoneum is reestablished and the intracorporeal pouch-anal anastomosis is completed, routine covering loop ileostomy is recommended. The pelvis is drained by the left iliac fossa 5 mm port. Before abolishing the pneumoperitoneum, it is important to replace the small bowel in the right upper abdominal cavity back into the center of the abdomen, as the patient is predominantly in a right-side down Trendelenburg position; otherwise the small bowel may herniate through the space lateral to the ileostomy, leading to intestinal obstruction in the early postoperative period (4).

SIMULTANEOUS LAPAROSCOPIC ABDOMINAL AND TRANSANAL EXCISION FOR LOW RECTAL TUMOURS

One of the technical challenges when operating on rectal tumors within 4 cm from anal verge is to obtain an adequate distal mural margin. We have employed a technique, known as simultaneous laparoscopic abdominal and transanal excision (SLATE), where an adequate distal margin can be safely achieved at the beginning of the operation (5). As the specimen is delivered per anum, the patient can enjoy the full benefits of minimally invasive surgery. Additionally, the simultaneous approach helps shorten the operative time. The abdominal and perineal surgeons perform the operation simultaneously. The abdominal team consists of a chief surgeon, an assistant surgeon, and a camera assistant, whereas the perineal surgeon operates at the table end. The positions of the surgeons are shown in Figure 34.6.

Abdominal Part

Having confirmed resectability of the tumor under the laparoscope, the abdominal surgeons proceed with laparoscopic TME using the technique previously described. Splenic flexure mobilization is first carried out. This is followed by sigmoid mobilization and

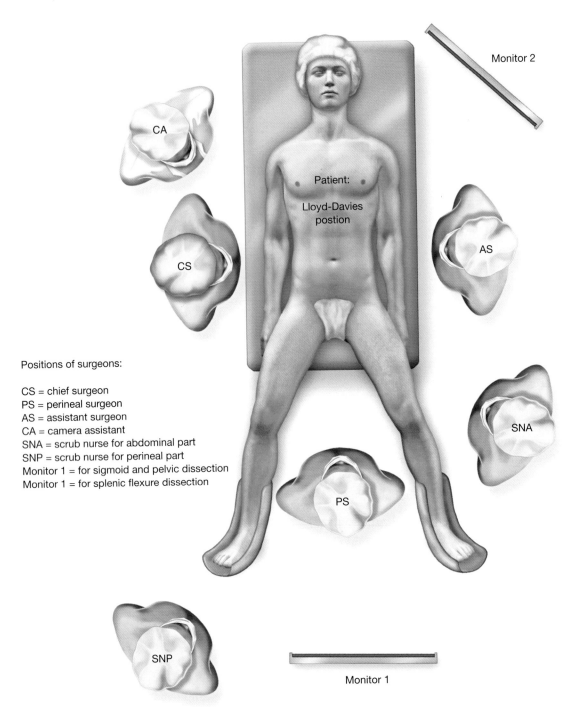

Positions of surgeons:

CS = chief surgeon
PS = perineal surgeon
AS = assistant surgeon
CA = camera assistant
SNA = scrub nurse for abdominal part
SNP = scrub nurse for perineal part
Monitor 1 = for sigmoid and pelvic dissection
Monitor 1 = for splenic flexure dissection

Figure 34.6 Positions of the patient and the surgical team in Simultaneous Laparoscopic Abdominal and Transanal Excision for low rectal tumours.

pelvic dissection, and after complete rectal and mesorectal mobilization, the large perineal gauze (see below) will be visible following division of the last few fascial strands around the anorectal junction, after which the distal transection is complete. The entire sigmoid and rectum, together with the specimen, is now delivered per anum to the perineal surgeon, caution being taken to avoid twisting of the colon. A covering loop ileostomy is routinely created and the pelvis is routinely drained.

Perineal Part

The perianal skin is retracted using a Lone Star retractor (Lone Star Medical Products, Stafford, USA) and a bivalved speculum is inserted into the anal canal to facilitate exposure of the lower rectum. The distal mucosal margin is circumferentially marked with cautery 0.5–1 cm above the dentate line. Before the dissection starts, a small gauze soaked with a cytotoxic agent such as 5% povidone iodine is packed into the anal canal below the tumor, and secured in place by sutures.

Starting at the diathermy mark, the mucosa is divided with cautery. Dissection is proximally undertaken in the intersphincteric plane until the anorectal ring is reached. Following this mobilization, lateral full-thickness dissection is performed proximally for about 2 cm. This dissection is largely facilitated by the use of bipolar scissors, which facilitates a bloodless field. The resultant rectal tube sleeve, with the povidine-iodine soaked gauze inside, is then distally closed with a running stitch. The stitch is left long at 3 and 9 O'clock positions to aid subsequent orientation. The cavity inside the anal canal is packed with a large gauze, which helps to mark the endpoint of pelvic dissection for the abdominal surgeons (see above).

After the abdominal surgeons have completed the pelvic dissection, the colon and rectum is delivered per anum. The specimen is excised and, with the help of abdominal surgeons, the orientation as well as the blood supply of the colon is checked. A colonic J-pouch is fashioned at the surgeon's preference. Hand-sewn, full-thickness coloanal anastomosis is then performed transanally using interrupted sutures. The sutures are left untied until all stitches have been placed. At the end of the operation, digital examination is carried out to ensure a widely patent lumen.

LAPAROSCOPIC-ASSISTED ABDOMINOPERINEAL RESECTION

Positioning of the Patient and Trocar Placement

The positions of the operating team are essentially similar to those already described for SLATE (Fig. 34.6). The perineal surgeon sits between the legs of the patient and operates with a headlight. Sacral support is used to facilitate perineal exposure and the legs of the patient are kept abducted and externally rotated. As a final check, one must make sure the tip of the coccyx is easily palpable before draping the patient.

The placement of the abdominal trocars is shown in Figure 34.2. As splenic flexure mobilization is usually not required, the right upper quadrant 5 mm trocar is unnecessary. One of the 5 mm ports in left iliac fossa is placed on the pre-marked stoma site; this is subsequently extended at the end of the operation, through which colostomy is raised.

Abdominal Part—Sigmoid and Pelvic Dissection

The sigmoid and upper rectal mobilization is undertaken as described above. In most cases, extensive mobilization of the descending colon is unnecessary. A proper and radical pelvic dissection should be undertaken since TME is contemplated in laparoscopic assisted abdominoperineal resection. Following complete pelvic dissection, the sigmoid colon is transected at a point chosen for colostomy, and the specimen is delivered to the perineal surgeon. Pneumoperitoneum is abolished and a sigmoid colostomy is raised through one of the extended 5 mm port over left iliac fossa; an abdominal drain is usually not required.

Perineal Part

Synchronous perineal dissection is undertaken once the abdominal surgeons have decided on a sphincter-ablating procedure. The technique is no different from open surgery. After division of anococcygeal ligaments posteriorly, the fascia of Waldeyer is divided under the guidance of abdominal surgeons, and communication with the peritoneal cavity is established. Lateral dissection is continued, and the specimen is delivered and excised

Part VII: Abdominoperineal Resection

from either the prostate or posterior vaginal wall anteriorly. Alternatively, a cuff of posterior vaginal wall is excised if the rectal tumor involves the anterior rectal wall. Hemostasis is checked, and the ischiorectal fat and skin are closed in layers around a vacuum drain.

RESULTS AND CONCLUSION

We reported the technique of laparoscopic TME in 2001 (6). Our data suggested that the technique was more recently associated with good short and medium term outcomes (7), and was oncologically sound (8). We have recently reported our long-term results of laparoscopic resection for rectal cancer (9), and we were able to achieve a local recurrence rate of 7.4% and an overall 5-year survival of 70%. These data suggest that laparoscopic resection for rectal cancer is safe and in fact the procedure of choice in selected patients.

Recommended References and Readings

1. Wong JC, Yau KK, Chung CC, Siu WT, Li MK. Endo-Lap OR: an innovative "minimally invasive operating room" design. *Surg Endosc* 2006;20(8):1252–56.
2. Chung CC, Kwok SP, Leung KL, Lau WY, Li AK. Use of a cotton tape tie in laparoscopic colorectal surgery. *Aust N Z J Surg* 1997;67(5):293–94.
3. Cheung HY, Chung CC, Wong JC, Yau KK, Li MK. Laparoscopic rectal cancer surgery with and without neoadjuvant chemo-irradiation: a comparative study. *Surg Endosc* 2009;23(1):147–52.
4. Ng KH, Ng DC, Cheung HY, et al. Obstructive complications of laparoscopically created defunctioning ileostomy. *Dis Colon Rectum* 2008;51(11):1664–68.
5. Wong CT, Chung CC, Li KW, et al. Simultaneous laparoscopic abdominal and transanal excision for low rectal tumors. *Surg Pract* 2007;11:76–80.
6. Chung CC, Ha JP, Tsang WW, Li MK. Laparoscopic-assisted total mesorectal excision and colonic J pouch reconstruction in the treatment of rectal cancer. *Surg Endosc* 2001;15(10):1098–1101.
7. Tsang WW, Chung CC, Li MK. Prospective evaluation of laparoscopic total mesorectal excision with colonic J-pouch reconstruction for mid and low rectal cancers. *Br J Surg* 2003;90(7):867–71.
8. Tsang WWC, Chung CC, Kwok SY, Li MKW. Laparoscopic sphincter-preserving total mesorectal excision with colonic J-pouch reconstruction: five-year results. *Ann Surg* 2006;243(3):353–58.
9. Ng KH, Chung CC, Li MKW, et al. Laparoscopic resection for rectal cancer: lessons learned from 579 cases. *Ann Surg* 2009;249:82–86.

35 Anterior, Posterior, Total

Martin R. Weiser, W. Douglas Wong, and Philip B. Paty

 ## INDICATIONS/CONTRAINDICATIONS

Exenterations or multivisceral/extended rectal resections are utilized as definitive surgical therapies for locally advanced primary rectal cancers that invade surrounding anatomical structures and for locally recurrent disease confined to the pelvis. These challenging procedures are associated with considerable morbidity and require extensive surgical planning. A multidisciplinary team including surgeons, medical and radiation oncologists, radiologists, intensivists, specialized nurses, and occupational and physical therapists should be assembled to address the multifaceted issues that are likely to arise. The expertise of the surgical team must be broad and should include specialists in colorectal, urologic, gynecologic, orthopedic, neurologic, and plastic/reconstructive surgery.

Locally Advanced Primary Rectal Cancer

Unlike many solid tumors, large locally advanced primary rectal cancers are not necessarily indicative of concurrent distant disease (1), and resection for cure is therefore potentially attainable (2). Nearly 15% of rectal cancers are adherent to adjacent pelvic organs. In this situation, it is critical that the surgeon anticipate a need for neoadjuvant therapy and multivisceral resection at the time of clinical presentation.

Furthermore, on surgical exploration, malignant infiltration cannot be clearly differentiated from inflammatory adhesion (3), so the surgeon must be prepared to aggressively resect adherent organs. Many studies have shown that en bloc resection of the surrounding anatomic structures invaded by tumor—*if* it results in clear (negative) margins—can lead to long-term survival (2–7). High-quality cross-sectional imaging, advanced planning, and strict adherence to the principals of surgical oncology are crucial in treating these difficult cases.

Recurrent Rectal Cancer

Following curative-intent resection of the primary lesion, rectal cancer recurs within the pelvis at a rate of 4–33%. Because uncontrolled pelvic recurrence can lead to disabling pain, bleeding, obstruction, and infection, an aggressive surgical approach is indicated when feasible. However, in recurrent disease, the surgical planes have been disrupted by initial pelvic resection of the primary tumor, making re-resection significantly more difficult. In light of the rigors and morbidity entailed by surgical therapy, careful patient selection is critical. Patients with significant comorbidities and poor performance status (ASA IV-V) are rarely candidates for the extensive surgery required.

Contraindications to exenteration also include the following:

- Unresectable extrapelvic metastases
- Sciatic pain and imaging evidence of sciatic nerve involvement
- S1 or S2 bony or neural involvement
- Circumferential pelvic sidewall involvement
- Bilateral ureteral obstruction

PREOPERATIVE PLANNING

Proper preoperative staging of locally advanced and recurrent rectal cancer is imperative when contemplating exenteration. One must identify those patients with distant metastases who should not undergo such potentially morbid treatment. Verification of recurrent disease (often by CT-guided biopsy) is recommended before undertaking any operation of this magnitude.

Physical Examination

Although many surgeons consider modern imaging modalities to be the most effective means of tumor staging, the importance of a proper physical examination, including detailed digital rectal and vaginal examinations, cannot be underestimated. Through physical examination, the experienced surgeon gains valuable information regarding the extent of a tumor and its fixation to adjacent organs and/or the bony pelvis. A thorough pelvic examination may be the simplest, most direct method of determining whether or not sphincter-sparing surgery is feasible, or multivisceral resection or exenteration necessary. Complete colonoscopy should also be done to exclude synchronous primary tumors (2).

Radiologic Imaging

Contrast-enhanced computed tomography (CT) scanning is the imaging modality most frequently used to assess extent of tumor and/or presence of metastatic disease. Although CT scans can provide an approximate idea of tumor size, however, they do not always enable accurate differentiation of tumor margins from the surrounding viscera. Thus, because obtaining an adequate circumferential resection margin is paramount to curative resection, CT evaluation is not always adequate in the setting of locally advanced or recurrent tumors. Magnetic resonance imaging (MRI) generally provides a more accurate indication of pelvic involvement and the potential need for multivisceral resection. The superiority of MRI in predicting extra-rectal involvement in primary disease has been supported by several comparative studies (6,8,9).

Endorectal ultrasound (EUS) is another imaging tool that can be used to assess the local extent of a primary rectal tumor. Early, mobile transmural bowel lesions can be gauged quite accurately by EUS (2). However, because of its limited depth of field, EUS tends to understage larger lesions and has less accuracy in the setting of locally advanced tumors (6,10). In addition, as is true of all imaging modalities, the accuracy of EUS in staging rectal cancer after radiation therapy is markedly reduced because of the presence of post-radiation edema, inflammation, necrosis, and fibrosis. Studies indicate that the accuracy of EUS in the evaluation of T-stage after radiotherapy is only 50%, with a 40% rate of overstaging (10); EUS is of even less utility in the setting of a large pelvic recurrence.

Fluorine-18 fluorodeoxyglucose positron emission tomography (FDG-PET), a powerful, noninvasive imaging modality for depicting tumor metabolic activity, is a valuable tool in the preoperative staging of locally advanced and recurrent rectal cancer. FDG-PET can be utilized to assess changes in tumor glucose metabolism (11) and is especially accurate in identifying recurrent disease. EUS, CT, and MRI have demonstrated poor accuracy in distinguishing viable tumor from scar or inflammatory tissue. However, FDG-PET appears to play a vital role in differentiating scar and viable tumor (11).

Neoadjuvant Therapy

The single-most important factor in curing rectal cancer is complete excision of the tumor with negative macroscopic and microscopic margins. Multimodality therapy, including chemoradiation, is often helpful in achieving this goal. In primary disease, preoperative chemoradiation has been shown to reduce local recurrence more effectively than postoperative therapy (12). A significant benefit of preoperative chemoradiotherapy is its potential to downsize the tumor (13), which may facilitate complete resection of locally advanced disease. Indeed, neoadjuvant chemoradiation has become standard practice in treating most locally advanced rectal cancers. Investigational approaches aimed at enhancing complete resection of advanced rectal cancer generally involve intensification of preoperative therapy. One such strategy is induction chemotherapy followed by standard chemoradiation. Chua et al. (14) reported on a phase II study of 105 poor-risk rectal cancer patients treated with induction capecitabine + oxaliplatin before receiving standard chemoradiation. "Poor-risk" was defined on MRI imaging as (a) tumor extending to within 1 mm of, or beyond, the mesorectal fascia; (b) T3 low-lying tumor at or below the levators; (c) tumor extending 5 mm or more into the perirectal fat; (d) T4 tumor. In the above-mentioned study, 93 of 97 patients eventually underwent complete negative-margin resections.

Patients with pelvic recurrence who have not previously received radiation should be considered candidates for preoperative chemoradiotherapy. Again, the goal is to downsize the recurrence in hopes of obtaining a complete negative-margin resection. In patients with history of limited radiotherapy, a modified regime may be possible. Patients who cannot undergo any additional radiation may be candidates for aggressive chemotherapy. In any case, if a patient has received preoperative chemotherapy and/or radiotherapy in the past, imaging should be done to exclude interval development of distant metastasis before subjecting that individual to radical resection re-staging.

Additional Studies

Preoperative evaluation, including physical examination and imaging, will determine the need for any additional studies such as pelvic ultrasound, cystoscopy, or dedicated sacral bone evaluation. Cystoscopy may be necessary before surgery, or it may be intraoperatively performed. Temporary ureteral catheters should be used liberally, especially in instances of recurrent disease, to help identify and protect the ureters.

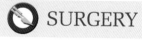 SURGERY

Surgical Technique

Rectal cancer spreading beyond the mesorectal plane adheres to and invades adjacent organs: the sacrum and sacral nerves posteriorly; the vagina and uterus or seminal vesicles and prostate, the bladder anteriorly; and the ureters, autonomic nerve plexus, internal iliac lymph nodes, and vessels laterally. As discussed earlier, any operation undertaken in this setting is extensive and complex, requiring careful selection of patients and the coordinated involvement of a multidisciplinary team of specialists. The surgical objective is to achieve complete resection of tumor with negative margins. In order to accomplish this goal, all organs involved by tumor must also be resected. At the same time, the surgical team should preserve as much healthy anatomy as possible. Extensive procedures of this nature often require surgical reconstruction.

Tumor adherent to regional anatomic structures is generally assumed to invade them; therefore, all or part of these organs must be removed en bloc with the tumor.

Focal invasion of adjacent organs, such as the seminal vesicles, vagina, bladder, ureter, or autonomic nerve plexus, and metastatic invasion of lymph nodes in the pelvic sidewall require extended rectal resection. The type of procedure—total pelvic exenteration, posterior exenteration, anterior exenteration, abdominoperineal resection (APR) with sacrectomy, sacropelvic exenteration—varies, depending on the extent of tumor spread into adjacent organs as well as the distance of tumor from the anal sphincter musculature.

Preoperative Regimen

Patients undergo bowel preparation the day before surgery. Placement of ureteral stents can be done preoperatively to help identify and protect the ureters. If an APR is planned, suturing of the anus will help prevent fecal contamination. Antibiotics are delivered in the operating room along with anesthesia. The patient is placed in the lithotomy position, giving the surgeon anterior access to the pelvis and the perineum. Surgery will be performed in one or two stages, depending on the type of resection.

Resection

The surgeon must first examine the abdomen for disseminated peritoneal disease and/ or for tiny hepatic metastases that may not have appeared on preoperative imaging studies, as detection of these would dictate a change in management. Following abdominal inspection, the origin of the inferior mesenteric artery (at the aorta) is dissected. The surgeon must examine the retroperitoneal lymph nodes for metastasis, the presence of which might indicate incurable disease, especially if the nodes cannot be easily removed. The ureters are identified and preserved; however, these are not transected until resectability is confirmed, enabling the surgical team to monitor output of urine. The inferior mesenteric artery is ligated and transected, and the rectosigmoid is subsequently transected about 10 cm proximal to the tumor. The surgeon dissects the rectum posteriorly, down to the levator ani, taking care to avoid the pelvic nerves whenever possible. The bladder is mobilized from the retropubic space. The lateral bladder pillars attached to the lateral pubic rami are ligated and transected. In a female patient, the cardinal ligaments supporting the vagina and cervix are ligated and transected at the pelvic sidewall. In a male patient, dissection continues anteriorly and includes the prostate.

An intraoperative decision must now be made: Will the surgical team proceed with a low anterior resection, or is an APR required? If an APR proves necessary, dissection must continue below the levator ani muscles. Following this, perineal dissection begins. The anal canal and the lower rectum are dissected and removed through the ischiorectal fossa and urogenital diaphragm. If the tumor is extensively invasive, removal of a female patient's vagina, vulva, and urethra may be required. The entire specimen may then be removed via an abdominal or perineal incision.

Types of Procedures (Figs. 35.1–35.4)

Total Exenteration is generally performed in the setting of large, bulky lesions that have spread into the bladder or prostate. Total pelvic exenteration entails removal of the rectum, bladder, vagina, uterus, cervix, and parametrium in female patients and removal of the rectum, bladder, prostate, and seminal vesicles in male patients.

Anterior Exenteration is undertaken when a sigmoid cancer invades the posterior bladder wall, anterior uterine wall, and organs located in the anterior plane of the pelvis.

Posterior Exenteration is performed in female patients when tumor involves the uterus. This procedure can be undertaken only if the bladder is free of tumor. Uterus,

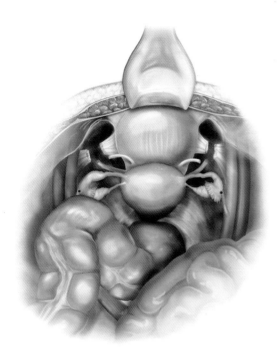

Figure 35.1 In total pelvic exenteration the lateral dissection begins on the common and external iliac vessels, which are lateral to the parietal layer of the endopelvic fascia. The internal iliac artery and vein are clamped, cut, and tied distal at their origin. The ureter is cut in the pelvis with care to preserve ureter length for reconstruction.

cervix, adnexa, and vagina (if required) are removed with the rectum. Posterior exenteration is similar to total exenteration; however, rather than performing dissection anterior to the bladder in the retropubic space, the peritoneum is incised over the bladder, and the bladder is dissected sharply off of the anterior surface of the cervix and the vagina down to or (depending on the level of the tumor) beyond the levator ani muscle. Distally, the ureters must be dissected free from the anterior parametria, over the ureteral tunnel running along the uterine artery.

APR/LAR with Partial Cystectomy or Vaginectomy may be considered if tumor does not extend far enough into the bladder (specifically involving the trigone) or the vagina

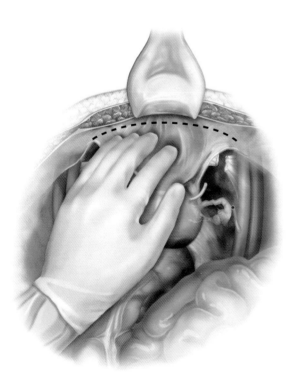

Figure 35.2 The surgeon may perform the dissection of the bladder before or after the posterior dissection of the pelvic organs. The bladder is dissected from the symphysis and pubic rami with dissection in the space of Retzius. The bladder is freed by dividing the lateral peritoneal attachments.

Part VIII: Pelvic Exenteration

Figure 35.3 Perineal dissection is required for total pelvic exenteration that includes the intra-levator organs (anal canal, labia majora, urethra). An elliptical incision is created from the tip of the coccyx to the pubic symphysis. In men, the incision ends at the bulb of the penis, with the urethra previously divided in the pelvis. The pelvic floor attachments are divided widely, freeing the urethra, vagina, and rectum.

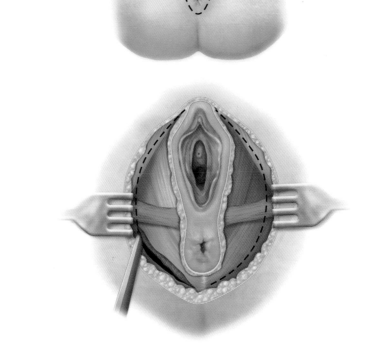

Figure 35.4 Following anterior dissection, the patient is placed prone for the sacral resection. A posterior sacral incision is made with excision of the anus. Flaps are raised to the lateral extent of the sacrum. The gluteus maximus and medius muscles are dissected from their sacral origins and the sciatic nerve is located by retracting the gluteus maximus and underlying piriformis muscle superiorly at the lateral aspect of the midsacrum. The nerve is superficial to the obturator internus muscle and courses inferolaterally between the ischial tuberosity and greater trochanter. The sacrotuberous and sacrospinous ligaments are incised at their attachments to the ischial tuberosity and ischial spine. A finger is inserted anteriorly from the medial aspect of the sciatic nerve. This facilitates dissection beneath the piriformis muscle and through the underlying endopelvic fascia. This exposure directs the sacral ostectomy and ensures adequate tumor clearance.

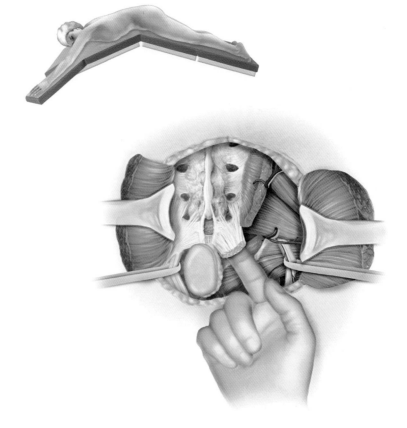

to warrant total removal of these organs. As regards the bladder, a partial cystectomy may be done and reimplantation of the ureters achieved with a psoas hitch reconstruction. If only part of the vagina is involved by tumor, local resection of the invaded portion may be appropriate; if the resulting vaginal defect is too large for primary closure, reconstruction can be achieved with a myocutaneous rectus abdominus flap.

Sacral Resections

Sacral resections are comparatively rare, and are generally done when rectal tumor invades or is broadly adherent to the sacrum or the coccyx.

APR with Sacrectomy begins in the same way as a total pelvic exenteration: anterior dissection takes place in the ventral plane, preserving bladder, female reproductive organs, or prostate when possible. Dissection is undertaken in a dorsal and dorsolateral fashion, following the presacral plane down to the level of the sacral transection. If transection of the sacrum at the S2/S3 level (or lower) is sufficient, the cancer is resectable. Using K-wire or osteotome, the level of sacral transection is marked on the anterior cortex of the sacrum. While the patient is turned and placed in the prone position, gauze may be packed into the presacral space to reduce bleeding. With the patient in the prone position, a dorsal longitudinal incision is made, starting at the level of L5 down to and around the anal canal. The gluteus maximus and gluteus minimus muscles are dissected from the sacrum and the flaps are bilaterally raised. Transection of the sacrotuberous and sacrospinous ligaments is done at the sacrum, facilitating access to the pelvic floor musculature and the infra-piriformis opening. Medial to the infra-piriformis, a finger can be inserted into the presacral space to identify the level of resection. The sacrum can be resected, with care taken to protect the nerve roots within the proximal (preserved) sacrum. Ultimately, the distal sacrum, lateral pelvic walls, and rectum are removed en bloc.

Sacropelvic Exenteration is a two-stage procedure in which the patient is turned and placed in the prone position for the second stage (15). This procedure involves the posterior dissection used for distal sacrectomy and the anterior dissection used in pelvic exenteration. It is done only in the setting of very bulky tumors involving the lower sacrum and invading the reproductive organs (in a female patient), the prostate (in a male patient), and the bladder (15). Following division of the sacrum (with the patient in the prone position) the rectum is removed in continuity with the sacrum and the resected visceral organs.

Pelvic Floor Reconstruction

Once surgical resection is completed, reconstruction can begin. Following these procedures there are often bowel, bladder, vaginal, and perineal defects that require reconstructive treatment. Reconstruction of the pelvis after extensive resection constitutes another facet of treatment for patients with recurrent rectal cancer. The major goals of reconstruction include optimizing healing, preventing perineal sepsis, and, in some patients, restoring function (16). The type of reconstruction is dictated by the type and extent of surgical resection. If the external sphincter musculature has been left intact, anastomosis of colon to the distal rectum or to the anal canal is possible. Because of the probability of anastomotic leak after such extensive surgery and neoadjuvant therapy, a defunctioning ileostomy is always recommended. In most cases, however, a rectal anastomosis is not possible, and a permanent colostomy is created. The surgeon then confronts a large irradiated pelvic "dead space": a space that is susceptible to abscess formation and prone to wound-healing complications. This "dead space" should be filled with omentum whenever possible. Restorative options include an omental pedicle graft and/or rotational myocutaneous flaps (6,16,17). Prosthetic or biological meshes have also been used. Reconstruction of large vaginal defects or defects in the perineal skin require myocutaneous flaps (17). If a cystectomy is performed, options for urinary diversion include the traditional ileal conduit or an orthotopic bladder substitution. Colon or ileum may be used for continent diversion (Indiana pouch, Mainz pouch,

Florida pouch, Miami pouch); or an ileal conduit, colonic conduit, or ureterocolostomy may be constructed for urinary diversion (15).

Intraoperative Radiation Therapy

Substantial progress has been made in recent years in the experimental, technical, and clinical application of intraoperative radiation therapy (IORT) as an intraoperative treatment modality for various cancers. A major goal of all radiation oncologists is to increase the dose delivered to tumor relative to the dose delivered to the normal adjacent tissues. As Willett and colleagues noted, this desire has led to the use of field-shaping techniques with multi-leaf collimation, multiple field techniques, and intensity-modulated radiation therapy, as well as intracavitary and interstitial brachytherapy (18). Intraoperative radiotherapy allows delivery of irradiation to the tumor bed while shielding normal tissue. Two alternative but complementary IORT techniques have evolved: intraoperative electron radiation (IOERT), which uses a linear accelerator to deliver electron particles, and high-dose-rate brachytherapy (HDR-IORT), which delivers an iridium seed (192-Ir) along after loading catheters. With either technique, normal tissues can actually be moved aside simultaneously or physically shielded. In addition, because the tumor can be visualized intraoperatively, it is possible to more accurately define areas at risk for tumor involvement (18).

In a study performed at the Massachusetts General Hospital, Nakfoor et al. assessed 101 patients with locally advanced primary rectal cancer who underwent preoperative radiation and IOERT. They found that patients with negative-margin (R0) resection had a 5-year local control rate of 89% and disease-specific survival of 63%. Patients with microscopically involved margins had a 5-year local control rate of 68%; patients with gross disease had a 5-year local control rate of 57% (19). A similar study at the Mayo Clinic demonstrated improvement in local control and survival with the addition of IOERT: 5-year overall survival was reportedly 46%, and 3-year overall survival improved from 24% to 55% (20).

The Memorial Sloan-Kettering Cancer Center (MSKCC) experience with intraoperative brachytherapy was reported by Alektiar et al. (21) in a study of 74 patients treated from 1992 to 1998. Median follow-up was 22 months. Of these, 50 patients underwent negative-margin (R0) resection. Five-year local control was 39%; 5-year disease-free and overall survival was 23%. Negative margins predicted local control: a 5-year rate of 43% in patients with R0 resection versus 26% in those with R1 resection. Patients with negative margins had a 5-year survival of 36% compared to only 11% in patients with positive margins. Morbidity in this series included wound complications (24%), ureteric stricturing (23%), bladder complications (20%), and peripheral neuropathy (16%).

 # COMPLICATIONS

Most modern series of exenteration have reported acceptable perioperative mortality but significant morbidity, including surgical site infection, sepsis related to the non-collapsible empty pelvis, and complications from urinary diversion. Gannon et al. reported an overall complication rate of 43% in their series of 72 patients undergoing exenteration for locally advanced rectal cancer. Thirty percent of the complications were major (enterocutaneous fistulae, respiratory failure with pneumonia, and urinary conduit leaks) resulting in >20-day length of hospital stay (22). Law et al. reported a 54% complication rate in their study of 24 patients undergoing exenteration for locally advanced rectal cancer, the majority of these related to the pelvis (23). In a series of 69 patients undergoing exenteration for a variety of malignancies, Ferenschild et al. reported 1% in-hospital mortality, and overall major and minor complication rates of 34% and 57%, respectively. (The majority of these complications involved wounds and urinary diversion (24).) Vermaas et al. reported 3% in-hospital mortality and 34% major morbidity (including a high proportion of problems related to urinary diversion) in 35 patients with primary and recurrent rectal cancer who underwent exenteration (25).

Complications and perioperative mortality increase when more radical procedures such as sacropelvic resection are undertaken. In 1994, Wanebo et al. reported 8.5% perioperative mortality in 47 patients undergoing exenteration for recurrent rectal cancer. The majority of patients suffered complications, most commonly related to perineal and abdominal wound sepsis (26). It should be noted that a significant proportion of these procedures involved relatively high sacrectomies (S1 and S2). Jimenez et al. reported on an MSKCC study involving 55 patients undergoing total pelvic exenteration between 1991 and 2000, 20 of whom had exenteration combined with sacrectomy. Overall 3-month mortality and overall morbidity were 5.5% and 78%, respectively. The rate of major complications was 40%, and the majority of complications were associated with perineal wound breakdown and sepsis (27).

Another detailed study from MSKCC, published in 2006, reported on complications following sacropelvic resection in 29 patients. Sacral resection was performed at the S2/S3 level in 55%, and at the S4/S5 level in 45% of the study cohort. Previous surgery predicted the type of salvage operation required: total exenteration with sacrectomy was performed in 69% of those who previously had APR; a less radical procedure was done for those who previously had sphincter-saving surgery. In 59% of patients, pedicle flaps were used to reconstruct the pelvis. The total complication rate was 59%; 45% of these complications were major, consisting mostly of perineal wound breakdown and pelvic sepsis. There was one perioperative death (28).

Oncologic Results

Salo et al. (29) completed a 10-year retrospective analysis of 131 patients with locally recurrent rectal cancer undergoing curative-intent surgery at MSKCC from 1986 to 1995. The goals of this study were to determine predictors of resectability and assess post-salvage survival. Resection proved possible in 79% of these patients. Median hospital stay was 14 days. Overall 5-year survival was 31%. Concomitant salvage procedures included sacrectomy (16 patients), partial vaginectomy (15), hysterectomy (9), and pelvic sidewall dissection (21). APR was performed in 46 patients; low anterior resection in 20; total pelvic exenteration in 18; Hartmann's resection in 11; perineal sacrectomy in 3; perineal excision in 3; and abdominal resection in 2. Fifty-two patients received IORT. The median survival in 71 patients, who had curative R0 resection, was 42 months; 3-year survival was 57%; and 5-year survival was 35%. In patients with R1 resection, median survival was 32 months; 3-year survival was 38%; and 5-year survival was 23%. In patients with an incomplete R2 resection (with gross residual disease), median survival was 27 months; 3-year survival was 36%; and 5-year survival was 9%. In the 28 patients who were not resected, median survival was 16 months; 3-year survival was 4%; and 5-year survival was 0% (29).

Similar trends were noted in the series of exenterations reported by Jimenez et al. and the series of sacropelvic resections published by Melton et al. Jimenez and colleagues noted a median disease-free survival of 53 months for patients undergoing negative-margin (R0) resection versus 32 months for those undergoing positive-margin (R1/R2) resection (27). For patients undergoing sacropelvic resection, Melton and colleagues reported a median disease-specific survival of 49 months with R0 resection, but only 23 months with R1/R2 resection (28).

Clearly, the necessity of a complete R0 resection cannot be overstated (21,30,31). There have been many efforts to identify factors associated with complete resection, in an attempt to help surgeons select patients who are truly suitable for exenteration. The length of time between resection of the primary rectal cancer and diagnosis of local recurrence is a prognostic factor: an interval of <1 year is indicative of a poor prognosis (which may reflect an inadequate original resection and/or aggressive tumor biology) (32). However, an isolated true anastomotic recurrence is a good prognostic factor. Central recurrences (as opposed to peripheral recurrences) are more amenable to resection with negative margins, and are therefore associated with a better surgical outcome. In an MSKCC study of 119 patients undergoing surgery and IORT for recurrent colorectal cancer from 1994 to 2000, Moore et al. (30) found that tumors confined to the axial location, or to the axial and anterior locations, were more likely to be completely resectable than tumors involving the pelvic sidewall or lateral structures. They reported that negative margins were achieved in 90% of patients who had axial recurrences only, and in 71% of patients who had axial and anterior recurrences only. Negative margins were also achieved in 64% of cases where there was no lateral involvement by tumor, and in 55% of cases where there was no iliac vessel involvement by tumor. However, negative margins were achieved in only 43% of cases in which the recurrence was located anywhere *but* axially and anteriorly. Where there was lateral involvement by tumor, negative margins were achieved in only 35%. If the iliac vessel was involved, negative margins were achieved in only 17%. In regards to long-term outcome, poor prognostic factors included type of original procedure (APR vs. sphincter-saving), elevated preoperative carcinoembryonic antigen, preoperative pain, vascular invasion, and short disease-free interval (for recurrent disease) (29,32,33). Ultimately, however, the surgeon must often explore the pelvis to determine resectability.

CONCLUSION

Pelvic exenteration is a very extensive and radical operation associated with high morbidity. It is generally undertaken only when cure is considered possible. Careful patient selection is critical. Good preoperative imaging with a high-resolution MRI scan will enhance planning of the appropriate surgical procedure. A multidisciplinary approach, involving a team of various specialists including not only colorectal surgeons, but also gynecologists, orthopedic surgeons, plastic and reconstructive surgeons, radiation oncologists, and medical oncologists is necessary to ensure proper preoperative planning and surgical implementation. Patients need to be psychologically prepared for extensive resections, prolonged hospital stays, and high incidence of morbidity. Input from stoma therapy nurses, dieticians, and preoperative counselors is helpful in preparing patents for the rigors of treatment. Even with neoadjuvant therapy and complementary use of IORT, complete R0 resection is essential if there is to be any possibility of cure (21,30,31).

Nevertheless, the feasibility of surgical exenteration means that carefully selected patients with rectal tumors extending into adjacent organs now have potentially curative treatment options. Following multimodality treatment and extended surgical resection, a 5-year survival of up to 60% can be achieved, with acceptable morbidity. The procedure should be performed in a specialty referral center in which sufficient experience and adequate multidisciplinary resources are available.

References

1. Spratt JS, Spjut HJ. Prevalence and prognosis of individual clinical and pathologic variables associated with colorectal carcinoma. *Cancer* 1967;20:1976–85.
2. Lopez MJ. Multivisceral resection for colorectal cancer. *J Surg Oncol* 2001;76:1–5.
3. Gebhardt C, Meyer W, Ruckriegel S, Meier U. Multivisceral resection of advanced colorectal carcinoma. *Langenbeck's Arch Surg* 1999;384:194–99.
4. Nakafusa Y, Tanaka T, Tanaka M, et al. Comparison of multivisceral resection and standard operation for locally advanced colorectal cancer: analysis of prognostic factors for short-term and long-term outcome. *Dis Colon Rectum* 2004;47:2055–63.
5. Lehnert T, Methner M, Pollok A, et al. Multivisceral resection for locally advanced primary colon and rectal cancer. An analysis of prognostic factors in 201 patients. *Ann Surg* 2002;235: 217–25.
6. Klaassen RA, Nieuwenhuijzen GA, Martijn H, et al. Treatment of locally advanced rectal cancer. *Surg Oncol* 2004;13:137–47.
7. Govindarajan A, Coburn NG, Kiss A, et al. Population-based assessment of the surgical management of locally advanced colorectal cancer. *J Natl Cancer Inst* 2006;98:1474–81.

8. Beets-Tan RG, Beets GL, Vliegen RF, et al. Accuracy of magnetic resonance imaging in prediction of tumor-free resection margin in rectal cancer surgery. *Lancet* 2001;357:497–504.
9. Mathur P, Smith JJ, Ramsey C, et al. Comparison of CT and MRI in the pre-operative staging of rectal adenocarcinoma and prediction of circumferential resection margin involvement by MRI. *Colorectal Dis* 2003;5:396–401.
10. Siddiqui AA, Fayiga Y, Huerta S. The role of endoscopic ultrasound in the evaluation of rectal cancer. *Int Semin Surg Oncol* 2006;3:36.
11. Cascini GL, Avallone A, Delrio P, et al. ^{18}F-FDG PET is an early predictor of pathologic tumor response to preoperative radiochemotherapy in locally advanced rectal cancer. *J Nucl Med* 2006;47:1241–48.
12. Sauer R, Becker H, Hohenberger W, et al. Preoperative versus postoperative chemoradiotherapy for rectal cancer. *N Engl J Med* 2004;351:1731–40.
13. Quah HM, Chou JF, Gonen M, et al. Pathologic stage is most prognostic of disease-free survival in locally advanced rectal cancer patients after preoperative chemoradiation. *Cancer* 2008;113:57–64.
14. Chua YJ, Barbachano Y, Cunningham D, et al. Neoadjuvant capecitabine and oxaliplatin before chemoradiotherapy and

total mesorectal excision in MRI-defined poor-risk rectal cancer: a phase 2 trial. *Lancet Oncol* 2010;11:241–48.

15. Smith JD, Paty PB. Extended surgery and pelvic exenteration for locally advanced rectal cancer. What are the limits? *Acta Chir Iugosl* 2010;57:23–27.

16. Madoff RD. Extended resections for advanced rectal cancer. *Br J Surg* 2006;93:1311–12.

17. Bell SW, Dehni N, Chaouat M, et al. Primary rectus abdominis myocutaneous flap for repair of perineal and vaginal defects after extended abdominoperineal resection. *Br J Surg* 2005;92:482–86.

18. Willett CG, Czito BG, Tyler DS. Intraoperative radiation therapy. *J Clin Oncol* 2007;25:971–77.

19. Nakfoor BM, Willett CG, Shellito PC, et al. The impact of 5-fluorouracil and intraoperative electron beam radiation therapy on the outcome of patients with locally advanced primary rectal and rectosigmoid cancer. *Ann Surg* 1998;228:194–200.

20. Gunderson LL, Nelson H, Martenson JA, et al. Locally advanced primary colorectal cancer: Intraoperative electron and external beam irradiation +/– 5-FU. *Int J Radiat Oncol Biol Phys* 1997;37:601–14.

21. Alektiar KM, Zelefsky MJ, Paty PB, et al. High-dose rate intraoperative brachytherapy for recurrent colorectal cancer. *Int J Radiat Oncol Biol Phys* 2000;48:219–26.

22. Gannon CJ, Zager JS, Chang GJ, et al. Pelvic exenteration affords safe and durable treatment for locally advanced rectal carcinoma. *Ann Surg Oncol* 2007;14:1870–77.

23. Law WL, Chu KW, Choi HK. Total pelvic exenteration for locally advanced rectal cancer. *J Am Coll Surg* 2000;190:78–83.

24. Ferenschild FT, Vermaas M, Verhoef C, et al. Total pelvic exenteration for primary and recurrent malignancies. *World J Surg* 2009;33:1502–08.

25. Vermaas M, Ferenschild FTJ, Verhoef C, et al. Total pelvic exenteration for primary locally advanced and locally recurrent rectal cancer. *Eur J Surg Oncol* 2007;33:452–458.

26. Wanebo HJ, Koness RJ, Vezeridis MP, et al. Pelvic resection of recurrent rectal cancer. *Ann Surg* 1994;220:586–95.

27. Jimenez RE, Shoup M, Cohen AM, et al. Contemporary outcomes of total pelvic exenteration in the treatment of colorectal cancer. *Dis Colon Rectum* 2003;46:1619–25.

28. Melton GB, Paty PB, Boland PJ, et al. Sacral resection for recurrent rectal cancer: analysis of morbidity and treatment results. *Dis Colon Rectum* 2006;49:1099–107.

29. Salo JC, Paty PB, Guillem J, et al. Surgical salvage of recurrent rectal carcinoma after curative resection: a 10-year experience. *Ann Surg Oncol* 1999;6:171–77.

30. Moore HG, Shoup M, Riedel E, et al. Colorectal cancer pelvic recurrences: determinants of resectability. *Dis Colon Rectum* 2004;47:1599–1606.

31. Mannaerts GHH, Rutten HJT, Martihn H, et al. Abdominosacral resection for primary irresectable and locally recurrent rectal cancer. *Dis Colon Rectum* 2001;44:806–14.

32. Park JK, Kim YW, Hur H, et al. Prognostic factors affecting oncologic outcomes in patients with locally recurrent rectal cancer: impact of patterns of pelvic recurrence on curative resection. *Langenbecks Arch Surg* 2009;394:71–77.

33. Shoup M, Guillem JG, Alektiar KM, et al. Predictors of survival in recurrent rectal cancer after resection and intraoperative radiotherapy. *Dis Colon Rectum* 2002;45:585–92.

36 Lateral Lymph Node Dissection for Rectal Carcinoma

Petr Tsarkov and Badma Bashankaev

Introduction/Objectives

Recent progress in rectal cancer staging, development of surgical procedures (e.g., total mesorectal excision [TME] and nerve-sparing TME), and advances in neo- and adjuvant therapy (such as chemotherapy and radiotherapy [RT]) has dramatically reduced loco-regional recurrence but still has not eliminated it (1). Local recurrences are likely to be a result of one of the following reasons—missed microscopic involvement of circular resection margin, rare involvement of distal mesorectum beyond "5 cm" barrier, lateral spread to pelvic lymph nodes beyond the mesorectum and possibly seeding of the pelvis during surgical dissection (2).

When reviewing series of patients who developed local recurrence after radical TME, lateral pelvic wall involvement is found in 20–80% of them (3–5). Thus, lateral lymph nodes (LLN) can be a potential site of locoregional recurrence even in the absence of circumferential margin involvement. Lateral lymph nodes recurrence (LLR) to pelvic sidewalls may be even higher (up to 83%) in patients with primary locally advanced rectal cancer (1). That phenomenon can be explained by recently found connections between the mesorectal and (lateral) extramesorectal lymph node system (6). The authors have suggested a hypothesis that a lymphatic fluid including cancer cells is squeezed into the LLN system. Since standard TME does not include lateral lymph node dissection (LLD) those nodes are not included in the standard surgical specimen. In addition lymph fluid might leak and form a presacral seroma that might also give a rise to local recurrence.

Unfortunately the widespread idea of relying on neoadjuvant therapy as a radiotherapy "mop" to sterilize low rectal cancer is currently accepted in Western countries. The use of preoperative RT as was shown in a large randomized Dutch study demonstrated a significant reduction of LLR in irradiated patients (7). The benefits of preop RT include about a 15–25% likelihood of complete pathologic response and tumor shrinkage and/or downstaging (8,9). But RT holds a significant potential risk of urinary and sexual dysfunction, and possible postoperative fecal incontinence (10–12).

There is no proven correlation between the regression of a primary tumor and the regression of regional nodal disease. The rate of pathologically proven metastatic mesorectal and lateral pelvic lymph nodes in low rectal cancer patients may be as high as 39% even after the completion of neoadjuvant RT (13).

Along with neoadjuvant chemoRT, surgical procedures to prevent LLN metastasis have been proposed, such as LLD. Although Western surgeons attempted LLD as early as the 1950s (14–16), this procedure is currently favored in East, mostly in Japan. The current approach towards LLNs in most Western colorectal centers, as noted by Yano and Moran, is to ignore their presence, or to treat obviously involved nodes with radiotherapy or chemoradiotherapy. More importantly, involved nodes are considered to be systemic disease (17).

The incidence of lateral nodal involvement in patients with lower rectal cancer has been reported as 16–23%. It has been demonstrated that in patients with pathologically proven lateral nodal involvement LLD results in a 5-year survival rate of 25–50%.

Mori has presented the data from Japanese registry, which showed that LLNs involvement was present in 1.1% of cases of T1 rectal cancers, 3.1% with T2 involvement, 11.6% with T4a penetration, and almost 15% in case of T4b invasion. Involvement of lateral nodes resulted in 32% 5-year survival rate in this group of patients (18).

In the review of neoadjuvant chemoRT and TME surgical treatment of 366 patients with rectal cancer, Kim et al. have reported that LLN metastasis is the major cause of locoregional recurrence (1).

Locoregional recurrence despite all modern trends of neoadjuvant chemoRT and TME attest to the need for more intense surgical research and/or technical improvements.

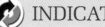 INDICATIONS/CONTRAINDICATIONS

Indications

The indications for LLD are still controversial even amongst Japanese surgeons.

Since preoperative imaging modalities are close to the desired predictive value for LLN only in few centers (19), the criteria for LLD are derived from analyzing other factors. There have been reported several risk factors predictive of lateral nodes involvement, some of which can be determined before operation.

The most predictive risk factors are as follow:

- **Tumor location below the level of peritoneal reflexion,** and the lower the tumor the higher the incidence of lateral node metastasis. Takahashi et al. (20) have demonstrated that in patients with rectal tumors above peritoneal reflexion the incidence of LLN involvement is 1.7%, while for the tumors below peritoneal reflexion this rate is 16.7% ($P < 0.001$), with maximum of 36.8% for tumors located just above the dentate line.
- **Depth of tumor invasion**—through bowel wall (T3) and infiltrating fascia propria of the rectum and adjacent organs (T4). The highest incidence of positive LLNs of 10.0–27.2% has been demonstrated for tumors invading mesorectal fat (T3) and 27.3–31.0% for cancer involving adjacent organs and structures (T4) (20,21). Multivariable analysis performed by Sugihara and colleagues (22) revealed that tumors below peritoneal reflexion as well as female sex, tumor size of more than 4 cm and T3/4 stage were significantly associated with an increased incidence of positive LLNs.
- **Tumor histological grade**—moderately and poorly differentiated adenocarcinomas have higher chances of metastases to LLNs.
- **Positive mesorectal lymph nodes**—several authors have shown that presence of positive lymph nodes in mesorectal fat is an important predictive factor of LLN involvement (22–24).

Based on results of multiple studies, the current Japanese decision concerning paraaortic and LLN dissection is determined by location of tumor, its histological grade, and stage of cancer (25). All patients with middle and lower rectal cancer classified as

Dukes' C undergo LLD. Prophylactic LLD is performed for Dukes' B tumors with G2 or G3 features (moderately and poorly differentiated adenocarcinomas) in order to remove LLNs with possible micrometastasis.

Precise preoperative diagnosis of both primary tumor characteristics and lateral nodal involvement, thus, define indications for LLD but remain difficult. The utility of endorectal ultrasound (US), computed tomography (CT), and magnetic resonance imaging (MRI) in predicting T-stage has been demonstrated in multiple studies, whereas the ability to evaluate lymph node status using these methods is relatively poor (26).

A recently published meta-analysis of 35 clinical trials of endorectal US in the diagnosis of nodal involvement in patients with rectal cancer demonstrated by pooled analysis sensitivity of 73.2% with a better ability to exclude rather than confirm nodal invasion (27). In a recent prospective study any visible mesorectal and LLNs on 5-mm thick section preoperative CT were recognized as positive, and postoperative histopathology assessment confirmed high sensitivity (95%) and specificity (96%) of CT in predicting LLN status. The new technique of visualizing metastatic mesorectal lymph nodes on MRI images after injection of USPIO (ultra-small particles of iron oxide) was assessed in several studies and showed promising preliminary results in revealing metastatic lymph nodes (26,27). Still there is no report on LLN assessment with the use of this technique.

Tan et al. reviewed more than 1,000 rectal cancer cases and found that when a combination of three or more variables was present—female sex, tumors that were not well differentiated, pathological T3 and above, positive microscopic lymphatic invasion, and positive mesorectal nodes—the odds of lateral node metastasis were more than 7.5 times higher ($P < 0.001$) than in cases when less than three variables were noted (28).

PREOPERATIVE PLANNING

Preoperative planning includes a thorough physical examination. Enlarged inguinal lymph nodes should be noted. Physical examination, including digital rectal examination, vaginal inspection, and regional lymph node assessment may help to assess the possible risk of LLN involvement.

Rigid proctoscopy is performed to assess the accurate distance from lower border of the tumor to the anal verge and/or dentate line. Colonoscopy is required to identify any synchronous lesions. However, barium or Gastrografin enema is helpful in cases with severe tumor stenosis.

Although some authors are not suggesting chest CT as a routine diagnostic tool (29), all our patients are undergoing chest CT in order to exclude pulmonary metastasis.

A routine examination list includes an abdominal US or an abdominal CT scan with intravenous contrast.

In cases with nonobstructing cancer a rectal US is performed to stage the lesion. A phased-array MRI is obtained by colorectal surgery-oriented radiologist is a vital part of the multidisciplinary approach to the treatment. MRI identification of LLN >5 mm with irregular borders, mixed MR-signal intensity, or both is considered as highly suspicious for tumor involvement. LLN location, number, and their relation to any neighboring anatomic structures should be clearly noted.

Positioning

The patient is positioned in Lloyd-Davies position in Allen stirrups. Safe positioning of the patient's bony prominent part is very important; padding of neurovascular bundles is performed to prevent their damage. The surgeon is initially positioned on the left side of the patient, the first assistant is positioned on the right side, and second assistant is positioned between the patient's legs. During surgery the surgeon can change sides several times as needed. After induction of anesthesia, an additional digital rectal examination is performed to verify the tumor location, height, mobility, and the involvement of any other organs.

Part VIII: Pelvic Exenteration

Technique

A laparotomy is performed through a lower midline incision; great care is taken not to damage the bladder, which is usually dissected and retracted to the left as the 2 cm above pubic bone is quite important to optimize adequate visualization of the lower pelvis. After the midline laparotomy and intra-abdominal inspection a wound retracting system is installed. The surgeon retracts the small bowel, right colon, omentum, and proximal left colon under the blades of the retractor in order to open the sigmoid colon and its mesentery. The optimal view should include the duodenum as an upper border, aorta and vena cava on the right side with the white line of Toldt on the left side.

The modern principles of extended upward and LLN dissection imply complete removal of all fatty tissue from the para-aortic and lateral pelvic areas with maximum preservation of pelvic autonomic nervous system in all levels.

According to Japanese concepts based on early anatomic studies of Senba (30) and Kuru (31), the rectal muscle tube is surrounded by three fat-tissue "spaces". The first space corresponds to mesorectum that is enveloped by rectal fascia propria. Two hypogastric nerves and the pelvic plexuses are attached to both postero-lateral sides of mesorectum. Adjacent to the nerves lie the right and left second fat-tissue spaces. Lateral borders are the internal iliac vessels and their visceral branches. The left and right third spaces are located lateral to internal iliac vessels in both obturator fossae. Since establishing as a standard in Japanese colorectal surgery, this three-space dissection around the rectum is considered essential to achieve complete pelvic lymph node dissection in all three areas.

We perform para-aortic lymphadenectomy on a routine basis for all rectal, sigmoid, and left colon cancers.

The usual way to enter the preaortic space is to lift the sigmoid mesocolon in lateral-to-medial direction. The white line of Toldt along sigmoid colon is incised with monopolar electrocautery starting above the promontorium and all way up to the descending colon. It is essential to enter the embryologic interfascial avascular layer between sigmoid mesocolon fascia propria and renal fascia. The method of traction and countertraction is helpful in achieving that. The first assistant lifts the sigmoid colon gently handling it in the middle while the operator is dissecting the back of sigmoid mesentery off the underlying tissues. This maneuver helps to maintain left ureter safe below the dissection plane and visualize autonomic nervous structures. As soon as the left hypogastric nerve or hypogastric plexus is reached, it is carefully peeled off from the mesentery surface and left intact on the aorta.

The sigmoid colon is moved to the left and drawn upwards, the operator incises peritoneum at the root of its mesentery above the aorta. Using fine forceps the first assistant lifts the medial edge of peritoneal incision in the countertraction way. Thus the preaortic space is entered from the medial side. The described lateral and medial incisions meet to form reach-through hole above the aorta just above the hypogastric plexus. The operator enters this space with left index finger and uses it like a hook to lift the dissected vascular bundle off the aorta (Figure 36.1.1). Due to this maneuver good exposure of autonomic nerves and left ureter is assured. The peritoneal incision is extended upwards until the third part of duodenum is reached. The latter is gently retracted cranially and carefully dissected off. So left angle incision is formed with vertical part

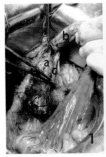 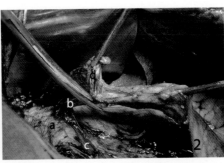

Figure 36.1 Paraaortic lymph node dissection. 1 – Vascular bundle containing IMA is pulled up above the aorta; 2 – IMA skeletonizing with scissors. a – aorta; b – IMA; c – left splanchnic lumbar nerve; d – paravasal fat tissue with apical lymph nodes.

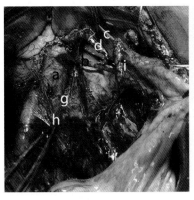
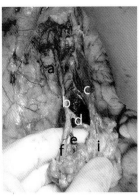

Figure 36.2 Paraaortic lymph node dissection. Skeletonized IMA and IMV. a – aorta; b – IMA; c – IMV; d – left colic artery; e – sigmoid arteries; f – superior rectal artery; g – left splanchnic lumbar nerve; h – hypogastric plexus; i – paravasal fat tissue with apical lymph nodes.

projecting to aorto-caval space and horizontal part—to lower border of duodenum. The origin of inferior mesenteric artery (IMA) is 2.5–3.0 cm lower the horizontal incision.

After that the preaortic fascia is opened and fat tissue surrounding the IMA root is cleared off the aorta between left and right splanchnic lumbar nerves leaving latter intact. It is preferably to use Harmonic scalplel (Ethicon Endo-Surgery, Inc., Cincinnati, OH) to reduce nerve damage at this step. The preaortic fat containing apical lymph nodes is cleared off the aorta surface in cranio-caudal and medial-lateral direction from the edges of peritoneal incision towards the origin of IMA. The fat envelope of IMA is incised up to vessel adventitia and dissected downward for a distance of a few centimeters. Using scissors of harmonic scalpel the IMA is freed circumferentially from paravasal fat all way down to the origin of left colic, sigmoid and superior rectal arteries (Figure 36.1.2). The mobilized preaortic and paravasal fat is moved down. This method of vessels "skeletizing" enables performing extended paraaortic lymph node dissection together with precise isolation and separate dissection of IMA branches without excessive colon resection.

To identify the trunk of inferior mesenteric vein (IMV) the peritoneal incision below the duodenum is prolonged further laterally. Extended paraaortic lymph node dissection is finished with clearing the space between IMA and IMV (Figures 36.2.1; 36.2.2). The LigaSure (Covidien, Norwalk, CT) is used to dissect the vessels: IMA right under the origin of left colic artery with its preservation, IMV – at the level of its conjoint with the trunk of left colic artery.

The mesentery is then divided with the LigaSure along the descending and sigmoid colon with preservation of the marginal artery and vein.

Once the level of intended proximal colon division is defined, the colon is freed and divided with a stapler. The proximal colon is wrapped with wet gauze and positioned under the left upper blade of wound retractor. The distal colon is used as retracting handle to enter the correct fascial plane of pelvis for TME start with hypogastric nerves being a key anatomic landmark.

The principles of careful dissection of the first pelvic fat-tissue space correspond to the TME technique that is described in several other chapters. The dissection plane lies in between the parietal (presacral) fascia and fascia propria of rectum with total preservation of hypogastric nerves and pelvic plexuses on both sides. When rectal excision is complete, the bowel wall is transected (or the perineal excision is completed in the case of an abdomino-perineal excision (APR)) and the specimen is removed, careful palpation of the lateral spaces on both sides is performed to reveal possible enlarged and/or indurated LLNs (Fig. 36.3). Intra-operative US of lateral spaces from the pelvic cavity can be helpful in identifying LLNs.

Unlike the preferences of some surgeons to perform LLD *en bloc* with the rectum or before its full extraction, we prefer to start the excision of LLNs after the rectal specimen is taken out. This method enables better access to this relatively small cavity and helps better control and preserve vessels and nervous structures throughout the procedure. Before the start of LLD, the ureter from the corresponding side of pelvis is medially retracted and fixed with a rubber loop to achieve good exposure. The following structures

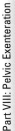

Part VIII: Pelvic Exenteration

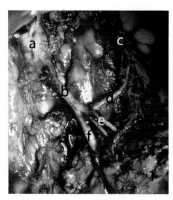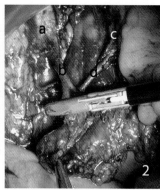

Figure 36.3 Paraaortic lymph node dissection. 1 – Skeletonized IMA and IMV; 2 – Division of IMA. a – aorta; b – IMA; c – IMV; d – left colic artery; e – sigmoid arteries; f – superior rectal artery.

are the anatomical landmarks for LLD: common iliac artery bifurcation cranially, bladder wall medially, external iliac vein laterally, and obturator muscle fascia from beneath.

Three ways to enter and clear the obturator (third) space can be implemented.

The first access option is the medial-to-lateral approach along the internal iliac vessels. First, the obturator fossa fat is gently peeled off the lateral wall of internal iliac artery up to the origin of the superior vesical artery. The latter is drawn medially and the peeling maneuver is continued down to the terminal branches of the internal iliac artery. For better exposure, the obturator vessels can be ligated and transected at this level. The obturator fat tissue is removed with preservation of obturator nerve that crosses the fossa in craniocaudal direction.

The second option is to enter the obturator space through paravesical approach. First, the lateral wall of internal iliac artery is cleared and then the peritoneum lateral to the bladder wall is additionally opened. In women this step demands transaction of the round ligament in that location. This technique allows entry of the obturator fossa from its distal part between the external iliac vessels and visceral branches of internal iliac vessels. The obturator fossa is cleared in caudal to a cranial direction with preservation of the obturator nerve.

Finally, the third technique that was developed by our group (32) allows better visualization and manipulation in the obturator space. The surgeon stands on the opposite side of the dissection. The paravesical space is entered and the peritoneal dissection is extended to the external iliac vessels. The peritoneum across external iliac artery is opened, the underlying vessels are freed (Fig. 36.4.1), and gently retracted medially with a rubber loop (Fig. 36.4.2). When the external iliac vessels are drawn medially, it helps access to the caudal part of obturator fossa which is hardly reached by conventional approach. The fat tissue is removed from the middle part of obturator fossa between the external iliac vessels medially and psoas muscle laterally (Figs. 36.4.3, 36.5.1, 36.5.2). The external iliac vessels are pulled back to the lateral side of the obturator fossa and the fat removal is finished.

After the obturator fossa (third space) is cleared out, lymph nodes from the second space are taken out. To perform that, the hypogastric nerve and pelvic plexus are gently drawn medially and fat tissue attached to their lateral border is peeled away down to the level of the pelvic plexus and sacral nerves. The complex of the visceral internal iliac branches forms the lateral border of second space. In case of advanced disease some of the vascular or nervous structures can be removed en bloc with the dissected fat tissue. In routine cases, a nerve-sparing LLD is performed (Figs. 36.5 and 36.6). Great care is taken to preserve major nerves branches.

LLD is a time-consuming procedure, which requires 20–30 minutes for each side even when performed by a high-volume rectal cancer surgeon. It can require several hours in complex cases or when undertaken by a low-volume colorectal surgeon in the beginning of learning curve. If required a contralateral LLD is performed in the same manner as a mirrored technique, resulting in bilateral lymph node dissection.

After LLD is complete a Blake drain is placed in the obturator fossa on each side and fixed to the skin of corresponding iliac region of abdominal wall. A pelvic drain is

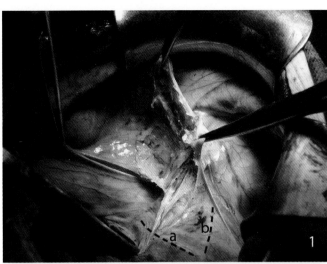

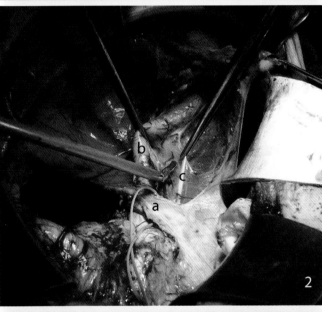

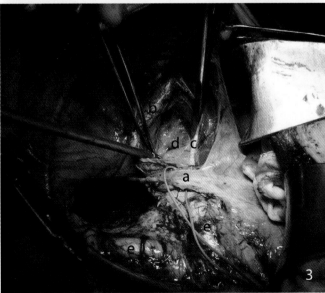

Figure 36.4 Right side LLD with external iliac artery retracted medially. 1 – Peritoneal incision along external iliac artery; 2 – Entering obturator space; 3 – Further developing of the obturator space. a – right ureter; b – right external iliac artery; c – branch of right femoral nerve; d – fat in right obturator space; e – common iliac arteries.

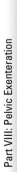

Figure 36.5 LLD with external iliac artery retracted medially. 1, 2 – Developing of the right obturator space; 3 – Demonstration of preserved pelvic nerves after left side lateral lymph node dissection. a – right ureter; b – right external iliac artery; c – right obturator nerve; d – ileopsoas muscle; e – left hypogastric nerve; g – left pelvic plexus.

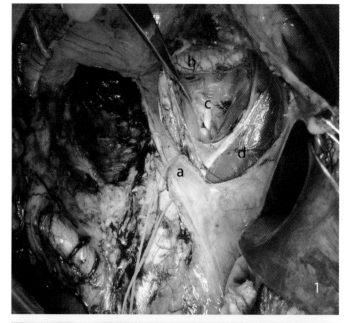

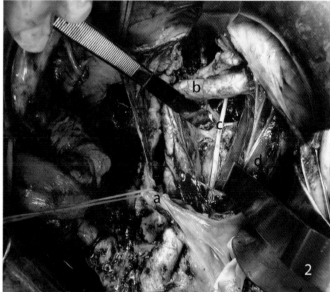

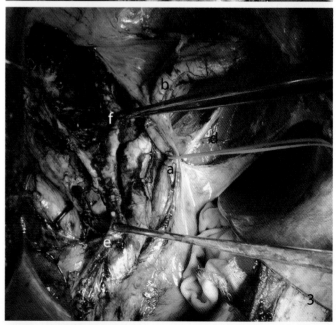

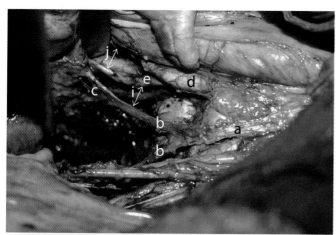

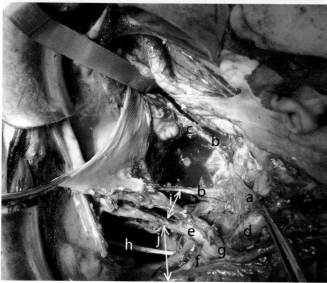

Figure 36.6 Nerve-sparing bilateral LLD. a – hypogastric plexus; b – hypogastric nerves; c – right pelvic plexus; d – common iliac artery; e – right internal iliac artery; f – external iliac artery; g - left ureter; h – left obturator nerve; i - "second space" (between pelvic plexus and internal iliac artery); j – "third space" (between internal and external iliac arteries).

also placed after the colorectal anastomosis is performed. We routinely perform stapled colorectal anastomosis with a diverting loop colostomy.

 ## POSTOPERATIVE MANAGEMENT

The patients after rectal excision with LLD are postoperatively followed in intensive care unit and when stable are transferred to the ward. The principles of early ambulation, analgesia, antibiotics, anticoagulant, infusion, and transfusion therapy don't differ significantly from conventional rectal cancer surgery. Extensive dissection of lymphatic tissue and cavity within the pelvis often leads to lymphorrhea of up to 500 ml/day from each side of the LLD but the amount gradually reduces usually within 2 weeks. It is essential to control and maintain adequate drainage from obturator spaces, to monitor vital signs and blood counts, perform pelvic US or CT scan if needed to detect fluid collections in the pelvis and to try to prevent infectious complications and lymphoceles. Maintaining a high protein diet as well as peanut oil consumption may make the exudate more viscous and help diminish lymphorrhea. In rare cases, a lymphocele demands percutaneous or transvaginal US-guided drainage. Drains from LLD areas are discharged once the output is <100 ml/day. An additional control US study is performed after the drains are removed.

The control of urinary function is another important part of postoperative management. In case of increased postvoiding residual urine volume (more than 200 ml) or patient inability to void spontaneously after bladder catheter is removed, pharmacological or electrostimulating therapy is attempted to restore bladder function. If these measures fail to rectify the problem trocar epicystotomy is performed.

 ## COMPLICATIONS

Efforts to improve survival by utilizing more radical lymphatic excision have been accompanied by increased morbidity. Additional pelvic dissection demands longer operative time, may cause additional blood loss and pelvic nervous system injury. Early reports of LLD indicated that implementation of this technique increased operative time and blood loss. Authors from the National Cancer Center Hospital from Tokyo (33) reported median operative times of 5 hours 17 minutes and 6 hours 33 minutes for standard and extended LLD, respectively. The median blood loss in their series was 1,528 ml and 2,128 ml for cases with standard and extended LLD, respectively. The same group had reported a high incidence of postoperative urinary and sexual dysfunction (34). Loss of bladder sensitivity and sexual impotency were reported in 39.4% of Dukes' B and 76% of Dukes' C patients from the LLD group and in 8.8% and 37.5% of the standard surgery group, respectively.

Further refinement of pelvic dissection based on recent anatomic clarification and the development of nerve-preserving techniques helped significantly reduce genitourinary complications of LLD. Recent results of partial autonomic nerve preservation demonstrated maintenance of bladder function in 74–100% of patients, while restoration of sexual function was not always successful and resulted in impotency and/or ejaculatory problems in 12–70% of male patients (5,34–37).

The results of the first detailed meticulous nerve-sparing LLD were presented by Moriya et al. (38) who described three types of nerve-preserving surgery: total autonomic nerve preservation, preservation of pelvic nerves, and partial pelvic nerve preservation. Improving skills in nerve-sparing LLD not only helped in maintaining urination in 84% of patients, but also reduced operative time to 334 minutes and blood loss to 935 ml. Further investigation led to a new national concept of nerve-preserving rectal cancer surgery in Japan (39). Pelvic autonomic nerve preservation is classified into four types based on the works of Hojo et al. (40), Moriya et al. (38), Sugihara et al. (41), and Takahashi et al. (20) complete preservation of autonomic nerves, preservation of autonomic nerves on one side, resection of hypogastric plexus, and resection of hypogastric plexus with unilateral pelvic plexus preservation. As demonstrated by Morita et al. (25) the extent of genitourinary dysfunction is directly related to the volume of nerve system preservation. Both total and unilateral preservation of the pelvic nervous system maintains urinary function, while subtotal pelvic nerve resection inevitably leads to functional impairment. Sexual function is preserved in 80% of patients with total or unilateral nerve-sparing surgery, while resection of the hypogastric plexus results in erectile dysfunction in 45% and most patients with subtotal nervous system resection never regain sexual function.

RESULTS

The number of English language studies devoted to evaluation of LLD effectiveness is very limited. Most studies originate from Japan and are retrospective, although they include large numbers of patients.

The Western experience with aortopelvic lymph node dissection comes back to late 1940s and early 1950s, when initial works of Gilchrist and David (42), Waugh and Kirklin (43), and Pfeifer and Miller (44) have revealed that lymph node involvement in patients with rectal cancer below the peritoneal reflexion was a significant predictor of poorer survival. The first results of extended APR with regional lymphatic removal were published by Deddish (15), Sauer and Bacon (14), Bacon et al. (45), and Sterns and Deddish (16). Although these works lack detailed depiction of the extent of LLD, they are likely to have been limited to internal iliac lymph node removal. These papers reported the incidence of LLN metastasis of 16-30% and a slight survival improvement in patients who underwent extensive surgery. The difference in 5-year survival was more evident in the subgroups of patients with Dukes' C lower rectal cancer (40% and 23% for extended and standard surgery, respectively) (16). Still the authors emphasized high morbidity rates following extensive surgery including intra-operative hemorrhage, bladder dysfunction, and prolonged hospitalization thus making the benefit of LLD questionable.

Based on these reports, Western surgeons abandoned further research of extensive LLD, until the published results from Memorial Sloan-Kettering Cancer Center demonstrated a significant survival advantage for patients with Dukes' C rectal cancer who underwent *en bloc* LLD as compared to standard resections (5). Still no influence on local control was achieved in this series. The authors performed limited pelvic lymphadenectomy (only removing the internal iliac nodes, no obturator space clearance, and no nerve preserving techniques) in 192 out of 412 rectal cancer patients and demonstrated 5-year survival rates of 63.8% and 54.3% for extended and standard operations, respectively. Among numerous factors involved in regression analysis, pelvic lymphadenectomy and distance from the anal verge demonstrated the strongest association with survival. The disappointing experience of iliac lymph node dissection for rectal cancer in St. Mark's hospital (37) showed no improvement in crude 5-year survival and even worse survival in patients after extended surgery for Dukes' C rectal cancer compared to standard operation. Another American paper from the University of Chicago revealed the benefit of LLD in decreasing local recurrence rate from 16.4% to 9.4%, though it was not statistically significant, and no influence on survival was reported (46).

Meanwhile, the extensive Japanese experience with LLD was more promising. The technique of meticulous lymph node dissection in three "spaces" (perirectal fat, tissue along pelvic plexus and obturator fossa fat) was established and practiced long before the first Japanese reports appeared in English language literature. The National Cancer Center Hospital presented the results of LLD in 423 patients operated on from 1969 to 1980 (47). The incidence of LLN metastasis in lower advanced rectal cancer group was 23% and these patients had the worst survival rate (16 of 17 patients died within 5 years of follow-up). A subsequent report from the same institution included analysis of 459 patients and demonstrated statistically significant improvement in 5-year survival for patients who underwent LLD over those who underwent the conventional approach (from 63.7% to 83.2% and 30.8% to 52.5% for Dukes' B and C patients, respectively) (48). The improvement in local control was also significant 5-year local recurrence rate decreased from 26.1% to 8.4% and from 44.3% to 24.5% for Dukes' B and C patients, respectively. A further report by the same group confirmed significant benefit of LLD in ameliorating LLR and 5-year survival in patients with Dukes' B and C stage low rectal cancer (34), but also stressed the increased incidence of voiding and sexual dysfunction after LLD. Loss of bladder sensitivity and sexual impotency was reported in 39.4% and 76% of patients from extended surgery group and 8.8% and 37.5% in standard surgery group, respectively.

Another analysis of these data (33) suggested that extended LLD was superior to standard LLD in terms of both 5-year disease-free survival (75.8% and 67.4%, respectively) and local recurrence rate (12% and 17%, respectively).

In the last 10 years several big studies addressed effectiveness of LLD in the Japanese population. Retrospective series of Takahashi et al. (20) and Ueno et al. (24) demonstrated evident correlation—the more distal the tumor is, the higher the risk of LLN involvement; specifically rates were 0.6–10.5% for tumors located above 6 cm from dentate line and 29.6–42.0% for those lesions at the level of dentate line. The study by Takahashi et al. (20) also suggested that LLD may be of extreme benefit for patients with isolated lateral nodes metastases only without affected mesorectal lymph nodes who demonstrate 5-year overall survival of 75% compared to 32% in patients with positive both lateral and mesorectal lymph nodes.

In a recent multicenter trial from Japan, a total of 2,751 patients were included in a retrospective analysis. Among them 35% received LLN dissection. The majority of them had tumors located below the peritoneal reflexion with 15% LLNs positivity. Although surprisingly patients without LLD showed significantly better prognosis than those who had undergone it, in Stage II the survival was significantly better in patients with LLD in those without it, and there was no difference of the survival between patients with Stage III disease. The authors concluded that the worse prognosis following lateral LLD may be because of a higher proportion of patients having more advanced stage disease in this group. The patients with positive LLN survived longer after lateral lymphadenectomy with a 5-year survival rate of 45%. LLN dissection might reduce local recurrence and improve the 5-year survival rate by removal of positive LLN, but not all positive LLN will present overt local recurrence and not all local recurrences will cause cancer death.

Another group of Japanese investigators have developed a new therapeutic measurement tool to estimate the benefit of LLN dissection (49). It is called therapeutic value index and is calculated by multiplying the frequency of metastasis to the area and the cancer-related 5-year survival rate of patients with metastasis to this area. In this study, lateral nodal involvement was observed in 17% of patients, a quarter of whom had no involved nodes in the mesorectum. The 5-year survival rate in patients having lateral nodal involvement was 41.6%, and their cumulative local recurrence-free 5-year survival rate was 59.0%. It was very interesting that patients who had positive lateral nodes but no nodes in the mesorectum had a 5-year survival rate of 78.7%. The therapeutic value index for survival benefit and the local control benefit by lateral dissection were calculated to be 7 points and almost 10 points, respectively. These values were comparable to the therapeutic index scores of lymphadenectomy of the mesorectum region dissection (7 points), and much higher than those obtained by lymphadenectomy of the superior rectal artery area (1.6 points) and those obtained by lymphadenectomy of the IMA area (0.4 points).

One of major reasons why Western colorectal surgeons abandoned LLD is wide adoption of preoperative radiation therapy as a noninvasive alternative to LLD. In case of suspected LLN metastasis, Japanese approach is to perform TME with LLD, while in Western countries the standard of care is neoadjuvant radio- or chemoradiotherapy followed by TME surgery. Thus, recent papers address comparison of preoperative RT and LLD in achieving local control and increasing survival rate.

A recent retrospective study from Japan evaluated the results of four different treatment options: RT together with LLD, RT alone, LLD alone, and neither RT nor LLD of these in 115 patients (50). There was no difference between the groups in terms of overall postoperative survival, disease-free survival, or recurrence. The authors suggested that preoperative radiotherapy can be an alternative to LLD.

The only randomized trial compared the results in two groups of patients who either underwent or did not undergo LLN dissection (13). It included only 45 patients and failed to show any benefit from LLD to either local control or disease-free survival. This study has certain limits. The first of which is the small cohort of patients included. The authors mentioned that six patients were excluded, but do not characterize these patients. Secondly, nerve-sparing techniques were not described and as already noted have a great impact on evaluation of functional outcome after LLD.

Our experience with LLD suggests that it requires an additional profound knowledge of lower pelvis anatomy with skills in extended dissection. The procedure has an obvious learning curve, and is clearly considered a complex pelvic surgery case. An additional problem is dissection in the deep fatty pelvis often encountered in the Caucasian population, which is associated with an increased operative time and blood loss. Our approach of LLD with medial retraction of external iliac vessels provides beneficial visualization of LLN, thus decreasing risk of trauma to the surrounding structures with an increased superior LLD. Nerve-sparing LLD in patients with no direct tumor invasion is valuable and important surgical approach which provides superior functional results and quality of life. Our experience showed that LLD is associated with 20% increase in 3-year overall survival and an 8% increase in 5-year overall survival without a decrease in distant metastasis.

CONCLUSIONS

LLN dissection for rectal carcinoma is a technically demanding and controversial surgical procedure. It is a feasible and safe tool, which should be included in the skills set of a rectal cancer surgeon. Our experience has shown that it might give some benefits to patients though it may be associated with increased operative time, blood loss, and overall morbidity.

Recommended References and Readings

1. Kim TH, Jeong SY, Choi DH, et al. Lateral lymph node metastasis is a major cause of locoregional recurrence in rectal cancer treated with preoperative chemoradiotherapy and curative resection. *Ann Surg Oncol* 2008;15(3):729–37.
2. Colquhoun P, Wexner SD, Cohen A. Adjuvant therapy is valuable in the treatment of rectal cancer despite total mesorectal excision. *J Surg Oncol* 2003;83(3):133–39.
3. Boyle KM, Sagar PM, Chalmers AG, et al. Surgery for locally recurrent rectal cancer. *Dis Colon Rectum* 2005;48(5):929–37.
4. Heriot AG, Byrne CM, Lee P, et al. Extended radical resection: the choice for locally recurrent rectal cancer. *Dis Colon Rectum* 2008;51(3):284–91.
5. Enker WE, Pilipshen SJ, Heilweil ML, et al. En bloc pelvic lymphadenectomy and sphincter preservation in the surgical management of rectal cancer. *Ann Surg* 1986;203(4):426–33.
6. Kusters M, Wallner C, Lange MM, et al. Origin of presacral local recurrence after rectal cancer treatment. *Br J Surg* 2010;97:1582–88.
7. Kapiteijn E, Marijnen CA, Nagtegaal ID, et al. Preoperative radiotherapy combined with total mesorectal excision for resectable rectal cancer. *N Engl J Med* 2001;345(9):638–46.
8. Hiotis SP, Weber SM, Cohen AM, et al. Assessing the predictive value of clinical complete response to neoadjuvant therapy for rectal cancer: an analysis of 488 patients. *J Am Coll Surg* 2002;194(2):131–35; discussion 135–36.
9. Wheeler JM, Dodds E, Warren BF, et al. Preoperative chemoradiotherapy and total mesorectal excision surgery for locally advanced rectal cancer: correlation with rectal cancer regression grade. *Dis Colon Rectum* 2004;47(12):2025–31.
10. Dahlberg M, Glimelius B, Graf W, et al. Preoperative irradiation affects functional results after surgery for rectal cancer: results from a randomized study. *Dis Colon Rectum* 1998;41(5):543–49; discussion 549–51.
11. Tsujinaka S, Kawamura YJ, Konishi F, et al. Long-term efficacy of preoperative radiotherapy for locally advanced low rectal cancer. *Int J Colorectal Dis* 2008;23(1):67–76.
12. Peeters KC, van de Velde CJ, Leer JW, et al. Late side effects of short-course preoperative radiotherapy combined with total mesorectal excision for rectal cancer: increased bowel dysfunction in irradiated patients—a Dutch colorectal cancer group study. *J Clin Oncol* 2005;23(25):6199–206.
13. Nagawa H, Muto T, Sunouchi K, et al. Randomized, controlled trial of lateral node dissection vs. nerve-preserving resection in patients with rectal cancer after preoperative radiotherapy. *Dis Colon Rectum* 2001;44(9):1274–80.
14. Sauer I, Bacon HE. A new approach for excision of carcinoma of the lower portion of the rectum and anal canal. *Surg Gynecol Obstet* 1952;95(2):229–42.
15. Deddish MR. Abdominopelvic lymph node dissection in cancer of the rectum and distal colon. *Cancer* 1951;4(6):1364–66.
16. Stearns MW Jr, Deddish MR. Five-year results of abdominopelvic lymph node dissection for carcinoma of the rectum. *Dis Colon Rectum* 1959;2(2):169–72.
17. Yano H, Moran BJ. The incidence of lateral pelvic side-wall nodal involvement in low rectal cancer may be similar in Japan and the West. *Br J Surg* 2008;95(1):33–49.
18. Mori T. Reply. *Langenbecks Arch Surg* 1999;384(4):407–08.
19. Akasu T, Iinuma G, Takawa M, et al. Accuracy of high-resolution magnetic resonance imaging in preoperative staging of rectal cancer. *Ann Surg Oncol* 2009;16(10):2787–94.
20. Takahashi T, Ueno M, Azekura K, et al. Lateral node dissection and total mesorectal excision for rectal cancer. *Dis Colon Rectum* 2000;43(10 Suppl):S59–68.
21. Mori T, Takahashi K, Yasuno M. Radical resection with autonomic nerve preservation and lymph node dissection techniques in lower rectal cancer surgery and its results: the impact of lateral lymph node dissection. *Langenbecks Arch Surg* 1998;383(6):409–15.
22. Sugihara K, Kobayashi H, Kato T, et al. Indication and benefit of pelvic sidewall dissection for rectal cancer. *Dis Colon Rectum* 2006;49(11):1663–72.
23. Ueno H, Yamauchi C, Hase K, et al. Clinicopathological study of intrapelvic cancer spread to the iliac area in lower rectal adenocarcinoma by serial sectioning. *Br J Surg* 1999;86(12):1532–37.
24. Ueno M, Oya M, Azekura K, et al. Incidence and prognostic significance of lateral lymph node metastasis in patients with advanced low rectal cancer. *Br J Surg* 2005;92(6):756–63.
25. Morita T, Murata A, Koyama M, et al. Current status of autonomic nerve-preserving surgery for mid and lower rectal cancers: Japanese experience with lateral node dissection. *Dis Colon Rectum* 2003;46(10 Suppl):S78–87; discussion S87–88.
26. Lahaye MJ, Engelen SM, Nelemans PJ, et al. Imaging for predicting the risk factors—the circumferential resection margin and nodal disease—of local recurrence in rectal cancer: a meta-analysis. *Semin Ultrasound CT MR* 2005;26(4):259–68.
27. Puli SR, Reddy JB, Bechtold ML, et al. Accuracy of endoscopic ultrasound to diagnose nodal invasion by rectal cancers: a meta-analysis and systematic review. *Ann Surg Oncol* 2009;16(5):1255–65.
28. Tan KY, Yamamoto S, Fujita S, et al. Improving prediction of lateral node spread in low rectal cancers—multivariate analysis of clinicopathological factors in 1,046 cases. *Langenbecks Arch Surg* 2010;395(5):545–49.
29. Grossmann I, Avenarius JK, Mastboom WJ, et al. Preoperative staging with chest CT in patients with colorectal carcinoma: not as a routine procedure. *Ann Surg Oncol* 2010;17(8):2045–50.
30. Senba Y. An anatomical study of lymphatic system of the rectum [in Japanese]. *J Hukuoka Med Coil* 1927;20:1213–68.
31. Kuru M. Cancer of the rectum [in Japanese]. *J Jpn Surg Soc* 1940;41:832–77.
32. Vorob'ev GI, Odariuk TS, Tsar'kov PV, Eropkin PV. Aortoiliopelvic lymphadenectomy in surgical treatment of rectal cancer. *Khirurgiia (Mosk)*. 1998;(4):4–8. [Article in Russian]
33. Moriya Y, Hojo K, Sawada T, et al. Significance of lateral node dissection for advanced rectal carcinoma at or below the peritoneal reflection. *Dis Colon Rectum* 1989;32(4):307–15.
34. Hojo K, Sawada T, Moriya Y. An analysis of survival and voiding, sexual function after wide iliopelvic lymphadenectomy in patients with carcinoma of the rectum, compared with conventional lymphadenectomy. *Dis Colon Rectum* 1989;32(2):128–33.
35. Enker WE. Potency, cure, and local control in the operative treatment of rectal cancer. *Arch Surg* 1992;127(12):1396–401; discussion 1402.
36. Michelassi F, Block GE. Morbidity and mortality of wide pelvic lymphadenectomy for rectal adenocarcinoma. *Dis Colon Rectum* 1992;35(12):1143–47.
37. Glass RE, Ritchie JK, Thompson HR, et al. The results of surgical treatment of cancer of the rectum by radical resection and extended abdomino-iliac lymphadenectomy. *Br J Surg* 1985;72(8):599–601.

38. Moriya Y, Sugihara K, Akasu T, et al. Nerve-sparing surgery with lateral node dissection for advanced lower rectal cancer. *Eur J Cancer* 1995;31A(7–8):1229–32.

39. Yasutomi M. Advances in rectal cancer surgery in Japan. *Dis Colon Rectum* 1997;40(10 Suppl):S74–79.

40. Hojo K, Vernava AM 3rd, Sugihara K, et al. Preservation of urine voiding and sexual function after rectal cancer surgery. *Dis Colon Rectum* 1991;34(7):532–39.

41. Sugihara K, Moriya Y, Akasu T, et al. Pelvic autonomic nerve preservation for patients with rectal carcinoma. Oncologic and functional outcome. *Cancer* 1996;78(9):1871–80.

42. Gilchrist D, David V. Prognosis of carcinoma of the bowel. *Surg Gynecol Obstet* 1948;86:359–71.

43. Waugh J, Kirklin J. The importance of the lesion in prognosis and treatment of carcinoma of the rectum and low sigmoid colon. *Ann Surg* 1949;129:22–3.

44. Pfeiffer D, Miller D. Cancer of the rectum; 5 and 10 year follow-up study of cases of cancer below the peritoneal reflexion. *Surg Gynecol Obstet* 1950;91:319–22.

45. Bacon H, Dirbas F, Myers T, et al. Extensive lymphadenectomy and high ligation of the inferior mesenteric artery for carci-noma of the left colon and rectum. *Dis Colon Rectum* 1958;1:457–65.

46. Michelassi F, Block G, Vanucci L, et al. A 5- to 21-year follow-up and analysis of 250 patients with rectal adenocarcinoma. *Ann Surg* 1988;208:379–89.

47. Hojo K, Koyama Y, Moriya Y. Lymphatic spread and its prognostic value in patients with rectal cancer. *Am J Surg* 1982;144(3):350–54.

48. Koyama Y, Moriya Y, Hojo K. Effects of extended systematic lymphadenectomy for adenocarcinoma of the rectum—significant improvement of survival rate and decrease of local recurrence. *Jpn J Clin Oncol* 1984;14(4):623–32.

49. Ueno H, Mochizuki H, Hashiguchi Y, et al. Potential prognostic benefit of lateral pelvic node dissection for rectal cancer located below the peritoneal reflection. *Ann Surg* 2007;245(1):80–87.

50. Watanabe T, Tsurita G, Muto T, et al. Extended lymphadenectomy and preoperative radiotherapy for lower rectal cancers. *Surgery* 2002;132(1):27–33.

37 The EXPRESS Procedures for Full Thickness Rectal Prolapse and Rectal Intussusception With or Without Rectocele Repair

Norman S. Williams and Christopher L.H. Chan

Introduction

Posterior pelvic compartment dysfunction is a challenging problem as appropriate therapies are limited. Management is often conservative, and surgery only indicated for very select groups including prolapsing disorders of the rectal wall. These disorders of the rectal wall: overt rectal prolapse, rectal intussusception (RI), and rectocele, are usually seen in females. The etiology is poorly understood but is likely to be associated with obstetric injury with pelvic tissue atrophy. One surgical strategy to correct these prolapsing disorders involves suspension of the rectum to a fixed point using synthetic or biological implants.

The EXPRESS procedure has been developed in an attempt to further improve outcomes following surgery in patients with prolapsing disorders of the rectal wall. It is a novel, relatively minimally invasive form of anterior rectopexy, using a perineal rather than abdominal approach, with the aid of a dermal porcine implant.

BIOLOGICAL IMPLANTS

The use of implants in surgery has become increasingly frequent over the last century, particularly polypropylene-based meshes in the management of abdominal wall defects/hernias. The disadvantage, however, of synthetic meshes in particular reference to colorectal surgery has been the well-documented risks of infection, extrusion, and fistulation (1,2). With these concerns biological implants have been introduced. They are predominantly derived from porcine dermis, due to its similarity in structure to human dermis.

One such commercially available porcine dermal implant is Permacol™ (Covidien, MA, USA), an acellular cross-linked porcine collagen. The cross linking prevents degradation by collagenases and it is therefore theoretically permanent once implanted. It also elicits a very mild inflammatory response, with minimal fibrosis, and can be successfully used to reconstruct defects within infected fields. In addition, histological studies have demonstrated the implant to be associated with ordered neocollagen deposition presumed to result in greater tissue strength than at the time of implantation (3). These characteristics make Permacol™ an ideal implant to utilize in surgery for pelvic disorders, particularly those of the posterior compartment, which require any implant to be placed in close proximity to the rectum.

RECTAL INTUSSUSCEPTION AND RECTOCELE

Rectal evacuatory disorder/dysfunction (RED) is a complex problem where the primary abnormality is the preferential storage of residue in the rectum for prolonged periods, with the inability to evacuate this residue adequately. The pathophysiologies that underlie RED are not well understood as the etiology is varied: anatomical disorders of the rectum, for example, megarectum and prolapsing disorders of the rectal wall, for example, RI and rectocele. Rectal intussusception can be defined as a full thickness invagination of the rectal wall, which is thought to cause symptoms by impeding the evacuation of the rectum either by occlusion of the rectal lumen (recto-rectal) or the anal canal (recto-anal). Furthermore, the presence of the intussusception, particularly in the upper anal canal, may result in a sense of incomplete evacuation despite adequate clearance of rectal contents. However, the significance of RI is not fully understood due to its presence in studies of asymptomatic volunteers, albeit in a less severe form (4). Commonly associated with RI is a rectocele, a ballooning of the anterior rectum into the posterior vaginal wall resulting in trapping of rectal contents thus contributing to symptoms of evacuatory dysfunction.

There are few described procedures for a surgical repair of RI (5), and can be divided into resectional, intra-rectal Delorme's, stapled transanal rectal resection (STARR) procedure, or suspensory techniques, such as the various forms of abdominal rectopexy. Most, however, are universally associated with poor functional outcomes (6), or serious complications (7,8).

With these limitations in mind we have developed an innovative minimally invasive technique that combines the advantages of abdominal rectopexy procedures, namely, lower recurrence rates, with the advantages of perineal approaches, lower morbidity, and ability to repair a coexistent rectocele. The **EX**ternal **P**elvic **RE**ctal SuSpension (EXPRESS) is essentially an anterior perineal rectopexy, which involves fixation of the rectum to the periosteum of the superior pubic ramus with or without simultaneous reinforcement of the rectovaginal septum with a Permacol™ patch, to correct any coexistent rectocele.

EXPRESS FOR RECTAL INTUSSUSCEPTION

Indications

Patients with severe rectal evacuatory dysfunction refractory to maximal conservative therapy and a normal colonic transit with:

i. Full-thickness internal rectal circumferential prolapse (rectal intussusception) (Shorvon grade 4 or more) impeding rectal emptying on defecography ± functional rectocele (more than 2 cm) containing residual barium termination of rectal evacuation during defecography.

ii. Patients with symptoms including tenesmus or the sensation of a lump within the rectum after defecation (in association with an intussusception) and/or an uncomfortable swelling within the vagina, or the need for vaginal digitation (in association with a rectocele) may also be considered for surgery.

Contraindications

Patients younger than age 18 years
Unfit for surgery
Delayed colonic transit and/or rectal hyposensitivity

Preoperative

Patients are carefully selected for the procedure on the basis of symptom profile, clinical examination, and indications stated above. Patients with severe RED (symptoms of tenesmus, something coming down, or a sensation of a lump within the rectum (associated with RI) and/or an uncomfortable swelling in the vagina or a need for vaginal digitation (in association with rectocele) are considered for the procedure only after concomitant organic pathology has been excluded.

Comprehensive anorectal physiologic investigations should be performed in all patients, to include diagnostic defecography and assessment of anal sphincter function and integrity, using manometry and endoanal ultrasound respectively. Rectal sensory thresholds to balloon distension, evaluation of pudendal nerve terminal motor latencies, and assessment of colonic transit using a simple radio-opaque marker study are undertaken.

In addition, all patients must have initially undergone a period of maximal conservative therapy tailored to their presenting symptoms and physiologic findings, which is coordinated by a nurse specialist. This incorporates psychosocial counseling, optimization of diet and lifestyle, optimization of medication, pelvic floor coordination exercises, and true biofeedback techniques (including balloon expulsion). Only patients who fail to respond to this therapeutic program are considered for surgery.

Surgery

Positioning

The patient is placed in a modified Lloyd-Davies position on the operating table, with pneumatic compression stockings to reduce the risk of thromboembolism. A urethral catheter is inserted to empty the bladder and the skin is prepared and draped to allow access to the perineum as well as the suprapubic region.

A convex crescentic incision is made between the rectum and the vagina/scrotum (Fig. 37.1). The skin and subcutaneous tissue are dissected from the underlying anterior sphincter complex so as to not damage the anterior aspect, thus enabling entry into the extra sphincteric plane. The plane between the posterior wall of the vagina and the anterior wall of the rectum is entered taking care not to injure the sphincter complex or buttonhole the rectum or vagina. Infiltration with saline solution aids in development of this plane. The dissection is continued cephalad as far as the posterior fornix of the vagina to the level of Denonvilliers' fascia (Fig. 37.2). Once the anterior plane has been dissected satisfactorily, the lateral wall of the rectum can be mobilized using blunt dissection.

Although the operation is much more commonly performed in women, the procedure can be applied to male patients. The dissection in the male resembles that of a perineal prostatectomy in which the rectourethral/prostatic plane is entered by dividing

Figure 37.1 A convex crescentic incision is made in the perineum.

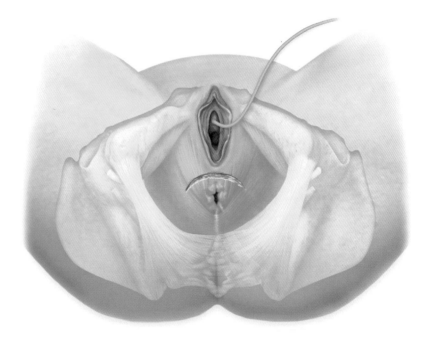

the rectourethralis muscle close to the rectum. The anterior rectal wall is then mobilized, using a combination of blunt and diathermy dissection, from the prostate in close proximity to the rectum to avoid damage to the neurovascular bundles located at the inferolateral aspect of the prostate.

The assistant makes two transverse incisions over the lateral aspects of the superior pubic rami 2–3 cm long. The dissection is deepened to gain access to the retropubic space bilaterally. A custom made tunneller is advanced through the perineal incision

Figure 37.2 The dissection is extended into the rectovaginal/ prostatic plane.

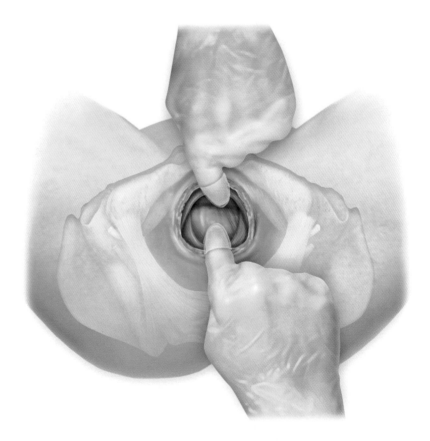

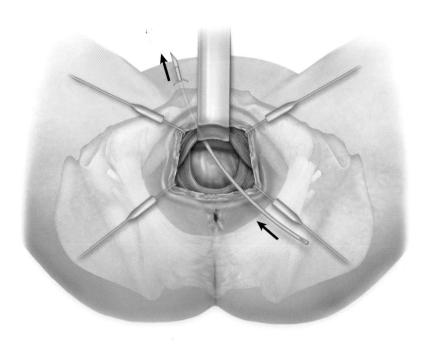

Figure 37.3 A sharp pointed tunneller is passed through the perineal wound retropubically and delivered through the suprapubic wound.

retropubically; care is taken not to damage the vagina at this point, and delivered through the suprapubic incisions (Fig. 37.3). Two T-shaped strips of Permacol™ are utilized for the rectal suspension. The corner of the transverse portion of the T-piece is sutured to a specially designed olive, which can be secured to the end of the tunnelling device and then delivered through the retropubic tunnel back into the perineal wound (Fig. 37.4).

The transverse portion of the T-piece should be sutured to the anterolateral rectal wall with its upper margin at approximately 8 cm from the upper margin of the external anal sphincter using 3.0 polydiaxone (PDS) interrupted sutures and involving the rectal serosa and muscle but not the mucosa. Once the transverse portions are secured

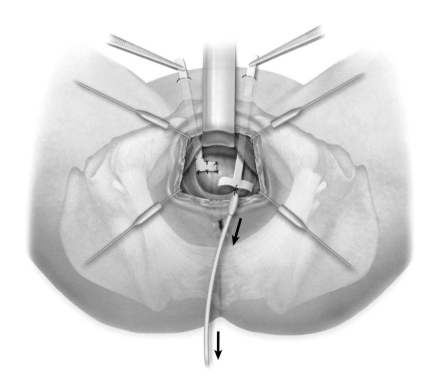

Figure 37.4 The T-strips of Permacol™ are drawn through the suprapubic wounds attached to the tunneller and delivered into the perineal wound. The transverse portion of the strip is sutured to the rectal wall.

Figure 37.5 Upward traction is delivered on the Permacol™ strips and they are secured to the periosteum of the pubis.

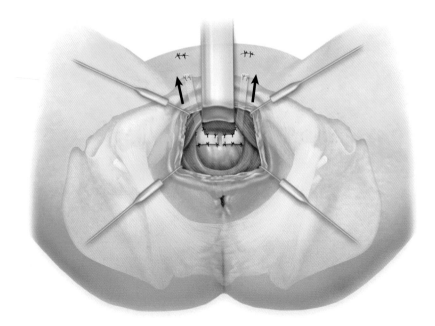

to the anterolateral wall, the assistant applies upward traction on the longitudinal portion of the T-strips through the suprapubic wounds (Fig. 37.5). The previously placed pubic rami sutures are then attached to the longitudinal aspect of the T-strip and tied resulting in suspension of the rectum to the superior pubic ramus.

Rectocele Repair

Any coexistent rectocele can now be repaired. Initially the redundant bulging anterior rectal wall is plicated with a 2-0 Vicryl. Inserting a custom designed square 5 by 5 cm Permacol™ patch with 5 by 2 cm wings then reinforces the rectovaginal septum (Fig. 37.6). The square portion of the patch is fixed to the anterior rectal wall with interrupted 2-0 PDS sutures and the winged portion is fixed to the periosteum of the ischial tuberosities again with 2-0 PDS. After hemostasis is secured, two suction drains are left *in situ*. The subcutaneous tissues are closed and the skin approximated with interrupted absorbable sutures.

Figure 37.6 Rectocele repair.

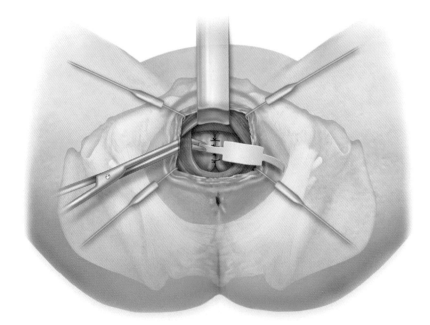

Postoperative

Patients are allowed to eat and drink on the first postoperative day as tolerated, during which time full mobilization is encouraged. After 48 hours, the urethral catheter and suction drains (if output is less than 30 ml) are removed.

Patients are discharged after the first bowel movement to be reviewed in the surgical outpatient clinic after 2 months.

Complications

Intraoperative

Inadvertent breaching of the vaginal wall during rectovaginal dissection. This can be easily repaired with direct suture with no subsequent complication.

Inadvertent breaching of the anterior rectal wall during rectovaginal dissection. This can be repaired by direct suture but may require subsequent drainage, and formation of a defunctioning stoma.

Postoperative

Self-limiting wound infection is common; usually settles with antibiotics or local surgical drainage.

Postoperative wound pain (n = 4)
Transient bladder dysfunction (n = 1)
Erectile dysfunction (temporary in male) (n = 1)
Dyspareunia (female) (n = 2)
Rectovaginal fistula (n = 1)
Rectoperineal fistula (n = 1)

Most complications are related to minor wound infections or erosions through the posterior vaginal wall. They can be treated conservatively and rarely require surgical drainage.

The Permacol™ implant is well tolerated on the whole but initially may result in some vaginal discharge, which typically settles after 6–8 weeks. This is more common if a rectocele repair has been performed and may result in dyspareunia, which is usually transient, but which patients should be warned about preoperatively.

The most significant complication is associated with inadvertent rectal perforation particularly if unnoticed at the time of surgery, as this is likely to result in sepsis within the rectovaginal plane with subsequent rectovaginal/perineal fistulation. The management of such a complication would be surgical drainage of the sepsis and temporary defunctioning stoma formation.

Results

Currently, we have follow-up data on the cohort of 22 patients (20F, 19/20 had concomitant rectocele repaired) for a median of 35 months (range 24–48 months) postoperatively. Symptoms of difficulty emptying and vaginal bulging improved significantly with a trend toward improvement in straining, digitation, passage of mucous, and a sense of blockage/obstruction. Any preoperative symptoms of fecal incontinence were unchanged.

Sixty five percent of patients appeared satisfied with the outcome of their surgery and 71% felt that they had sustained an improvement in symptoms following their operation.

Physiological and Proctographic Assessment

There were no changes in manometric assessment of maximum anal canal resting or squeeze pressures from those recorded preoperatively. Evacuatory function appeared to significantly improve (i.e., decrease in overall time to evacuate). There was a significant reduction in rectocele size in those requiring a concomitant repair. Intussusception grade showed a significant improvement, but deteriorated in two patients and remained the same in one.

OVERT RECTAL PROLAPSE

Surgery

The optimum surgical management for rectal prolapse remains unclear as anatomical abnormalities often occur together. Operations for this condition, although numerous, basically fall into two main categories: those performed by a perineal approach and those conducted through the abdomen. Abdominal rectopexy involves fixation of the mobilized rectum to the sacrum. Although it has a relatively low recurrence rate, it suffers from all the risks of major abdominal surgery. In addition, there is a small risk of damage to the pelvic autonomic nerves, which might result in bladder, bowel, and sexual disturbances. Furthermore, an abdominal rectopexy often causes or exacerbates constipation, a reason that has led some surgeons to combine it with a sigmoid resection, which has the potential to increase morbidity, or advocate an anterior dissection only. For these reasons abdominal rectopexy is not usually recommended for the elderly, infirm patient or increasingly for the young male patient for risk of impotence. The perineal procedures fall into two main categories: Délorme's procedure and the Altemeier operation (proctosigmoidectomy). The Délorme's involves a rectal mucosectomy, and has a low morbidity but high recurrence rate, which may approach 50% (9). The Altemeier procedure involves a rectosigmoid resection and colorectal anastomosis, and has a higher morbidity than Délorme's procedure, yet the recurrence rate is claimed to be lower (10). The ideal operation for rectal prolapse should be safe, minimally invasive, improve function, and have a low recurrence rate. Délorme's procedure more or less fits the first three categories but not the latter. Our initial aim, therefore, was to modify the operation in a relatively minimally invasive manner in an attempt to deal with its Achilles heel, namely, the high recurrence rate.

It is unclear why recurrence occurs after Délorme's procedure, but one likely possibility is that the old apex lengthens once again and descends out of the anus. If this is so, attaching a series of "guide wires" around the apex of the prolapse, exerting upward tension on these, and then attaching them to a fixed point might prevent it. As described previously, the properties of Permacol™ make it an ideal implant to suture to the rectum without the usual concerns that are prescient with the use of synthetic implants.

EXPRESS FOR OVERT RECTAL PROLAPSE

Surgery

Positioning

Prior to surgery, all patients are counseled extensively by a member of the surgical team and informed consent obtained. All patients undergo a full bowel preparation (e.g., sodium picosulfate). Antibiotics and thromboprophylaxis are administered at the time of anesthetic induction. The procedure is performed under epidural anesthesia or full general anesthetic with muscle relaxation.

Surgical Technique

The patient is placed in the Lloyd-Davies position and after urethral catheterization, the rectum and vagina are copiously lavaged with dilute Betadine® (The Purdue Frederick Company, Norwalk, CT) and after appropriate skin preparation, the patient is draped, exposing the perineum and the suprapubic regions.

The prolapse is everted maximally with Babcock's forceps and the submucous plane is infiltrated with a 1 in 300,000 adrenaline/saline solution. A mucosectomy is performed circumferentially with a hand-held diathermy commencing 1–2 cm proximal to the dentate line and continuing over the exposed part of the prolapse and extending for 3–4 cm beyond the apex on its intraluminal surface (Fig. 37.7). Two semi-circumferential incisions measuring approximately 4–5 cm are then made with the diathermy through

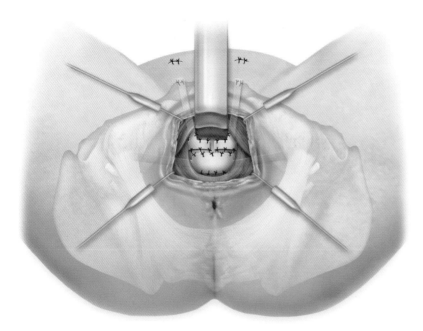

Figure 37.7 Final appearance following combined EXPRESS and rectocele repair.

the denuded muscle of the apex of the prolapse in the right and left anterolateral quadrants to expose the inner surfaces of the rectal serosa. A purpose-designed sharp, pointed tunneller is then passed through the right incision in an upward direction (Fig. 37.8). This tunneller is passed between the layers of the prolapsed rectal wall, above the external anal sphincter through the pelvic floor, and continued in the subcutaneous layer of the skin, skirting the lateral aspect of the labia or scrotum to emerge through a previously made short incision overlying the lateral part of the right superior pubic ramus, taking care to remain superficial to the adductor longus tendon. The detachable needle-point of the tunneller is removed and replaced with a small plastic olive.

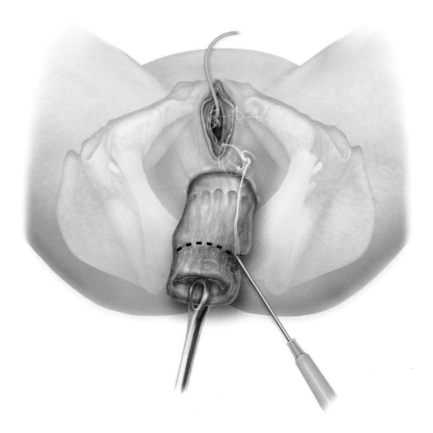

Figure 37.8 A mucosectomy is performed circumferentially 1–2 cm proximal to the dentate line and extending 3–4 cm beyond the apex.

Figure 37.9 A sharp pointed tunneller is passed between the layers of the prolapse to emerge from the suprapubic wound.

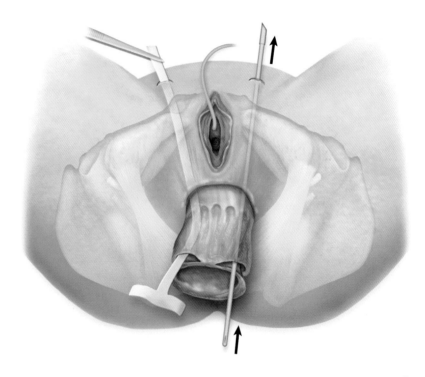

The apex of the T part of the Permacol™ strip is then attached to the olive with a 1-0 nylon suture (Fig. 37.9). The tunneller is drawn downward by the perineal operator to emerge through the apex of the denuded prolapse, bringing with it the T part of the Permacol™ strip (Fig. 37.10). The strip is detached from the tunneller by cutting the nylon suture. Great care is exercised during this maneuver to ensure aseptic technique and to avoid any contamination. Thus, the Permacol™ is soaked in gentamicin solution before use and a second surgeon prepares the suprapubic wounds and handles the Permacol™ with separate sterile instruments. The same maneuver is repeated on the left anterolateral segment of the prolapse. The T parts of the Permacol™ strips are next

Figure 37.10 A plastic olive replaces the sharp point of the tunneller and the Permacol™ strip is attached.

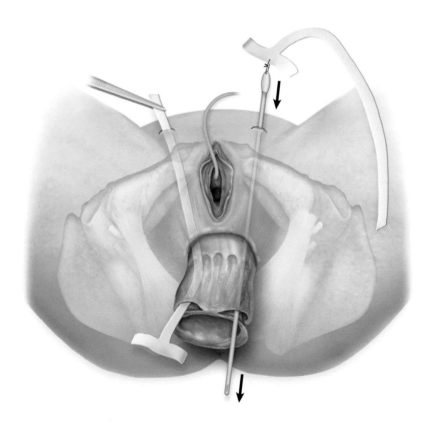

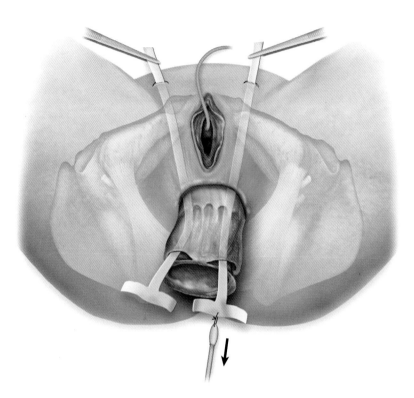

Figure 37.11 The tunneller is drawn downward by the perineal operator to emerge through the apex of the denuded prolapse, bringing with it the T part of the Permacol™ strip.

sutured within the two muscle layers of the apex of the prolapse with interrupted 2-0 PDS sutures so each T part of each strip occupies nearly half of the circumference of the denuded apex (Fig. 37.11). The result is that the incision in the apex of the prolapse is closed and the Permacol™ is buried in the muscle of the apex. This suture line is then buried by a second layer of interrupted PDS sutures (Fig. 37.12). The mucosal

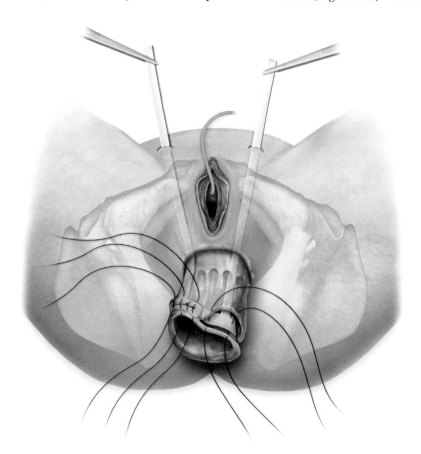

Figure 37.12 The T parts of the Permacol™ strips are sutured within the two muscle layers of the apex of the prolapse so that the T part of each strip occupies nearly half of the circumference of the denuded apex.

Figure 37.13 The suture line is then buried by a second layer of sutures.

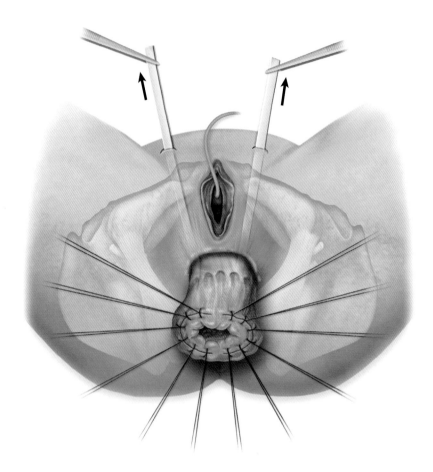

defect is then closed circumferentially with interrupted 20 Monocryl sutures and the prolapse is reduced back into the rectal lumen. The second surgeon then exerts upward traction on the Permacol™ strips through the suprapubic wounds, and with the patient head down each Permacol™ strip is sutured to the underlying periosteum of the pubic tubercle with two interrupted 1-0 PDS sutures under moderate tension (Fig. 37.13). The suprapubic wounds are closed with subcuticular Monocryl and dressed (Fig. 37.14).

Figure 37.14 The rectoanal mucosal defect is repaired, the prolapse is reduced, and upward traction is exerted on the Permacol™ strips, which are then sutured to the underlying periosteum of the pubis.

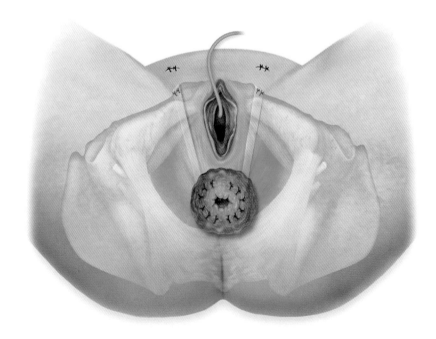

Postoperative Management

There are no specific dietary restrictions postoperatively and bowel confinement is not necessary, because the patient's bowel wall is not breached. Patients are encouraged to take a high-fiber diet as soon as they feel ready to eat (after anesthesia) and laxatives are given (e.g., macrogols, magnesium salts, and ispaghula husk) to promote stool softening, and hence reduce the incidence of straining in the early postoperative period (when analgesics can lead to constipation). Discharge from hospital is usually based on the resumption of bowel opening and good recovery after surgery.

Complications

To date there has been no mortality associated with this procedure (n = 20). Major complications are rare, and all known complications encountered are listed below.

> Minor wound sepsis (n = 3)
> Wound sepsis requiring surgical drainage (n = 1)

Results

Currently, we have follow-up data on the cohort of 20 (18F) patients for a median 14 months (range 10–14 months). Three patients developed a full thickness recurrence (15%), however, only two had further surgery, one on Altimeter's procedure and one had a further EXPRESS, which was successful.

Functional Outcome

The operation improves symptoms related to difficulty in evacuation, the sensation of prolapse, as well as the quality of life (11).

DISCUSSION

The EXPRESS procedure is a safe and relatively minimally invasive procedure that can be used for intrarectal and external rectal prolapse. It appears to have a superior recurrence rate to Delorme's, though long term data is not yet available. The EXPRESS procedure improves evacuatory symptoms, which is maintained at 3 years, and the majority of patients appear satisfied with their surgery.

One particular advantage of the EXPRESS procedure is that it can be easily combined with other perineal or abdominal repairs for other pelvic organ prolapses. This technique thus provides coloproctologists with another surgical option in the treatment of this often crippling problem. Other techniques such as the stapled transanal rectal resection procedure are based on removal/excision of tissue (12). Recent reports have expressed concern over its high morbidity (7). The concept of the EXPRESS procedure is different, in that the principle is to reinforce and reconstruct tissue. We believe that this is a very important consideration in the long term. In our series, Permacol™ is the material used in the reconstruction but other available biological materials may also be suitable. It is, however, very important to use materials that are resistant to infection and do not erode the bowel.

CONCLUSION

The EXPRESS procedure can improve symptoms of evacuatory dysfunction and prolapse, consistent with improvement in anatomic severity of the RI and rectocele (13). Medium follow-up data suggest that the improvement of symptoms are maintained in the majority of patients and are satisfied with the outcome of the EXPRESS procedure. The EXPRESS procedure is a relatively minimally invasive technique and appears equivalent to other surgical options for the management of rectal prolapse, intussusception, and rectocele in terms of symptom, quality of life, physiological and anatomical changes, and long-term morbidity.

Recommended References and Readings

1. Voyles CR, Richardson JD, Bland KI, Tobin GR, Flint LM, Polk HC Jr. Emergency abdominal wall reconstruction with polypropylene mesh: short-term benefits versus long-term complications. *Ann Surg* 1981;194(2):219–23.
2. Kaufman Z, Engelberg M, Zager M. Fecal fistula: a late complication of Marlex mesh repair. *Dis Colon Rectum* 1981;24(7):543–4.
3. Hammond TM, Chin-Aleong J, Navsaria H, Williams NS. Human in vivo cellular response to a cross-linked acellular collagen implant. *Br J Surg* 2008;95(4):438–46.
4. Shorvon PJ, McHugh S, Diamant NE, Somers S, Stevenson GW. Defecography in normal volunteers: results and implications. *Gut* 1989;30(12):1737–49.
5. Briel JW, Schouten WR, Boerma MO. Long-term results of suture rectopexy in patients with fecal incontinence associated with incomplete rectal prolapse. *Dis Colon Rectum* 1997;40(10): 1228–32.
6. Schultz I, Mellgren A, Dolk A, Johansson C, Holmström B. Long-term results and functional outcome after Ripstein rectopexy. *Dis Colon Rectum* 2000;43(1):35–43.
7. Naldini G. Serious unconventional complications of surgery with stapler for haemorrhoidal prolapse and obstructed defecation due to rectocele and rectal intussusception. *Colorectal Dis* 2011;13(3):323–7.
8. Binda GA, Pescatori M, Romano G. The dark side of double-stapled transanal rectal resection. *Dis Colon Rectum* 2005;48(9): 1830–31; author reply 31–2.
9. Watts AM, Thompson MR. Evaluation of Delorme's procedure as a treatment for full-thickness rectal prolapse. *Br J Surg* 2000; 87(2):218–22.
10. Williams JG, Rothenberger DA, Madoff RD, Goldberg SM. Treatment of rectal prolapse in the elderly by perineal rectosigmoidectomy. *Dis Colon Rectum* 1992;35(9):830–34.
11. Williams NS, Giordano P, Dvorkin LS, Huang A, Hetzer FH, Scott SM. External pelvic rectal suspension (the Express procedure) for full-thickness rectal prolapse: evolution of a new technique. *Dis Colon Rectum* 2005;48(2):307–16.
12. Boccasanta P, Venturi M, Stuto A, et al. Stapled transanal rectal resection for outlet obstruction: a prospective, multicenter trial. *Dis Colon Rectum* 2004;47(8):1285–96; discussion 96–7.
13. Williams NS, Dvorkin LS, Giordano P, et al. EXternal Pelvic REctal SuSpension (Express procedure) for rectal intussusception, with and without rectocele repair. *Br J Surg* 2005;92(5): 598–604.

38 Reconstruction of the Pelvis: Muscle Transfer

Martin I. Newman

 ## INDICATIONS/CONTRAINDICATIONS

Muscle flap reconstruction of the perineum may be necessary following radical ablative procedures, such as abdominoperineal reconstruction. The indications to proceed with reconstruction may include the inability to close the pelvic floor and/or perineum following resection at the time of the initial procedure or the anticipated inability of the wound to heal normally secondary to active infection, previous surgery, or irradiation. In addition, radical surgery for malignant colorectal neoplasms may also involve resection of a portion of the vagina or labia as is often seen when malignancies extend to and invade these structures. In these cases a single well designed and inset pedicle muscle or myocutaneous flap may be used to reconstruct the vagina as well as the perineum. In other cases, a combination of flaps may help the reconstructive surgeon to achieve the desired goal.

Several pedicled muscle and myocutaneous flap options exist for pelvic reconstruction and include, but are not limited to, the right or left rectus abdominus and/or the right and left gracilis. Such flaps offer excellent options for reconstruction following the ablation of primary, recurrent, or persistent lower gastrointestinal tumors. In individuals in whom these donor options are not available, alternatives do exist in the form of pedicled or free muscle, myocutaneous and fasciocutaneous flaps. Additional options such as these are described in a variety of texts and journals dedicated to the reconstructive surgeon. This chapter will focus primarily on the vertical rectus abdominus myocutaneous (VRAM) flap, which is our preferred option.

There are few if any contraindications to proceeding with flap reconstruction of pelvic defects in this context. However, hemodynamic instability at operation may be an indication for the surgeon to defer reconstruction, as it is with most reconstructive procedures. Few defects cannot be temporized with dressings or negative pressure devices while patients regain stability. In contrast, certain situations such as congenital anomalies, previous surgeries, and/or trauma have implications in the design of the reconstruction. A previous ostomy that has been placed through the rectus muscle may compromise the perfusion to the distal portion of rectus abdominus based flap and may stimulate the reconstructive surgeon to seek alternative options. Previous cosmetic procedures, too, may have implications. In these cases a VRAM flap would not be possible. However, it is not a contraindication to perform a muscle only flap that may serve to achieve all or part of the desired reconstructive goals. Notwithstanding, previous ligation or obliteration of the deep inferior epigastric pedicle is a contraindication to the utilization of that particular rectus muscle, although it does not preclude the use of the contralateral rectus muscle if its vascular pedicle is intact. Similarly, previous surgeries or traumas that have ablated the cutaneous perforators overlying the gracilis muscle or previous obliteration or ligation of the major vascular pedicle to the muscle itself may impose limits on this potential donor site as an option. Congenital anomalies of these structures are rare, but should also be considered in surgical planning. Previous irradiation is also a factor for consideration. Previous irradiation of a donor muscle and skin, as opposed to irradiation of the recipient site, should stimulate the surgeon to consider other options. Although flaps may be irradiated following transposition and inset with satisfactory results, a previously irradiated flap as a donor can be problematic. Potential issues with this approach include difficulty raising the flap in the altered bed, viability of the flap following harvest, closure and healing of the donor site, and performance of the flap following transposition and inset.

Relative contraindication such as obesity, poor nutritional status, history of smoking, or steroid and antimetabolic medications (among others) are well appreciated by the reconstructive surgeon. However, in major ablative colorectal ablative procedures for active malignant neoplasms, surgeons may not have the luxury of deferring intervention until these factors can be adequately corrected. Thus, patient specific characteristics such as those described serve more so as indicators of potential postoperative complications rather than contraindication to reconstruction.

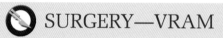

SURGERY—VRAM

Initial Intraoperative Evaluation & Positioning

The most common indication for muscle flap reconstruction of the perineum as described above in our practice is an abdominoperineal resection (APR) in a previously irradiated patient. The typical scenario is a patient who has a persistent or recurrent neoplasm following chemotherapy and radiation. The radical nature of the APR often leaves patients with an appreciable defect of the pelvic floor and the surrounding perineal skin. In our practice, in most patients, optimum results are achieved using a right VRAM flap that is based on the right deep inferior epigastric pedicle. Thus, this flap will be the focus of this chapter. The right muscle is preferred as it preserves the left rectus muscle for the intended colostomy. Of course, situations such as those described above including previous ligation of the right deep inferior epigastric vascular pedicle should stimulate the reconstructive surgeon to consider the left rectus abdominus muscle or the gracilis muscles as excellent alternatives.

Assuming normal anatomy, the operation begins at the conclusion of the oncologic resection. The distal descending colon is left stapled closed and the midline incision is left open (if incomplete, it should be extended to the xiphoid process). The umbilicus should be preserved on the left side of the abdominal incision. The patient is already positioned in lithotomy, with the medial thighs prepped and draped in case a gracilis muscle is required. The defect is evaluated by the plastic surgery team. To raise the right rectus flap, the surgeon is positioned on the patient's left; a headlight is helpful.

Elevation of the VRAM Flap

We begin the procedure with evaluation of the deep inferior epigastric pedicle on the right. Assuming that the native vasculature is intact, we proceed with the design of the myocutaneous flap. This process begins with a semilunar incision parallel and to the right of the midline incision made on the skin overlying the right rectus muscle extending from the pubis to the xiphoid process. At its widest point, the semilunar incision should be between 8–10 cm lateral to the midline. Dissection continues through the soft tissue straight down to the anterior rectus fascia, which is preserved. Within this crescent of skin overlying the rectus muscle, at the most superior third, an ellipse is designed with the intention of preserving the skin, the underlying subcutaneous tissue, and the associated cutaneous perforators that arise from the underlying rectus muscle. The balance of the skin and subcutaneous tissue within the crescent is débrided. The purpose of designing the flap as a crescent and débriding the skin and subcutaneous tissue not to be included in the transposition is to provide the patient with a well-balanced skin edge for closure later in the case. Irregularly shaped incisions leave patients with an undesirable abdominal contour deformity following complete healing.

Following the debridement of nonessential skin and subcutaneous tissue the remaining skin paddle to be preserved is secured to the anterior rectus muscular fascia with approximately eight 2-0 Vicryl sutures at the points of the compass. The purpose of this maneuver is to reduce the risk of perforator avulsion during transposition and has proven extremely helpful in our experience. Bites are taken through the skin paddle and the underlying anterior rectus fascia, taking care not to strangulate the muscle's blood supply. The tails of these sutures are left long and will be removed following transposition. The skin and subcutaneous tissue overlying the right external oblique is then dissected away from the anterior abdominal wall fascia along that plane, in a medial-to-lateral fashion, to the level of the anterior axillary line. The purpose of raising this flap is to correct for the loss of skin and subcutaneous tissue over the rectus. At closure, later in the case, this dissection will facilitate advancement of the flap in a lateral-to-medial direction and a tension free closure at the midline. During elevation of this flap, care is taken to control the numerous perforators encountered to reduce the risk of postoperative hematoma. Smaller perforating vessels may be controlled with simple electrocautery. However, larger perforators, as are often seen in obese patients, may respond better to medium vascular clips.

Next, the muscle is meticulously dissected from the anterior rectus sheath. Care is taken to preserve the skin paddle, the associated subcutaneous tissue, and the associated anterior rectus fascia underlying the skin paddle. This tissue, including the anterior rectus fascia directly underneath the skin paddle, should be preserved with the flap. The purpose of this maneuver is to preserve the perforating vessels arising from the rectus muscle perfusing the overlying soft tissue and skin paddle. Naturally, this maneuver will create a defect in the anterior abdominal wall fascia. However, in our practice this defect is effectively repaired with mesh; our preference is a biologic mesh in these clean-contaminated cases. Dissection of the muscle from the anterior sheath is facilitated by fine dissection technique utilizing a combination of blunt and sharp dissection performed with sharp tenotomy scissors, needlepoint electrocautery, and micro-bipolar The latter is especially helpful in controlling bleeders on the muscle belly itself. The goal of this dissection is to separate the rectus muscle from the anterior rectus sheath while preserving the muscle fibers and overlying skin panel with its associated subcutaneous tissue and fascia. This is a critical portion of the case, for damage to the rectus muscle at any point along its course may interfere with the blood supply that arises inferiorly from the deep epigastric artery and courses superiorly through the muscle belly. It is especially critical to preserve the muscle at the inscriptions where the blood supply and girth of the muscle is the thinnest. Should the fascia be densely adherent to the inscription, and impossible to safely dissect from the inscription or muscle proper, it is preferable to sacrifice the fascia (as opposed to the muscle) and primarily repair the resultant fascial defect.

Once the muscle has been separated from the anterior rectus sheath, carefully preserving the fascia underlying the skin paddle, the flap is elevated. To achieve this goal, the muscle is divided along the costal margin; this step is facilitated with electrocautery and vascular clips. It is critical to identify and securely control the superficial epigastric artery and vein on the proximal and distal ends to reduce the risk of unwanted postoperative bleeding.

Once the superior blood supply has been divided, the skin paddle and muscle are elevated en-block as the flap is raised and pealed away from the posterior rectus sheath in a superior-to-inferior direction. This maneuver is facilitated with a combination of sharp and blunt dissection and monopolar and bipolar cautery. Care is taken to control the lateral muscular perforating vessels that are encountered at the most lateral aspect of the rectus sheath. Bipolar cautery is helpful in this respect. The dissection proceeds in this manner inferiorly, towards the inferior third, approximately to the level of the arcuate line. At this point, the surgeon will begin to note small branches arising from the more distally apparent deep inferior epigastric artery and vein, which arise from the lateral inferior corner and course along the posterior margin of the muscle. It is critical to preserve these structures as they represent the blood supply to the flap. Dissection slows and becomes more meticulous at this point. We find it helpful to use a moist gauze to help separate the vascular pedicle from the posterior rectus sheath here. In this manner, dissection continues in a superior-to-inferior direction to the tendinous, most inferior portion of the rectus muscle. Following complete elevation, the flap is ready for transposition.

Transposition and Inset of the VRAM

To facilitate trauma free transposition, a St. Mark's retractor is utilized to displace pelvic structures inferiorly and anteriorly, while the assistant—who stands on the right of the patient—retracts the bowel and omentum superiorly. Standing on the left side of the patient, the surgeon places the flap and skin paddle in the right-hand and reaches over to place their left hand within the perineal defect. The flap is passed from above taking care to push the flap through the pelvis from above and not to pull on the flap from below. The left hand helps control the course of the flap as it passes through the pelvic defect. Undue tension, as is caused by pulling from below, may avulse the perforators and should be avoided. Also care should be taken not to twist or kink the flap, as doing so would compromise the blood supply. Following this maneuver the surgeon changes the left glove.

At this point the surgeon should reevaluate the dissection along the proximal aspect of the flap as it arises from its pubic origin. Should any adhesions or attachments to the anterior or posterior rectus sheath be noted, they should be released to provide the most tension free result. In rare cases, the muscle may need to be released further. For example, when a large fibrotic uterus obstructs the course of the flap, the muscle can be released from its pubic insertion preserving the deep inferior epigastric pedicle. This maneuver, however, should be performed by the experienced surgeon only, for tension on the vessels themselves may compromise the flap.

Following the transposition, the reconstructive surgeon may position themselves between the legs for inset of the flap, while the colorectal surgeon matures the ostomy. Towards this goal, the skin paddle is manipulated into the defect and evaluated. Any redundant or nonviable appearing skin should be débrided at this time. Once the fine adjustments have been made to the skin paddle, the broad rectus muscle is manipulated to reestablish the pelvic floor. This reestablishment of the pelvic floor can be achieved by securing the edges of the rectus to the remaining levator muscles with 2-0 Vicryl sutures. When placing sutures through the rectus muscle, care is taken not to compromise the blood supply by placing the sutures at the most lateral edges of the muscle. The skin paddle is inset with a combination of 2-0 polydioxanone (PDS) sutures placed deep in the dermis in interrupted fashion and 2-0 Vicryl sutures placed in interrupted fashion to approximate the skin. Prior to final closure, a number 19 round channel drain is placed alongside the muscle flap and deep into the pelvis. It is brought out through the soft tissue of the buttocks and secured with a zero silk suture and ultimately the flap is coated with bacitracin ointment.

Abdominal Wall Closure

As indicated above, harvest of this flap results in a defect of the skin, subcutaneous tissue, and fascia overlying the previous location of the right rectus muscle. To facilitate a durable closure, the remaining anterior and posterior rectus sheath are approximated to each other and closed along the midline to the intact left side. We perform this closure with a running looped #1 PDS suture. This closure is begun at the pubis and advanced to the superior one-third of the midline where primary closure is often impossible secondary to the harvest of the anterior rectus sheath at this level. To repair this defect biologic mesh is utilized in routine fashion. Although this has resulted in "bulging" in rare cases, it is more often not an issue. We have found bovine pericardium-based mesh to be helpful with these repairs. The previous elevation of the right skin flap will allow primary closure of the skin and subcutaneous tissue in a tension free manner. In our experience, a primary closure of the skin has been possible in all cases. Closure of the skin and subcutaneous tissue is facilitated by placing 2-0 PDS sutures in interrupted fashion through Scarpa's fascia and finally the skin is closed with staples. However, prior to final closure, the wound is irrigated with copious amounts of antimicrobial solution and a number 19 round channel drain is placed underneath the right skin flap and brought out through the right lower quadrant, which is secured with a zero silk suture.

Vaginal Reconstruction

As previously indicated, ablation may also involve a portion of the vaginal canal and labia. In our practice, the VRAM design and technique described above has been modified in an effort to repair both the perineal defect as well as the vaginal defect utilizing this single myocutaneous flap. The modifications primarily involve the design of the skin flap and the manner in which the muscle and skin are inset.

The skin paddle is modified early in the case and designed to be longer than the one used to repair the perineal defect only. The portion of the skin paddle intended for perineal repair remains the same. However, superior to this, an additional 3–4 cm of skin is preserved and de-epithelized.

The inset of the muscle is modified as well. After transposition, the broad flat belly of the muscle (previously the posterior margin of the muscle) is approximated against the posterior vaginal wall. Small defects can simply be "patched" with the muscle, while larger, more complete defects of the vaginal canal can be repaired by approximating the lateral muscle edges along the remaining walls of the canal. The repair of these more complete defects utilizes the muscle to reconstruct the proximal three-fourth of the posterior wall, while the remaining one-fourth of the wall is repaired with the skin flap as discussed below. Repair is facilitated with the placement of 2-0 Vicryl sutures in interrupted fashion along the most lateral margin of the rectus taking care not to strangulate the blood supply to the flap as discussed above. One or two interrupted sutures may also be required to approximate the muscle to the cervix for defects that require this.

Following inset of the muscle, the perineal skin flap is inset as described above. However, the modification of the skin flap provides approximately 3–4 cm of de-epithelized skin at the posterior commissure of the labia, the most anterior part of the skin flap. This de-epithelized skin is pushed inward and posteriorly and approximated to the muscle and the remaining lateral vaginal canal walls. Should the posterior commissure require repair, this may be achieved with 2-0 PDS sutures in the deep dermis, while the labia are approximated with 2-0 Vicryl sutures. Bacitracin ointment is used to coat all intravaginal exposed muscles and de-epithelized skin that will mucosalize.

 POSTOPERATIVE MANAGEMENT

Following completion of the surgery, the patient is placed on an air-fluid bed with an abduction pillow placed between the knees. Bacitracin ointment is placed on the incision sites and on the intravaginal flap if one was created three times each day, for a period of 3 days only. The air-fluid bed is also maintained for 3 days during which time the patient may lie on their back or side, but may not sit on the flap. On the third postoperative day, the bacitracin is discontinued, and the patient is transferred to an air-bed designed to add low-air-loss therapy. Physical therapy is helpful in teaching patient bed-to-standing maneuvers and assistance with initial ambulation, for on post operative day (POD) number 3, the patient begins to ambulate. For the next 3 weeks, the patient may stand, walk, lie on their back or their side, but may not sit on the flap. Once this time frame has transpired, they may begin to sit, for short periods of time, on an air doughnut advancing as tolerated. Drain care is routine. The patient is instructed to avoid heavy lifting or exercise for up to 6 months to help prevent injury to the reconstructed abdominal wall.

 COMPLICATIONS

Complications in the immediate postoperative phase include, among others, flap failure, persistent postoperative bleeding, and hematoma. Flap failure may be partial or complete; if the entire flap fails, debridement is recommended and an alternative reconstructive plan is designed. In contrast, if a portion of the skin paddle appears ischemic in the immediate postoperative phase, certain measures may be taken prior to debridement. These steps include the removal of a few sutures, and conservative wound care. If ischemia progresses to complete necrosis, debridement may proceed, usually within the first several days to weeks following surgery. During this waiting period the necrosis is allowed to demarcate and temporized with an antimicrobial dressing such as silver sulfadiazine.

Significant bleeding from any of the named of vessels described above may very well likely require return to the operating room for control. Hematomas, if small, may be conservatively treated. However, large hematomas may compromise the venous return to the flap and may require operative drainage.

Further out, infection and wound issues are the most likely complications encountered. The most common place for infection is posterior to direct this muscle deep within the pelvis and is often identified by erythema, leucocytosis, pyrexia, and chills. Computerized axial tomography scan is helpful in making the diagnosis, and many of these may be amenable to drainage by interventional radiology. However, should a collection be refractory to percutaneous drainage, operative drainage may be necessary.

Wound healing issues are common, in fact minor superficial skin dehiscence is very common but fortunately responds well to routine wound care. However, a major dehiscence may occur secondary to the noncompliant patient sitting on the flap prior to complete healing, or it may occur for some other reason. A major dehiscence may require operative debridement and/or more aggressive wound management such as negative pressure therapy.

For those patients undergoing vaginal reconstruction, long-term complications may include inability to participate in intercourse or hygiene problems. In our practice, through quality of life surveys, we note approximately 50% of our patients who undergo this portion of the procedure to be sexually active. Hygiene issues can usually be corrected at a revision of surgery designed to restore the normal labial anatomy.

 RESULTS

Preoperative and postoperative photographs (Figs. 38.1–38.3). The results obtained from this procedure are most often satisfactory for the surgeon and are usually associated with a high patient satisfaction. Following reconstruction as described in this chapter, patients can walk, stand, and sit in a normal fashion without pain. Some females, whose tumor has invaded the vaginal walls, can even go on to have intercourse in a relatively normal fashion. Patient satisfaction is noted to be higher in patients who have personal experience with the loss of these everyday functions, for the reconstruction restores the "norm" they have come to expect. This includes many of the patients who have lost the ability to enjoy a "normal" life secondary to pain or bleeding associated with anal or low rectal tumor recurrence in a previously irradiated field.

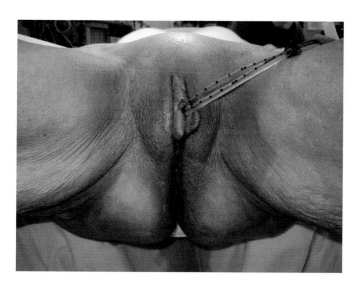

Figure 38.1 Preoperative appearance of perineal area prior to ablation. Urinary catheter and stents in place.

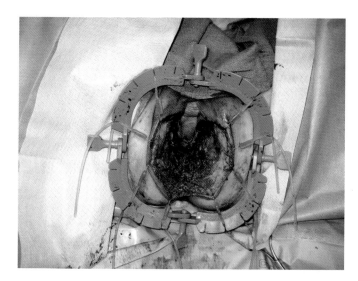

Figure 38.2 Intraoperative appearance of perineal area following ablation. Remaining and visible are the anterior vaginal wall and cervix, only.

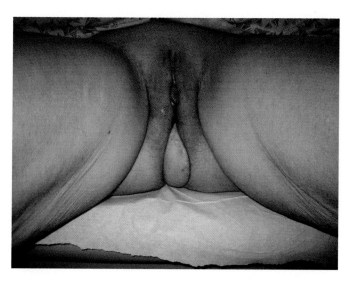

Figure 38.3 Postoperative appearance 7 months following procedure. This patient sits and participates in intercourse without restriction.

✸ CONCLUSIONS

In summary, the right vertical rectus abdominus myocutaneous flap is an excellent option for reconstruction of pelvic defects in the technique described. This flap is a robust flap with an exceptionally good blood supply and bulk. Additionally it is versatile and can be used not only to reconstruct the perineal defect but the pelvic floor and the vagina as well. Long-term follow-up of our patients demonstrates durability and high satisfaction.

Suggested Readings

Banzet P. Vaginal reconstruction by rectus abdominis musculocutaneous flap after pelvic cancer: report of 11 cases. *Plast Reconstr Surg* 1996;97(1):263.

Mathes SJ, Nahai F. Reconstructive Surgery: Principles, Anatomy, & Technique. St. Louis, MO: QMP, 1997.

Moon HK, Taylor GI. The vascular anatomy of rectus abdominis musculocutaneous flaps based on the deep superior epigastric system. *Plast Reconstr Surg* 1988;82(5):815–29.

Nelson RA, Butler CE. Surgical outcomes of VRAM versus thigh flaps for immediate reconstruction of pelvic and perineal cancer resection defects. *Plast Reconstr Surg* 2009;123(1): 175–83.

Segre D, Landra M. Vaginal reconstruction with vertically oriented rectus abdominus myocutaneous (VRAM) flap following APR for locally advanced rectal cancer. *Tech Coloproctol* 2005;9: 267.

39 Open

John Migaly

 ## INDICATIONS/CONTRAINDICATIONS

The importance of appropriate planning and technique in the formation of a colostomy is often underestimated; however, it should be noted that a significant number of elective colostomies and urgent colostomies tend to be permanent. Despite the impromptu circumstances of many colostomies, a thoughtful and consistent approach toward colostomy creation can avoid a problematic ostomy, which can be equivalent of a "life sentence" for the patient if the ostomy is poorly fashioned.

Colostomies may be created for one of a variety of elective, semielective, or urgent indications. Colostomies are created in cases where diversion of the fecal stream may be necessary in distal colitis, and for diversion in cases of intra-abdominal catastrophes such as diverticular perforation, ischemic necrosis of the colon, or iatrogenic perforation. Proximal diversion may be necessary for debilitating fecal incontinence, in cases of necrotizing soft tissue infection or sacral decubitus where patients may have large, nonhealing perineal or sacral wounds. Stomas may be useful adjuncts for complex repair of rectovaginal or rectourethral fistulas.

Ostomies are very often performed in cases of large bowel obstruction secondary to neoplasia or to protect a distal rectal or coloanal anastomosis. In cases of colonic obstruction where proximal diversion may be necessary, quite often an ileostomy is not appropriate as a form of diversion, because although it will divert the fecal stream, it may or may not decompress the colon depending on whether the patient has a competent ileocecal valve. In cases where the ileocecal valve is competent, the cecum can still become distended, ischemic, and subsequently perforate; therefore a colostomy may be more appropriate.

The indications for open rather than laparoscopic colostomies are primarily situational. In many instances the patients may have had multiple prior abdominal surgeries and thus a laparoscopic approach may not be advisable or feasible. Very often, obesity and body habitus may dictate the choice of the procedure. In situations where there is acute large and/or small bowel dilatation, laparoscopy may not be practical because of the lack of intra-abdominal domain; therefore an open technique is utilized.

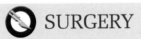 PREOPERATIVE PLANNING

Choosing a Site for a Colostomy

One of the most important aspects involved in the creation of a colostomy is choosing an appropriate position on the abdominal wall for the colostomy. The siting of an ostomy is quite important for the obese patient and for the thin patient alike. The patient should be marked for the stoma in both the standing and the seated position. Often times a stoma site will be ideal in the standing position and not in the seated position. Folds of skin may be far more prominent in the seated position than in the standing position. These folds should be avoided as it is very difficult to maintain a seal with the colostomy appliance when the stoma is seated in a fold. Care should be taken to choose a site for the stoma that is within the body of the rectus and not lateral to the rectus sheath. This positioning can often be quite deceiving in obese patients as the landmarks can be obscured by the patient's pannus. A stoma that is lateral to the rectus sheath can predispose the patient to a parastomal hernia. Another important factor in marking someone for a stoma is the belt line. Ideally, stomas should be sited above the belt line, but there are some patients who have relatively high belt lines where a high or above the belt line stoma is not practical.

In patients that have had multiple abdominal procedures, the site of the stoma does not necessarily have to be away from prior incisions unless there is significant skin dimpling, retraction, or excavation of that segment of the abdominal wall. In fact it might be cosmetically preferable for that particular patient to avoid an additional incision.

Bowel Preparation

In urgent or emergent cases where a stoma is needed, bowel preparation is usually not safe, feasible or necessary. In fact, most elective colostomies do not merit a mechanical bowel preparation.

SURGERY

Positioning

Traditionally, we position the overwhelming majority of patients scheduled to undergo colorectal surgery, including colostomies, in the low lithotomy position. This position allows access to the anus for proctoscopy, colonoscopy or any other adjunctive anorectal procedures. It also allows better visualization and manipulation of the upper abdomen from a low incision; this is particularly useful in cases where splenic flexure mobilization is necessary. In these cases, standing between the patient's legs can be advantageous.

Technique

End Colostomy

An end colostomy is most commonly placed in the left lower quadrant and is usually created after an abdominoperineal resection or a Hartmann's procedure. After the resection is completed, the colostomy is created by mobilizing the left colon such that there is adequate reach for the colostomy to come out of a left lower quadrant aperture. Quite often, it is necessary to mobilize the splenic flexure in order to have adequate reach to the left lower quadrant and to be delivered through a thick abdominal wall. If reach is still a problem, then the root or base of the left colon mesentery can be mobilized as long as the vascular arcades are not disrupted.

Part X: Colostomy

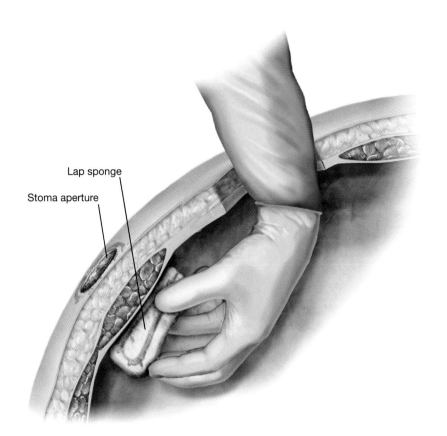

Stoma aperture

Lap sponge

Figure 39.1 A folded up lap pad is placed on the underside of the abdominal beneath the stoma site to prevent injury to the bowel during entry into the abdomen.

As previously described, the ostomy site should lie in the rectus sheath lateral to the midline. The fascia to the midline incision and the skin are clasped at its free edges and drawn medially. Exquisite care must be taken in order to ensure that the entire dissection from the skin incision to the posterior rectus sheath proceeds in a perpendicular plane and that the dissection is not inadvertently beveled toward the midline, thus creating a colostomy that is too close to the midline of the fascia.

A folded lap pad is placed on the underside of the abdominal beneath the stoma site and pushed upwards (Fig. 39.1). At the skin level, a marking pen is used to mark out a circular incision on the skin about the size of a quarter for the ostomy aperture. This disk of skin is removed using the knife or electrocautery.

The electrocautery is used to dissect through the subcutaneous fascia until the fascia (anterior rectus sheath) is encountered. The author does not "de-fat" the subcutaneous tissues of the stoma site in order to avoid retraction of the stoma and parastomal hernia. Once the anterior rectus sheath is encountered, a vertical incision is made in the fascia. Cruciate incisions are avoided in order to reduce the likelihood of a parastomal hernia.

Once the rectus muscles are encountered, the muscles are not divided, but rather split between Kelly clamps. The rectus muscles are retracted to either side using Army-Navy retractors to expose the posterior rectus sheath. With the lap pad being held up against the abdominal wall to protect the underlying bowel, the cautery is used to divide the posterior rectus sheath and the peritoneum until the previously mentioned lap pad is encountered. Through this hole, a large Kelly clamp is placed into the abdomen and the tip is pulled upward, thus exposing the abdominal aspect of the colostomy aperture, allowing the surgeon to ensure hemostasis. The fascial aperture is enlarged to allow two fingers to comfortably enter the abdomen (Fig. 39.2).

A Babcock is placed through the ostomy aperture into the abdomen and the ostomy is slowly brought through the colostomy site and out to the skin surface. If the ostomy is too bulky, to come through the aperture easily, the epiploic appendages can be removed from the distal colon. It is not advisable to strip the mesentery, particularly in obese patients, because of concerns for adequate blood supply. Similarly one should

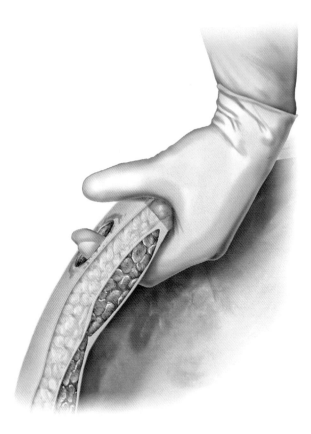

Figure 39.2 The fascial aperture is enlarged to allow two fingers to comfortably enter the abdomen.

resist the urge especially in obese patients to significantly enlarge the size of the fascial aperture. Once the colon is brought through the stoma aperture, it is important to ensure that the colon and mesentery are in the correct orientation and to secure the colon to the aperture by keeping a Babcock on the edge of the colon.

Colostomy Maturation

Once the fascia and skin have been closed, the stapled end of the colon is opened and the edges of the stoma are sutured to the skin using 3-0 polyglactic acid suture (Vicryl). In contrast to an ileostomy, a colostomy does not need to be everted because the effluent from a colostomy is not as caustic to the peristomal skin as is the effluent from an ileostomy.

Loop Colostomy

A transverse loop colostomy can sometimes be a quick, efficient, and minimally invasive choice for diversion. An open transverse colostomy can be performed through a single, left upper-quadrant incision.

A 4-cm transverse incision is made in the left upper quadrant overlying the rectus sheath. The incision is extended into the subcutaneous tissue and the fascia. The rectus muscles are split and retracted between Army-Navy retractors; the posterior fascia and peritoneum are entered carefully and sharply. The aperture is subsequently enlarged to accommodate two fingers into the abdomen. A Babcock is placed into the abdomen and the transverse colon is brought out of the incision. The omentum is dissected from the transverse colon and a window is made under the transverse colon at its junction with the transverse mesocolon. A colostomy bridge or red rubber catheter is placed under the loop stoma and fastened to the skin to prevent retraction. The colostomy is then matured in the standard fashion described above.

A loop sigmoid colostomy is also fairly easy to create but usually requires some mobilization of the colon and lends itself to a laparoscopic approach which is described elsewhere.

Figure 39.3 End-loop colostomy.

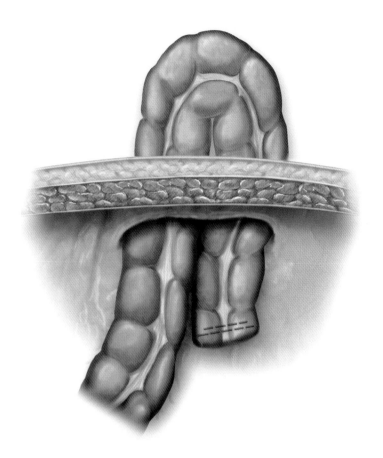

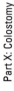

Divided End-Loop Colostomy

Occasionally, despite adequate mobilization of the colon, it may still be difficult to bring the stoma through the aperture; this often happens in obese patients, and is usually due to a combination of the patient's thick abdominal wall and the fact that sometimes the mesentery just does not have ample length to allow for reach through the aperture. In cases such as this, a divided end-loop colostomy may be a good alternative. Instead of bringing the end of the colon through the aperture, folding the colon into an end-loop can sometimes take the tension off of the colon mesentery to allow for adequate reach through the mesentery (Fig. 39.3). An end-loop colostomy is matured in the same manner as described above.

Mucous Fistula

A mucous fistula is created when the distal end of the divided bowel is brought out through a skin incision and a portion of this end is matured to the skin. This procedure might be employed if there is a question of distal obstruction despite proximal diversion. The corner of the distal staple line may be delivered out through the midline incision or through the same aperture as the proximal stoma. In cases where the proximal versus distal end may not be obvious, the use of proctoscopic or transanal sigmoidoscopic insufflation can assist in identification of the distal limb.

 POSTOPERATIVE MANAGEMENT

Diet can be advanced as tolerated. In cases where there has been an extensive adhesiolysis, there may be an associated prolonged ileus.

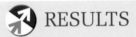

COMPLICATIONS

There are several complications associated with stoma creation; in cases where the stoma is placed in a less than ideal position, the seal with the appliance can be less than ideal. This problem can be quite troublesome and can significantly interfere with activities of daily life.

Retraction of the stoma is usually associated with tension on the mesentery of the colon or obesity where the distance between skin and rectus muscle is greater than the available blood supply to the colon.

Stenosis of the stoma is usually associated with poor blood supply to the stoma. Less often the stenosis is purely at the skin level. In these cases a skin level release is usually sufficient as opposed to a formal revision.

A stoma is technically a purposeful creation of a hernia. A parastomal hernia is the herniation of omentum or bowel through the fascial aperture of the stoma. These hernias can be symptomatic and can be the cause of significant pain or obstruction.

Stomal prolapse is not uncommon with loop stomas, but can also occur with end stomas. In loop stomas, it is commonly the distal limb that prolapses. The more proximally along the colon the stoma is constructed, the likelihood of prolapse increases.

RESULTS

Preoperative planning, appropriate stoma sighting, and precise operative technique have resulted in relatively low complication rates from stoma creation.

CONCLUSIONS

The creation of a stoma is relatively straightforward; however, a poorly constructed stoma can significantly affect a patient's quality of life, therefore all efforts should be made to plan and create an effective colostomy.

Recommended References and Readings

1. Shellito PC. Complications of abdominal stoma surgery. *Dis Col Rect* 1998;41(12):1562–72.
2. Doberneck RC. Revision and closure of the colostomy. *Surg Clin North Am* 1991;71(1):193–201.
3. Nasmyth DG. Stomas in colorectal surgery: options and alternatives. *Digest Dis* 1990;8(4):240–52.
4. Devlin HB. Colostomy. Indications, management and complications. *Ann R Coll Surg Engl* 1973;52(6):392–408.
5. Boman-Sandelin K, Fenyo G. Construction and closure of loop transverse colostomy. *Dis Col Rectum* 1985;28:772–4.
6. Prasad ML, Pearl RK, Abcarian H. End-loop colostomy. *Surg Gynecol Obstet* 1984;158(4):380–382.
7. Bass EM, Del Pino A, Tan A, et al. Does perioperative stoma marking and education by the stoma therapist affect outcome? *Dis Colon Rect* 1997;40:440–2.
8. Mirelman D, Corman ML, Veidenheimer MC, Coller JA. Colostomies-indications and contraindications: Lahey Clinic experience 1963–1974. *Dis Colon Rect* 1978;21:172–6.
9. Smit R, Walt AJ. The morbidity and cost of the temporary colostomy. *Dis Colon Rect* 1978;21:558–61.
10. Hulten L. Enterostomies—technical aspects. *Scand J Gastroenterol Suppl* 1988;149:125–35.

40 Laparoscopic

Charles B. Whitlow and David E. Beck

 INDICATIONS/CONTRAINDICATIONS

Colostomy formation is a procedure particularly well suited to laparoscopic techniques since there is no requirement for specimen extraction. While it is not as technically challenging as colectomy, it involves some of the same steps as colectomy and attention to detail is mandatory to ensure optimal results. This admonition is especially true for patients in whom a permanent stoma is being created, which may not always be known at the time of stoma formation.

There are numerous indications for colostomy, all with the ultimate need to divert the fecal stream from its normal anatomic egress. These indications include fistulizing perineal Crohn's disease, rectovaginal fistula, diseases which require wide perianal skin excision with or without skin grafting, such as hidradenitis suppurativa, Buschke-Lowenstein type anal condyloma, and decubitus ulcers, fecal incontinence, radiation proctitis, obstructing/unresectable rectal cancer, anorectal trauma, and urethrorectal fistula.

For most indications, a sigmoid colostomy is superior to a colostomy created from more proximal colon. The ease with which the transverse colon can be delivered as a stoma is more than offset by the difficulty of ostomy care experienced by patients. In some cases ileostomy (described in a separate chapter) may be more appropriate or preferred to a colostomy. However, the surgeon should remember that in cases of distal obstruction, performing an ileostomy for diversion may not relieve the obstruction due to competency of the ileocecal valve.

Contraindications for laparoscopic procedures include the need for an open procedure or a history of extensive adhesions encountered during previous procedures. A history of previous abdominal surgery does not portend the presence of extensive adhesions.

 PREOPERATIVE PLANNING

One of the most important considerations for colostomy formation is proper siting of the stoma. Ideally the site is preoperatively marked with the assistance of an enterostomal therapist or wound ostomy continence nurse. The goals of siting are to select a location within the borders of the rectus abdominis muscle, on a flat surface, which the patient can see. In many individuals this position will be at the cephalad apex of the infraumbilical fat pad. A location above or below the belt line is also dependent on the type of clothing that the patient typically wears. Additionally, the stoma should be away from scars, skin folds, and bony prominences. The proposed location must be verified with the patient supine, sitting, and standing and then marked. The marking technique will vary according to the urgency of the surgery and from the use of indelible markers or tattooing to mark the site.

Standard bowel preparation is not mandatory. However, because the empty colon intraoperatively handles better than the stool filled colon, it is the authors' preference to have patients who can tolerate a preparation, ingest a limited isotonic lavage prep (one-quarter to half gallon of a polyethylene glycol solution). Patients are instructed to limit diet to only clear liquids the day prior to surgery. Oral antibiotics are not prescribed but standard intravenous broad-spectrum antibiotics are given within 1 hour of skin incision. Deep vein thrombosis prophylaxis is also ordered. Informed consent should include the potential for conversion to an open procedure.

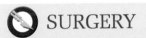

SURGERY

Patient Positioning and Preparation

The patient is initially placed supine on a beanbag, gel pad, or cushion. After induction of general anesthesia, an orogastric tube and indwelling urinary bladder catheter are placed. The patient is then placed in modified lithotomy position with the thighs even with the hips and pressure points appropriately padded. One or both arms may be adducted to facilitate securing the patients for the extremes of positioning used during laparoscopy. The patient is then secured to the table, usually with tape. Rectal irrigation with tap water is performed until clear unless the patient has an obstructing lesion. The skin is prepped with antiseptic solution and draping is undertaken in a standard fashion.

Instrument/Monitor Positioning

The primary monitor is placed on the patient's left near the level of the hip. A secondary monitor can be placed at the left shoulder or at an alternate site viewable by the surgical technician. Insufflation tubing, suction tubing, cautery power cord, laparoscopy camera wiring, and a laparoscope light cord are brought off the patient's left side if possible. A 10 mm laparoscope with a 30-degree lens is preferred.

Port Selection and Placement

An umbilical or supraumbilical location is used for placement of a 10/11 mm port (Fig. 40.1). The port is placed using an open (modified Hasson) technique. Specifically, a vertical skin incision with a scalpel is followed by dissection down to the linea alba. An Ochsner clamp is used to elevate the midline at the level of the umbilical stump and the linea alba is then incised. S-shaped retractors are helpful in exposing the midline. Entry into the peritoneum is accomplished either bluntly with a Kelly clamp or sharply. A more cephalad midline or right upper quadrant site may be necessary if the selected stoma site is less than one hand's breadth from the umbilicus or the patient has had multiple previous midline incisions. Once entry into the peritoneal cavity is obtained, a 10/11 mm blunt-tip balloon trocar is placed and secured. Alternatively, a 0 polyglycolic acid suture is placed into the fascia in a purse-string manner with which a standard 10/11 mm trocar is secured (12 mm if an end colostomy is planned).

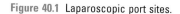

Figure 40.1 Laparoscopic port sites.

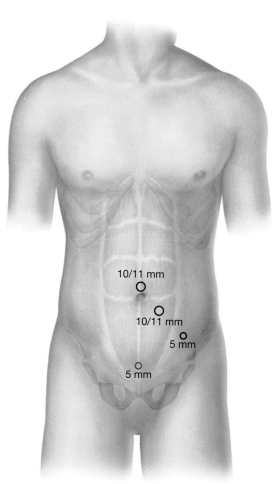

10/11 mm

10/11 mm

5 mm

5 mm

Laparoscopic inspection of the peritoneal cavity is undertaken to exclude any unsuspected pathology. This time is also the time to identify if the patient has a redundant/mobile colon that does not require further mobilization. A second 10/11 mm port is then placed at the preoperatively marked stoma site. This port can be placed with a standard vertical skin incision or a 2 cm disk of skin can be excised prior to placement of the stoma-site trocar. A grasper is inserted and the sigmoid colon is identified and grasped. If the colon has sufficient mobility and reaches the abdominal wall with the pneumoperitoneum intact, then there is usually adequate redundancy to create a loop stoma. If this situation is identified, then the port at the preselected ostomy site is all that is needed.

If the colon requires mobilization and/or if adhesiolysis is required, additional ports are placed under laparoscopic visualization. A 5 mm port is placed in the right lower quadrant and if necessary a second 5 mm port is placed in the suprapubic or right upper quadrant.

Mobilization and Transection

Simple mobilization of the sigmoid and descending colon is usually adequate for a loop colostomy. This mobilization is accomplished by incision along the lateral attachment of the left colon mesentery using electrocautery shears and then bluntly dissecting the mesentery off of the retroperitoneum (Fig. 40.2). Care is taken to protect the retroperitoneal structures including the ureter and gonadal vessels. With medial retraction, the peritoneum is incised and using blunt dissection the colonic mesentery is freed from

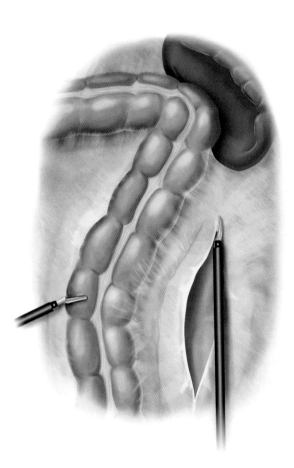

Figure 40.2 Sigmoid colon is retracted medially and peritoneal reflection is incised.

the retroperitoneum. This step is accomplished easily if the correct plane is used. Mobilization should be performed until the sigmoid colon can be brought up to the abdominal wall without tension, with the pneumoperitoneum intact. In the case of end colostomy the mesentery is divided using a hemostatic energy source (ultrasonic shears or bipolar vessel sealing device). Moreover, this can be performed above the inferior mesenteric artery as high ligation of this vessel is not necessary for this procedure. If the inferior mesenteric artery is to be divided, the left ureter should be identified and protected prior to division. If additional length is needed the splenic flexure should be mobilized by further dividing the attachments of the colon along the left retroperitoneum, the splenocolic attachments, and the omentum. A laparoscopic bowel stapler is used to divide the colon at the point at which the mesentery is divided. Additional proximal mesenteric division is performed until adequate length is obtained, taking care to preserve the marginal artery blood supply.

Creation of Aperture

The colon to be brought out for the stoma is grasped with an atraumatic clamp (Fig. 40.3). The subcutaneous fat is incised followed by vertical incision of the anterior rectus sheath. The rectus abdominis muscle is then bluntly spread and retracted with appendiceal retractors. The pneumoperitoneum is released after which the peritoneal opening is enlarged by dividing the posterior fascia and peritoneum and the bowel is brought through the aperture. Proper orientation is ensured by examining the proximal and distal limbs and the absence of twists. In the case of loop colostomy we prefer to secure the loop with a plastic rod placed underneath the colon and secured to the adjacent skin with nylon or absorbable suture. Laparoscopic verification of appropriate anatomic orientation of the afferent and efferent limbs should be undertaken. In addition, proctoscopy or flexible sigmoidectomy may be undertaken to verify orientation.

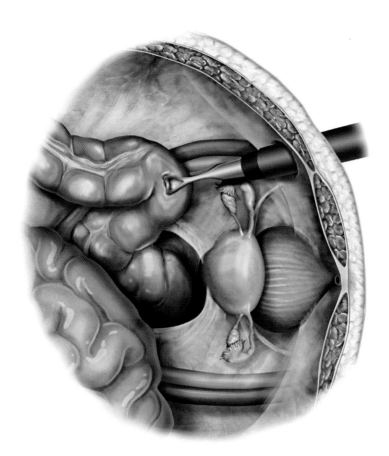

Figure 40.3 Laparoscopic colostomy. Bowel is manipulated to the stomal opening using a laparoscopic Babcock grasper.

Closure of Port Sites/Stoma Maturation

The umbilical port site fascia is closed with interrupted 0 polyglycolic acid suture and skin wound are closed with subcuticular 4-0 absorbable suture. In the case of loop colostomy, 75% of the colon circumference is divided. Both ends are then matured with interrupted 3-0 polyglycolic acid or chromic sutures. An end loop colostomy can be created by stapling off the distal limb. The proximal (functional limb) is matured and the stapled closed limb left in the subcutaneous fat. The defunctionalized limb can be identified by insufflating air by a proctoscope and/or by flexible sigmoidoscopy.

 ## POSTOPERATIVE MANAGEMENT

The orogastric tube is removed prior to extubation and the Foley catheter is removed later in the day or the next morning. Patients are supported with intravenous fluids and offered liquids when they are hungry. Patients resume intestinal activity and diet very quickly, often eating the evening of, or the day following, surgery. Solid food is started when flatus is expressed from the stoma. Pain management is usually provided by patient controlled analgesia supplemented with Ketorolac. The patient is switched to oral pain medication when they are taking fluids and early ambulation is encouraged. Patients are ready for discharge when they can care for their stoma, tolerate a diet, and have evidence of bowel function.

 ## COMPLICATIONS

Laparoscopic ostomy procedures retain most of the potential complications associated with open procedures including, skin problems, excessive output, retraction, prolapse, ischemia, stenosis, necrosis, hemorrhage, and hernia. Preoperative planning and good technique will prevent most of these problems.

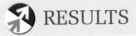

RESULTS

Multiple studies have attested to the safety and advantages of laparoscopic assisted colostomy creation (1–15). Success rates have been high and if patients are properly selected, conversion rates are low.

CONCLUSIONS

Although colostomies are becoming less common than they were several decades ago, they remain a life altering event for the patients in whom they are created. As such all efforts should be made to limit physiologic and psychological trauma; patients and many are suitable for laparoscopic techniques. Attention to preoperative planning and operative technique can produce a well functioning stoma and increase patient acceptance of their stoma.

Recommended References and Readings

1. Orkin BA, Cataldo PA. Intestinal stomas. In: Wolff BG, Fleshman JW, Beck DE, et al. eds. *The ASCRS Textbook of Colorectal Surgery*. New York: Springer-Verlag, 2007:622–42.
2. Hyman N, Nelson R. Stomal complications. In: Wolff BG, Fleshman JW, Beck DE, et al. eds. *The ASCRS Textbook of Colorectal Surgery*. New York: Springer-Verlag, 2007:643–52.
3. Lange V, Meyer G, Schardey HM, Schildberg FW. Laparoscopic creation of a loop colostomy. *J Laparoendosc Surg* 1991;1(5): 307–12.
4. Romero CA, James KM, Cooperstone LM, Mishrick AS, Ger R. Laparoscopic sigmoid colostomy for perianal Crohn's disease. *Surg Laparosc Endosc* 1992;2(2):148–51.
5. Ludwig KA, Milsom JW, Garcia-Ruiz A, Fazio VW. Laparoscopic techniques for fecal diversion. *Dis Colon Rectum* 1996; 39:285–88.
6. Oliveira L, Reissman P, Nogueras J, Wexner SD. Laparoscopic creation of stomas. *Surg Endosc* 1997;11:19–23.
7. Boike GM, Lurain JR. Laparoscopic descending colostomy in three patients with cervical carcinoma. *Gynecol Oncol* 1994;54 (3):381–84.
8. Fuhrman GM, Ota DM. Laparoscopic intestinal stomas. *Dis Colon Rectum* 1994;37(5):444–49.
9. Hashizume M, Haraguchi Y, Ikeda Y, Kajiyama K, Fujie T, Sugimachi K. Laparoscopy-assisted colostomy. *Surg Laparosc Endosc* 1994;4(1):70–72.
10. Hollyoak MA, Lumley J, Stitz RW. Laparoscopic stoma formation for faecal diversion. *Br J Surg* 1998;85(2):226–28.
11. Young CJ, Eyers AA, Solomon MJ. Defunctioning of the anorectum: historical controlled study of laparoscopic vs. open procedures. *Dis Colon Rectum* 1998;41(2):190–94.
12. Marquis P, Marrel A, Jambon B. Quality of life in patients with stomas: the Montreux Study. *Ostomy Wound Manage* 2003; 49(2):48–55.
13. Wirsching M, Druner HU, Herrmann G. Results of psychosocial adjustment to long-term colostomy. *Psychother Psychosom* 1975;26(5):245–56.
14. Devlin HB. Colostomy: past and present. *Ann R Coll Surg Engl* 1990;72:175.
15. Rosito O, Nino-Murcia M, Wolfe VA, Kiratli BJ, Perkash I. The effects of colostomy on the quality of life in patients with spinal cord injury: a retrospective analysis. *J Spinal Cord Med* 2002;25(3):174–83.

41 Laparoscopic Ileostomy

Bradford Sklow and William J. Peche

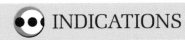 INDICATIONS

Laparoscopic ileostomy for fecal diversion is minimally invasive and can be accomplished with minimal morbidity (1–3). The laparoscopic approach offers the advantages of decreased pain, smaller incision, quicker return of bowel function, and shorter hospital stay. Most of the time a diverting loop ileostomy is constructed, but an end ileostomy can also be easily performed using the laparoscopic approach. The indications for performing a laparoscopic ileostomy for fecal diversion include fecal incontinence, rectovaginal fistula, perianal Crohn's disease, obstructing unresectable colon cancer, and anastomotic leak (4). There are no absolute contraindications to performing a laparoscopic ileostomy, even in patients who are considered high risk or who have had previous abdominal surgery (5,6).

 PREOPERATIVE PLANNING

No bowel prep is needed or indicated. The patient should meet with an enterostomal therapy (ET) nurse to be marked with a permanent marker on their abdomen at the site for the planned ileostomy to ensure proper stoma location. Any questions can be answered and concerns addressed during that visit with an ET nurse. Preoperatively meeting with an ET nurse has been shown to reduce postoperative complications and problems with stomas, especially ileostomies (7,8).

 SURGERY

The patient is positioned in the supine position on the operating room table. A beanbag is optional, but usually unnecessary for this procedure as long as the patient has been carefully secured to the table. Preoperative antibiotics consisting of a second-generation cephalosporin are administered within 1 hour of skin incision. The site of the planned ileostomy is scratched with a small needle as the marker ink can be wiped off during the prep of the skin. The operating surgeon stands on the left side of the table and a

Figure 41.1 Laparoscopic port placement. Hassan trocar is shown at the umbilicus.

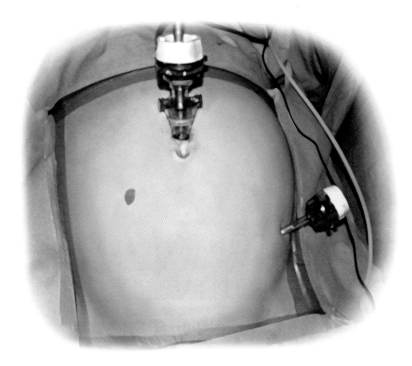

5-mm trocar is placed superior to the umbilicus after pneumoperitoneum is established using a Veress needle. A 5-mm, 30-degree laparoscope is inserted through the supraumbilical port. Alternatively, a 10-mm trocar can be placed using a direct Hassan technique above the umbilicus, and a 10-mm, 30-degree laparoscope is used (Fig. 41.1). An additional 5-mm port is placed on the left side of the abdomen two fingerbreadths medial and superior the left iliac crest (Fig. 41.1). An optional third 5-mm port can be placed through the planned ileostomy site on the right side of the abdomen (Fig. 41.2). Mobilization of the terminal ileum may be facilitated by releasing the lateral attachments along the pelvic brim up to the right gutter. The site of the stoma is chosen approximately

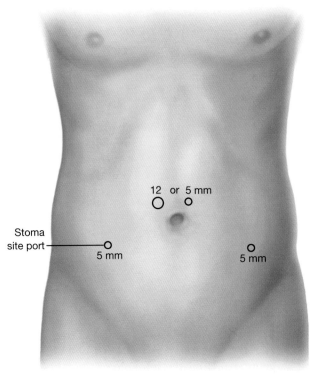

Figure 41.2 Port placement with optional 5-mm port through the planned stoma site.

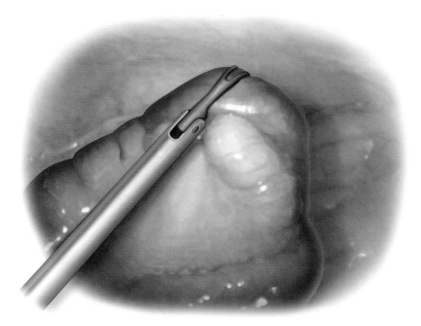

Figure 41.3 Loop of ileum is delivered up to the abdominal wall.

30–40 cm proximal to the ileocecal valve and grasped with an atraumatic bowel grasper (Fig. 41.3). The ileum is oriented with the grasper as not to twist the loop of ileum. The preselected stoma site on the right side of the abdomen is prepared by making a 2-cm diameter skin opening. The rectus muscle is opened to allow two fingers to pass with a muscle-splitting technique. The loop of ileum is delivered through the rectus muscle above the level of the skin (Fig. 41.4). A stoma rod may or may not be required to suspend the loop depending on the body habitus of the patient. The abdomen is then re-insufflated and the loop of ileum is visualized going into the stoma site to ensure that the ileostomy was not twisted during delivery through the abdominal wall. The distal limb is placed inferiorly and the functioning and is placed superiorly. At this point the ileum can be divided using an open surgical linear cutter to create a divided and loop stoma and the distal end tucked back into the abdomen below the fascia. This has the advantage of being completely diverting. The laparoscopic ports are removed, and the

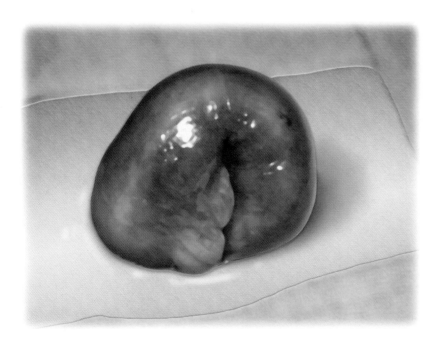

Figure 41.4 Loop of ileum before opening and maturing the stoma.

Figure 41.5 The incision is made in the ileum closer to the distal end.

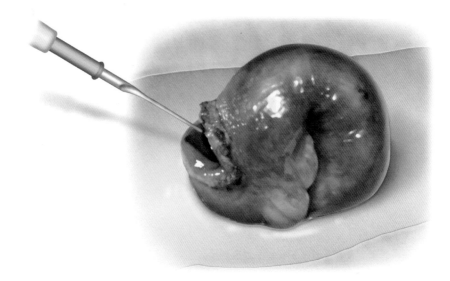

port site incisions are closed with absorbable, subdermal sutures. Sterile dressings are applied prior to maturing the ileostomy. If a loop ileostomy is performed, an incision is made 80% around the circumference of the ileum. The proximal limb of the ileum will be everted as the functioning limb (Fig. 41.5). The proximal aspect of the stoma is Brooked above the level of the skin to the dermis with 3-0 absorbable sutures and the distal end is sutured flush to the dermis of the skin gathering the bowel wall to a small portion of the circumference of the skin opening at the most inferior part of the stoma site (Figs. 41.6 and 41.7). Ultimately, a stoma appliance is applied.

 ## POSTOPERATIVE MANAGEMENT

After creation of a laparoscopic loop or end ileostomy, diet can be advanced as tolerated. Return of bowel function usually occurs within 48–72 hours. Once bowel function has resumed, the ileostomy output may be high initially. Patients must consume an adequate amount of fluids to keep up with the stoma output and avoid dehydration.

Figure 41.6 Maturing the ileostomy using absorbable sutures.

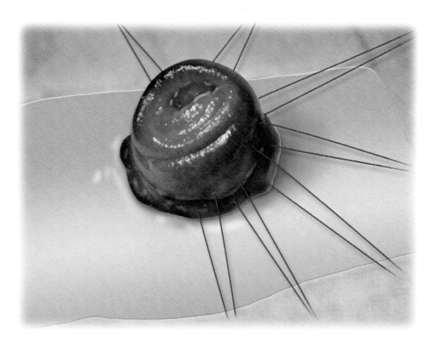

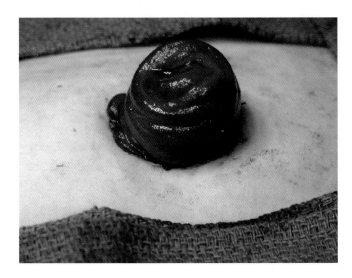

Figure 41.7 Brooked ileostomy ready for stoma appliance.

Electrolyte abnormalities are common, and patients with high-output ileostomies should have their electrolytes checked. Output should be less than 1,500 ml/day prior to discharge. If the stoma output remains high, there are various medications that can help to reduce the effluent. Fiber supplementation, Imodium, Lomotil, tincture of opium, and codeine are helpful. If a patient still has high output despite the use of antidiarrheal medications, they may need to be discharged on intravenous (IV) fluids. Over a period of weeks, the ileostomy output will decrease to between 500 and 800 ml/day. If a stoma rod was used for a loop ileostomy, it can be removed on postoperative day 3–5. Peristomal skin care is paramount in the postoperative period. Proteolytic enzymes and the high alkaline content of the stoma effluent are responsible for significant skin irritation (8). Care of the patient should involve close cooperation between the surgeon and enterostomal therapist. Stoma care teaching by an enterostomal therapist is helpful in educating patients on the care of their ileostomy.

COMPLICATIONS

The laparoscopic approach lends itself to all the complications associated with laparoscopy in general. The most common access injury is small-bowel injury from trocar or Veress needle insertion (0.13%) (9). Extra care must be taken to avoid the complication of twisting the ileostomy. Tactile sensation and visualization are reduced with the laparoscopic approach and an instrument can over grasp or release without warning (10). The incidence of complications rates for ileostomy formation is variable in the literature, ranging from 24% to 69% (8,11–15). The largest study by Park et al. reported a complication rate of 34% in 1,616 patients with both ileostomies and colostomies performed at Cook County hospital over a 20-year period (8). This study also demonstrated the highest complication rate of 75% in loop ileostomies. Arumugam et al. performed a prospective study demonstrating that body mass index, diabetes, and emergency surgery were associated with complications on multivariate regression analysis (11). Complications are generally classified as being early or late. Early complications include peristomal dermatitis, dehydration, necrosis/ischemia, retraction, and infection. The most common complication was peristomal dermatitis or irritation and has a reported incidence of 15–42% (15,16). Placing the ileostomy in the proper location along with adequate skin care in conjunction with an ET nurse will help minimize this complication. Dehydration combined with electrolyte abnormalities is also very common following construction of a new ileostomy and up to 20% of patients require either hospital readmission or IV fluids as an outpatient (17). A small percentage of patients may require IV fluid supplementation at home following creation of a new ileostomy. Peristomal infections and abscess are uncommon with a reported incidence of 2–15% (8,11,12). An abscess must be surgically drained at the mucocutaneous junction or outside the border of the stoma appliance. The subsequent development of a fistula is not uncommon, and if persistent, it often requires new stoma formation.

Late complications include parastomal hernia, bowel obstruction, stenosis, nephrolithiasis, and stomal prolapse (10,18). The incidence of paraileostomy hernia ranges from 1.8% to 28.3% for end ileostomy and 0–6.2% for loop ileostomy (19–22). Risk factors for parastomal hernia include obesity, poor nutrition, steroid therapy, wound infection, and chronic cough (23–25). Parastomal hernias are generally asymptomatic and should be managed conservatively. Pain, difficulty with fitting the stoma appliance, bowel obstruction, strangulation, and perforation are indications for repair of the hernia. The results of parastomal hernia repair are disappointing with high recurrence rates (23). Options include primary suture repair, repair with prosthetic or biologic mesh, and stoma relocation (18).

RESULTS

Laparoscopic ileostomy is safe with low conversion rates. Swain and Ellis retrospectively reviewed 53 laparoscopic loop ileostomy procedures. There were no conversions. The average duration of the surgery was 47 minutes and there were no early complications reported (2). Other series have included laparoscopic end and loop colostomies and ileostomies with conversion rate between 2.4% and 15.6% and early complications related to the operation of 6–9.5% (1,3). These studies concluded that laparoscopic stoma creation is safe and effective.

CONCLUSIONS

- Ileostomy construction is well suited for the laparoscopic approach with low conversion rates and short operative times.
- Preoperative appointment with an ET nurse is important for proper ileostomy location selection and to minimize postoperative complications.
- The majority of postoperative complications are stoma related and not due to the laparoscopic technique itself.

References

1. Schwandner O, Schiedeck T, Bruch H. Stoma creation for fecal diversion: is the laparoscopic technique appropriate? *Int J Colorectal Dis* 1998;13(5–6):251–5.
2. Swain B, Ellis N. Laparoscopic-assisted loop ileostomy an acceptable option for temporary fecal diversion after anorectal surgery. *Dis Colon Rectum* 2002;45(5):705–7.
3. Oliveira L, Reissman P, Nogueras J, Wexner SD. Laparoscopic creation of stomas. *Surg Endosc* 1997;11(1):19–23.
4. Joh YG, Kim SH, Hahn KY, Stulberg J, Chung CS, Lee DK. Anastomotic leakage after laparoscopic proctectomy can be managed by a minimally invasive approach. *Dis Colon Rectum* 2009;52 (1):91–6.
5. Marks JH, Kawun UB, Hamdan W, Marks G. Redefining contraindications to laparoscopic colorectal resection for high-risk patients. *Surg Endosc* 2008;22(8):1899–904.
6. Offodile AC, Lee SW, Yoo J, et al. Does prior abdominal surgery influence conversion rates and outcomes of laparoscopic right colectomy in patients with neoplasia? *Dis Colon Rectum* 2008;51(11):1669–74.
7. Bass EM, Pino AD, Tan A, Pearl RK, Orsay CP, Abcarian H. Does preoperative stoma making and education by the enterostomal therapist affect outcome? *Dis Colon Rectum* 1997;40(4):440–2.

8. Park JJ, Del Pino A, Orsay CP, et al. Stoma complications: the Cook County experience. *Dis Colon Rectum* 1999;42(12):1575–80.
9. Van der Voort M, Heijnsdijk EAM, Gouma DJ. Bowel injury as a complication of laparoscopy. *Br J Surg* 2004;91:1253–8.
10. Ng KH, Ng DCK, Cheung HYS, et al. Obstructive complications of laparoscopically created defunctioning ileostomy. *Dis Colon Rectum* 2008;51:1664–8. 17.
11. Arumugam PJ, Bevan L, Macdonald L, et al. A prospective audit of stoma: analysis of risk factors and complications and their management. *Colorectal Dis* 2003;5(1):49–52.
12. Robertson I, Leung D, Hughes D, et al. Prospective analysis of stoma-related complications. *Colorectal Dis* 2005;7:279–85.
13. Londono-Schimmer EE, Leong AP, Phillips RK. Life table analysis of stomal complications following colostomy. *Dis Colon Rectum* 1994;37(9):916–20.
14. Pearl RK, Prasad ML, Orsay CP, et al. Early complications from intestinal stomas. *Arch Surg* 1985;120(10):1145–7.
15. Duchesne JC, Wang YZ, Weintraub SL, Hunt JP. Stoma complications: a multivariated analysis. *Am Surg* 2002;68(11):961–6.
16. Hellman J, Lago CP. Dermatologic complications in colostomy and ileostomy patients. *Int J Dermatol* 1990;29(2):129–33.
17. Feinberg SM, McLeod RS, Cohen Z. Complication of loop ileostomy. *Am J Surg* 1987;153(1):102–7.
18. Shabbir J, Britton DC. Stoma complications: a literature overview. *Colorectal Dis* 2009. [Epub ahead of print].

19. Williams JG, Etherington R, Hayward MWJ, Hughes LE. Paraileostomy hernia: a clinical and radiological study. *Br J Surg* 1990; 77:1355–7.

20. Rullier E, Le Toux N, Laurent C, et al. Loop ileostomy versus loop colostomy for defunctioning low anastomosis during rectal cancer surgery. *World J Surg* 2001;25:274–8.

21. Edwards DP, Leppington-Clarke A, Sexton R, et al. Stoma related complications are more frequent after transverse colostomy than loop ileostomy: a prospective randomized clinical trial. *Br J Surg* 2001;88:360–3.

22. Thalheimmer A, Bueter M, Kortuem M, et al. Morbidity of temporary loop ileostomy in patients with colorectal cancer. *Dis Colon Rectum* 2006;49(7):1011–17.

23. Shellito PC. Complications of abdominal stoma surgery. *Dis Colon Rectum* 1998;41:1562–72.

24. Leslie D. The parastomal hernia. *Surg Clin North Am* 1984;64: 407–15.

25. Pearl RK. Parastomal hernias. *World J Surg* 1989;13:569–72.

Part XI: Ileostomy

42 Continent Ileostomy

Victor W. Fazio and Myles R. Joyce

Introduction

The continent ileostomy (K-pouch) emerged in response to patient's desire to avoid an end ileostomy. Patients cited difficulties with leakage; others complained of psychological and body image problems with application of an external device. The planned intermittent evacuation of the continent ileostomy provided a significant improvement in quality of life for motivated patients. However, the popularity for formation of this internal reservoir attenuated with the emergence of ileal pouch-anal anastomosis (IPAA) as the gold standard when desiring restoration of intestinal continuity and continence (1,2). The ileal pouch allows restoration of the normal defecatory pathway. Thus, K-pouch formation is now mainly confined to a few specialized centers. In essence, it is an internal reservoir that stores intestinal contents. It has a nipple valve that prevents leakage of gas and feces. The stoma aperture should be flushed with the skin. It is emptied by interval intubations of the pouch using a soft plastic tube. Since its original description by Nils Kock in 1969 (3), there have been several modifications principally directed at stabilization of the nipple valve.

Most patients who have a continent ileostomy are extremely satisfied with the quality of life it offers and are willing to undergo multiple revisions if it avoids returning to a conventional ileostomy (4). However, it is an operation that should not be entered into lightly by the patient and the surgeon as it is technically challenging, utilizes 40–60 cm of small bowel for construction, requires significant maintenance, and leaves the patient prone to potential fluid and electrolytic disturbances if the reservoir requires subsequent removal.

INDICATIONS/CONTRAINDICATIONS

Indications and Contraindications for Continent Ileostomy Formation

Current indications for formation include patients requiring total proctocolectomy (TPC) with sphincter dysfunction who wish to avoid an end ileostomy; patients with an existing ileostomy who wish to convert to an internal reservoir; patients in whom excision of the sphincter complex is required as part of an oncological resection (selected patients); and those with a failed pouch in whom salvage pouch surgery (redo pouch) is not feasible or has a low potential for success. Converting a failing ileal pouch to a K-pouch theoretically ensures bowel preservation. In addition, we counsel patients undergoing a planned IPAA of this alternative option if reach is going to be an issue, despite the use of all techniques to ensure that the ileal pouch reaches the anal canal in a tension-free manner. We are particularly conscious of this problem in patients undergoing salvage pouch surgery for pelvic sepsis, tall male patients, and those with a foreshortened mesentery. Patients considering a continent ileostomy should be carefully counseled preoperatively as to the inherent risks and understand that a conventional end ileostomy is associated with fewer problems. Ideally, they should be provided with the option of speaking to patients who have had both a good and a bad result from K-pouch formation. However, it is our experience that the majority of patients, who seek a K-pouch have researched all aspects of care and potential complications. A significant proportion of work in the Cleveland Clinic, Ohio, consists of K-pouch revisions principally for nipple valve dysfunction, which despite improvements remains the Achilles' heel of the procedure.

Contraindications to continent ileostomy formation include patients who have lost a significant proportion of small bowel from preceding surgery, those with recrudescent Crohn's disease, those with psychological problems, and those who are excessively obese. Obese patients often have a shortened, thickened mesentery, which is a problem when creating the nipple valve and is a risk factor for valve slippage. In addition, the increased abdominal girth gives problems with reach when creating the exit conduit. The presence of intra-abdominal desmoid disease in patients with familial adenomatous polyposis (FAP) is also a contraindication.

PREOPERATIVE PLANNING

The technique and pouch design for K-pouch construction often varies among institutions and depends on whether one is forming a *de novo* pouch following TPC or whether one is converting an existing failed pouch to continent ileostomy. The majority of techniques have evolved with time. The overall goal is to create a functional reservoir with an eventual capacity of 500–1,000 ml, which is continent to gas and feces. The exit conduit should be easily intubated to empty reservoir contents. CT enterography will help to exclude proximal small-bowel Crohn's disease, especially in patients with indeterminate colitis.

The patient requires marking by the surgeon or an experienced enterostomal therapist. In contrast to an end ileostomy, the stoma may be placed relatively low in the abdomen. The chosen site is most often below the belt line and above the pubic hairline, as when successful it does not require an external appliance. The patient is either placed supine or in a modified lithotomy position depending on the indication for surgery. Ureteric catheters are placed in patients undergoing redo pelvic surgery where we insert ureteric stents. In patients with an existing K-pouch undergoing salvage surgery the K-pouch is emptied of all contents. This measure reduces the potential for intraoperative spillage when mobilizing or opening the pouch, which is risky as the pouch wall is generally very thin.

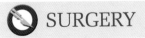 SURGERY

Surgical Technique

The abdomen is entered via a lower midline laparotomy incision taking care to avoid enterotomies. In patients with preceding surgery and dense adhesions, hydrodissection may be required to identify tissue planes, reducing potential for enterotomies. The traditional technique for pouch construction used two 12–15-cm loops of terminal ileum.

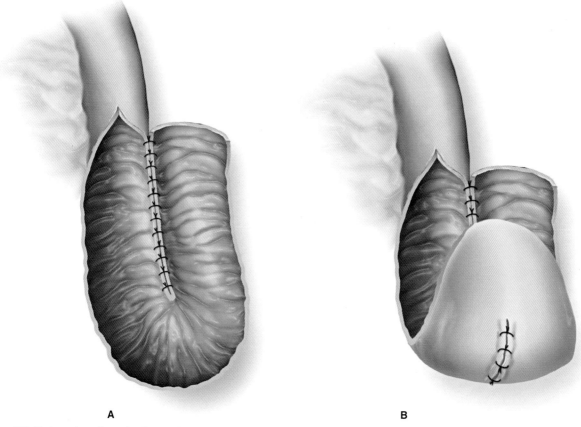

A   B

Figure 42.1 U-shaped configuration for continent ileostomy formation.

An additional 15 cm of ileum was used distal to the pouch with 12 cm used for nipple valve intussusception and remainder was used to construct the exit conduit. The bowel loops are aligned in a U-shaped fashion with approximation of the antimesenteric borders performed using continuous 2-0 chromic catgut or polyvinyl suture (5). The limbs are then opened on the antimesenteric borders with the posterior wall constructed using a second layer of continuous absorbable suture to approximate the mucosa (Fig. 42.1).

The authors favor an S-shaped reservoir, which requires the addition of a third limb (Fig. 42.2) (6). In considering the S-pouch design, we believe that separating the afferent limb from the exit conduit allows for easier pouch rotation if needed in the future. We devote 20 cm of the terminal ileum to the nipple valve and exit conduit. Intussuscepting 12 cm of the efferent limb gives a 6 cm valve with 8 cm remaining for the exit conduit. Similar to the U-shaped design the three limbs are opposed with seromuscular sutures, bowel is opened on the antimesenteric border, and mucosal approximation is completed (Fig. 42.3 A and B).

It took Nils Kock several years and some modifications before discovering that intussusception of a component of the exit conduit achieved continence. In the original design no valve was created and later attempts involved mobilizing the rectus abdominus muscle to produce functional obstruction. The original technique for keeping the valve intussuscepted consisted of inserting several rows of sutures through the two limbs over a Hegar's dilator. There have been several modifications since including the Barnett continent ileostomy (7). The authors' technique consists of intussuscepting a portion of the exit conduit using a Babcock forceps, to create the nipple valve, which is approximately 6 cm in length. Prior to intussusception the peritoneum of the efferent limb is stripped from its adjacent mesentery, which may also be defatted using electrocautery. This reduces its bulk and improves the ability to intussuscept the future valve.

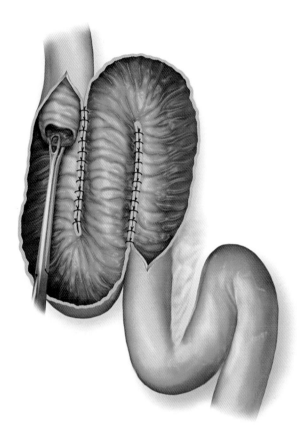

Figure 42.2 S-pouch configuration for continent ileostomy formation as favored by authors.

The critical step then involves stabilization of the valve, which the authors perform using three to four applications of a transverse stapler (reusable PI 55, Covidien, Norwalk, CT) (Fig. 42.4 A and B) (8). The pin must be removed from the stapler as if left in place it will likely give rise to a fistula. Care must be taken not to damage the blood supply to the nipple. The anterior portion of the pouch is then closed starting at the apex of the nipple valve. The authors use 2/0 Vicryl sutures and incorporate the anterior portion of the nipple valve in the initial part of the anterior closure. When the anterior closure reaches the apex of the nipple valve we provide further stabilization by the application

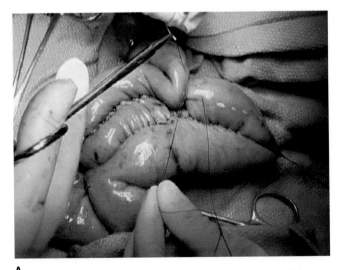

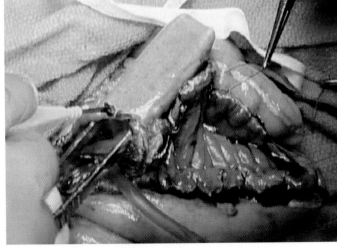

A   B

Figure 42.3 A. Aligning the three limbs of the S-pouch. **B.** Opening the aligned loops on the antimesenteric border.

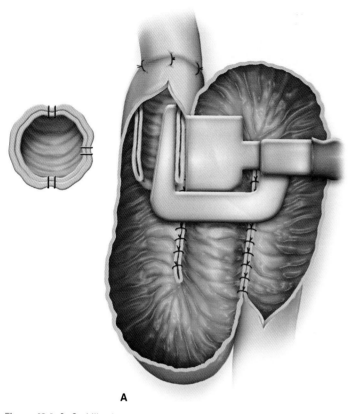
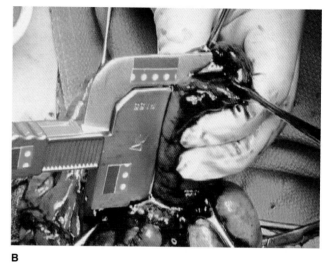

A   **B**

Figure 42.4 **A.** Stabilization of the nipple valve using three to four applications of a stapler. **B.** Intraoperative image of the TX stapler used to stabilize the nipple valve.

of an additional fire of the transverse stapler over the sutured layer (Fig. 42.5). Anterior closure of the pouch is then completed. A silicone catheter tube is then inserted into the pouch and the capacity plus valve integrity is tested (Fig. 42.6). Anchoring sutures secure the pouch lateral to the stoma opening through the posterior fascia. The exit conduit is delivered and a more medial set of sutures then inserted (Fig. 42.7 A and B). The aperture of the exit conduit should be a snug fit as too tight risks ischemia and lax risks valve prolapse and parastomal herniation. The exit conduit is sutured flush with

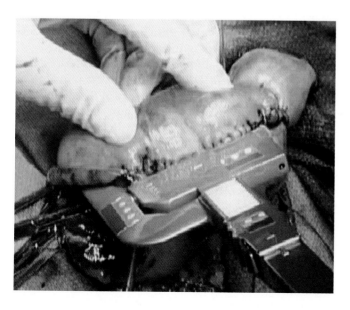

Figure 42.5 Application of PI 55 stapler over the anterior portion of the nipple valve that has already been stabilized with sutures to anterior portion of pouch.

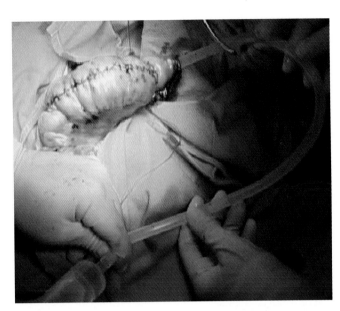

Figure 42.6 Testing pouch capacity plus valve integrity.

the stoma opening using absorbable sutures inserted in an interrupted fashion (Fig. 42.8). It is critically important that the tube can be inserted without difficulty or need for excessive angulation (Fig. 42.9).

The distance between the abdominal wall orifice and pouch should be kept as short as possible to facilitate ease of intubation. At the end of the procedure, we secure the tube in place using tripod sutures, which prevent tube slippage or advancement into the pouch (Fig. 42.10). The tube tip is placed midway between the valve entrance in the pouch and the pouch wall. It is then allowed to drain by gravity.

Conversion of a Failed Ileal Pouch-Anal Anastomosis to Continent Ileostomy

The possibility for converting a pelvic pouch to continent ileostomy was initially reported by Ecker et al. (9) in 1996 and then by Behrens et al. (10) in 1999. They reported excellent retention rates with an overall improvement in quality of life. Conversion of a pelvic pouch to continent ileostomy may be technically challenging. In some cases the existing pouch may be unusable, especially if the cause for pouch failure was pelvic sepsis. Patients must be counseled that if the component of the operation requiring pouch excision is prolonged, associated with significant blood loss or is technically difficult then surgically it may be more prudent to initially create an end ileostomy. In 6–12 months one may covert the end ileostomy to a continent ileostomy.

Patients are placed in a modified lithotomy position and bilateral ureteric stents are inserted. The existing ileal pouch is circumferentially mobilized to the pelvic floor taking care to preserve its blood supply. In most cases, the mesentery of the pouch lies in the sacrum but some surgeons position the mesentery anteriorly and thus, the pouch itself may be fused to the sacrum, increasing the risk of damage with mobilization. If the ileal pouch is successfully mobilized, one often finds that the cause of preceding pelvic sepsis originated at the old pouch-anal anastomosis. This distal segment may be sacrificed which still leaves a very healthy, viable pouch proximally. The small bowel is then divided approximately 20 cm upstream from the pouch and this is used to create the nipple valve and exit conduit as previously described. Thus, in the majority of cases creating a two-loop continent ileostomy if the original ileal pouch had a J-configuration. The pouch is rotated and the proximal small bowel is anastomosed to the old apex. In the majority of cases we place Seprafilm® (Genzyme, Cambridge, MA) to reduce the potential for intra-abdominal adhesions, especially given the potential need for further surgeries.

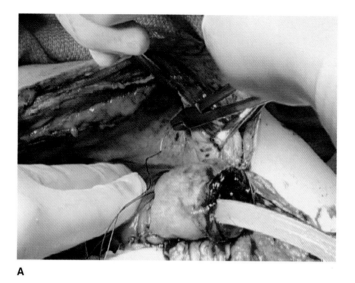

A

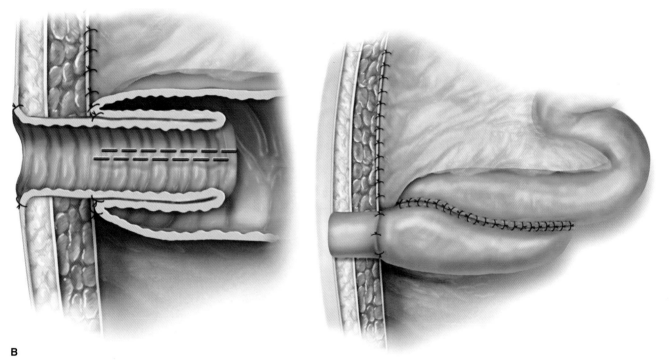

B

Figure 42.7 **A.** Anchoring the fundus of the pouch lateral to the stoma opening. **B.** Anchoring fundus of pouch and closure of parastomal space.

POSTOPERATIVE MANAGEMENT

In addition to the standard postoperative care for those undergoing major abdominal surgery continent ileostomy, patients require a specialized nursing plan (11). The patient will arrive on the floor with a drainage catheter tube held in place by tripod sutures and the pouch draining via gravity. The nurse will be given orders to gently irrigate the pouch using 30 cc normal saline. This will begin in the recovery room and be performed every 2 hours initially until return of intestinal function. If resistance is encountered, irrigated solution does not return freely, or if the stoma appears ischemic, then the surgeon is contacted. Often simple mobilization of the drainage tube is all that is required to achieve adequate irrigation. The tip of the catheter may have migrated becoming

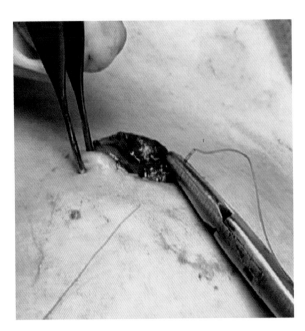

Figure 42.8 Exit conduit is sutured flush with the stoma opening.

adherent to the pouch wall or valve. Within 24–48 hours an enterostomal therapist will cut the stabilizing tripod sutures and apply a faceplate. Our preference is to leave the catheter *in situ* for 4–6 weeks to facilitate reservoir drainage and lessen pouch distension. This reduces the potential for suture breakdown during the healing phase.

There is a strong onus on the patient to take active care of the pouch. The patient and their family must be educated on how to irrigate the pouch and reposition the catheter if drainage is inadequate. We also encourage them to follow a low-residue diet and to avoid any foods that have the potential to block the pouch. We prefer to remove

Figure 42.9 Drainage tube must pass easily and without excessive angulations into the pouch.

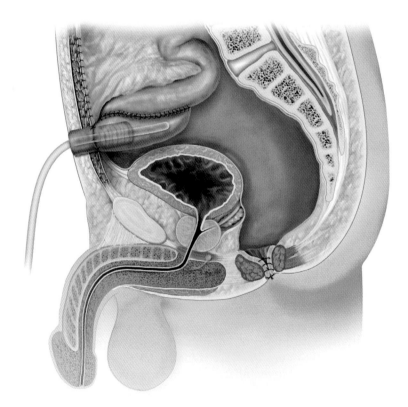

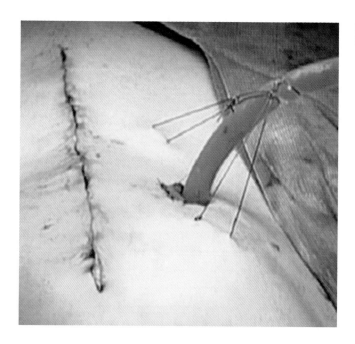

Figure 42.10 Tripod sutures secure the draining tube.

the *in situ* catheter at an office visit. This allows us to reinforce the technique for pouch drainage and intubate the pouch if any difficulty arises. The patient then intubates the pouch under supervision. As a rule the pouch should be allowed to distend gradually and thus, initial pouch intubations are required more frequently than at a later stage. Ultimately, the pouch should acquire a capacity of 800–1,200 ml without any restrictions on patients' food intake. They receive intensive enterostomal therapy care on how to manage problems. If there is difficultly with intubation the patient is advised to relax their abdominal muscles by lying supine and flexing the right knee. The catheter is then lubricated with traction placed on the peristomal skin to facilitate insertion. Under no circumstance should the catheter be forced as this carries the risk of pouch perforation.

COMPLICATIONS

Early complications include anastomotic leakage, intra-abdominal abscess, necrosis of the nipple valve, and intraluminal pouch hemorrhage. Failure to progress in a timely manner, prolonged ileus, leukocytosis, persistent pyrexia, and systemic or local sepsis are often manifestations of a pouch problem in the postoperative period. An intra-abdominal abscess may be treated by CT-guided percutaneous drainage. However, the majority of these complications require relaparotomy and proximal defunctioning loop ileostomy (12). If luminal bleeding is significant enough to cause hemodynamic compromise or a significant drop in hemoglobin, then the first step involves endoscopic evaluation of the pouch. Often a bleeding point may be localized to a suture line and is amenable to endoscopic clipping or injection with an adrenaline-based solution. The surgeon must ensure that there is no associated coagulation abnormality. Diffuse ooze without localized bleeding may be treated by irrigating the pouch using an epinephrine enema. If the patient has necrosis of the nipple valve, one should perform a flexible pouchoscopy to determine its extent. If necrosis involves tip of only the exit conduit, conservative management such as continuous damage is appropriate although it may lead to a stricture amenable to local revision in 3 months. If nipple valve necrosis is more extensive, the patient will at a minimum require a defunctioning ileostomy with revision of the valve in 3–6 months. We explain to the patient the importance of liaising with our institute if they are readmitted to an outside hospital with pouch pathology. When a surgeon is not familiar with the index surgery encounters an anastomotic leakage or other continent ileostomy problem

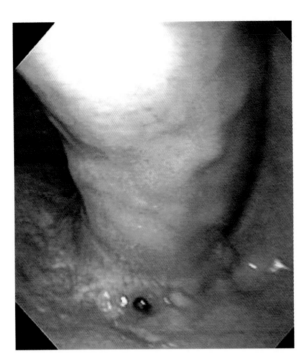

Figure 42.11 Fistula arising from the base of nipple valve giving rise to incontinence.

postoperatively, there is an inherent tendency to resect the pouch when a proximal defunctioning ileostomy would suffice.

Long-term complications are mainly related to problems with the nipple valve and thus, several modifications have been added to the original procedure to try and minimize this difficulty. Nipple valve slippage may involve a full de-intussusception in which the entire valve unravels lengthening the efferent limb, which may become kinked giving problems with intubation. This tends to originate on the mesenteric side and is radiologically identifiable by lengthening of the efferent limb. On occasion, the patient may present as an emergency because of failure to intubate. The pouch becomes overdistended and one needs to decompress the reservoir typically using an ileoscope or pediatric scope. A catheter is then inserted into the pouch under direct vision and fixed in place. This is left *in situ* until the patient can be scheduled for an appropriate procedure to correct the valve slippage. On one occasion the authors encountered a patient who lost their medina catheter within the reservoir, which could not be removed despite multiple endoscopic attempts. The patient needed a laparotomy to retrieve the catheter and correct the valve slippage. In many incidences the valve de-intussusception is associated with a fistula in the base of the valve (Fig. 42.11). The underlying etiology is not completely understandable, but many authors believe that it is an ischemic phenomenon related to some form of pressure effect from the de-intussuscepting valve. Endoscopy is a very effective method for identifying a fistula and requires retroflexion within the pouch to allow adequate visualization of the valve. Modifications performed in an attempt to attenuate the incidence of valve slippage include myotomy or serial diathermy serosal incisions on the two ileal surfaces in an attempt to get the ileal surfaces to stick. However, there was no great change in the incidence of valve slippage with these modifications. Reducing the mesenteric bulk with rotation of the mesentery of the intended intussuscepted valve was found to be more successful. This technique involved peritoneal stripping and mesenteric defatting as previously described. Another modification included the application of a collar in an attempt to stabilize the two ileal limbs. Initial materials used include polytetrafluoroethylene and Marlex. However, in keeping with the authors' experience, the high incidence of associated fistulae meant that wherever feasible one should avoid using foreign materials in association with continent ileostomy construction (4). Other continent ileostomy-related problems include parastomal herniation, pouchitis, fistulization, hemorrhage, detachment of the pouch from the anterior abdominal wall, and volvulus of the pouch (13).

Technical Considerations When Considering Salvage Continent Ileostomy Surgery

In patients with parastomal herniation, a skin-level stricture, or other efferent limb problems, a local surgical procedure may be feasible (14). This involves carefully mobilizing the exit conduit to the fascial level. In the case of a skin-level stricture, the efferent limb is dissected to healthy tissue. In patients with parastomal herniation and poor quality tissues we may elect to use biological material for the hernia repair, bringing the exit conduit through the center of this material.

In many cases a laparotomy is required to definitively deal with pouch problems. The pouch must be emptied of any contents. In keeping with all repeat abdominal surgeries there is the risk for enterotomies and it may be practical to enter at a site removed from existing scar tissue. Our initial plan is to divide all attachments to the pouch and achieve 360 degree control around the efferent limb. It is critical that one avoids any damage to the exit conduit or its blood supply as this may be used again. If the problem is valve slippage then we open the pouch at the side on which one intends to fix the valve. Provided there is sufficient length the existing valve can be further intussuscepted and stabilized as previously described (7). If this technique is not suitable then a new valve may have to be created using the proximal ileum of the afferent limb. The pouch is rotated and the proximal edge of the ileum is anastomosed to the reservoir, generally at the site of the old conduit.

Patients with Crohn's disease often manifest with pouch strictures commonly at the afferent limb. If amenable we would consider a strictureplasty using the traditional Heineke-Mikulicz technique. On occasions we have encountered patients with a very distorted afferent limb and chose to perform a bypass of healthy afferent limb to the pouch. While not ideal it preserves pouch function for a period of time reducing the incidence of pouch loss.

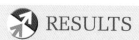 RESULTS

Quality of Life After Continent Ileostomy

In 2006, we reported on the institute's long-term outcomes for patients undergoing continent ileostomy formation with the overall aim of identifying factors associated with adverse outcomes and to compare changes in quality of life after reservoir removal (4). Three hundred and thirty patients who underwent continent ileostomy formation between 1974 and 2001 were identified. Quality of life was evaluated using the continent ileostomy surgery follow up questionnaire and the Cleveland Clinic Global Quality of Life (CGQL) scale. The CGQL scoring system measures the patient's current quality of life, current quality of health, and current energy level on a scale of 0-10 (0, worst; 10, best). The scores are added and divided by 30, giving a final CGQL score.

The preferred surgical technique (S-pouch configuration) used for pouch creation was as described in the operative section. Prior to 1984, Marlex or Mersilene mesh was used in 73 patients to stabilize the valve and aid fixation of the pouch to abdominal wall. This technique was subsequently abandoned due to the high fistula rate associated with the use of mesh (42.5%). Patients were followed up for a median of 11 (range, 1–27) years. Pouch excision rate was 16.6%. The 10- and 20-year continent ileostomy survival rates for ulcerative colitis (UC) and FAP was 92.5% and 83.3%, respectively. As expected those with a diagnosis of Crohn's disease or indeterminate colitis had a lower K-pouch survival rate at 10 and 20 years (i.e., 58.4% and 39.1%, respectively). When performing a Cox proportional hazard model to test factors associated with pouch failure, the likelihood of pouch failure was three times higher for those who developed a pouch-related fistula, 2.4 times higher for female patients, and 1.8 times higher for every 5-unit increase in body mass index (BMI). Patients with Crohn's disease or indeterminate colitis were 4.5 times more likely to undergo pouch failure in comparison to their UC and FAP counterparts.

In this study, quality of life was also compared between those with continent ileostomy and those who required removal of the reservoir with conversion to an end ileostomy. Patients with an end ileostomy were more likely to report social, work, and sexual restrictions in comparison to those with a retained K-pouch.

Conversion of a Failed Ileal Pouch-Anal Anastomosis to Continent Ileostomy

The authors have recently reported on their outcomes in 64 such patients covering the time frame from 1982 to 2007 (15). Septic complications after the index ileal pouch surgery accounted for 56.3% of this patient group. This encompassed pelvic sepsis, perianal abscess, and pouch fistula. Other indications for pouch failure necessitating conversion included persistent anal pain, dysplasia, poor pouch function, resistant pouchitis, stricture formation, irritable pouch syndrome, and others. In four patients it was not feasible to create a primary IPAA and thus, the alternative decision was to proceed with a continent ileostomy. All patients were counseled preoperatively as to the potential need for a change in intraoperative strategy. Three pouches left *in situ* were later used for reconstruction, high lightening the importance of considering future strategies in patients with a failing pouch when one is contemplating pouch excision versus end ileostomy. We would consider Crohn's disease as a contraindication to pouch construction except in uncommon circumstances. However, in a small percentage of patients, Crohn's disease is only diagnosed on histopathological examination of the excised colon or when the patient presents with pouch or small bowel complications attributed to Crohn's disease. Despite this problem the continent ileostomy pouch retention rate for such patients was reasonably good.

The overall rate of long-term complications in this series was 60.9%, with 46.9% having more than one complication. Twenty-nine patients (45.3%) required revisional surgery with 17 (58.6%) undergoing revision within 1 year. At a median follow up of 5 years (range, 1–19), three patients required pouch excision. Underlying pathology was fistulizing Crohn's disease, recurrent parastomal abscess, and pouch dysfunction despite multiple revisions. Overall functional outcomes and quality of life was good. Fifty-nine of the 61 patients with a retained pouch (*n* = 64) were functional with a median pouch intubation frequency of four times per day (range, 2–10) and median night time requirement for emptying of once (range, 0–2). The median CGQL score was 0.77.

We appreciate that this selected group is extremely motivated to avoid an end ileostomy and was willing to undergo further continent revisions. Nonetheless, it highlights that in keeping with all series, a failing ileal pelvic pouch may be converted to a viable continent ileostomy in appropriately counseled patient (9,10,15,16).

✸✷ CONCLUSION

It is the authors' belief that the continent ileostomy will continue to have a role in the management of patients wishing to avoid an end ileostomy. The ileal pouch anal anastomosis still remains the gold standard for patients desiring restoration of intestinal function. However, in those patients with sphincter dysfunction, a failing ileal pouch, significantly reach problems at the time of primary ileal pouch creation, or those wishing to convert from an end ileostomy, the continent ileostomy should be considered as a viable option. It is technically challenging and should only be performed by surgeons with appropriate experience with the technical aspects of construction and the ability to deal with associated complications.

Recommended References and Readings

1. Parks AG, Nicholls RJ. Proctocolectomy without ileostomy for ulcerative colitis. *Br Med J* 1978;2:85–88.
2. Fazio VW, Ziv Y, Church JM, et al. Ileal pouch-anal anastomoses complications and function in 1005 patients. *Ann Surg* 1995;222:120–27.
3. Kock NG. Intra-abdominal "reservoir" in patients with permanent ileostomy. Preliminary observations on a procedure resulting in fecal "continence" in five ileostomy patients. *Arch Surg* 1969;99:223–31.
4. Nessar G, Fazio VW, Tekis P, et al. Long-term outcome and quality of life after continent ileostomy. *Dis Colon Rectum* 2006;49:336–44.
5. Dozois RR, Dozois EJ. The continent ileostomy. In: Baker RJ, Fischer JE, eds. *Mastery of Surgery*. 5th ed, Vol. 2. Philadelphia, PA: Lippincott Williams & Wilkins, 2001:1425–34.
6. McLeod RS, Fazio VW. The continent ileostomy: an acceptable alternative. *J Enterostomal Ther* 1984;11:140–46.
7. Barnett WO. Continent ileostomy reservoir. *South Med J* 1987; 80:1262–65.
8. Fazio VW, Tjandra JJ. Technique for nipple valve fixation to prevent valve slippage in continent ileostomy. *Dis Colon Rectum* 1992;35:1177–79.
9. Ecker W, Haberer M, Feifel G. Conversion of the failing ileoanal pouch to reservoir-ileostomy rather than to ileostomy alone. *Dis Colon Rectum* 1996;39:977–80.
10. Behrens DT, Paris M, Luttrell JN. Conversion of a failed ileal pouch-anal anastomosis to a continent ileostomy. *Dis Colon Rectum* 1999;42:490–95.
11. Church JM, Fazio VW. The continent ileostomy: indications, techniques for construction, and management of complications. *Sem Colon Rectal Surg* 1991;2:102–10.
12. Hultén L. The continent ileostomy—management of complications in current therapy in colon and rectal surgery. 2nd ed. Philadelphia: Elsevier, Mosby, 2005:235–40.
13. Wasmuth HH, Svinsa M, Trano A, et al. Surgical load and long-term outcomes for patients with Kock continent ileostomy. *Colorectal Dis* 2007;9:713–17.
14. Gottlieb LM, Handelsman JC. Treatment of outflow tract problems associated with continent ileostomy (Kock pouch). Report of six cases. *Dis Colon Rectum* 1991;34:936–40.
15. Lian L, Fazio VW, Remzi FH, et al. Outcomes for patients undergoing continent ileostomy after a failed ileal pouch-anal anastomosis. *Dis Colon Rectum* 2009;52:1409–16.
16. Börjesson L, Oresland T, Hultén L. The failed pelvic pouch: conversion to a continent ileostomy. *Tech Coloproctol* 2004;8: 102–05.

43 Repair of Stomal Stenosis

Jared C. Frattini and Jorge E. Marcet

Introduction

Intestinal stomas have been used for decades as a means of temporary or permanent diversion of the fecal stream in the setting of colorectal cancer, inflammatory bowel disease, diverticulitis, and trauma. A colostomy or ileostomy can be a loop, end, or end loop with each type of stoma having advantages and disadvantages. Creation of intestinal stomas is often thought of as a common and basic procedure and is frequently left to be created by a less experienced member of the surgical team (1). Complications resulting from a poorly fashioned stoma can negatively impact not only the patient but the health care system (2).

The complication rate associated with stomas ranges between 20–60% (2,3). These complications are characterized as early and late; the time period of greatest risk is within the first 5-years postoperatively (1,2). Various complications include poor location, stenosis, prolapse, parastomal herniation, retraction, necrosis, and skin excoriation. (Table 43.1) The rate of stomal complications is equivalent regardless of the nature of surgery, elective or emergent and regardless of the type of stoma, colostomy, or ileostomy (1). When an enterostomal therapist is involved with preoperative and postoperative stoma teaching and care, the complication rate is significantly reduced (3,5). In one study of 164 patients, an enterostomal therapist reduced stomal complications by six fold (3).

STOMAL STENOSIS

Stomal stenosis or narrowing of the stomal lumen has been reported to occur in 2–17% of intestinal stomas and can occur at the fascial or skin level (1,3,4). It is considered to be a late complication of stoma creation. Stenosis can be caused by ischemia, a small fascial or skin opening, tension, obesity, prolonged peristomal excoriation, peristomal sepsis, or peristomal Crohn's disease. (4) (Table 43.2) Several studies have demonstrated an increase in stoma stenosis in patients with Crohn's disease compared to those with

TABLE 43.1	Common Complications of Stomas
1) Poor location	5) Retraction
2) Stenosis	6) Necrosis
3) Prolapse	7) Skin excoriation
4) Parastomal herniation	

ulcerative colitis when a permanent ileostomy was created (6,7). Generalized symptoms of stomal stenosis can be obstructive in nature or constipation followed by large volume output. Symptoms of stomal stenosis at the skin or fascial level include narrow stools, pain upon evacuation, and excessive, explosive, high-pitched gas (4) (Table 43.3).

Stomal Stenosis: Management

The management of stomal stenosis can be based upon the severity of the symptoms and degree of stenosis. The degree or severity of stenosis can easily be assessed by digital exam. The stenosis can be managed conservatively or operatively; with either a local procedure or with relocation of the stoma. If the symptoms of stenosis do not interfere with stoma care or with the patient's quality of life then conservative management can be applied. Conservative management can include a low residue diet and stool softeners or laxatives to allow adequate flow through the stenosis (4). There are no good data to suggest the efficacy of conservative management or the time until which surgical management should be employed.

If conservative measures fail to satisfactorily improve the symptoms, there are several repair techniques that can be employed. Table 43.4 Dilation of the stenosis can be performed as the next step in treatment. Dilation can be done with either a digit or with Hegar dilators (Fig. 43.1). Dilation with a digit is performed with the smallest digit first which is passed through the stenosis and kept in place for 10 seconds. A stepwise sequential progression of larger finger size is used to sequentially dilate the stenosis. Hegar dilators can also be used in the same stepwise fashion to dilate the stenosis. Regardless of the method, several sessions may be necessary to achieve success. Dilation is a controversial method because there are reports that chronic dilation can cause the stenosis to progress rather than regress (4). In addition, dilation can result in perforation.

Another dilation method that has been successfully used to treat stenosis is the use of stomal plugs. Stomal plugs are commonly used to control stoma output and to aid in concealing the stoma; once a plug is inserted into the stomal aperture it expands to seal the stoma. A report documents the successful use of a plug to dilate the colostomies of two patients. The method of action is believed to be a constant radial dilating force thus increasing the stomal aperture and avoiding the need for future surgical intervention (8). Unfortunately, stomal plugs are not commercially available in the USA.

A technique of subcutaneous fasciotomy has been described to repair ileal stenosis secondary to fascial compression in newly created ileostomies (Fig. 43.2). With the ostomy appliance still in place, small incisions are created caudad and cephalad outside the border of the stoma appliance. Scissors are then inserted into the incision such that the bottom blade is underneath the fascia and then the fascia is opened toward the

TABLE 43.2	Etiology of Stomal Stenosis
1) Ischemia	5) Prolonged peristomal excoriation
2) Obesity	6) Peristomal sepsis
3) Small fascial or skin opening	7) Peristomal Crohn's disease
4) Tension	

TABLE 43.3	Symptoms of Stomal Stenosis
1) Obstruction 2) Constipation 3) Narrow stools	4) Pain upon evacuation 5) Excessive, explosive, high-pitched gas

TABLE 43.4	Techniques to Repair Stomal Stenosis

1) Dilation
   a) Hegar dilators
   b) Stomal plug
2) Subcutaneous fasciotomy
	3) W-plasty
	4) Z-plasty
	5) Open revision

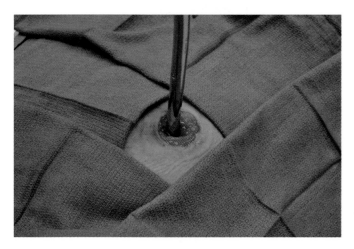

Figure 43.1 Stomal stenosis can be treated with sequential dilation with Hegar dilators.

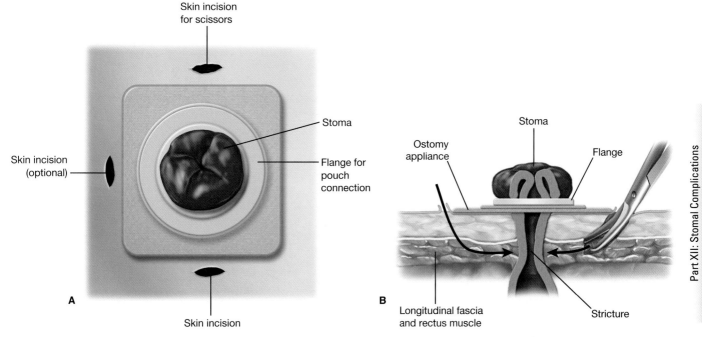

Figure 43.2 **A,B.** Subcutaneous fasciotomy.

serosa of the bowel. This maneuver is done is the same manner as fasciotomies are done for the compartments of the lower leg. While performing the fasciotomy, a finger is kept in the stoma to determine the limit of the fasciotomy by palpating the tip of the scissors through the bowel wall and to help prevent injury to the bowel wall. The fascia should be incised through the stoma aperture already present in the fascia. If these two incisions and resultant fasciotomies are not sufficient to relieve the stenosis, a third incision is created laterally. This fasciotomy is more difficult due to the fact that the incision is against the fibers of the rectus sheath (9).

Stenosis occurring at the skin level can be treated by employing techniques commonly used by our plastic surgery colleagues. These techniques avoid the necessity of performing a laparotomy to revise and/or resite the stoma. The W-plasty and Z-plasty have both been described for the treatment of skin level stenosis (10,11). To perform the W-plasty, the stoma is mobilized beyond the fascia into the peritoneal cavity by an incision around the mucocutaneous junction (Fig. 43.3A). The skin is marked as to

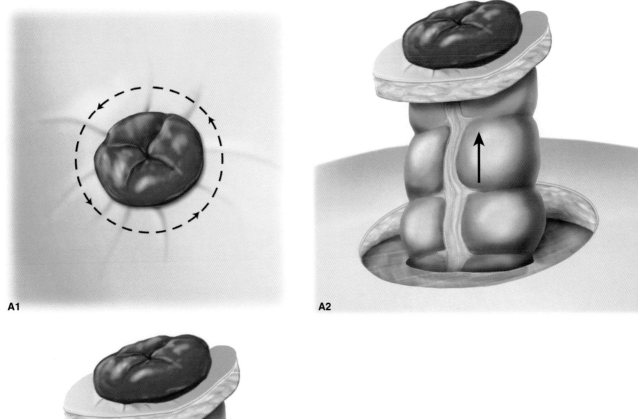

A1

A2

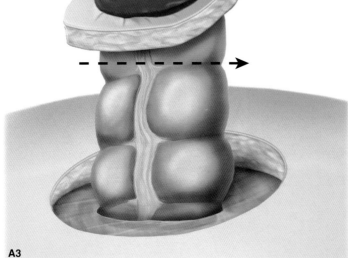

A3

Figure 43.3 **A.** Mobilization of stoma with excision of stenosis. **B.** Incision of skin and mucosa in "W" fashion. **C.** Final appearance. (*continued*)

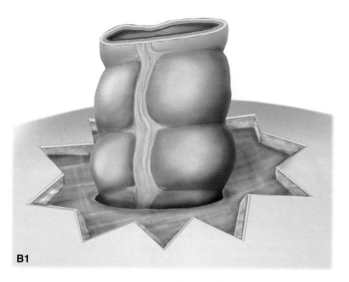

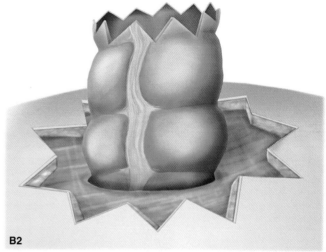

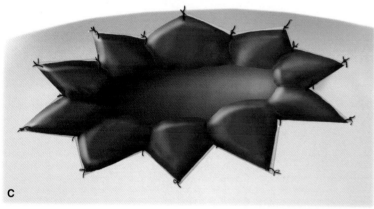

Figure 43.3 (*Continued*)

where the triangular flaps will be incised using a no. 11 blade. Vertical flaps are made at right angles to the dermis with sides or no more than 6 mm with corners of 90 degree or less. The mucosa of the stoma is then incised to fit into the pattern made on the skin (Fig. 43.3B). The stoma is then matured using a Gillies' corner stitch (Fig. 43.3C). This technique was used in four patients with stenotic colostomies and all were patent at a median of 12.5 months postoperatively (11).

The Z-plasty is another common plastic surgery technique that has been used to treat stenosis at the skin level. An incision is made at the mucocutaneous junction being sure to include the scar and the bowel is mobilized into the peritoneal cavity (Fig. 43.4A). The corners of the skin incision (dermis) and bowel (serosa) are secured by a mattress suture (Fig. 43.4B). A skin incision approximately 1.5 cm in length is made at an angle of 60 degree to the skin edge. A corresponding incision of the same length is made full thickness through the bowel and is 1.5 cm from the skin incision (Fig. 43.4C). The stoma is then matured by suturing the labeled areas accordingly (Fig. 43.4D/E). This technique was used in six patients with colostomies in which three patients had a Z-plasty performed on both sides of the stoma and three had the Z-plasty performed on only one side of the stoma. There was no evidence of recurrent stenosis after up to 6 years of follow-up (10).

Less commonly, stenosis caused by retraction or ischemia may require an in-depth revision with laparotomy and mobilization of additional length of bowel. Before undertaking such an approach conservative measures should be tried and sufficient time given for healing of the previously constructed stoma. The intent of surgery is to dissect a sufficient length of bowel so that a tension free ostomy is created. Achieving this goal may require mobilization of the splenic flexure for left-sided colostomies. Division of the inferior mesenteric vessels may also be necessary, leaving a well-vascularized pedicle

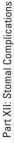

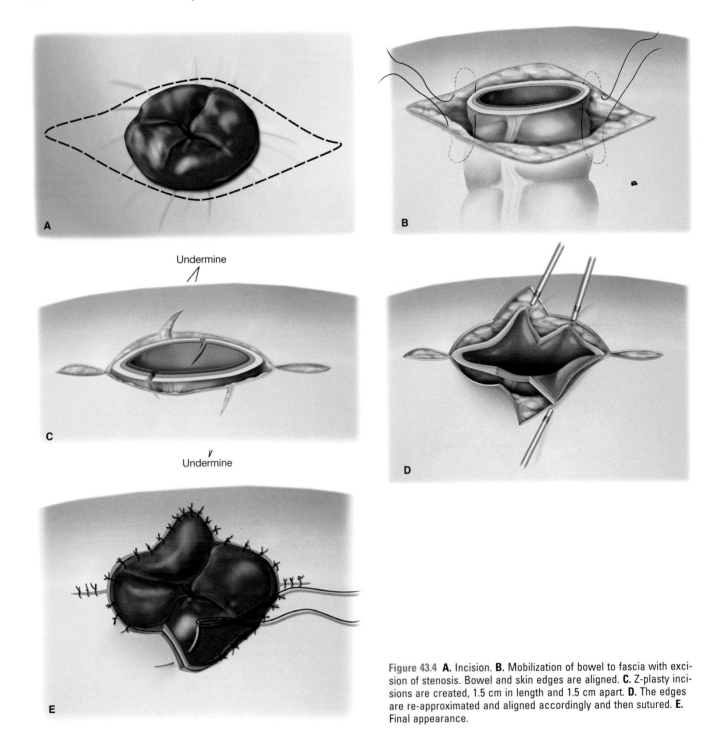

Figure 43.4 A. Incision. **B.** Mobilization of bowel to fascia with excision of stenosis. Bowel and skin edges are aligned. **C.** Z-plasty incisions are created, 1.5 cm in length and 1.5 cm apart. **D.** The edges are re-approximated and aligned accordingly and then sutured. **E.** Final appearance.

based upon the marginal blood supply, to develop enough length of bowel to reach the abdominal wall.

A similar approach is taken when a major revision of an ileostomy is required. Dissection of the ileal mesentery is done with judicious ligation of the mesenteric vessels, if necessary, to develop a well-vascularized pedicle of sufficient length to reach the skin and allow for eversion of the ileostomy.

When possible, the same skin opening of the previously stenotic ostomy is used after a major revision. The skin opening may simply be made larger by excising a wider disc of skin. However, in some cases, relocation of the stoma more cephalad on the abdominal wall may be dictated by the inability of the mesentery to reach the previous stoma site. Additionally, before any in-depth revision of an ostomy, proper siting of the previous ostomy should be ascertained and relocation of the stoma is done as necessary to enable proper stoma care.

✦ CONCLUSION

The etiology of stomal stenosis is multifactorial; the best preventative measure is careful attention to surgical technique. Avoiding ischemia and tension and siting the stoma appropriately in combination with both preoperative and postoperative enterostomal therapist teaching are paramount. Following these techniques will aid in preventing stomal stenosis and in avoiding the resultant impact on the patient's quality of life and the financial burden on the health care system. The best way to manage stomal stenosis is conservatively with nonoperative measures. The next step would be the least invasive and least complex surgical procedure. If one is not familiar with the techniques of Z-plasty, W-plasty, or subcutaneous fasciotomy, an open procedure should be the technique of choice. If the stoma does require relocation, mobilization through the stoma hole without a midline laparotomy may be successful (12).

Recommended References and Readings

1. Shellito P. Complications of abdominal stoma surgery. *Dis Colon Rectum* 1998;41:1562–72.
2. Robertson I, Leung E, et al. Prospective analysis of stoma-related complications. *Colorectal Disease* 2005;7:279–85.
3. Duchesne J, Wang Y, et al. Stoma complications: a multivariate analysis. *Am Surg* 2002;68:961–66.
4. Barr J. Assessment and management of stomal complications: a framework for clinical decision making. *Ostomy Wound Management* 2004;50:50–52.
5. Park J, Del Pino A, et al. Stoma complications: the Cook County Hospital experience. *Dis Colon Rectum* 1999;42:1575–80.
6. Takahashi K, Funayama Y, et al. Stoma-related complications in inflammatory bowel disease. *Dig Surg* 2008;25:16–20.
7. Carlsen E, Bergan A. Technical aspects and complications of end-ileostomies. *World J Surg* 1995;19:632–36.
8. Riaz AA, Jeetle SS, Bobb KA, Jones PW, Thompson HH. Stomal plugs: a novel treatment option for stomal stenosis. *Techn Coloproctol* 2005;9:172.
9. Malt RA, Bartlett MK, Wheelock FC. Subcutaneous fasciotomy for relief of stricture of the ileostomy. *Surg Gynecol Obstet* 1984;159:175–76.
10. Lyons A, Simon B. Z-plasty for colostomy stenosis. *Ann Surg* 1960;151:59–62.
11. Beraldo S, Titley G, Allan A. Use of W-plasty in stenotic stoma: a new solution for an old problem. *Colorectal Dis* 2006;8:715–16.
12. Baig MK, Larach J, Chang CC, et al. Outcome of parastomal hernia repair with and without midline laparotomy. *Tech Coloproctol* 2006;10:282–86.

44 Parastomal Repair: Open Techniques

Terry C. Hicks

THE BACKGROUND PARAGRAPH

Parastomal hernia describes a hernia beside a stoma, which may be clinically diagnosed by palpating a bulge adjacent to the stoma and confirmed by CT scan, which demonstrates intraabdominal contents protruding along an ostomy (1).

The rate of Parastomal hernia has been reported to range between 5–52%. The great variance reported has been attributed to the utilization of different definitions of hernia and a wide range of follow-up criteria for patients (2–4).

INDICATIONS

Absolute indications for Parastomal hernia repair include patients with obstruction or incarceration with strangulation. Relative indications for repair include difficulty with appliance management, pain, cosmesis, and patients who have difficulty with irrigation. Multiple risk factors associated with the development of parastomal hernias have been identified. Patient specific factors include obesity, advanced age, malnutrition, chronic respiratory disorders that are associated with increased intra-abdominal pressure, immunosuppression, and wound infection. Other suggested factors include stoma placement outside the rectus muscle and creation of an excessively large fascial opening.

Open techniques for parastomal hernia repair include direct local tissue repair, relocating the intestinal stoma with the closure of the primary aperture, and application of prosthetic material around the stoma at different levels upon or within the abdominal wall. This chapter will discuss these three open surgical approaches.

PREOPERATIVE PLANNING

Once the patient has completed an appropriate preoperative medical clearance, consideration should be given to a standard bowel preparation. Although recent literature has suggested that standard bowel prep is not mandatory, it is the author's preference as the cleansed colon is technically easier to manipulate when it does not have a significant fecal load. For those patients who can tolerate an oral preparation, an iso-osmotic lavage prep is suggested (polyethylene glycol solution). An appropriate broad-spectrum antibiotic should be administered intravenously, within 1 hour prior to the initial incision. As with other abdominal operations, routine venous thrombosis prophylaxis is utilized. The consent form should include information concerning the utilization of prosthetic materials in the management of the repair, as well as a clear discussion of alternatives, and reasonable clinical expectations.

 SURGERY

After adequate general anesthesia has been obtained, the patient is placed in the lithotomy or supine position with the extremities appropriately padded. The utilization of an oral gastric tube and urinary bladder catheter are routine. The patient may need some rotational adjustment to provide the best exposure to the ostomy site.

Operative Technique

Direct Fascial Repair

An arched incision is made through the skin around the hernia site. With careful retraction, the hernia sac is excised, the contents reduced, and the peritoneum suture closed. The edges of the fascial defect are then approximated with a series of interrupted, nonabsorbable sutures to reduce the opening to two finger breadths. The subcutaneous space may be drained if there is more than a small amount of bleeding during the procedure (Figs. 44.1 and 44.2).

Relocation of Stoma

Preoperative marking of a new stoma site in another abdominal quadrant is important. This is usually the side opposite to the current site. After skin preparation and patient positioning, the existing ostomy is carefully isolated from the abdominal wall, and the stomal lumen is sutured closed or stapled to prevent any contamination of the field.

Figure 44.1 True parastomal hernia.

True Parastomal Hernia

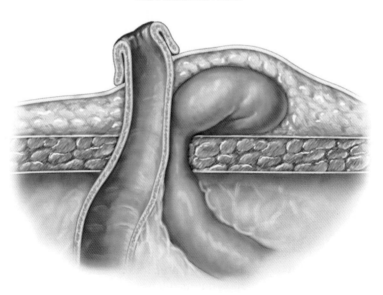

Open Underlay Technique

Open Underlay Technique

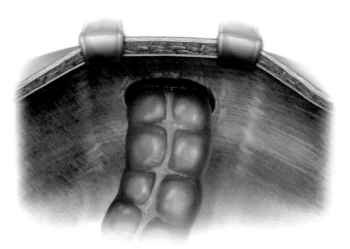

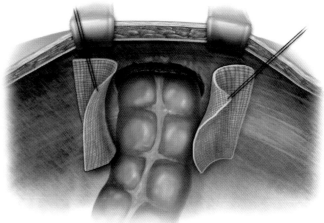

Open Underlay Technique

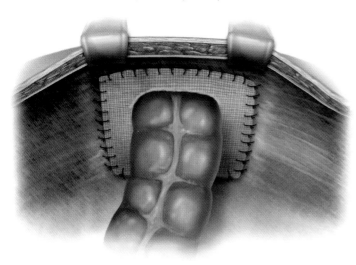

Figure 44.2 Open underlay technique for parastomal hernia repair.

The hernia is reduced and the hernia sac is excised. A small midline incision is utilized to enter the abdominal cavity for adhesiolysis and exposure to both the new and old sites. The new ostomy site is created and the bowel is carefully brought through the new fascial opening without rotation or compromise to lumen or blood supply. Once the stoma has been mobilized and in the abdominal cavity, the remaining hernia site is repaired with interrupted fascial sutures. It may be desirable to place prosthetic material in the sublay position under the muscle and external to the peritoneum to ensure an adequate repair for large hernia defects. Finally, the abdominal wound is closed, and the new stoma is matured at the skin level: with a 2.5 cm spigot for ileostomy and flush for colostomy.

An alternative to the use of a midline wound is possible with large parastomal hernias. The initial incision is around the stoma to free the bowel from the skin and hernia sac. With this technique, the hernia defect is used to gain access to take down the abdominal wall adhesions and accomplish the necessary bowel mobilization. The new stomal site can also be created using the hernia opening and a midline incision is avoided. After delivery the bowel through the new stomal opening, the hernia is repaired as described above; ultimately the stoma is matured (Fig. 44.3).

Part XII: Stomal Complications

Figure 44.3 Open relocation technique.

Open Relocation Technique

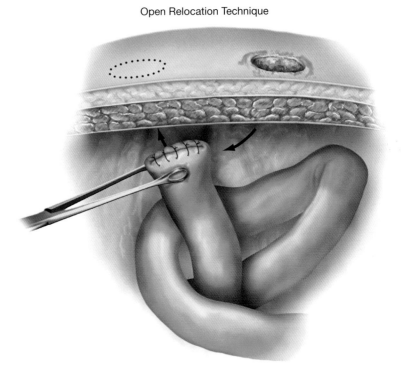

The Open Onlay Procedure

A large semicircular incision is made at an appropriate distance from the stoma, and with adequate exposure, the subcutaneous tissues are dissected free from the fascia. The hernia sac is identified, the contents are reduced, and the peritoneum is closed. The edges of the fascial defect can then be re-approximated with interrupted sutures after which the repair is reinforced with a prosthetic material, which is wrapped around the subcutaneous portion of the colon, and sutured into place. Some surgeons place closed suction drains in the subcutaneous position exiting the skin outside of where the stomal appliance adheres to the skin (Fig. 44.4).

Figure 44.4 Open onlay technique (after reduction of Hernia).

Open Onlay Technique

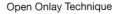

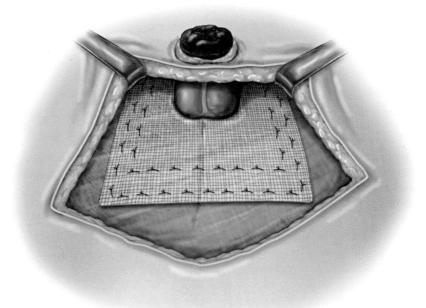

The Underlay Repair

The ostomy site is initially covered with a protective barrier to avoid contamination of the field, and then a laparotomy is performed using a length of the existing midline incision away from the stoma just adequate to approach the hernia defect. The hernia sac and its contents are then identified, and reduced into the peritoneum, after which the edges of the fascial defects are gently re-approximated using interrupted suture technique. The sublay procedure is then performed with the utilization of a prosthetic material. It is important that it be cut so that it can surround the colon, and extend at least 5 cm past the edge of the abdominal wall defect. The mesh can be sutured in place with interrupted or running technique, and then the abdominal cavity can be closed in a routine fashion.

Special Considerations

Because the direct facial technique has a recurrence rate of approximately 68%, this technique has been recently abandoned, and considered by most to be only of historical significance. Clinical trials have shown that stoma relocation provides better clinical results than the direct fascial repair technique. The sublay and/or onlay procedure with prosthetic material has proven to provide the best statistical results. The utilization of prosthetic material has been associated with complications inherent with utilization of a foreign body. Multiple surgical experiences have been reported utilizing mesh materials including absorbable, nonabsorbable, partly absorbable, and acellular collagen matrix meshes. Although composite meshes are presently available, most recent authors championed the use of biological meshes.

Postoperative Management

Routine postoperative care includes orogastric tube removal prior to extubation in the operating room. Bladder catheter removal is dependent upon the patient's anesthetic requirements in the postoperative period. Re-institution of diet is usually held until flatus has passed through the stoma, but is clinician dependent. A visit from the stomal nurse is a productive clinical tool prior to the patient's discharge.

 COMPLICATIONS

Infection is of major concern with the opened technique, because the case is considered "contaminated." Thus, care always must be taken to isolate any stomal contents from its surrounding tissues. Infection and potential hernia recurrence are the main undesired outcomes.

 RESULTS

After relocation the risk of recurrent parastomal hernia at new sites is at least as high as after the primary enterostomy; recurrence rates range from 24–86%. Parastomal hernia repair with prosthetic mesh is reported to produce lower recurrence rates when compared to relocation or direct suture repair of the stoma where at the present time, large randomized studies are not available (3,5,6).

 CONCLUSIONS

Parastomal hernia repair represents a major surgical challenge presenting in up to 50% of patients receiving a colostomy. There are several nonlaparoscopic techniques that have been attempted for repair. Significant recurrence rates are associated with relocation of the stoma and direct suture repair of the fascia. Lower recurrence rates have been reported with prosthetic material repairs, but more studies of randomized trials with longer term follow-up will be necessary to identify which prosthetic material repair will ultimately be defined as the gold standard.

Recommended References and Readings

1. Cingi A, Cakir T, Sever A, et al. Enterostomy site hernias: a clinical and computerized tomographic evaluation. *Dis Colon Rectum* 2006;49(10):1559–63.
2. Carne PW, Robertson GM, Frizelle FA. Parastomal hernia. *Br J Surg* 2003;90(7):784–93.
3. Devlin HB, Kingsnorth A. Parastomal hernia. In: Devlin A. Kingsnorth A, eds. *Management of Abdominal Hernias*. 2nd ed. London: Butterworths, 1998:257–66.
4. Everingham L. The Parastomal hernia dilemma. *World Council of Enterostomal Therapists J* 1998;18:32–34.
5. Rubin MS, Schoetz DJ Jr, Matthews JB. Parastomal hernia. Is stoma relocation superior to fascial repair? *Arch Surg* 1994;129(4):413–18.
6. Rieger N, Moore J, Hewett P, et al. Parastomal hernia repair. *Colorectal Dis* 2004;6(3):203–205.

Suggested Readings

Amin SN, Armitage NC, Abercrombie JF, et al. Lateral repair of parastomal hernia. *Ann R Coll Surg Engl* 2001;83(3):206–08.

Birolini C, Utiyama EM, Rodrigues AJ Jr, Birolini D. Elective colonic operation and prosthetic repair of incisional hernia: does contamination contraindicate abdominal wall prosthesis use? *J Am Coll Surg* 2000;191:366–72.

Catena F, Ansaloni L, Gazzotti F, et al. Use of porcine dermal collagen graft (Permacol) for hernia repair in contaminated fields. *Hernia* 2007;11:57–60.

Cengiz Y, Israelsson LA. Parastomal hernia. *Eur Surg* 2003;35:28–31.

Cheung MT, Chia NH, Chiu WY. Surgical treatment of parastomal hernia complicating sigmoid colostomies. *Dis Colon Rectum* 2001;44(2):266–70.

de Ruiter P, Bijnen AB. Successful local repair of paracolostomy hernia with a newly developed prosthetic device. *Int J Colorectal Dis* 1992;7(3):132–34.

Hsu PW, Salgado CJ, Kent K, et al. Evaluation of porcine dermal collagen (Permacol) used in abdominal wall reconstruction. *J Plast Reconstr Aesthet Surg* 2008.

Kasperk R, Klinge U, Schumpelick V. The repair of large parastomal hernias using a mid-line approach and a prosthetic mesh in the sublay position. *Am J Surg* 2000;179(3):186–88.

Kish KJ, Buinewicz BR, Morris JB. Acellular dermal matrix (AlloDerm): new material in the repair of stoma site hernias. *Am Surg* 2005;71(12):1047–50.

Leslie D. The parastomal hernia. *Surg Clin North Am* 1984;64(2):407–15.

Londono-Schimmer EE, Leong AP, Phillips RK. Life table analysis of stomal complications following colostomy. *Dis Colon Rectum* 1994;37(9):916–20.

Longman RJ, Thomson WH. Mesh repair of Parastomal hernias-a safety modification. *Colorectal Dis* 2005;7(3):292–94.

Martin L, Foster G. Parastomal hernia. *Ann R Coll Surg Engl* 1996;78(2):81–84.

Morris-Stiff G, Hughes LE. The continuing challenge of Parastomal hernia: failure of a novel polypropylene mesh repair. *Ann R Coll Surg Engl* 1998;80(3):184–87.

Pearl RK, Sone JH. Management of peristomal hernia: techniques of repair. In: Greenburg AG, ed. *Nyhus and Condon's Hernia*. 5th ed. Philadelphia: Lippincott Williams & Wilkins, 2002: 415–22.

Rubin MS, Schoetz DJ Jr, Matthews JB. Parastomal hernia: is stoma relocation superior to fascial repair? *Arch Surg* 1994;129:413–18.

Saclarides TJ, Hsu A, Quiros R. In situ mesh repair of Parastomal hernias. *Am Surg* 2004;70(8):701–05.

Schumpelick V, Klinge U. Incisional abdominal hernia: the open mesh repair. *Langenbecks Arch Surg* 2004;389:1–5.

Schumpelick V, Klosterhafen B, Muller M, et al. Minimized polypropylene meshes for preperitoneal mesh plasty in incisional hernia. *Chirurg* 1990;70:422–30.

Steele SR, Lee P, Martin MJ, et al. Is parastomal hernia repair with polypropylene mesh safe? *Am J Surg* 2003;185(5):436–40.

Stelzner S, Hellmich G, Ludwig K. Repair of paracolostomy hernias with a prosthetic mesh in the intraperitoneal onlay position: modified Sugarbaker technique. *Dis Colon Rectum* 2004;47(2):185–91.

Taner T, Cima RR, Larson DW, et al. The use of human acellular dermal matrix for Parastomal hernia repair in patients with inflammatory bowel disease: a novel technique to repair fascial defects. *Dis Colon Rectum*. 2009;52:349–54.

45 Parastomal Hernia: Underlay Technique

David E. Beck

 ## INDICATIONS/CONTRAINDICATIONS

Parastomal hernia is one of the more common complications of an ostomy (1). Indications for repair include bowel obstruction, incarceration, or enlargement of the hernia to the point where it interferes with maintenance of an appliance and/or if. the hernia is unsightly. Laparoscopic repair is suitable when the patient's stoma is appropriately sited, the patient lacks a history of extensive adhesions, and their hernia is not too large. Large parastomal hernias are often more appropriately repaired with an open technique. Obtaining good results with underlay mesh usually requires a mesh with at least a 3–5 cm overlap of the mesh beyond the edges of the hernia. This goal is difficult to achieve laparoscopically in patients having large hernias. Another relative contraindication to a laparoscopic approach is the need for an associated open procedure. Both ileostomies and colostomies are suitable for laparoscopic procedures and several techniques of repair have been described (2–6). This chapter will discuss the underlay technique. A similar procedure using an open technique was described by Sugarbaker in 1980 (7). The technique eliminates some of the technical and physiologic problems associated with a "key hole" technique of mesh placement.

 ## PREOPERATIVE PLANNING

Preoperative Preparation

Standard bowel preparation is not mandatory. However, because the empty colon intra-operatively handles better than the stool filled colon, it is the author's preference to have patients who can tolerate a preparation, ingest a limited isotonic lavage prep (one-fourth to half gallon of a polyethylene glycol solution). Patients are instructed to take only clear liquids the day prior to surgery. Oral antibiotics are not prescribed but standard intravenous broad-spectrum antibiotics are given within 1 hour of skin incision; deep vein prophylaxis is also ordered. Informed consent should always include the potential for conversion to an open procedure and for stoma relocation.

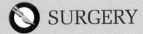 SURGERY

Patient Positioning and Preparation

After induction of general endotracheal anesthesia, an orogastric tube and indwelling urinary bladder catheter are placed. The patient is then placed in modified lithotomy position with the thighs even with the hips and pressure points appropriately padded. One or both arms may be adducted to facilitate securing the patient for the extremes of positioning used during laparoscopy. If only one arm is adducted, it should be on the side opposite the side of the hernia and stoma. The patient is then secured to the table, usually with tape. If one or both arms are kept out the tape is placed in a "cross your heart" manner. The skin is prepped with antiseptic solution and draping is done in a fashion to provide for lateral exposure for ports, especially on the side opposite the hernia and stoma. One author (Muysoms) has suggested covering the abdominal wall with an adhesive drape to limit potential contamination of the mesh (2).

Instrument/Monitor Positioning

The primary surgeon usually stands on the patient's side opposite the stoma or between the patient's legs (Fig. 45.1). The primary monitor is placed on the patient's side that contains the stoma near the level of their hip. A secondary monitor can be placed at the patient's shoulder or at an alternate site viewable by the assistant or surgical technician. Insufflation tubing, suction tubing, cautery power cord, laparoscopy camera wiring, and a laparoscope light cord are brought off the patient's side. A 10 mm laparoscope with a 30-degree lens is preferred.

Port Selection and Placement

A 10/11 mm port is placed using an open (modified Hasson) technique in the left lateral abdomen on the side opposite the ostomy and hernia. Laparoscopic inspection of the peritoneal cavity is performed looking for unsuspected pathology and identifies the patient with dense extensive adhesions that would make a laparoscopic approach

Figure 45.1 Positioning and port placement for laparoscopic assisted colostomy.

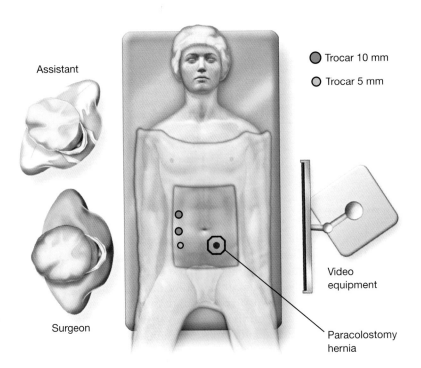

problematic. If the abdomen is suitable, additional ports are placed under laparoscopic visualization at the locations described in Figure 45.1. Unless a quality 5 mm camera and mesh fixation devise (tacker) are available, one of the ports needs to be at least 10 mm in diameter. The exact port placement will vary depending on adhesions and the location and size of the hernia. In general, ports are placed a hand's width apart and on the side of the abdomen opposite the hernia (Fig. 45.1—left sided stoma). If the stoma is located on the right side of the abdomen, the port placement locations are reversed.

Operative Technique

Division of Adhesions and Reduction of Hernia

Adhesions to the anterior abdominal wall are divided with sharp dissection and traction. This step can often be tedious and has the potential for bowel injury, especially true if previous repairs have employed mesh. Extensive dense adhesions may require conversion to an open technique. Bowel loops are gently reduced from the hernia using traction and carful division of adhesions. Alternate energy sources may be helpful for some vascular adhesions, but are not a substitute for careful dissection. When the entire bowel has been reduced, the bowel leading to the stoma will remain; the peritoneal sac is left in place. The underlay technique requires that the bowel has adequate laxity to allow the bowel to track between the mesh and abdominal wall. Reduction of the hernia will usually provide adequate laxity. Additional mobilization of the bowel may be necessary to allow adequate lateralization of the bowel. The ostomy bowel is retracted and delivered intra-abdominally, to reduce any prolapse. The ostomy bowel is then pulled to the lateral or superior edge of the hernia defect. The bowel serosa can be sutured to the peritoneum with absorbable sutures at the edge of the defect. The abdominal wall is also inspected for additional hernias that need repair.

A piece of mesh is selected that will cover the hernia defect with a 5 cm overlap. It is often helpful to compare the mesh on the outer abdominal wall. To minimize the risk of contamination, the mesh should not touch the stoma itself and contact with the skin should be avoided. Several types of mesh have been used, including nonabsorbable, absorbable, partly absorbable, and acellular collagen matrix meshes.

If peripheral tacking sutures are to be used, they are placed at the edges of the mesh. The mesh is then tightly rolled and inserted through one of the larger trocars into the abdomen. Here it is unrolled and moved toward the stoma and hernia and oriented. After orienting the mesh, the traction sutures are extracted with a "suture passer" technique through small separate skin incisions. The sutures are tied down to the anterior abdominal fascia, creating transabdominal fixation. Authors have used a variable number of these traction/fixation sutures ranging from one suture every 5 cm to just four sutures. As tacking devices have improved, the number of traction/fixation sutures has been reduced or eliminated such that the author currently uses four sutures. After the sutures are secured, a mechanical fixation device (e.g., SorbaFix™ [Davol Inc, Warwick, UK] or ProTack™ [Covidien, Mansfield, MA, USA]) is used to place "tackers" at the margin of the mesh and along the bowel tract and edge of the fascial defect. Care is taken to produce appropriate tension on the mesh and to avoid putting the tackers into the ostomy bowel or mesentery. Enough laxity is provided for the ostomy bowel to exit the mesh. After mesh fixation, the bowel is again inspected to exclude any unsuspected injury or bowel compression (Figs. 45.2, 45.3).

 ## POSTOPERATIVE MANAGEMENT

The orogastric tube is removed prior to extubation. The Foley catheter is removed later in the day or the next morning. Patients are supported with intravenous fluids and offered liquids when they are hungry. Solid food is started after flatus is passed from the stoma. Pain management is usually provided by patient controlled analgesia

Figure 45.2 Fixation of mesh in a laparoscopic hernia repair.

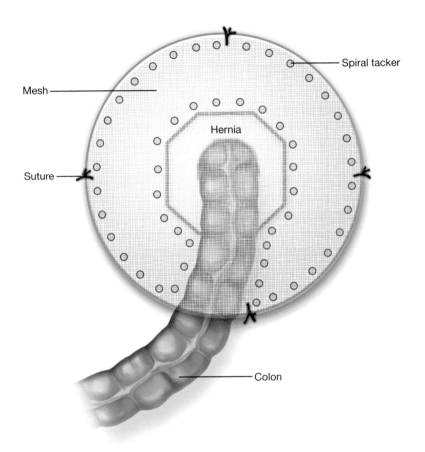

supplemented with ketorolac. The patient is switched to oral pain medication when taking fluids. Early ambulation is encouraged. Patients are ready for discharge when they can care for their stoma, tolerate a diet, and have evidence of bowel function. As the bowel is not detached from its skin attachment and stomal education is not required, recovery is usually rapid.

Figure 45.3 Intra-abdominal view of hernia repair.

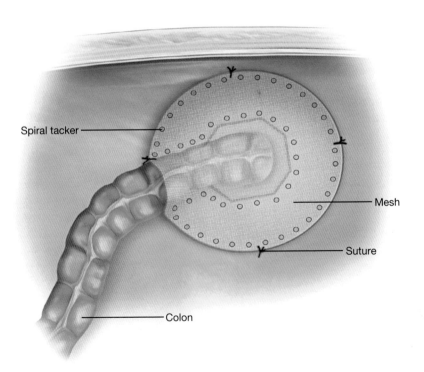

COMPLICATIONS

Early complications include unsuspected bowel injury, infection, or obstruction of the colon. Longer term complications include hernia recurrence, bowel erosion, and rarely pain.

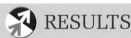 RESULTS

A number of small series have been published with short follow-ups. Recurrences have been reported in 7 out of 72 patients (8–12). A laparoscopic technique is not feasible in all patients and in one study 15% of 55 procedures had to be converted to an open operation (11). In two studies of 59 patients, bowel injury occurred in 22% of patients (8,11). In another study of 47 patients in which polytetrafluorethylene (ePTFE) mesh was used, infection resulted in mesh removal in 9% of patients (11).

 CONCLUSIONS

Parastomal hernia repair is feasible as well as safe. Increasing experience and randomized controlled trials will be needed to define the optimal technique of repair. Until such information is available, laparoscopic repair with an underlay technique is a viable option in selected patients.

References

1. Israelsson LA. Parastomal hernias. *Surg Clin North Am* 2008; 88(1):113–25.
2. Muysoms F. Laparoscopic repair of parastomal hernias with a modified Sugarbaker technique. *Acta Chir Belg* 2007;107: 476–80.
3. Craft RO, Huguet KL, McLemore EC, Harold KL. Laparoscopic parastomal hernia repair. *Hernia* 2008;12(2):137–40.
4. Mancini GJ, McClusky DA III, Khaitan L, et al. Laparoscopic parastomal hernia repair using a nonslit mesh technique. *Surg Endosc* 2007;21(9):1487–91.
5. Jani K, Palanivelu C, Parthasarathi R, Madhankumar MV. Laparoscopic repair of a paracolostomy hernia: secure reinforced closure of the defect prevents recurrence. *J Laparoendosc Adv Surg Tech A* 2007;17(2):216–18.
6. Ballas KD, Rafailidis SF, Marakis GN, et al. Intraperitoneal ePTFE mesh repair of parastomal hernias. *Hernia* 2006;10(4):350–53.
7. Sugarbaker PH. Prosthetic mesh repair of large hernias at the site of colonic stomas. *Surg Gynecol Obstet* 1980;150(4): 576–78.
8. LeBlanc KA, Bellanger DE, Whitaker JM, Hausmann MG. Laparoscopic parastomal hernia repair. *Hernia* 2005;9(2):140–44.
9. Kozlowski PM, Wang PC, Winfield HN. Laparoscopic repair of incisional and parastomal hernias after major genitourinary or abdominal surgery. *J Endourol* 2001;15:175–79.
10. Safadi B. Laparoscopic repair of parastomal hernias: early results. *Surg Endosc* 2004;18(4):676–80.
11. Hanssom BM, de Hingh IH, Bleichrodt RP. Laparoscopic parastomal hernia repair is feasible and safe: early results of a prospective clinical study including 55 consecutive patients. *Surg Endosc* 2007;21:989–93.
12. Muysoms EE, Hauters PJ, Van Nieuwenhove Y, et al. Laparoscopic repair of parastomal hernias: a multi-centre retrospective review and shift in technique. *Acta Chir Belg* 2008;108(4): 400–404.

46 Parastomal Hernia: Laparoscopic Sugarbaker Repair

Brent D. Matthews and Arthur L. Rawlings

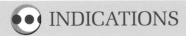 INDICATIONS

Indications for Repair

The indications for repair of a parastomal hernia are pain, persistent dermatitis from leakage of a poorly fitting stoma appliance, obstruction, strangulation, and poor cosmesis. Laparoscopic repair can be considered unless the patient has minimal working space from a large incisional or parastomal hernia, has abdominal distention due to intestinal obstruction, is in extremis from intestinal strangulation, or cannot tolerate pneumoperitoneum due to premorbid medical conditions. Relocation instead of repair should be considered if the stoma was poorly located the first time or is compromised due to a mesenteric volvulus or intestinal strangulation.

 PREOPERATIVE PLANNING

Patients with a colostomy or an ileal conduit may be considered for preoperative bowel preparation, although such preparation is not always necessary. They, along with patients with an ileostomy, can usually just be placed on a clear liquid diet for a few days before surgery.

The operation is performed under general anesthesia with endotracheal intubation. A single dose of an appropriate preoperative antibiotic is given. Sequential compression devices are placed and a Foley catheter is inserted unless the patient has an ileal conduit. An orogastric tube is inserted for gastric decompression. The patient is positioned supine with arms tucked and padded. Colostomies and ileostomies are over sewn with a 2-0 silk suture and covered with a clear, occlusive bandage. Urinary stomas have a 16 French Foley catheter inserted, the balloon is gently inflated, and it is draped off with a clear, occlusive bandage. The abdomen is prepped with Chloraprep or Betadine solution and an Ioban occlusive drape is placed over the whole abdomen.

Port Placement

The initial ports are placed contralateral to the stoma site. A cutdown technique to establish access and pneumoperitoneum utilizing "S" retractors is excellent for gaining exposure sequentially to each fascial layer through the skin incision. The fascia is elevated and opened between two pediatric Kocher clamps. The initial entry point is usually on the contralateral upper abdomen. A 10-mm trocar is inserted and a pneumoperitoneum of 15 mm Hg is obtained. The abdomen is inspected with a 30-degree 10 mm scope for injury to any intraabdominal structures and is assessed for adhesions. Two 5-mm ports are placed under direct visualization ipsilateral to the initial 10-mm port as far laterally as reasonably possible. One is usually about the level of the umbilicus while the other one is about 5-7 cm lower. Some adhesions may need to be taken down prior to inserting any of the additional ports to create working space in the abdomen.

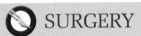 SURGERY

Once the three ports are placed, careful adhesiolysis and reduction of the hernia begins. This maneuver is performed sharply with very judicious, if any, use of electrocautery or ultrasonic energy. This step can be the most tedious and time-consuming part of the operation as great care must be taken to avoid an enterotomy. Multiple reinspections of the operative field and intestine during and after adhesiolysis are mandatory. Loops of incarcerated bowel must be distinguished from the loop of bowel ending in the ostomy. The bowel mesentery must be preserved. An ostomy with a compromised blood supply will not serve the patient well. The stoma mesentery can also help serve as a guiding structure while trying to sort out multiple small intestinal loops incarcerated into a large hernia defect. The hernia contents must be reduced, but there is no need to excise the hernia sac itself. The afferent limb of the stoma is mobilized to allow for lateralization of the stoma limb as required for the Sugarbaker technique.

After the hernia contents are reduced, the facial defect is measured. There are a few techniques available. A spinal needle is placed through the abdominal wall perpendicular to the edge of the defect and marked on the abdominal wall. After all edges of the defect are marked, the size of the defect is measured after the abdomen is deflated so as not to overestimate its size. One can also cut a plastic ruler lengthwise and introduce it into the abdomen through the 10-mm trocar. This can be held up against the defect for measurement. This is handy when the defect is small, but is impractical if the defect is larger than the length of the ruler. Finally, a piece of cord tape or suture can be stretched across the defect intracorporally, withdrawn, and measured extracorporally. Regardless of the approach, an accurate measurement in the vertical and horizontial axes is essential to a good repair.

A dual-sided expanded polytetrafluoroethylene (ePTFE) mesh (Dual-Mesh, W.L. Gore, Flagstaff, AZ) is appropriately sized to cover the stoma as well as 5 cm beyond the facial defect. This dual-sided microporous mesh prevents erosion of the biomaterial into the afferent limb of the stoma as it tunnels laterally against the abdominal wall. The orientation is marked on the mesh to facilitate orientation intracorporally. Sutures are placed on the four sides of the mesh while keeping in mind the path the bowel will take as it exits the mesh laterally. Prior to inserting the mesh, two 5-mm trocars are placed ipsilateral to the stoma under direct visualization. These ports are used to view the mesh and as working ports for placing tacks along the medial edge of the mesh.

The camera is switched to an ipsilateral port with a 30-degree 5-mm scope. A locking grasper is introduced into the abdomen through an ipsilateral 5-mm port and the tip is directed out of the abdomen through the 10-mm contralateral port. The mesh is rolled, the 10-mm port is removed, and the mesh is pulled into the abdomen through the 10-mm trocar site with the locking grasper. Although some have expressed concern with contaminating the mesh by pulling it through the skin incision, we have not found this fear to be supported. The camera is replaced with the 10-mm scope through the 10-mm port. The mesh is unrolled and oriented correctly in the abdomen.

A full 5 cm overlap beyond the defined edges of the fascia is assured by intracorporeal measurement. A helpful approach is to pass a spinal needle through the abdominal wall at the edge of the facial defect and to perform the intracorporeal measurement with a bowel grasper. The authors' bowel graspers open to 4 cm and have a 4.5 cm bare area that allows intraabdominal horizontal and vertical measurement. Typically, the superior stitch location is measured and placed; a suture passer is inserted transabdominally through a small stab incision at the appropriate location. Each suture is pulled through the stab incision. Care is given to obtain a 1 cm purchase on the fascia with the stitch. The lateral stitch is measured and placed next in a similar manner. These two stitches are tied in place. The inferior and medial stitches are not measured. Instead, the mesh is elevated to the abdominal wall and placed on tension with a grasper. The suture passage through the fascia is determined with a spinal needle. A stab incision is made at that location and the suture passer is used to retrieve the sutures. These stitches are pulled through the abdominal wall and tied.

Spiral tacks are deployed at 1 cm intervals around the edge of the mesh except where the bowel exits the mesh laterally. A second row of tacks is deployed 3 cm from the edge of the mesh in a "double crown" technique as well as a row on each side of the bowel as it exits the mesh. One of the keys of a good repair is having a properly sized tunnel for the bowel. In order to better assess the size of the tunnel, the intraabdominal pressure is reduced to 8 mm Hg. This maneuver relieves some of the tension on the abdominal wall while still giving enough space to place the tacks on each side of the bowel as it exits the mesh. Finally, transabdominal 1-0 Prolene sutures are placed every 4 cm around the circumference of the mesh. A spinal needle is used to identify the location of each suture, which is placed through the mesh with a suture passer.

The abdomen is inspected one last time for hemostasis and enterotomies. The abdomen is deflated and the trocar sites are closed in normal fashion.

POSTOPERATIVE MANAGEMENT

Patients are usually admitted to the floor unless there are other compelling reasons for a monitored care bed. Orders include ambulation as soon as possible, patient-controlled analgesic, prophylaxis against deep venous thrombosis, and antiemetics. There is no routine use of a nasogastric tube or of postoperative antibiotics. Diet is started as soon as there is evidence of return of bowel function. Patients are released from the hospital when they are tolerating a diet, have their pain controlled with oral analgesics, and demonstrate a functioning ostomy, typically on postoperative day 4.

COMPLICATIONS

Obstruction

One of the technical challenges of the modified Sugarbaker repair is in sizing the tunnel for the loop of bowel leading to the ostomy. The mesh is placed when the abdomen is distended making accurate sizing difficult. Too large of a tunnel provides space for a loop of bowel to insinuate itself into the defect and become obstructed between the mesh and the abdominal wall. Too small of a tunnel can actually obstruct the bowel leading to the ostomy. Both of these can present the surgeon with a diagnostic challenge postoperatively. Does the patient have a postoperative ileus or an obstruction from the mesh? The latter requires immediate surgical revision while the former can be managed conservatively. When faced with this dilemma, placing a digit in the stoma to evaluate the tunnel aperture and/or a CT scan can be extremely helpful in deciding on patient management.

Infection

Infection of port sites can generally be treated with local opening, draining, and packing. Antibiotics are advised if there is extensive cellulitis. Infected mesh generally cannot be treated conservatively, especially ePTFE. Although drainage by interventional radiology and a long course of antibiotics can be attempted to salvage the repair, one must be prepared to return to the operating room and explant the mesh if that fails.

Enterotomy

If the enterotomy is detected at the time of the operation, it is repaired laparoscopically or in an open fashion depending on its extent and the skill of the surgeon. Our practice would be to repair the enterotomy, complete the lysis of adhesions and hernia reduction, and repair the hernia at a later date. The adhesions are much less at the second laparoscopic procedure and the repair can be performed safely. If there is the misfortune that the enterotomy is missed at the time of the operation, the patient requires an urgent return to the operating room where the mesh is removed, the enterotomy is repaired, and the hernia is fixed with a biological mesh, in a primary fashion, or left to be repaired at a later date.

Fistula formation caused by erosion of mesh or tacks into adherent loops of bowel is a severe, late complication to this procedure. The editors have been the recipients of these patients, in whom mesh removal and bowel resection are required. Even with good patient selection and perfect technique, one may experience this complication and need to remove the mesh and resect the bowel.

Recurrence

There is scant literature on the repair of parastomal hernia recurrences after a laparoscopic repair. Our experience is limited to three patients. All patients had undergone a laparoscopic parastomal repair with a keyholed mesh. The parastomal hernia repair recurred due to a separation of the mesh along the keyhole slit. Zacharakis et al. (1) reported on one case where a revisional repair was done 3 months after the primary laparoscopic repair. At the revision, the original mesh was noted to have migrated into the hernia defect. This was one of four repairs done by this group and was the only mesh placed with spiral tacks and no transfascial sutures. At the repair, the original mesh was not removed. An appropriately sized Dual-Mesh was placed over the existing mesh and defect in a keyhole fashion. There was no statement about long-term follow-up.

✥ CONCLUSION

Parastomal hernias are a frequent complication. There are several open and laparoscopic repairs available. Unfortunately, there are no large randomized controlled trials comparing the various techniques and no one method has clearly become the standard for repair. As small case series of laparoscopic repairs accumulate in the literature, the trend has recently been toward a modified Sugarbaker repair with ePTFE mesh. This is the repair that we described here which the authors will continue to use until more convincing scientific evidence directs them otherwise.

Recommended Readings

Berger D, Bientzle M. Laparoscopic repair of parastomal hernias: a single surgeon's experience in 66 patients. *Dis Colon Rectum* 2007;50(10):1668–73.

Bickel A, Shinkarevsky E, Eitan A. Laparoscopic repair of paracolostomy hernia. *J Laparoendosc Adv Surg Tech A* 1999;9(4):353–5.

Carne PW, Robertson GM, Frizelle FA. Parastomal hernia. *Br J Surg* 2003;90(7):784–93.

Craft RO, Huguet KL, McLemore EC, Harold KL. Laparoscopic parastomal hernia repair. *Hernia* 2008;12(2):137–40.

Devlin HB, Kingsnorth A. Parastomal hernia. In: Devlin A, Kingsnorth A, eds. *Management of Abdominal Hernias*. 2nd ed. London: Butterworths, 1998:257–66.

Hansson BM, Bleichrodt RP, de Hingh IH. Laparoscopic parastomal hernia repair using a keyhole technique results in a high recurrence rate. *Surg Endosc* 2009;23(7):1456–9.

Hansson BM, de Hingh IH, Bleichrodt RP. Laparoscopic parastomal hernia repair is feasible and safe: early results of a prospective clinical study including 55 consecutive patients. *Surg Endosc* 2007;21(6):989–93.

Hansson BM, van Nieuwenhoven EJ, Bleichrodt RP. Promising new technique in the repair of parastomal hernia. *Surg Endosc* 2003;17(11):1789–91.

LeBlanc KA, Bellanger DE. Laparoscopic repair of paraostomy hernias: early results. *J Am Coll Surg* 2002;194(2):232–9.

LeBlanc KA, Bellanger DE, Whitaker JM, Hausmann MG. Laparoscopic parastomal hernia repair. *Hernia* 2005;9(2):140–44.

Mancini GJ, McClusky DA III, Khaitan L, et al. Laparoscopic parastomal hernia repair using a nonslit mesh technique. *Surg Endosc* 2007;21(9):1487–91.

Muysoms EE, Hauters PJ, Van Nieuwenhove Y, Huten N, Claeys DA. Laparoscopic repair of parastomal hernias: a multi-centre retrospective review and shift in technique. *Acta Chir Belg* 2008; 108(4):400–4.

Porcheron J, Payan B, Balique JG. Mesh repair of paracolostomal hernia by laparoscopy. *Surg Endosc* 1998;12(10):1281.

Safadi B. Laparoscopic repair of parastomal hernias: early results. *Surg Endosc* 2004;18(4):676–80.

Shabbir J, Britton DC. Stoma complications: a literature overview. *Colorectal Dis* 2010;12(10):958–64.

Shellito PC. Complications of abdominal stoma surgery. *Dis Colon Rectum* 1998;41(12):1562–72.

Sugarbaker PH. Prosthetic mesh repair of large hernias at the site of colonic stomas. *Surg Gynecol Obstet* 1980;150(4):576–8.

Reference

1. Zacharakis E, Shalhoub J, Selvapatt N, Darzi A, Ziprin P. Revisional laparoscopic parastomal hernia repair. *JSLS* 2008;12(4): 403–6.

47 Open Hartmann's Reversal

Roberta L. Muldoon

Introduction

The majority of diseases of the colon can be managed with a single-stage procedure. There are, however, still circumstances in which the operating surgeon is concerned about performing a primary anastomosis after having completed a segmental resection of the left colon, and feels that stool diversion is in the best interest of the patient. Severe inflammation or gross contamination of the abdominal cavity may preclude primary anastomosis. The most common scenarios in which Hartmann's procedures are performed are cancer and perforated diverticulitis with abdominal sepsis. A Hartmann's procedure leaves the patient with an end colostomy as well as a rectal stump. Ideally, over time the inflammation or primary condition resolves, and Hartmann's reversal or colostomy takedown can be considered. This procedure is known for its high morbidity, so caution should be exercised in preparing for this procedure.

 ## INDICATIONS/CONTRAINDICATIONS

A number of factors should be kept in mind when deciding to proceed with Hartmann's reversal. These factors will impact the likelihood of a patient having a complication either during or after the procedure. By optimizing the condition of the patient, one may be able to decrease the morbidity associated with this procedure.

The timing of the reversal has been examined, but there is no clear consensus as to when it is appropriate to proceed. Aydin et al. studied 121 patients who underwent successful Hartmann's reversal. They found that patients undergoing reversal at 4 months after the primary procedure were 2.5 times more likely to have a surgical complication when compared with those who had the reversal done within 4 months of the primary procedure. Those patients who underwent reversal at 8 months after the primary procedure were 5.5 times more likely to have a surgical complication when compared with patients who had reversal within the 4-month window (1). This finding suggests that closure within 4 months is the safest time to proceed. Pearce et al. reviewed 145 patients who underwent Hartmann's reversal and found that 6 out of 12 patients (50%) who underwent reversal in under 3 months from the time of the primary surgery suffered an anastomotic leak. Twenty-eight patients underwent reversal between 3 and 6 months after their initial surgery. Of these, seven patients (25%) suffered an anastomotic leak. Forty patients had their reversal after 6 months from the original surgery, and all healed well without evidence of leak (2). This paper suggests that a waiting period of 6 months is the safest for the patient. When Keck et al. reviewed their data of 111 Hartmann's reversals, they found no difference in morbidity, mortality, or complication rates between those patients who had their takedown early (before 15 weeks) or late (after 15 weeks). They did find that patients whose reversals were done early did have longer hospitalizations, and that the operations were perceived by the surgeon as being more difficult (3). It is important to note that none of these papers specifically looked at the severity or complexity of the original operation. This status would clearly affect the recovery time of the patients and would clearly have an effect on the ease and success of the reversal procedure.

It is generally accepted that early reversal (<3 months) may lead to complications secondary to adhesions and residual inflammation still present from the inciting process and the original surgery. This can lead to more difficult, prolonged surgeries, with increased blood loss and prolonged hospitalization. On the other end of the spectrum, it is thought that waiting too long may lead to difficulty in mobilizing and anastomosing the rectal stump, which decreases in size over time due to lack of use. It is important when reviewing this literature to consider the effect of the original operation on the outcome. None of these papers specifically evaluated at the complexity or indication for the original operation. Perhaps the increase in complications that is sometimes seen with waiting may be a reflection of the difficulty of the original operation, the severity of the disease process, patient comorbidities, and a prolonged recovery time from a difficult original surgery, rather than a reflection of just the passage of time.

The decision as to the appropriate timing of the reversal needs to be made on an individual basis. First and foremost, the patient must be in overall good condition with recovery from the primary surgery and able to undergo a second operation. Consideration of the original disease process, the operative intervention itself, as well as how the recuperation progressed will be a helpful information in planning when to proceed with the reversal. Ideally, the patients should be at or close to their premorbid state with regard to ambulation, nutrition, and overall strength. If they needed to be placed on steroids for treatment of their disease process, these should be weaned if possible prior to colostomy takedown. The initial inciting event should have resolved, and enough time given to have resolution of the inflammatory process. Finally, there should be no sign of ongoing infection, which could lead to an increased risk of wound infection or intra-abdominal abscess formation.

PREOPERATIVE PLANNING

Preoperative evaluation includes assessment of the remaining colon as well as the rectal stump. The colon should be endoscopically evaluated to exclude cancer or other possible pathology of the colon. The rectal stump should also be viewed. This exclude associated rectal pathology, as well as to give an indication as to the length of the rectal stump. Knowledge of the length can be helpful in determining where to look for the proximal end in a pelvis that may have a significant amount of scar tissue present. It is very helpful also to review the operative note of the primary surgery, especially if you did not perform the original operation. Knowing, for example, that the bowel was tacked to the anterior abdominal wall or that a stitch had been placed at the proximal end of the bowel can be a valuable information. It is also helpful to know where the proximal end of the bowel might be located, so that it is not injured either with entry into the abdominal cavity or while lysing pelvic adhesions.

Patients should undergo a full bowel preparation prior to the surgery. If inspissated mucus is found at the time of endoscopic evaluation of the rectum, then enemas per rectum can be given to clear this prior to the surgery. Lastly, the need for the use of ureteral stents should be considered. Although the use of stents does not eliminate the risk of ureteral injury, it has been shown to improve early detection, which is associated with decreased morbidity associated with this complication (4). The decision to use stents is based, in part, on the severity of the disease at the original operation as well as the difficulty of the primary operation. The time interval between the two surgeries, the patient's history of prior operations, and the patients' body habits should also be considered when making this decision.

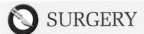# SURGERY

Technique

The patient should be positioned in the modified lithotomy position. Deep venous thrombosis prophylaxis should be administered as well as a dose of preoperative antibiotics. A bladder catheter should be inserted and stents placed at this time if desired. The stoma can be sutured closed to minimize any contamination during the case. The stoma is then covered with sterile gauze to collect any fluid that might leak out from the stoma, and then the entire abdomen covered with an antimicrobial adhesive covering. After the abdomen is prepped and draped in the usual sterile manner, lower midline incision is made. Upon entering the abdomen, care should be taken to avoid injury of small-bowel loops that may be adherent to the anterior abdominal wall. All adhesions in and around the stoma should be carefully divided so that there is clear visualization of the distal colon exiting the anterior abdominal wall. Once the distal colon is circumferentially freed at the fascial level, the bowel can be divided. A GIA stapler is positioned just beneath the anterior abdominal wall with the intention of preserving as much of the bowel length as possible (Fig. 47.1). Once the colon is divided, it is usually easier to complete the remainder of the adhesiolysis. A retractor system can now be put into place. It is important to assess which vessels were divided at the primary operation and which vessels are still intact. This knowledge will be important, not only in assessing the remaining colon's blood supply, but may also play a key role in the mobility of the colon reaching down to the proximal end of the rectum. The small bowel needs to be freed out of the pelvis and packed into the upper abdomen. The distal colon

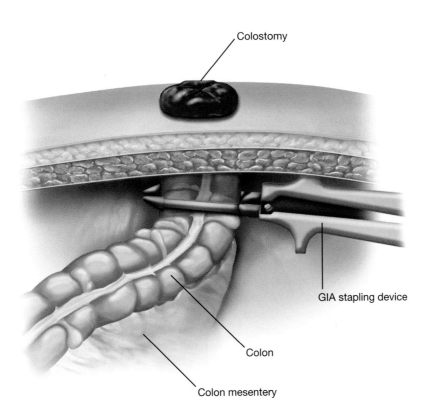

Colostomy

GIA stapling device

Colon

Colon mesentery

Figure 47.1 Abdominal wall with colostomy in place. Stapler aligned just beneath abdominal wall ready to fire.

can also usually be temporarily packed into the upper abdomen. It is the editor's preference to first mobilize the stoma, and resect and close the proximal segment usually over a circular stapler anvil prior to reopening the laparotomy incision.

With good visualization of the pelvis, the rectal stump can be identified and mobilized. If at the original surgery the rectal stump was long and sutured to the anterior or lateral wall, the localization is usually fairly straightforward. More often though, the case is that the rectal stump is shorter and has retracted into the pelvis with reperitonealization, making location more challenging. If it is difficult, the following maneuvers can be helpful. Air can be gently insufflated with a rigid proctoscope to help identify the rectum. The rectal sizers can also be used to stent the rectum, thus giving some direction as to its location and boundaries. The rigid proctoscope can also be inserted and advanced under direct visualization to help identify the most proximal end. The amount of mobilization necessarily depends on the length of the rectum, the type of anastomosis planned (stapled vs. hand-sewn), and the angulation of the rectum. If the rectum is straight, only the most proximal end needs to be mobilized ensuring that the edges are cleared for a "clean" anastomosis. If, however, the rectum has folded back on itself or has significant angulation present and you are planning a stapled anastomosis, then further mobilization will be necessary for safe insertion of the stapler from below. It is imperative that the rectum be adequately dissected free from bladder in the male and from the vagina in the female. It is sometimes difficult to assess the exact plane between the rectum and the vagina. In this case, it is often helpful to place either a finger or the rectal sizers in the vagina. The vagina can then be retracted anteriorly, which can assist in developing the plane between these two structures.

Once the rectum has been mobilized it must be assessed for suitability for anastomosis. The original etiology needs to be contemplated, and adequacy of the primary resection assessed. At times, in the setting of acute perforated diverticulitis, the perforated and most diseased portion of the colon is resected leaving behind a portion of the sigmoid colon down in the pelvis. In this setting, the distal portion of sigmoid needs to be resected, so the anastomosis is performed to the top of the true rectum. Likewise, if the pathology had revealed cancer with inadequate margins, addition resection might be merited. Once the rectum is assessed and ready for anastomosis, the distal colon needs to be assessed and prepared for anastomosis. The proximal colon must be anastomosed to the rectum and not to the distal sigmoid colon.

The proximal colon should be assessed for suitability for anastomosis. The distal margin should have healthy tissue with a good blood supply. It should reach down to the pelvis without any tension. Toward this end the splenic flexure should be mobilized by medially retracting the colon and incising along the white line of Toldt. The plane between the colon mesentery and the retroperitoneum should be identified and developed medially and superiorly toward the splenic flexure. The splenocolic ligaments are divided. With difficult splenic flexures, it is sometimes beneficial to approach the flexure from medial to lateral. In this case, the omentum is retracted superiorly and the transverse colon inferiorly. The omentum is dissected from the transverse colon, thus allowing entry into the lesser sac. This plane can then be developed toward the splenic flexure until it is completely mobilized. If after mobilization of the splenic flexure there still seems to be undue tension when the colon is assessed for anastomosis, then the blood vessels should be assessed. The inferior mesenteric artery and vein should be divided if they were not divided during the original operation. Care must be taken when taking these vessels that the marginal artery is preserved since this will be the blood supply to the distal colon.

Once adequate length and viability have been attained, the anastomosis can be performed (Fig. 47.2). The anastomosis can be undertaken with either a stapling technique or suture. Docherty et al. performed a prospective randomized trial comparing hand-sewn anastomoses to stapled anastomoses. They found that though there was a significantly higher rate of radiologic leak noted in the hand-sewn group, there was no difference in clinical anastomotic leak rates, morbidity, or mortality when comparing the two different methods (5). The hand-sewn technique can be challenging when performed deep in the pelvis. The authors and the editors prefer a stapled anastomosis.

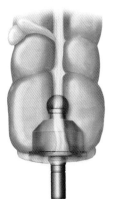

Figure 47.2 Colon aligned with stapler in place.

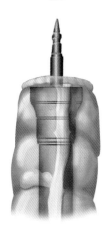

The distal end of the colon is prepared first by clearing any excess fat from the distal 1 cm, which may interfere with clear visualization of the colon or with the anastomosis. Towels should be placed around the bowel to maintain the sterility of the field. A purse-string stitch is then placed at the distal end of the colon. A permanent monofilament stitch on a straight needle is then passed through the purse-string instrument after which the staple line is then excised. The purse-string device is then removed and the anvil to the stapler is then placed into the lumen of the bowel. The purse string is then tightened around the anvil. Care should be taken to make sure that there is a cuff of bowel present and that the purse string does not leave any gaps around the anvil (Fig. 47.3A). The distal end of the bowel with the anvil should be carefully examined to ensure that there are no diverticulum present, which could cause problems with the anastomosis and that there is minimal fat or additional tissue that may potentially interfere with the staple line. Alternatively, the double-stapled technique may be employed using the original rectal stump staple line. However, great care must be taken to ensure that all distal sigmoid are resected during the original operation.

The circular end-to-end anastomotic (EEA) stapler is then inserted into the rectum and carefully advanced to the proximal end of the rectum. If resistance is encountered, the stapler should be removed and either the dilators can be passed or the rectum can be endoscopically visualized. Excessive force should not be utilized in an attempt to advance the stapler, because such force can result in tearing of the rectal wall. Most of the time the problem will be that the stapler is caught on a valve and simple dilation with the sizers will correct this problem. The stapler can then be reinserted and carefully advanced to the proximal end of the colon. Care should be taken to make sure that the stapler has reached the proximal end and that the rectum is lying flat over the stapler mechanism. The spike is then deployed, aiming to have it come out either just above or just below the middle of the staple line. Once the spike is fully deployed, the anvil is attached, making sure that the colon has not been twisted. It is imperative that no adjacent tissue is caught in the stapler. In the female, it is imperative that the vagina be separated from the rectum and retracted

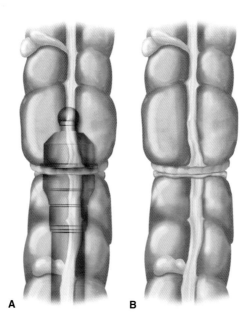

Figure 47.3 **A.** Stapler closed and fired. **B.** Anastomosis removal of stapler.

so as not to be incorporated into the staple line to avoid the complication of a rectovaginal or colovaginal fistula. Once the entire circumference of the anastomosis is cleared, the stapler is then closed and fired (Fig. 47.3B). The stapler is the opened, rotated, and gently removed. The tissue from the stapler should be removed and examined to see if complete rings are present. Lack of complete rings could signify a problem with the anastomosis.

The anastomosis is assessed for leaks by gently clamping the colon with a noncrushing bowel clamp above the anastomosis. Saline is instilled into the pelvis so that the anastomosis is submerged. An endoscope is inserted into the rectum and air is gently insufflated until the colon is dilated. The anastomosis should be assessed for escaping air bubbles. If none is seen, the air can be removed from the colon and the saline can be removed from the pelvis. If bubbles are seen, it signifies a leak at the anastomosis, which will require repair or takedown and re-creation of the anastomosis.

After completion of the anastomosis, the abdomen is closed and the end of the stoma excised. Prior to closing the midline wound, the stoma site should be checked to make sure that there are no adhesions on small bowel, which might still be attached to this portion of the bowel. It is also helpful to free this small remaining piece of bowel from the fascia prior to closing, since this will assist in ease of removal from the exterior approach once the abdomen has been closed. The midline fascia and skin are then closed and a dressing placed.

The remaining small portion of bowel and the stoma can be removed. A circular incision is made at the mucocutaneous junction. This incision is then taken down separating the small remnant of bowel from the subcutaneous tissue and the fascia. Once the bowel is removed, the fascia is closed. The wound is irrigated. The stoma site is partially closed by placing a 3-0 absorbable monofilament purse string at the dermal level. A small Penrose drain is placed in the center of this wound as the purse string is tied down. A dressing is placed over this wound.

POSTOPERATIVE MANAGEMENT

The bladder catheter is generally removed the morning after surgery unless the anastomosis is deep in the pelvis. The patients are allowed clear liquids until the time that they have some bowel function at which time they are advanced to a low-residue diet. The Penrose drain from the stoma site is removed when the patient is discharged from the hospital. A clean dry dressing is placed over the stoma site and this is allowed to granulate closed.

COMPLICATIONS

Overall mortality for this procedure ranges from 0% to 3.7% and, as would be expected, is related to age (2,3,6–9). Salem et al. noted that their overall mortality rate was 0.4%. In young patients the mortality rate was extremely low; however, this rate increased to 2.6% in patients older than 77 years (10).

The Hartmann's reversal procedure has a known high morbidity rate that ranges from 25% to 48.5% (1,3,7–9,11). These complications should be seriously considered in the first place, when one is deciding to do the Hartmann's procedure. These risks need to be weighed against the benefits of doing this procedure. The most common complications associated with this procedure are wound infections. The rate ranges from 12.9% up to 21% (6,9,11). Careful attention to detail can lower the risk of this complication. The second most common complication seen with this procedure is ileus, which can occur up to 18% of the time (11). Anastomotic leak can also occur and has been found to range from 3.3% to 4%, and is comparable to other procedures with colonic anastomosis (1,3,8). Other complications associated with colostomy takedown are bleeding, dehiscence, rectovaginal fistula (3.7%), stricture formation (3.7%), pneumonia (5%), urinary tract infection (3%), and hernia formation either at the midline incision or at the stoma site (2,11). Schmeizer et al. analyzed their data and found that the only predictive risk factor for postoperative morbidity was hypoalbuminemia (9).

RESULTS

It is important to realize that a large number of patients who have a Hartmann's procedure will never have their stoma taken down. It has been shown that only 54–59% of patients have a reversal performed (1,2,7,10,12). Younger patients are more likely to have their stomas taken down, as are male patients (13). The disease process that required the stoma in the first place does play a role in the likelihood of having the stoma taken down. Mealy et al. noted that patients who had a stoma created secondary to diverticulitis were much more likely to have their stoma reversed than those that had a stoma creased secondary to cancer, 84.6% versus 48.3%, respectively (7). Age also plays a role in the likelihood of reversal. Salem et al. looked at those patients who had a colostomy creased secondary to diverticulitis. Eighty percent of patients younger than 50 years had their stoma reversed compared to only 30% of those who were older than 77 years (10).

One must also consider those patients who have reversal attempted but the procedure is not successful, and the patient is left with a permanent colostomy. Boland et al. reviewed 39 Hartmann's reversals. They found that 10 patients (26%) had stomas at the time of discharge from their reversal operation. Of these patients, three were intended to be permanent and seven were temporary. Of these seven temporary stomas, three were closed, three were pending closure at the completion of the study, and one was a failure of the anastomosis and became a permanent stoma. Based on these numbers, they had a 10% failure rate at reversal of the Hartmann's procedure (11). Mealy et al. also reviewed their data with regard to this issue. They found that 11.2% (8 out of 71) of the patients who underwent attempted colostomy reversal had additional stomas created. Of these eight patients, two patients eventually had their stomas reversed for an overall failure rate of 8.4% (7). These failures also have to be added to the already large group that never comes to attempted Hartmann's reversal.

Considerations

Because of the high morbidity rate, as well as the high rate of patients who never undergo colostomy reversal, it is important to consider options at the initial operation to avoid this circumstance if possible. There are certainly instances where sound surgical judgment dictates that the best option for the patient is to have a Hartmann's procedure. Another option to consider is primary anastomosis and diverting loop ileostomy. Patients with a diverting loop ileostomy are five times more likely to have their stomas reversed compared to those patients with a colostomy (12). Ileostomy takedown is an easier procedure with a shorter operative time, making it an attractive option. Bell et al. compared complications associated with colostomy reversal to those associated with ileostomy reversal. They found that the overall morbidity from a Hartmann's reversal was 55% compared to 20% for an ileostomy reversal. Of these complications, 20% required operative intervention for the colostomy reversal group, whereas only 5% required operative intervention for the ileostomy reversal group (14).

CONCLUSION

Hartmann's reversal is a procedure known to have a high morbidity rate. All options should be considered at the time of the initial operation, carefully weighing the risks and benefits of the Hartmann's procedure. There will still be cases where the Hartmann's procedure is the safest option for the patient. In this case, thoughtful consideration needs to be given to the ideal time for colostomy closure. The difficulty of the initial operation, severity of disease, the patient's recuperation period, and comorbidities all play an important role in deciding when to proceed. Finally, careful attention to detail during the procedure can minimize complication from this procedure.

Recommended References and Readings

1. Aydin H, Remzi F, Tekkis PP, Fazio VW. Hartmann's reversal is associated with high postoperative adverse events. *Dis Colon Rectum* 2005;48:2117–26.
2. Pearce N, Scott S, Karran SJ. Timing and method of reversal of Hartmann's procedure. *Br J Surg* 1992;79:839–41.
3. Keck J, Collopy B, Ryan PJ, Fink R, Mackay JR, Woods RJ. Reversal of Hartmann's procedure; effect of timing and technique on ease and safety. *Dis Colon Rectum* 1994;37:243–48.
4. Bothwell W, Bleicher R, Dent TL. Prophylactic ureteral catheterization in colon surgery. A five year review. *Dis Colon Rectum* 1994;37:330–34.
5. Docherty J, McGregor J, Akyol AM, Murray GD, Galloway DJ. Comparison of manually constructed and stapled anastomoses in colorectal surgery. *Ann Surg* 1995;221:176–84.
6. Ghorra S, Rzeczycki T, Natarajan R, Pricolo VE. Colostomy closure: impact of preoperative risk factors on morbidity. *Am Surg* 1999;65:266–69.
7. Mealy K, O'Broin E, Donohue J, Tanner A, Keane FB. Reversible colostomy—what is the outcome? *Dis Colon Rectum* 1996;39:1227–31.
8. Roe A, Prabhu S, Ali A, Brown C, Brodribb AJ. Reversal of Hartmann's procedure: timing and operative technique. *Br J Surg* 1991;78:1167–70.
9. Schmelzer T, Mostafa G, Norton HJ, et al. Reversal of Hartmann's procedure: a high risk operation? *Surgery* 2007;142:598–607.
10. Salem L, Anaya D, Roberts KE, Flum DR. Hartmann's colectomy and reversal in diverticulitis: a population-level assessment. *Dis Colon Rectum* 2005;48:988–95.
11. Boland E, Hsu A, Brand MI, Saclarides TJ. Hartmann's colostomy reversal: outcome of patients undergoing surgery with the intention of eliminating fecal diversion. *Am Surg* 2007;73:664–68.
12. Daluvoy S, Gonzalez F, Vaziri K, Sabnis A, Brody F. Factors associated with ostomy reversal. *Surg Endosc* 2008;22:2168–70.
13. Maggard M, Zingmond D, O'Connell JB, Ko CY. What proportion of patients with an ostomy (for diverticulitis) gets reversed? *Am Surg* 2004;70:928–31.
14. Bell C, Asolati M, Hamilton E, et al. A comparison of complications associated with colostomy reversal versus ileostomy reversal. *Am J Surg* 2005;190:717–20.

48 Laparoscopic Colostomy Reversal

Floriano Marchetti and Abdullah Al Haddad

In 1923, Henry Hartmann introduced the concept of colonic resection and diversion for the treatment of cancers of the distal colon (1). Since that time, this operation has been employed to treat a variety of conditions, mainly of the left colon such as complicated diverticulitis with peritonitis, trauma, obstructing or perforated neoplasms of the left colon or rectum, as well as volvulus or ischemia.

While this procedure has proven effective in reducing mortality in such conditions, the reversal of the end colostomy remains a major surgical procedure associated with significant surgical morbidity up to 50–60%, and mortality as high as 5–10% (2–5).

Furthermore, this operation is burdened by a usually lengthy hospital stay and prolonged convalescence with significant socioeconomical cost.

Once laparoscopy was introduced to colon and rectal surgery, it was only natural to try to use a minimally invasive approach also for this operation with the goal of reducing morbidity, mortality, and especially hospital stay and convalescence.

In fact, early results were encouraging. In one of the earliest reports of laparoscopic colostomy reversal, Sosa et al. found that laparoscopic-assisted Hartmann's reversal results in comparable morbidity, but may be associated with shorter hospital stay when compared to laparotomy (6).

Since then, laparoscopic colostomy reversal has been evaluated in many studies, which have indicated this approach to be safe and have shown results not only comparable to the open technique, but also, in some cases, superior, particularly in terms of time to recovery (7). Rosen et al. in 2006 reported the advantage of laparoscopic Hartmann's reversal in the way of a shorter hospitalization and shorter time to bowel function (4).

Many authors have reported the advantages of laparoscopic colostomy reversal in terms of lower morbidity. A recent meta-analysis of 12 studies (8) comparing open (OHR) versus laparoscopic Hartmann reversal (LHR) found the following in the LHR group:

- Overall morbidity was lower (mean 12.2% LHR vs. 20.3% OHR). Complications included, wound infection (10.8% vs. 14.2%), anastomotic leakage (1.2% vs. 5.1%), and cardiopulmonary complications (3.6% vs. 6.9%).
- Length of hospital was shorter (mean 6.9, range 3–11 vs. 10.7 days, range 3–18 days).
- Rate of reoperation was lower (3.6% vs. 6.9%).

However, it should be noted that to date, the available studies are all retrospective series with small numbers of patients (7–71 patients). Therefore, the impact of selection bias in these results remains to be determined. Furthermore, the statistical power of such studies is objectively limited.

On the other hand, LHR is a technically demanding operation with a steep learning curve and conversion rates are as high as 22% (8). Khaikin et al. reported that laparoscopic colostomy reversal was technically challenging, and required more operative time than did open technique (9).

However, despite these limitations, in the hands of experienced laparoscopic surgeons, laparoscopic HR appears safe and associated with a reasonably low conversion rate. Furthermore, it is possible that newer prospective studies will confirm the relatively low morbidity rate, shorter hospital stay, and earlier return to bowel function. In fact, with the expansion and further development of minimally invasive surgery, morbidity and conversion rates may be reduced further. The advantage of smaller incisions, decreased postoperative pain, shorter recovery time, and early return to normal activity have been well described (10–14).

INDICATIONS/CONTRAINDICATIONS

Depending on the original surgical indication for the stoma and if the disease process has been resolved, the stoma can be reversed.

Indications

All Hartmann's resections conducted on the left colon are amenable to a laparoscopic reversal attempt. Complicated diverticulitis remains the most frequent indication to a Hartmann procedure, followed by obstructed or perforated left-sided colon cancer. Trauma, volvulus, and ischemia are less frequent indications.

A laparoscopic approach may also be attempted for patients with long Hartmann's pouches such as after segmental transverse colectomies or right colectomies with end ileostomies.

It is possible to speculate that patients who have undergone Hartmann operations performed laparoscopically are the ideal candidates for subsequent laparoscopic HR. However, most colorectal surgeons will have to manage patients who underwent open resections and were possibly operated in emergency by other surgeons. If the patient was operated elsewhere or by another surgeon, the operative note should be reviewed.

- Use of adhesion barriers: it is possible that such patients will present with less adhesions and, therefore, be better candidates for laparoscopic reversal. Although the real advantages remain controversial the use of such materials has been shown to be beneficial in decreasing postoperative adhesion formation.
- The presence of markers on the stapled end of the rectum: the identification of the rectal stump can be challenging. The presence of nonabsorbable suture near the staple line aids in the identification of the rectum. In several series, the inability to identify the rectal stump was one of the most frequent reasons for conversion (4,6,9,15,16). In one series, this was the reason for seven of the eight conversions (7).
- The length of rectum or recto-sigmoid stump: a longer stump is usually more promptly identified both at laparoscopy and at laparotomy.
- The presence of an intact superior rectal artery may help to prevent the recoil of the rectum in the pelvis.
- The presence of the uterus in female patients: the rectum may retract behind the uterus and form with it dense adhesions, which will render the dissection more complicated.

Contraindications

Contraindications of stoma reversal include the following:

- Patient preference
- Unresolved disease process such as carcinomatosis, persistent inflammation, or ischemia

- Incontinence or expectation of incontinence
- Distal obstruction
- The presence of medical conditions and comorbidities, which may also be contraindications to open surgery.

Contraindications to Laparoscopic Hartmann's Reversal

- Technically unfeasible cases such as abdomens with extensive adhesions, or in presence of extensive radiation changes.
- Hostile anatomy: the rectal stump or the ureter is not identified with certainty.

 # PREOPERATIVE PLANNING

Since most of these patients underwent emergency surgery without any preoperative screening, most surgeons prefer to evaluate the colon prior to the colostomy reversal by either colonoscopy or barium enema. In our practice, if a patient is 50 or older, or if he/she has increased risk factors for colorectal cancer, the preferred option is a colonoscopy through the stoma and a flexible sigmoidoscopy of the rectal stump. We also obtain a contrast study with water-soluble contrast to assess two important parameters such as the length and the shape of the rectal stump and the level of the splenic flexure. Younger patients without risk factors for colorectal cancer may undergo only the contrast study with hydro-soluble contrast.

If the index procedure was done for cancer, a complete staging workup should be done to assess recurrent or metastatic cancer. Computed tomography as well as a carcinoembryonic antigen (CEA) would serve well for this. PET/CT scan should be reserved when CT scan findings are unclear.

Patients are instructed to fast for the night prior to surgery. The issue of mechanical bowel preparation remains controversial. Multiple reports have now questioned the benefits of such practice. A recent Cochrane database review of 13 randomized studies involving 4,777 patients concluded that there is no statistically significant evidence to prove that patients benefit from bowel preparation (17). However, our preference is to perform a mechanical bowel preparation the day before surgery and two phosphate enemas on the morning of surgery. The rationale is to allow an easier manipulation of the bowel during the laparoscopic handling of the colon, which could be rendered quite difficult in the presence of varying amounts of hard stool. In addition, the presence of stool in the rectal stump would be a problem when an end-to-end or a side-to-end colorectal anastomosis is performed with the circular stapler or the anvil advanced through the rectum. Therefore, two phosphate enemas of the rectal stump should be given to the patient prior to surgery, particularly if no endoscopic examination of the stump has been performed prior to surgery. Furthermore, all our patients undergoing a colorectal anastomosis with a circular stapler introduced per rectum also undergo a rectal lavage at the time of surgery, using a large bore Pezzer drain, saline, and Betadine.

Intravenous antibiotics should be given within 1 hour of the incision and oral antibiotics preparation is not often used. However, all our patients receive oral Metronidazole and Neomycin the day prior to the surgery.

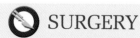 # SURGERY

Surgery and Technique

There are different types of colostomies depending on the indication for diversion and the surgeon's preference, such as end and loop colostomies. However, in this chapter, we will review the laparoscopic techniques for reversal of end colostomies typical of Hartmann's operations.

There are three different approaches to a laparoscopic reversal of colostomy:

- Laparoscopic Hartmann's reversal
- Hand-assisted Hartmann's reversal
- Single-port incision Hartmann's reversal

Laparoscopic Hartmann's Reversal

After general endotracheal anesthesia is induced and a bladder catheter is placed, the patient will be placed in lithotomy position using Allen stirrups (Allen Medical Systems; Hill-Rom Holdings, Inc., Batesville, Indiana) ensuring easy access to the anus. (**Pitfall:** a patient not properly positioned at the edge of the table will preclude access to the anus when introducing the circular stapler for the anastomosis.) Thus, it is crucial that the patient is well secured to the bed, not only for obvious safety reasons, but also because the steep Trendelenburg position often necessary for laparoscopic cases may lead to major cephalad shifting of the body. The consequence is that the buttocks may shift over the table, and, therefore, render transanal access quite difficult.

Both arms have to be tucked along the sides of the patient to ensure that adequate padding and protection are provided. In the rare cases that the anesthesiologists require access to one arm, the left arm can be left out given the need for tilting the bed toward the right side when the stoma is on the left side.

Next, as discussed above, the patient needs to be secured to the bed, given the extreme positions the bed will assume during the operation (steep Trendelenburg and tilt). This maneuver is usually accomplished with a beanbag. However, our preference is to use multiple strips of 3″ cloth adhesive tape to strap the patient to the bed. The skin of chest, breasts on female patients will have to be protected with towels and pads as necessary. Particular care needs to be taken to pad the arms to avoid compression of the radial nerve with subsequent risks of wrist drop. The patient is then prepped and draped in sterile fashion.

For the typical Hartmann reversal, where the colostomy is usually on the left side, the operation is conducted with the surgeon and assistant standing on the right of the patient with the monitor on the left side. The nurse stands in between the legs of the patient or on the right side of the patient as well.

The initial port placement depends on patient factors and surgeons preferences. As suggested by Rosen et al. (4), in presence of a midline scar extending to the epigastrium the first port should be placed at the level of the colostomy, which should therefore be taken down. Alternatively, a Hasson open technique could be used to place the initial port in the right upper quadrant (6,9). In presence of a lower midline incision a 5- or 10-mm port could be placed above the upper extent of the midline incision (6,18), or in the right upper quadrant.

In our practice, the operation starts usually by circumferentially mobilizing the stoma with preservation of the mesentery. The colon is then trimmed to healthy tissue. A purse-string device or a purse-string suture is used before the insertion of the anvil of the end-to-end anastomosis (EEA) stapling device in the colon. The purse-string is then closed and tied and the colon then dropped back into the abdomen. A 12-mm trocar is inserted through the colostomy site for pneumoperitoneum and secured at the fascia either by running a purse-string on the fascia and the rectus muscle or by placing figure-of-eight sutures on the fascia to ensure a good seal around the port.

Prior to inserting the remaining ports, the abdominal cavity should be carefully inspected. The pneumoperitoneum helps separate the intra-abdominal structures and place the adhesions under tension allowing for visualization of the right side of the abdomen. If the visualization across the midline of the abdomen is satisfactory, then we proceed to place the other ports in the right upper quadrant and in the right iliac fossa. Obviously, the presence, the extension, and the locations of the adhesions with the anterior abdominal wall will affect the positioning of the other trocars. The camera can be carefully used to take down some of these adhesions in order to free space for the port insertion. However, in case visualization is completely obstructed by the adhesions, one alternative is to place one or more ports on the left side where it is safe, to facilitate the lysis of the adhesions with the anterior abdominal wall. This step is followed by the placement of ports on the right side as previously described. If this is not feasible, we place a port using an open technique on the right upper quadrant. The camera can then be moved to this port and a second port placed in the right lower quadrant. It is possible to use 5-mm ports in all cases. The use of bladeless ports is mandatory, particularly in this procedure.

The patient is positioned in Trendelenburg position and tilted to the right so that the left side of the patient is up.

The first phase is usually the presence of adhesions involving the small bowel, the omentum, and the descending colon. Therefore, methodical and careful dissection is initiated.

- There are usually several loops of small bowel adherent to the pelvic structures. These adhesions need to be carefully mobilized to provide access to the rectal stump.
- Next, the attention should be turned to free the left gutter and the descending colon.
- Adhesiolysis should be limited to what is necessary to provide good exposure of the left-sided pelvic structures.

Once this maneuver has been completed, there is no need to continue to divide other adhesions that will not interfere with the planned surgery.

At this point, the attention is directed toward the pelvis to identify the rectal stump. This maneuver can be quite difficult especially if no nonabsorbable sutures were left on the staple line and/or if the superior rectal vessels were divided. Therefore, if no sutures are found, the insertion of dilators, stapling devices, rigid or flexible sigmoidoscopy, or insufflation of air using a syringe (4,19) is recommended. In this case, a 25-mm EEA sizer or a similar size Hegar dilator can be used.

However, our preference is to perform a rigid proctoscopy. In fact, particularly if the index surgery was done >6 months before, the rectum becomes more friable and rigid. The natural bends of the rectum might become more acute due to some pelvic fibrosis and, therefore, more difficult to negotiate with a rigid instrument. Therefore, introducing blindly a sizer or a dilator or even the stapler itself may result in a partial or full-thickness injury to the rectal stump. This problem is especially acute when the rectal stump is long and includes part of the sigmoid colon.

The rectal stump is then dissected from the surrounding adhesions as needed. Particular care is to be taken in identifying the left ureter and the iliac vessels, which should be always identified and kept out of harm's way.

A frequent situation is represented by the presence of extensive adhesions with the posterior wall of the bladder. In this case, it is usually necessary to fill the bladder with 250–300 cc of saline in order to better visualize the bladder and possibly find a safe plane for dissection. In women, the rectum may be found retracted and contracted in the pelvis behind the uterus. Usually, the introduction of rectal dilators as described above will help the visualization.

In the case when the original surgery was done for diverticulitis, any remnant of sigmoid colon still present, should be dissected and transected using an Endo GIA, making sure that the anastomosis is to the rectum and not to the remnant sigmoid colon. The 12-mm port at the colostomy site can then be used to introduce the endoscopic GIA to transect the colon at the rectosigmoid junction. Alternatively, the 5-mm port on the right iliac fossa can be switched to a 12-mm one. Passing the endoscopic stapler from the right lower quadrant port may result to be simpler and straightforward. Therefore, many surgeons prefer to start the case with a 12-mm port in this position. To extract the specimen, the 12-mm port at the stoma site may need to be removed and the purse-string opened.

At this point, the anvil of the EEA stapler is grasped and the descending colon is lowered down to the pelvis. If there is tension or the anvil does not reach the top of the rectal stump, the descending colon has to be mobilized more proximally. The splenic flexure is mobilized only if a tension-free colorectal anastomosis cannot be achieved.

The circular stapler is then very carefully advanced through the rectum. This is indeed a very delicate time of the procedure. As stated above, it could be very difficult to advance the stapler in a rectum that has become more rigid and tortuous and at the same time more fragile after months of fecal diversion. One should avoid, at all costs, forcing the stapler through this resistance. While an intraperitoneal tear of the rectum could be repaired, an extraperitoneal injury to the rectum could have disastrous consequences especially if overlooked at the time of surgery.

It is beneficial to free the rectum of secondary adhesions with the pelvic walls that formed as a consequence of the previous inflammation and surgery. At times, this maneuver helps. More frequently, however, the use of progressive sizers or Hegar dilators is necessary. Once again, we recommend the use of a rigid proctoscope prior to using any of these tools that will be pushed blindly against the rectal walls. In the worst cases, where the stapler cannot reach the top of the rectal stump, the spike is pushed through the rectal wall distal and anterior to the staple line resulting in an end-to-side anastomosis. A small blind pouch of the rectum will be usually well tolerated. However, if a larger pouch is left behind, this will have to be resected by firing another load of the endoscopic linear stapler.

An end-to-end colorectal anastomosis is then undertaken with direct vision by deploying the trocar through the top of the rectal stump. It is very important to deploy the trocar completely through the rectum to ensure a watertight closure of the stapler. Furthermore, it is important to ensure that the spike is not accidentally pulled back into the rectum, since this could lead to two separate openings on the rectal top, thus increasing the chances of a leak, if one of the openings falls outside the anastomosis area.

The anvil in the descending colon is held using endoscopic Babcock. (**Tip:** some surgeons find helpful to place the camera in the right iliac fossa port to facilitate the connection of the anvil with the spike.) After securing the anvil to the spike, and prior to closing the stapler, one should ensure that the colon is not rotated. The stapler is then closed under direct vision ensuring that no surrounding structure such as ureter, bladder, gonadal vessels, hypogastric nerves, and in some cases, vagina are not accidentally grasped and pulled into the anastomosis.

The EEA device is then fired and carefully removed. The completeness of the two donuts is verified. The anastomosis is then tested: the colon is clamped with a bowel clamp proximal to the staple line and saline is placed in the pelvis to submerge the anastomosis. The rectum is then insufflated either with a rigid proctoscope or using an Asepto syringe. The absence of air bubbling from the anastomosis will confirm a good seal. If air bubbles are seen, one should first locate the area or areas of leak, and then perform a repair instantly using endo-stitch devices or freehand suturing.

Hand-assisted Hartmann's Reversal

The use of the surgeon's trained hand during this particularly challenging operation may facilitate the successful completion of laparoscopy by reducing the technical difficulty of the operation. In fact, this could additionally expedite the case, therefore, avoiding excessive operating time while possibly maintaining the benefits of a smaller incision. It is also conceivable that in cases which are particularly intricate laparoscopically, converting to a hand-assisted technique might avoid to proceed to a full laparotomy. The use of hand-assisted laparoscopy in Hartmann reversal may also be seen as a bridge to full laparoscopic cases by providing a tactile feedback during the learning curve of advanced laparoscopic colorectal surgery. Conversely, one might argue that using a blunt dissection in a limited, fibrotic space during Hartmann reversal could lead to excessive bleeding. In addition, the recommended minimal 7-cm incision necessary to accommodate a hand (for 7½ glove) compares poorly to the fascial defect left by the previous colostomy, which should be limited to 2–3 cm (18).

In 2000, Lucarini et al. described the hand-assisted Hartmann reversal by using the Dexterity® Pneumo Sleeve™ (20). Today, the procedure can be more simply performed by using the GelPort (Applied Medical).

Similarly to the laparoscopic reversal, the operation begins by mobilizing the colostomy. This is done by extending the incision transversely for about 7 cm. The descending colon is completely mobilized and brought into the operative field. The anvil is placed within the colon, secured, and then returned into the abdomen; the GelPort is then placed. An initial exploration of the abdomen can be done at this time by carefully introducing the hand. If the area near the umbilicus appears free of adhesions the Hasson trocar can be placed at this time. If there is no space to place the trocar or if extensive local adhesions prevent further progress, we normally place trocars through the GelPort including the camera and generate the pneumoperitoneum. Two working ports and the camera port are helpful to start mobilizing the adhesions from the anterior abdominal wall. In a few lucky cases, the entire operation could be completed through this access. However, in general as soon as possible, the Hasson trocar is placed at the umbilicus and one or two ports are placed on the right side. In the original technique (20), the authors recommend to have the surgeon stand on the left side of the patient and uses his/her left hand through the sleeve. If the surgeon has difficulty working against the camera, he/she could move to the right side of the patient.

In this procedure, the hand can be used to assist in the dissection of the rectal stump or in the mobilization of the splenic flexure particularly in cases where considerable difficulty is encountered. The use of the hand could be particularly helpful in case of very extensive adhesions and in morbidly obese people (20).

Alternatively, the hand-assisted device could be inserted using a Pfannenstiel incision, which allows for an unobstructed view of the rectum and direct access to the colorectal anastomosis.

Once the rectum is identified and the descending colon properly mobilized, the operation can be completed as described previously. If a Pfannenstiel incision had been made, the colorectal anastomosis can be done under direct view and in case of air leaks, the anastomosis can be reinforced in an "open" fashion.

Single-Port Laparoscopic Hartmann's Reversal

The reduction in number of port access to the abdomen and the absence of incision may not be a simple cosmetic advantage, which in these patients who already have a midline incision might be relative, but may minimize the risks of wound infections as well as incisional hernia, and improve postoperative pain (21).

However, as of today, the use of single-port technique in the reversal of Hartmann has not gained popularity. According to Leroy et al., in a systematic review of the English literature from July 2008 to July 2010, 29 articles, and one systematic review, a total of 149 patients have been reported as undergoing colorectal single-port procedures (21). Not a single case of Hartmann reversal was found in this review.

We have performed four cases of single-port reversal of Hartmann. Three of these cases were done by using the colostomy site for the placement of a single-port device.

There are many commercial single port laparoscopic devices and the selection depends on the surgeon's preference and comfort.

The single-port device is inserted through the stoma site after taking down the stoma and inserting the anvil as described above. After inserting the single port, the 5-mm Olympus EndoEYE™ Surgical Videoscope is used as a camera. The patient needs to be tilted to the right and in a Trendelenburg position. After positioning of the patient, the mobilization of the left colon is started. One can use a 5- or 10-mm sealing device and bowel grasper for the dissection. In some single-port devices, you have the ability to use a 4th port. Given the small size of the incision, however, in some cases another port could become more a hindrance than a help. The lysis of adhesions is undertaken, at least initially, by standing on the left side of the patient.

Subsequently, during the mobilization of the descending colon the surgeon may find it helpful to stand in between the legs of the patient. The dissection is started via a lateral to medial approach extended all the way to the splenic flexure using a 5-mm sealing device of choice or the electrocautery. By retracting the colon medially, the ureter and the gonadal vessels are visualized and protected. The mesentery is also mobilized toward the midline from the retroperitoneum and the Gerota's fascia. The splenic flexure is then mobilized as needed. This will be helped by placing the patient in a reverse Trendelenburg position.

Once this part is completed, I return to the left side of the patient and the bed is returned to a Trendelenburg position.

The rectal stump is subsequently mobilized in the same manner as described above. If a remnant sigmoid colon needs to be resected, an Endo GIA can be used to resect the remnant and the specimen is extracted through the single port. The colorectal anastomosis is then carried out in the same fashion as described above.

 POSTOPERATIVE MANAGEMENT

In our practice, the patient is usually placed on a fast track regimen, which includes removal of the orogastric or the nasogastric tube at the end of surgery and placing the patient on a clear liquid diet the day of surgery or on postoperative day 1. The patient is offered a solid diet on postoperative day 2, and the bladder catheter is removed on postoperative day 1; drains are not routinely used. The exception is represented by extensive pelvic dissection of the rectum, potentially associated with more bleeding. DVT prophylaxis is always implemented until discharge.

In our practice, the patient is discharged home when tolerating a solid diet and after a bowel movement. However, it is becoming more common among colorectal surgeons to discharge the patient even without a bowel movement if he/she tolerates a solid diet and is passing flatus.

 COMPLICATIONS

Wound infection was found to be one of the most common complications of laparoscopic HR (10.8%). Early complications include also anesthesia and cardiopulmonary complications. These are followed by other common postoperative complications such as anastomotic leak, abscess, postoperative bleeding, and prolonged postoperative ileus.

Two meta-analyses available in the literature did show a benefit in terms of complications in the LHR group (8,22). Both reviews showed a lower rate of perioperative complications, and a shorter postoperative stay. Van de Wall et al. found an overall morbidity rate of 12.2% in LHR versus 20.3% in OHR (16). In this review, the decrease in complication rate was mainly found for wound infection (mean 10.8% vs. 14.2%), anastomotic leakage (mean 1.2% vs. 5.1%), and cardiopulmonary complications (mean 3.6% vs. 6.9%). In addition, a lower incidence of reoperation was found in LHR versus OHR (mean 3.6% vs. 6.9%). However, the other meta-analysis by Siddiqui et al. found no difference in infection rates, ileus, and leak rates. Conversely, this review found a statistically significant reduction in blood loss in the LHR ($P < 0.001$).

Late complications are adhesions, small-bowel obstruction, and stricture. No significant data is available to show any difference in terms of incidence of late complications between LHR and OHR.

 RESULTS

Based on the data available it appears that laparoscopic Hartmann's reversal is safe and results in fewer complications and shorter hospital stays compared with open reversal. The operation is obviously burdened by a considerable technical complexity. Conversion rates of up to 22%, and a limited number of series available in the literature reflect this (8). In addition, these series tend to comprise a limited number of patients. Therefore, selection biases may have had a role in the results presented in these series. Van de Wall found, for example, that patients treated with LHR were slightly younger (55 vs. 61), tended to have different indications for the original surgeries, and had a shorter mean interval between the Hartmann procedure and its reversal, compared to those who underwent OHR (8). In this analysis, 12 series comprising a total of 396 patients in the LHR group versus 5,853 patients in the OHR were reviewed.

In a more recent meta-analysis by Siddiqui et al. (22), eight studies were included in the final analysis and reviewed, with a total of 450 patients. There were only 193 patients in the laparoscopic group and 257 in the open group. Interestingly, in this review, OHR appeared to have longer operative times than LHR, although this was not statistically significant. Conversion rate was around 10% (19). Faure et al. reported a conversion rate of 14.28% of laparoscopic Hartmann's reversal with a shorter operating time and less morbidity compared with open Hartmann's reversal (23). The learning curve may now be to the point where a shorter operative time may direct more patients to undergo LHR. This may hopefully facilitate randomized studies with larger cohorts of patients.

To date, the data available show that patients undergoing OHR do not appear to fare better than patients treated with LHR and that LHR is comparable or even superior to OHR (22) in terms of shorter hospital stay, reduced complications rate, reduced postoperative pain, and earlier return to normal activity. Therefore, LHR is feasible and safe to do but does require experience and is not one of the easiest laparoscopic cases to do.

References

1. Hartmann H. Nouveau procede d'ablation des cancers de la partie terminale du colon pelvien. *Trentieme Congress de Chirurgie. Strasbourg France* 1923;411–13.
2. Bell C, Asolati M, Hamilton E, et al. A comparison of complications associated with colostomy reversal versus ileostomy reversal. *Am J Surg* 2005;190(5):717–20.
3. Vermeulen J, Coene PP, Van Hout NM, et al. Restoration of bowel continuity after surgery for acute perforated diverticulitis: should Hartmann's procedure be considered a one-stage procedure? *Colorectal Dis* 2008;11:619–24.
4. Rosen MJ, Cobb WS, Kercher KW, Heniford BT. Laparoscopic versus open colostomy reversal: a comparative analysis. *J Gastrointest Surg* 2006;10(6):895–900.
5. Keck JO, Collopy BT, Ryan PJ, et al. Reversal of Hartmann's procedure: effect of timing and technique on ease and safety. *Dis Colon Rectum* 1994;37(3):243–48. Review.
6. Sosa JL, Sleeman D, Puente I, et al. Laparoscopic-assisted colostomy closure after Hartmann's procedure. *Dis Colon Rectum* 1994;37(2):149–52.
7. Mazeh H, Greenstein AJ, Swedish K, et al. Laparoscopic and open reversal of Hartmann's procedure—a comparative retrospective analysis. *Surg Endosc* 2009;23(3):496–502.
8. Van de Wall BJM, Draaisma WA, Schouten ES, et al. Conventional and laparoscopic reversal of the Hartmann procedure: a review of literature. *J Gastrointest Surg* 2010;14:743–52.
9. Khaikin M, Zmora O, Rosin D, et al. Laparoscopically assisted reversal of Hartmann's procedure. *Surg Endosc* 2006;20(12):1883–86.
10. Alves A, Panis Y, Slim K, et al. Association Français de Chirurgie French multicentre prospective observational study of laparoscopic versus open colectomy for sigmoid diverticular disease. *Br J Surg* 2005;92(12):1520–25.
11. Schwenk W, Haase O, Neudecker J, Müller JM. Short term benefits for laparoscopic colorectal resection. *Cochrane Database Syst Rev* 2005;(3):CD003145. Review.
12. Braga M, Vignali A, Gianotti L, et al. Laparoscopic versus open colorectal surgery: a randomized trial on short-term outcome. *Ann Surg* 2002;236(6):759–66; discussion 767.
13. Degiuli M, Mineccia M, Bertone A, et al. Outcome of laparoscopic colorectal resection. *Surg Endosc* 2004;18(3):427–32. Epub Feb 2, 2004. Review.
14. Braga M, Vignali A, Zuliani W, et al. Laparoscopic versus open colorectal surgery: cost-benefit analysis in a single-center randomized trial. *Ann Surg* 2005;242(6):890–95, discussion 895–96.
15. Regadas FS, Siebra JA, Rodrigues LV, et al. Complications in laparoscopic colorectal resection: main types and prevention. *Surg Laparosc Endosc* 1998;8:189–92.
16. Vacher C, Zaghloul R, Borie F, et al. Laparoscopic re-establishment of digestive continuity following Hartmann's procedure. Retrospective study of the French Society of Endoscopic Surgery. *Ann Chir* 2002;127:189–92.
17. Guenaga KK, Matos D, Wille-Jørgensen P. Mechanical bowel preparation for elective colorectal surgery. *Cochrane Database Syst Rev* 2009;(1):CD001544.
18. Rosen MJ, Cobb WS, Kercher KW, et al. Laparoscopic restoration of intestinal continuity after Hartmann's procedure. *Am J Surg* 2005;189:670–74.
19. Anderson CA, Fowler DL, White S, Wintz N. Laparoscopic colostomy closure. *Surg Laparosc Endosc* 1993;3(1):69–72.
20. Lucarini L, Galleano R, Lombezzi R, et al. Laparoscopic-assisted Hartmann's reversal with the Dexterity Pneumo Sleeve. *Dis Colon Rectum* 2000;43(8):1164–67.
21. Diana M, Dhumane P, Cahill RA, et al. Minimal invasive single-site surgery in colorectal procedures: current state of the art. *J Minim Access Surg* 2011;7(1):52–60.
22. Siddiqui M, Sajid M, Baig M. Open versus laparoscopic approach for reversal of Hartmann's procedure: a systematic review. *Colorectal Dis* 2010;12(8):733–41.
23. Faure JP, Doucet C, Essique D, et al. Comparison of conventional and laparoscopic Hartmann's procedure reversal. *Surg Laparosc Endosc Percutan Tech* 2007;17(6):495–99.

49 Hand-Assisted Hartmann's Reversal

David E. Rivadeneira and Thomas E. Read

 ## INDICATIONS/CONTRAINDICATIONS

Indication

The benefits of laparoscopic techniques in colon and rectal surgery have been extensively reported and include a reduction in hospital stay, postoperative pain, and narcotic requirements with improvements in gastrointestinal function. A reduction in postoperative convalescence, improved cosmesis, reduction in postoperative wound complications, and decrease in adhesion formation have also been reported as advantages of laparoscopic approach (1–5).

Often the largest incision in laparoscopic colon and rectal procedures is usually dictated by the size of the specimen being removed, or the extraction site. In straight laparoscopic or laparoscopic-assisted methods, the extraction site, which often measures from 3 to 10 cm is often performed after a substantial amount of time and effort, has been expended in identifying vital structures, dissecting soft tissue planes, isolation and ligation of mesenteric vessels, and transaction of bowel wall. Often this approach seems counter-intuitive, in that a surgeon would spend a significant amount of time and effort to perform a minimally invasive laparoscopic colon and/or rectal resection and then at the end of the case to create a much larger incision for an extraction site in order to complete the procedure. Excluded from this discussion are those surgeons who perform laparoscopic colon and rectal resections via a transrectal or transvaginal extraction site. The utility and adoption of these natural orifice extraction sites are still in progress and will need some time to mature.

Hand-assisted laparoscopic surgery (HALS) is a method in which the surgeon is able to place an entire hand at times during the operation into the abdomen through a specially designed hand-assisted device or port while maintaining pneumoperitoneum. The benefit of HALS is that the extraction site can be used from the outset of the operation and will allow the return of tactile sensation, improved spatial relationships, allows for rapid exploration of the abdomen, enabling palpation of intra-abdominal organs and masses, offers excellent assistance with retraction and nontraumatic retraction of tissue planes, and blunt finger dissection. Introduction of the hand-assisted method can assist in dealing with a hostile abdomen with inflammatory processes or patients with extensive adhesions; in addition, it can allow for rapid control of hemorrhage and may overall allow laparoscopic completion of a procedure that otherwise would be converted (6–14).

The most common indication for a laparoscopic approach to the restoration of intestinal continuity is colostomy takedown and construction of coloproctostomy following sigmoid colectomy for complicated diverticular disease or "Hartmann reversal." The hand-assisted laparoscopic method can be an ideal approach in certain patients undergoing a Hartman's reversal (15). During the operation the colostomy site on the abdominal wall can be used as the entrance site for the hand-assisted laparoscopic device, in addition a substantial amount of adhesiolysis and mobilization can often be performed through the stoma incision, facilitating the entire procedure. Often a parastomal hernia is present which makes the placement of a hand through the incision much easier. The hand-assisted method can aid in blunt dissection and mobilization of the descending colon and splenic flexure in anticipation for a colorectal anastomosis. Mobilization of the stoma itself prior to establishing laparoscopic access also allows for the surgeon to assess intraperitoneal conditions and make a decision on whether laparoscopy is appropriate or not. If the laparoscopic equipment is kept unopened in the operating theatre prior to this assessment, cost savings can be realized in patients who require formal laparotomy, in that laparoscopy is never utilized and thus no conversion occurs. This is a similar concept to the "Peek Port" method that has been described for patients with complex colorectal disease who are contemplated for laparoscopic colectomy (16).

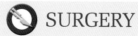

PREOPERATIVE PLANNING

Patients undergoing a hand-assisted Hartman's reversal should undergo all the necessary preoperative preparations that most patients undergoing open or laparoscopic methods. These include the following:

- Preoperative imaging studies, which may include CT scans of the abdomen and pelvis
- Retrograde contrast studies through the rectum and colostomy site
- Colonoscopy if clinically indicated

These studies should indicate to the surgeons the length and quality of the rectal/ Hartman's stump and position of the splenic flexure. Prior to embarking on a laparoscopic reversal of a Hartmann's procedure performed for diverticular disease, the surgeon should consider that it may be necessary to resect the retained sigmoid colon and mobilize the splenic flexure to allow soft descending colon to reach easily into the pelvis for a colorectal anastomosis. Preoperative evaluation of the colon and distal rectal stump with endoscopy and/or contrast enema will help the surgeon plan the operative procedure and exclude alternative diagnoses. In addition, patients should undergo proper mechanical bowel preparation and DVT and antibiotic prophylaxis.

SURGERY

Positioning

Patients are positioned on an electric bed in the modified Lloyd-Davis/lithotomy position, or in the supine position on a split leg table. A proctosigmoidoscopy is performed to assess the rectal stump and to provide a wash-out of any retained stool or mucus. After the abdomen is prepped with chloraprep or betadine, a large sheet of antibiotic-impregnated adhesive draped (Ioban) is placed over the entire abdomen with a folded 4 × 4 gauze over the colostomy site. This will allow for minimal cross contamination to other areas of the abdominal wall. Laparoscopic monitors are placed to the right and left side of the patient. The use of standard bowel graspers, dissectors, sheers/scissors, and energy-based devices will be used during the procedure as in other laparoscopic procedures.

Technique

There are several approaches to a hand-assisted reversal of a Hartman's procedure. The one that makes the most sense and we recommend is using the colostomy site as the hand-assisted assess area. The colostomy is dissected away from the mucocutaneous junction, with an incision that extends both medially and laterally around the colostomy for several centimeters. Detaching the colon from the subcutaneous tissue is often a fairly unencumbered dissection due to the high incidence of a paracolostomy hernia. Entrance into the abdomen and placement of the hand through the hand-assisted device is often aided by the presence of a parastomal hernia and its fascial separation. Direct visualization into the abdomen can be performed very well from the incision and local adhesions can be dealt with effectively, particularly those intimate with a previous midline incision from the initial operation. Once the colostomy has been detached from the abdominal wall and the colon resected to a healthy segment, it is then prepared with a purse-string suture and placement of the anvil part of the stapling device and returned into the abdomen. The hand-assisted device or port is placed into the colostomy site incision and pneumoperitoneum is achieved. The addition of one to three 5-mm trocars are placed in the right lateral abdomen and suprapubic area, and will be used for the laparoscope/camera and the laparoscopic instruments. The surgeon can approach the operation from a position in between the legs and place the right hand through the hand-assisted device and use the left hand with a laparoscopic dissector or energy-based device through the right-sided trocars. The assistant can stand on the patient's right side and can hold the camera through a trocar on that side. Conversely, the surgeon can stand on the patient's right side and reach over to the hand device with either hand and dissect through trocars on the right side or suprapubic area with the remaining hand.

Once dissection of the left/descending colon and splenic flexure is performed, the rectal or Hartman's stump is identified and prepared. At times, it may be necessary to remove partial or complete remnant sigmoid colon which can be achieved expediently and safely with the hand-assisted method. The surgeon stands on the patients left hand side and can insert the right hand through the device grasp the sigmoid colon or rectal stump. Additional dissection can be undertaken with the right hand with laparoscopic instruments through the trocars on the right side. The specimen is extracted through the hand port. A standard stapled anastomosis is created with a circular stapler.

POSTOPERATIVE MANAGEMENT

The postoperative management of patients undergoing a hand-assisted reversal of a colostomy should follow the same protocols as those undergoing open or straight laparoscopic methods.

COMPLICATIONS

To our knowledge there are no intrinsic complications attributed to the hand-assisted approach. Postoperative complication will mirror those as performed in open or laparoscopic methods.

RESULTS

Although there is extensive data in regards to hand-assisted laparoscopic colon and rectal operations, there is a paucity of data specifically dealing with hand-assisted methods in this procedure. Currently, there does not exist any prospective, randomized studies looking at the laparoscopic versus hand-assisted methods in Hartman's reversals. Anecdotally, both authors have used a hand-assisted approach on many patients undergoing Hartmann's reversal with very positive outcomes.

References

1. Kennedy GD, Heise C, Rajamanickam V, et al. Laparoscopy decreases postoperative complication rates after abdominal colectomy: results from the national surgical quality improvement program. *Ann Surg* 2009;249(4):596–601.
2. Allardyce RA, Bagshaw PF, Frampton CM, et al. Australasian Laparoscopic Colon Cancer Study shows that elderly patients may benefit from lower postoperative complication rates following laparoscopic versus open resection. *Br J Surg* 2010;97(1):86–91.
3. Veldkamp R, Kuhry E, Hop WC, et al. Laparoscopic surgery versus open surgery for colon cancer: short-term outcomes of a randomised trial. *Lancet Oncol* 2005;6(7):477–84.
4. Weeks JC, Nelson H, Gelber S, et al. Clinical Outcomes of Surgical Therapy (COST) Study Group. Short-term quality-of-life outcomes following laparoscopic-assisted colectomy vs open colectomy for colon cancer: a randomized trial. *JAMA* 2002;287(3):321–28.
5. Lee SW. Laparoscopic procedures for colon and rectal cancer surgery. *Clin Colon Rectal Surg* 2009;22(4):218–24.
6. Orenstein SB, Elliott HL, Reines LA, Novitsky YW. Advantages of the hand-assisted versus the open approach to elective colectomies. *Surg Endosc* 2011;25(5):1364–68.
7. Litwin DE, Darzi A, Jakimowicz J, et al. Hand-assisted laparoscopic surgery (HALS) with the HandPort system: initial experience with 68 patients. *Ann Surg* 2000;231:715–23.
8. Hand-assisted laparoscopic surgery vs standard laparoscopic surgery for colorectal disease: a prospective randomized trial. HALS Study Group. *Surg Endosc* 2000;14:896–901.
9. Targarona EM, Gracia E, Garriga J, et al. Prospective randomized trial comparing conventional laparoscopic colectomy with hand-assisted laparoscopic colectomy: applicability, immediate clinical outcome, inflammatory response, and cost. *Surg Endosc* 2002;16:234–39.
10. Rivadeneira DE, Marcello PW, Roberts PL, et al. Benefits of hand-assisted laparoscopic restorative proctocolectomy: a comparative study. *Dis Colon Rectum* 2004;47:1371–76.
11. Kang JC, Chung MH, Chao PC, et al. Hand-assisted laparoscopic colectomy versus open colectomy: a prospective randomized study. *Surg Endosc* 2004;18:577–81.
12. Marcello PW, Fleshman JW, Milsom JW, et al. Hand-assisted laparoscopic versus laparoscopic colorectal surgery: a multicenter, prospective, randomized trial. *Dis Colon Rectum* 2008;51:818–26.
13. Rivadeneira DE, Marcello PW. Current status of hand-assisted laparoscopic colon and rectal surgery: do we need a hand? *Semin Colon Rectal Surg* 2003;14:154–60.
14. Pietrabissa A, Moretto C, Carobbi A, et al. Hand-assisted laparoscopic low anterior resection: initial experience with a new procedure. *Surg Endosc* 2002;16:431–35.
15. Lucarini L, Galleano R, Lombezzi R, et al. Laparoscopic-assisted Hartmann's reversal with the Dexterity Pneumo Sleeve. *Dis Colon Rectum* 2000;43:1164–67.
16. Read TE, Salgado J, Ferraro D, et al. "Peek port": a novel approach for avoiding conversion in laparoscopic colectomy. *Surg Endosc* 2008;23(3):477–81.

50 Abdominal Surgery for Rectal Prolapse

Laurence R. Sands

Introduction

Rectal prolapse remains a relatively rare colorectal problem that is seen more often in women than in men. It has been associated with a lack of fixity of the rectum to the sacrum, a deep rectovaginal or rectovesical pouch, poor lateral rectal attachments, and a weakened pelvic floor musculature (1).

Rectal prolapse is a completely benign disease process. However, it often causes significant disability and anxiety to those affected. Many chronically affected patients simply achieve spontaneous reduction of the prolapse; however, other individuals require daily manual reduction. In addition, some patients may present with incarceration of the prolapse that may require emergent surgical repair. Long term complications from prolapse may also result in anal sphincter laxity, which may result in varying degrees of fecal incontinence.

One of the more contentious debates in colon and rectal surgery arises from the proper way by which to repair rectal prolapse. There have been numerous procedures described to surgically fix this problem, which must make both the patient and surgeon wary that no one has ever found the perfect operation for this condition. This situation is in part due to the fact that there is a general lack of consensus on the etiology of rectal prolapse. As such each operation is designed to address a particular aspect of the theorized to cause rectal prolapse.

The debate generally focuses on either abdominal or perineal repairs. The abdominal procedures will be the focus of this chapter. The basic premise behind all of these approaches is to lift the rectum and fixate it to the sacrum. This manouvre may be combined with resection of a portion of redundant sigmoid colon as well.

 ## INDICATIONS AND CONTRAINDICATIONS

The indications for surgery for rectal prolapse are quite simple: the mere existence of prolapse is an indication for repair since there is no non-surgical remedy for this problem. Therefore the most important aspect for the surgeon is to be certain of the diagnosis prior

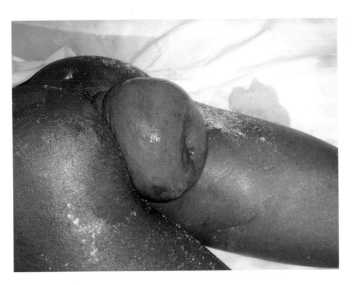

Figure 50.1 Full thickness rectal prolapse.

to attempting repair. The most commonly confused diagnosis that may resemble full thickness rectal prolapse is severe hemorrhoidal disease. In fact, at many institutions the emergency room physicians commonly refer to prolapsing internal hemorrhoids as rectal prolapse. It requires a more experienced clinician to determine the difference between these two entities because the therapies for each condition are quite different.

First the history may lend itself to establishing the diagnosis. The chronicity, the timing of the prolapse (whether it occurs spontaneously or with a bowel movement), and the degree of prolapse about which the patient complains may allow the physician to distinguish between the two entities. A detailed history of stool control and constipation, if any, should also be elicited.

Physical examination is confirmatory as the appearance of full thickness rectal prolapse is often very obvious and distinct from hemorrhoidal disease (Fig. 50.1).

It often has characteristic concentric rings as opposed to the wedge shaped abnormalities associated with prolapsing hemorrhoids (Fig. 50.2). Rectal prolapse may not be visible on initial examination of the patient and it may require the patient squatting on the toilet to reproduce the prolapse. This assessment should be part of the physical exam if the prolapse is not immediately obvious. In addition, one should assess sphincter tone and whether the anus appears patulous at the time of the physical exam, often a sign of chronicity of the condition.

The reasons not to repair prolapse may vary, but may be as simple as the patient not wishing to have the surgery or the patient being too ill with many comorbidities

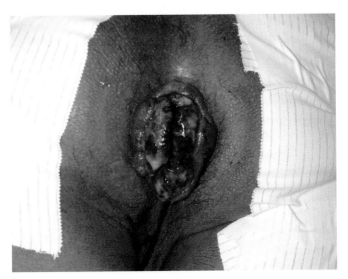

Figure 50.2 Incarcerated grade four hermorrhoids.

making the patient a prohibitively high operative risk. As this condition is more often found in the aging population, more conservative surgical approaches may be considered in view of the inability for these sicker patients to tolerate a major surgical procedure. As such these patients traditionally undergo a perineal procedure for prolapse. Abdominal procedures for prolapse have been preferred by many surgeons due to their durability, low recurrence rates, and correction of many of the anatomic deficiencies that may have caused the prolapse in the first place.

 PREOPERATIVE PLANNING

The essential element in planning for surgery includes deciding on the proper approach to repair the prolapse. A recent review of the Cochrane Database relating to rectal prolapse makes this decision even more difficult. A detailed review of the literature in this database found 12 randomized controlled trials relating to rectal prolapse surgery; one trial compared abdominal with perineal approaches for surgery, three trials compared different fixation methods, three trials reviewed division of lateral ligaments, one trial compared techniques of rectosigmoid resection, two trials compared laparoscopic with open surgery, and two trials compared resection with no resection and rectopexy. The reviewers concluded that there were insufficient data to determine whether abdominal or perineal approaches for rectal superior. They found no differences in the various techniques used for rectopexy but did see lower recurrence rates with division of the lateral ligaments but with increased incidences of constipation. Lower constipation rates were noted in those who underwent segmental resection. In addition, laparoscopic cases had fewer complications and shorter hospital stays (2).

One study attempted to demonstrate a clinical exam that may help determine whether a patient should undergo abdominal or perineal repair of the prolapse. These authors describe a "hook test" based on rectal examination to decide whether patients have a low-type of prolapse or a high type. They claim that better results may be obtained with a perineal procedure for low type prolapses (3).

A single surgeon experience over 21 years evaluated and compared those patients with external rectal prolapse who underwent either transperineal or transabdominal repair of the prolapse. He found that those patients undergoing an abdominal procedure had a significantly lower recurrence rate, an improved incontinence score, but a higher constipation rate. He concluded that one must consider the alternatives in repair and tailor them to the individual patient based on the presenting patient's overall degree of fitness and functional disorders (4).

As previously mentioned, if the patient is younger and generally fit, an abdominal procedure is ideal. Once this decision has been made, one must then choose which abdominal procedure to actually perform. A basic list of the procedures includes:

- Sigmoid resection and rectopexy with or without the use of the laparoscope
- Rectopexy alone with or without the use of the laparoscope

In addition, the rectopexy may be done in many different ways including the use of straight nonabsorbable suture material or the use of prosthetic products such as a mesh. Others have advocated simply mobilizing the rectum in the presacral space and allowing natural scar tissue to form, thereby preventing recurrence of the prolapse.

The decision to combine colon resection with rectopexy is made prior to surgery. This decision is often made based on the patient's history and preoperative physiologic studies. Patients with fecal incontinence or constipation are often evaluated preoperatively with anal manometry and colonic transit studies. Those with severe constipation are generally offered concomitant segmental colon resection while those with incontinence, diarrhea, or normal function may be safely offered rectopexy without sigmoid resection (5).

Rectal mobilization should be preoperatively planned as well since many surgeons differ in their approach of mobilizing the rectum. While many surgeons perform a posterior mobilization, many others oppose this approach for fear of injuring presacral nerves and veins and leaving the patients with sexual and urinary complications. Some surgeons divide the lateral ligaments while others leave them intact. Still others prefer to mobilize the rectum circumferentially to lift the rectum as high as possible out of the pelvis.

As in every case of abdominal surgery, the patient should be deemed medically fit to undergo the procedure, and the patients should receive both antibiotic prophylaxis to cover gram-negative organisms and anaerobes as well as prophylaxis to prevent deep vein thrombosis.

The planning steps for this procedure may be summarized as follows:

- Careful history and physical examination
- Fecal incontinence score
- Assess for signs and symptoms of constipation
- If constipation is present then perform anorectal physiologic studies and colonic transit study:
- Assess sphincter tone
- Preoperative clearance and surgical risk assessment
- Decide on abdominal versus perineal procedure
- Abdominal procedures
  - Open resection with rectopexy
  - Open rectopexy (no suture, suture, prosthetic material)
  - Laparoscopic resection with rectopexy
  - Laparoscopic rectopexy (no suture, suture, prosthetic material)

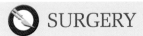 SURGERY

Patient Positioning and Preparation

The patient is placed under general anesthesia and then in a low-lying lithotomy position. The arms may be tucked at each side in the event laparoscopy is being done. The rectum may be irrigated in preparation for a rectal anastomosis if sigmoid resection is contemplated.

Surgical Technique

The use of laparoscopy in the treatment of rectal prolapse may have far greater benefit in the event that sigmoid resection is not planned. The rational is that the sigmoid colon is often very redundant and the resection requires that an incision be made to extract the specimen. The resection is often easy to perform through this rather small incision thereby obviating the need for the laparoscope, thus potentially saving time and operative expense.

Once the incision has been made, the presacral space may be easily entered through lateral windows, taking care not to injure the superior rectal vessels. The dissection may be continued posteriorly all the way to the pelvic floor. This space is an avascular plane and the mobilization should be performed to the tip of the coccyx. The surgeon must decide whether to leave the lateral ligaments of the rectum attached; many surgeons feel that these attachments prevent recurrent prolapse. However, there are other surgeons who circumferentially mobilize the entire rectum to be sure that the rectum is lifted up as high as possible prior to suturing and securing it to the presacral fascia. This fixation may be done with simple sutures or may be performed with prosthetic material such as mesh. The sutures are placed in the lower aspect of the mesorectum and sutured to the fascia overlying on the top of the sacral promontory. One must be careful not to injure the presacral veins, the nerves overlying the promontory, or the ureters when placing these sutures. At least two such stitches are placed, one on each side of the mesorectum.

The original procedure described by Ripstein involved mobilizing the rectum down to the coccyx and then placing a piece of mesh around the anterior aspect of the rectum at the level of the peritoneal reflection and then suturing this mesh to the presacral fascia. He felt that by changing the angle of the rectum with this type of anterior sling, recurrent prolapse would be prevented. He reported his series of 289 patients in 1972 and demonstrated just one death and no recurrences with this technique (6).

Gordon and Hoexter later reported a review of many other colorectal surgeons utilizing this approach in over 1,000 patients. While they showed a recurrence rate of only 2.3%, they did find considerable morbidity with a complication rate of 16.6%, the most common of which was fecal impaction possibly related to the sling being too tight or the angle of the rectum being too acute. Mesh erosion was also noted in a very small percentage of patients (7).

The procedure described by Wells using an Ivalon (polyvinyl alcohol) sponge was adopted in the United Kingdom. This procedure mobilizes the rectum, fixes the sponge posteriorly to the mesorectum, and then attaches the sponge to the presacral fascia. The advantage of this technique is that the anterior rectal wall is not wrapped as in Ripstein's procedure and thus the rectal lumen is not narrowed. This narrowing was felt to be the main cause of constipation and fecal impaction that was seen in the Ripstein procedure (8). The worst complication of the Well's procedure is pelvic abscess, which may require sponge removal. Abscess rates as high as 16% have been reported with this technique (9) and the procedure is no longer performed.

Frykman introduced the idea of sigmoid resection combined with rectopexy in 1955 (10). He described the procedure removing the redundant sigmoid colon after adequate mobilization to create a tension free anastomosis to the high rectum, full rectal mobilization to the pelvic floor lifting the rectum and suturing the lateral ligaments to the periosteum of the sacrum, and then suturing the endopelvic fascia anteriorly to obliterate the deep pelvic cul-de-sac. Goldberg popularized this procedure and it is now more commonly referred to as the Frykman-Goldberg procedure for prolapse. Recurrence rates have generally been reported between 0 and 9% but with operative morbidity varying from 0–23%.

Other techniques for rectal prolapse repair include the use of laparoscopy. True benefits in the management of many colonic diseases have been clearly demonstrated with laparoscopy. Doctors Senagore and Delaney have shown shorter hospital stays, lower wound infection rates, and improved postoperative cardiopulmonary status after performing 1,000 laparoscopic colectomies for various pathologies in a single institution (11). The laparoscopic approach for prolapse may include rectal mobilization, mesh placement, sutured rectopexy, sigmoid colectomy, and any combination of these procedures.

Alternatively, exclusion procedures have also been rarely done to treat rectal prolapse, and they are mentioned in this chapter merely for completeness. The technique as described by Lahaut is performed by mobilizing the rectosigmoid colon and then implanting it within the posterior rectus sheath. Thirty-four patients who underwent this type of surgery reported no recurrent prolapse although one patient died postoperatively. Eleven out of twelve patients reported improvement in continence with this procedure (12).

Postoperative Management

The patient is admitted to a regular surgical floor immediately after the recovery room. Nasogastric tubes are not routinely used and orders are written for a clear liquid diet after immediate recovery from surgery. Patients are generally offered regular food once they have passed flatus or stool. Foley catheters are typically left in place for a day or two after surgery to monitor urinary output. Because of the pelvic dissection, urinary retention may occur upon bladder catheter removal; if this occurs, the catheter is replaced for several more days. The patients are considered ready for discharge home once they start tolerating a regular diet and are able to have a normal bowel movement.

Some centers have even questioned the need for hospital admission to treat this condition. A recent publication suggested that a laparoscopic rectopexy may be performed as an outpatient. The surgeons specifically selected 12 patients for this type of surgery based on their personal motivation, younger age, and generally overall fit state. Only one of the patients required a return visit to the emergency room for diarrhea while many others were able to stop analgesia soon after surgery. The patients were so pleased with the procedure that most would even have recommended this to other patients needing this type of surgery. The authors demonstrated a significant cost savings with this approach (13).

Complications

Immediate operative complications of bleeding or injuring other intraabdominal structures during surgery are quite rare. Meticulous hemostasis along with identifying all anatomical structures should always be performed. The left ureter should be seen crossing the pelvic brim so as to not injure it during the procedure. In addition, thermal injury from the harmonic scalpel or bipolar device must be considered when nearing the pelvic sidewall structures.

Delayed complications such as wound infection and anastomotic leak present themselves as they do in any other major abdominal procedures. Anastomotic leak, although relatively rare for high colorectal anastomoses, may be completely avoided in those patients merely undergoing rectopexy without resection. The use of laparoscopy has been shown to minimize the risk of wound infection as well.

Recurrence, while not an immediate complication after abdominal procedures for prolapse, remains relatively low.

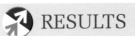 RESULTS

The results of abdominal procedures for rectal prolapse are quite good. While the procedures generally carry a higher morbidity than perineal procedures, they do seem to withstand the test of time and have fewer recurrences of the prolapse overall. The results however, are difficult to summarize and compare since there have been so many different abdominal procedures done for prolapse. However, a recent study from Norway clearly demonstrated the superiority of long-term patency of abdominal procedures for this condition. In their retrospective review, they demonstrated a 5-year patency of abdominal procedures of 93% with improved continence and stool evacuation. All patients undergoing either a Delorme or Thiersch procedure recurred within 5 years. They reported no recurrences after mesh rectopexy and concluded that abdominal procedures for prolapse are far more durable (14).

Some surgeons have advocated anterior rectal dissection and rectopexy rather than posterior or full thickness rectal mobilization in an effort to minimize sexual and urinary dysfunction. This ventral rectopexy procedure was performed in 65 consecutive older patients with full thickness rectal prolapse through a laparoscopic approach with improvement in fecal incontinence scores as well as constipation in the majority of patients. Only one patient recurred their rectal prolapse. The authors felt that even older patients may benefit from this procedure with a low morbidity and avoid the risk of bowel resection and anastomosis (15).

Another study from Belgium of 109 consecutive patients with full thickness rectal prolapse underwent laparoscopic ventral rectopexy avoiding posterior dissection and risk of injuring presacral nerves and vessels. The authors applied an anterior mesh to prevent intussusception and recurrent prolapse. Four patients underwent conversion to open surgery with an overall recurrence rate of 3.6% (16).

Another study evaluating the long-term outcome of laparoscopic compared to open repair for rectal prolapse reported similar recurrence rates long term but shorter hospital stays with the laparoscopic patients. Continence and constipation was generally improved in each group (17).

Other surgeons have also claimed that the need and risk of resection may not be necessary. In a recent publication, 70 patients with rectal prolapse and normal preoperative transit studies underwent suture fixation of the rectum alone after mobilizing the rectum but leaving the lateral stalks intact. These procedures were all done through a low-lying left lower quadrant incision exposing the presacral space. While they reported a recurrence rate of 7%, they also showed that no patients became constipated after surgery and 81% of patients had improvement in fecal control with a significant improvement in both anal canal manometric resting and squeeze pressures (18).

An Australian group compared their results of laparoscopic rectopexy to those procedures done in an open fashion. They found that five patients of the 126 (4%) who underwent laparoscopic rectopexy developed recurrence compared to one patient of the 46 in the open group (2.4%). These results did not reach statistical significance and they concluded that a laparoscopic approach to treat rectal prolapse was reasonable and safe (19).

The issue of whether abdominal surgery for prolapse is well tolerated in the older and infirmed patients was evaluated in a study from Finland. These authors performed either laparoscopic or open abdominal procedures for prolapse with half of the patients having an ASA class of III or IV. There was no mortality and only minor morbidity and operative times were similar for both laparoscopic and open rectopexy. Each surgical approach improved fecal control and nearly all of the patients were pleased with their results. There were only two recurrences of the 75 patients treated in total. The majority of the patients underwent laparoscopic surgery with a shorter hospital stay than those undergoing open surgery (20).

In summary, abdominal procedures for rectal prolapse are well tolerated even amongst the elderly. These approaches provide an excellent solution for a socially debilitating problem with good long-term outcome. They remain the approach of choice to which all other methods need be compared.

Suggested Readings

Gordon PH, Nivatvongs S. Principles and Practice of Surgery for the Colon, Rectum, and Anus: Quality Medical Publishing

Keighley MRB and Williams NS. Surgery of the Colon Rectum and Anus: WB Saunders.

Recommended References and Readings

1. Keighley MRB, Williams NS. *Surgery of the Anus Rectum and Colon.* Philadelphia, PA: WB Saunders, 1997:794.
2. Tou S, Brown SR, Malik AI, Nelson RL. Surgery for complete rectal prolapse in adults. *Cochrane Database Syst Rev* 2008;(4):CD001758.
3. Marzouk D, Ramdass MJ, Haji A, Akhtar M. Digital assessment of lower rectum fixity in rectal prolapse (DALR): a simple clinical anatomical test to determine the most suitable approach (abdominal versus perineal) for repair. *Surg Radiol Anat.* 2005; 27(5):414–19.
4. Pescatori M, Zbar AP. Tailored surgery for internal and external rectal prolapse: functional results of 268 patients operated upon by a single surgeon over a 21 year period. *Colorectal Dis* 2009;11(4):410–19.
5. Delaney CP. Laparoscopic management of rectal prolapse. *J Gastrointest Surg* 2007;11(2):150–52.
6. Ripstein CP. Definitive corrective surgery. *Dis Colon Rectum* 1972;15:334–46.
7. Gordon PH, Hoexter B. Complications of ripstein procedure. *Dis Colon Rectum* 1978;21:277–80.
8. Wells C. New operation for rectal prolapse. *Proc R Soc Med* 1959;52:602–03.
9. Kupfer CA, Goligher JC. One hundred consecutive cases of complete prolapse of the rectum treated by operation. *Br J Surg* 1970;57:481–87.
10. Frykman HM. Abdominal proctopexy and primary sigmoid resection for rectal procidentia. *Am J Surg* 1955;90:780–89.
11. Senagore AJ, Delaney CP. A critical analysis of laparoscopic colectomy at a single institution: lessons learned after 1000 cases. *Am J Surg* 2006;191(3):377–80.
12. Mortensen NJ, Vellacott KD, Wilson MG. Lahaut's operation for rectal prolapse. *Ann R Coll Surg Engl* 1984;66(1):17–18.
13. Vijay V, Halbert J, Zissimopoulos A, et al. *Surg Endosc* 2008;22(5):1237–40.
14. Hoel AT, Skarstein A, Ovrebo KK. Prolapse of the rectum, long-term results of surgical treatment. *Int J Colorectal Dis* 2009; 24(2):201–07.
15. Boons P, Collinson R, Cunningham C, Lindsay I. Laparoscopic ventral rectopexy for external rectal prolapse improves and avoids de novo constipation. *Colorectal Dis* 2009;12(6): 526–32.
16. D'Hoore A, Penninckx F. Laparoscopic ventral recto(colopo) pexy for rectal prolapse: surgical technique and outcome for 109 patients. *Surg Endosc.* 2006;20(12):1919–23.
17. Kariv Y, Delaney CP, Casillas S, et al. Long-term outcome after laparoscopic and open surgery for rectal prolapse; a case control study. *Surg Endosc* 2006;20(1):35–42.
18. Liyanage CA, Rathnayake G, Deen KI. A new technique for suture rectopexy without resection for rectal prolapse. *Tech Coloproctol* 2009;13(1):27–33.
19. Byrne CM, Smith SR, Solomon MJ, Young JM, Eyers AA, Young CJ. Long-term functional outcomes after laparoscopic and open rectopexy for the treatment of rectal prolapse. *Dis Colon Rectum* 2008;51(11):1597–604.
20. Carpelan-Holmstrom M, Kruuna O, Scheinin T. Laparoscopic rectal prolapse surgery combined with shorter hospital stay is safe in elderly and debilitate patients. *Surg Endosc* 2006;20 (9);1353–59.

51 Open Rectopexy

Sarah W. Grahn and Madhulika G. Varma

 INDICATIONS/CONTRAINDICATIONS

Rectal prolapse involves circumferential full-thickness protrusion of the rectal wall through the anal orifice (1). If the rectal wall has prolapsed but does not protrude through the anus, it is often referred to as occult prolapse or internal intussusceptions (1). It is important to distinguish between mucosal prolapse and full-thickness rectal prolapse; the former is characterized by protrusion of the mucosal layer whereas the muscle layer remains in the normal anatomic location. In contrast, full-thickness rectal prolapse is associated with the following anatomic features: a deep cul-de-sac, a redundant sigmoid, a lack of normal fixation of the rectum, laxity of the levator ani, and weakness of the internal and external sphincter, which is often associated with pudendal nerve dysfunction (1).

Diagnosis and Workup

The diagnosis of full-thickness rectal prolapse is a clinical diagnosis and patients often report a wide variety of associated symptoms including bleeding, pain, urge to defecate, mucous drainage, protrusion of a mass, constipation, and incontinence. Given that these symptoms are characteristic not only of prolapse but other anorectal conditions as well, a thorough evaluation to confirm the diagnosis is warranted. Colorectal cancers and colitides are important to exclude. To identify such cases, taking a detailed history and performing a physical exam and colonoscopy is imperative on all patients who are presumed to have rectal prolapse.

To assess the prolapse, it is often useful to examine the patient sitting on the toilet. The ability to sit on the commode and strain or evacuate stool often makes it easier for the patient to produce the prolapse, thus allowing the physician to ascertain its extent and differentiate between full-thickness and mucosal prolapse. The classic finding for true rectal prolapse is protrusion of circumferential folds, oftentimes accompanied by a sulcus between the prolapsed rectum and the anal opening. In contrast, mucosal prolapse lacks a sulcus and exhibit protruding tissue with radial folds.

Constipation occurs in 25–50% of patients (2), whereas 40–70% of patients experience fecal incontinence (3). Anal manometry is useful to assess sphincter function as chronic prolapse may lead to sphincter dysfunction, particularly of the internal sphincter. The decreased pressure of the internal sphincter may be the result of chronic trauma or may be associated with reversible activation of the rectoanal inhibitory reflex resulting from rectal distention by the prolapsed tissue (4). In addition, the rectoanal inhibitory reflex may be delayed or absent (5,6). Pudendal motor nerve latency testing may identify those patients with neurogenic fecal incontinence and endoanal ultrasound can help to distinguish between functional and anatomic etiologies (7). Given that 54% of patients with incontinence will have improvement of function with repair of their rectal prolapse, while a small percentage get worse, these tests help guide postoperative expectations (8). For patients with a history of constipation, electromyography should be obtained for those individuals with a history of severe straining and obstructive defecation as this may identify a subset of patients with puborectalis dysfunction who would benefit from biofeedback after surgery. Colonic transit studies can also identify those with colonic inertia who may benefit from an associated colonic resection at the time of prolapse repair.

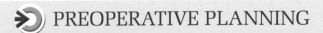

PREOPERATIVE PLANNING

Choice of Procedure

Although this chapter focuses specifically on open abdominal rectopexies, there are certain key decisions that must be made prior to counseling a patient to undergo treatment of their rectal prolapse. Open abdominal rectopexy is an excellent operation for those patients with full-thickness rectal prolapse without significant constipation.

Abdominal or Perineal

Surgical management is aimed at correcting the prolapse, improving continence and/or constipation while minimizing morbidity, mortality, and recurrence rates.

Factors that influence the choice of procedure include the patient's age, gender, comorbid conditions, functional status, and bowel function. In general, given the higher rates of recurrence for perineal procedures (16%) compared to abdominal approaches (5%), perineal procedures are reserved for elderly patients and those who have a significant perioperative risk for an adverse event (9). Because these procedures can often be completed with regional anesthesia, the lower risk of perioperative complications outweighs the increased recurrence rates in these high-risk patients. However, for patients who are healthy enough for general anesthesia, an abdominal approach is preferred.

Resection or Not

If the patient has chronic constipation, a sigmoid resection should be considered in addition to the rectopexy. If colonic transit times are very prolonged, a subtotal colectomy or sigmoid resection should be considered as part of the operative plan as preoperative retention of markers indicates an increased risk of postoperative constipation (10). Resection with rectopexy is associated with lower rates of postoperative constipation (11–13), as rectopexy alone may lead to worsening constipation (11,12).

Extent of Dissection

The extent of pelvic dissection during an abdominal rectopexy, including the lateral ligaments is a subject of debate. There is concern that division of the lateral stalks denervates the rectum and left colon increasing transit time and decreasing rectal sensation, both of which may contribute to increased postoperative constipation (14,15). However, this was challenged by Mollen and colleagues in a study of posterior rectopexy with Teflon mesh, with or without division of the lateral ligaments (16). While the postoperative colonic transit time overall was significantly increased compared to pre-operative values, the postoperative increase did not differ significantly between groups. The authors concluded that division of the lateral ligaments did not significantly influence postoperative functional outcome (16). In addition, other small studies of posterior mesh rectopexy have shown decreased recurrence rates with division of the lateral stalks (15). These studies are difficult to interpret, however, because the use of mesh, be it anterior as described by Ripstein or posterior as described by Wells, may contribute to decreased rectal capacity and constipation (14). Although the results of studies that preserve the lateral ligament are conflicting, there is a trend toward reduction in constipation (17). No randomized study of suture rectopexy alone with or without division of the lateral stalks has been published.

Lap Versus Open

The decision for open versus laparoscopic, with or without resection, depends on the surgeons' preference as well as patient factors such as previous pelvic surgery, concomitant vaginal prolapse, and associated symptoms of constipation or incontinence. Compared to laparotomy, laparoscopic rectopexy has the advantages of reduced pain, shortened hospital stay, early recovery, and earlier return to work (18). Laparoscopic rectopexy is now a widely used approach; however, for patients who have had extensive prior pelvic surgery or those individuals with concomitant vaginal prolapse requiring a combined procedure, an open rectopexy may be preferable.

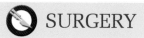 **SURGERY**

Positioning and Incision

All patients should have a full mechanical bowel preparation with parenteral preoperative antibiotics.

The patient is supine for induction of anesthesia, and then placed in low lithotomy with all pressure points padded; an orogastric tube and a bladder catheter are placed. The abdomen and perineum are both prepped and either a vertical lower midline or a pfannenstiel incision can be used. Careful attention is paid to avoid injury to the bladder. A radially expanding wound retractor is used. The patient is then placed in Trendelenburg position and the small bowel packed into the upper quadrants exposing the sigmoid colon and the rectum.

Dissection

Dissection begins by laterally mobilizing the sigmoid colon to allow visualization of the peritoneal attachment of the sigmoid mesentery to the presacral tissues. The sigmoid is then retracted cephalad and to the left to identify the contour of the superior hemorrhoidal vessel as it arches into the pelvis. The peritoneum on the right side of the rectosigmoid mesentery is incised and this opening is extended down along the sacral promontory into the pelvis. Similarly, the peritoneal attachments on the left side of the sigmoid mesentery are incised. The dissection is extended under the superior hemorrhoidal vessel to join the dissection done from the right side.

■ It is important to carefully identify and preserve the presacral nerves to maintain sexual and bladder function.

With a window created posterior to the superior hemorrhoidal vessel, the rectum can be anteriorly retracted to expose the plane between the fascia propria of the mesorectum and the presacral tissues. Using electrocautery, the avascular, filmy tissues can be sharply incised all the way down into the pelvis. It is important to stay within the proper plane, close to the mesorectum, to leave the presacral tissues intact.

▓ Careful attention in this region helps to avoid presacral venous bleeding that can be difficult to manage.

This dissection is extended down deep into the pelvis, beyond the distal extent of the mesorectum posteriorly to the level of the levator ani muscles. Once the posterior attachments have been divided, the peritoneum on the right and left sides of the rectum extending toward the anterior peritoneal reflection is divided.

▓ The anterior peritoneal reflection is often very low in patients with rectal prolapse.

The anterior peritoneal reflection may be even deeper and somewhat distorted in patients who have had a hysterectomy and there is often peritonealization of the vaginal cuff. With careful dissection anterolaterally, the lateral edges of the vaginal cuff can be identified. The anterior peritoneal reflection between the rectum and the vagina is then divided staying close to the vagina. Deep renal vein retractors are used to retract the vagina, and a plane between the vagina and the rectum is developed, extending anteriorly to the anal canal.

After the anterior and posterior planes are developed, the lateral attachments are partially divided to allow mobilization of the rectum.

▓ It is important to leave a part of the lateral attachment to maintain innervation for the rectum and the anus to minimize constipation.

After mobilizing the rectum and sigmoid, the region of the prior anterior peritoneal reflection is brought up toward the sacral promontory. The amount of tension is assessed and a site on the mesentery is selected that will eliminate any rectal redundancy in the pelvis and allow the rectum to rest on the sacral promontory so that it is straight but without excessive tension.

Suture Fixation

Once the site for the sutures is indentified on the rectum, the sacral promontory is prepared for the sutures. The tissues are cleared off of the anterior surface of the sacral promontory for 1–2 cm in a vertical fashion to expose the periosteum.

▓ It is important to avoid the presacral nerves and veins during this part of the dissection; thus, a vertical incision is made and the tissues are spread laterally.

The 0- or 2-0 nonabsorbable sutures placed using a medium Mayo needle that can be reloaded. First, the stitches are placed through the periosteum of the sacrum, then through the right side of the rectal mesentery at the level of the anterior reflection in a mattress fashion.

▓ It is important to maintain the proper orientation of the rectum to avoid torsion.
▓ It is important to ensure that the sutures are going through the lateral mesentery and peritoneum, but *not* through the rectal wall.

After both sutures are placed, but before securing them down, inspect for hemostasis as this area is difficult to assess once the rectopexy is complete. The sutures are secured. The abdomen is closed.

 POSTOPERATIVE MANAGEMENT

The patient is hospitalized for about 4 to 5 days. The morning after surgery, the patient is encouraged to ambulate and start liquids. However, patients with chronic constipation may have a prolonged ileus and thus, the decision to start oral intake must be assessed. The diet is advanced over the 24–48 hours and the bladder catheter is removed. In one study of open rectopexy, the mean length of stay was 5 days for cases done since 1999 (19).

COMPLICATIONS

Overall complication rates are difficult to assess given that most of the reports are retrospective small series, but reported complication rates range from 10–20%. Complications include small-bowel obstruction, antibiotic-associated colitis, iliofemoral DVT, pulmonary, urinary tract, and wound infections (20,21).

 RESULTS

Main outcomes after surgery for rectal prolapse include changes in constipation, changes in continence, and recurrence of rectal prolapse. More than 50% of patients with rectal prolapse have preoperative constipation. The influence of rectopexy on constipation is variable; while 30–83% of patients experience an improvement in constipation (19,22,23), symptoms worsen in 17–31% of patients (19,21,22).

Continence is improved in 35–75% of patients (19,20,22–24), and worsened in 12–18% (19,22).

Recurrence rates for abdominal suture rectopexy range from 0% to 9% (19,20,23,25). In one study, none of the patients developed a recurrence of complete prolapse of the rectum but 5% developed mucosal prolapsed (23).

 CONCLUSIONS

Although full-thickness rectal prolapse can be both debilitating and a source of embarrassment, it is rarely a medical emergency. This feature permits time for a complete preoperative evaluation. The operative plan can be tailored to the patient, taking into account the patient's medical comorbidities, bowel function, and status of fecal continence, thereby balancing the extent of the procedure, potential morbidity, and impact on continence and constipation with the potential recurrence. Surgeon's familiarity and comfort level with the myriad of surgical options also affects the choice of procedure.

Open rectopexy is a durable operation with acceptable morbidity and low recurrence rates making it an excellent choice for patients who are healthy enough to tolerate general anesthesia that may not be good candidates for a laparoscopic approach due to extensive prior pelvic surgery or need for combined gynecological procedures.

Part XIV: Abdominal Operations for Rectal Prolapse

References

1. Karulf RE, Madoff RD, Goldberg SM. Rectal prolapse. *Curr Probl Surg* 2001;38(10):771–832.
2. Madden MV, Kamm MA, Nicholls RJ, Santhanam AN, Cabot R, Speakman CT. Abdominal rectopexy for complete prolapse: prospective study evaluating changes in symptoms and anorectal function. *Dis Colon Rectum* 1992;35(1):48–55.
3. Brown AJ, Anderson JH, McKee RF, Finlay IG. Surgery for occult rectal prolapse. *Colorectal Dis* 2004;6(3):176–79.
4. Farouk R, Duthie GS, MacGregor AB, Bartolo DC. Rectoanal inhibition and incontinence in patients with rectal prolapse. *Br J Surg* 1994;81(5):743–46.
5. Spencer RJ. Manometric studies in rectal prolapse. *Dis Colon Rectum* 1984;27(8):523–25.
6. Hiltunen KM, Matikainen M, Auvinen O, Hietanen P. Clinical and manometric evaluation of anal sphincter function in patients with rectal prolapse. *Am J Surg* 1986;151(4):489–92.
7. Groenendijk AG, Birnie E, Boeckxstaens GE, Roovers JP, Bonsel GJ. Anorectal function testing and anal endosonography in the diagnostic work-up of patients with primary pelvic organ prolapse. *Gynecol Obstet Invest* 2009;67(3):187–94.
8. Delaini GG, Scaglia M, Hulten L. Abdominal rectopexy in the treatment of rectal prolapse: how to foresee the functional result. *Ann Ital Chir* 1994;65(2):183–87.
9. Kim DS, Tsang CB, Wong WD, Lowry AC, Goldberg SM, Madoff RD. Complete rectal prolapse: evolution of management and results. *Dis Colon Rectum* 1999;42(4):460–66; discussion 466–69.
10. Schultz I, Mellgren A, Oberg M, Dolk A, Holmström B. Whole gut transit is prolonged after Ripstein rectopexy. *Eur J Surg* 1999;165(3):242–47.
11. McKee RF, Lauder JC, Poon FW, Aitchison MA, Finlay IG. A prospective randomized study of abdominal rectopexy with and without sigmoidectomy in rectal prolapse. *Surg Gynecol Obstet* 1992;174(2):145–48.
12. Sayfan J, Pinho M, Alexander-Williams J, Keighley MR. Sutured posterior abdominal rectopexy with sigmoidectomy compared with Marlex rectopexy for rectal prolapse. *Br J Surg* 1990;77(2):143–45.
13. Luukkonen P, Mikkonen U, Jarvinen H. Abdominal rectopexy with sigmoidectomy versus rectopexy alone for rectal prolapse: a prospective, randomized study. *Int J Colorectal Dis* 1992;7(4):219–22.
14. Scaglia M, Fasth S, Hallgren T, Nordgren S, Oresland T, Hultén L. Abdominal rectopexy for rectal prolapse. Influence of surgical technique on functional outcome. *Dis Colon Rectum* 1994;37(8):805–13.
15. Speakman CT, Madden MV, Nicholls RJ, Kamm MA. Lateral ligament division during rectopexy causes constipation but

prevents recurrence: results of a prospective randomized study. *Br J Surg* 1991;78(12):1431–33.

16. Mollen RM, Kuijpers JH, van Hoek F. Effects of rectal mobilization and lateral ligaments division on colonic and anorectal function. *Dis Colon Rectum* 2000;43(9):1283–87.

17. Madiba TE, Baig MK, Wexner SD. Surgical management of rectal prolapse. *Arch Surg* 2005;140(1):63–73.

18. Kellokumpu IH, Vironen J, Scheinin T. Laparoscopic repair of rectal prolapse: a prospective study evaluating surgical outcome and changes in symptoms and bowel function. *Surg Endosc* 2000;14(7):634–40.

19. Kariv Y, Delaney CP, Casillas S, et al. Long-term outcome after laparoscopic and open surgery for rectal prolapse: a case-control study. *Surg Endosc* 2006;20(1):35–42.

20. Blatchford GJ, Perry RE, Thorson AG, Christensen MA. Rectopexy without resection for rectal prolapse. *Am J Surg* 1989; 158(6):574–76.

21. Novell JR, Osborne MJ, Winslet MC, Lewis AA. Prospective randomized trial of Ivalon sponge versus sutured rectopexy for full-thickness rectal prolapse. *Br J Surg* 1994;81(6): 904–06.

22. Graf W, Karlbom U, Påhlman L, Nilsson S, Ejerblad S. Functional results after abdominal suture rectopexy for rectal prolapse or intussusception. *Eur J Surg* 1996;162(11):905–11.

23. Khanna AK, Misra MK, Kumar K. Simplified sutured sacral rectopexy for complete rectal prolapse in adults. *Eur J Surg* 1996; 162(2):143–46.

24. Briel JW, Schouten WR, Boerma MO. Long-term results of suture rectopexy in patients with fecal incontinence associated with incomplete rectal prolapse. *Dis Colon Rectum* 1997; 40(10):1228–32.

25. Carter AE. Rectosacral suture fixation for complete rectal prolapse in the elderly, the frail and the demented. *Br J Surg* 1983; 70(9):522–23.

52 Laparoscopic Rectopexy

Howard M. Ross

 ## INDICATIONS

Laparoscopic rectopexy is an important technique for the treatment of rectal prolapse. Laparoscopic rectopexy can be combined with sigmoid resection or performed alone as a means of treating full thickness rectal prolapse when resection is not desired. Laparoscopic rectopexy without resection is especially useful when patients have problems with fecal incontinence or when a patient or surgeon does not want to accept the risk of an anastomotic leak (1).

 ## PREOPERATIVE PLANNING

It is this authors and the editors' practice to utilize a preoperative mechanical bowel preparation the evening prior to surgery. The mechanical preparation facilitates physical manipulation of the rectum with laparoscopic instruments.

 ## SURGERY

Laparoscopic rectopexy is a relatively easily performed technique which includes full circumferential mobilization of the rectum to the level of the pelvic floor. Surgeons should be facile with endoscopic suturing techniques and have equipment which will permit the secure attachment of the mesorectum to the presacral fascia.

Positioning

Patients should be placed in supine position in stirrups. The patient's thighs should be parallel to the torso to enable the unencumbered motion of the surgeon's arms. Generally a camera port is placed at the superior edge of the umbilicus, with two lateral 5 mm ports in both the right and left lower quadrants. A 30-degree telescope enables lateral viewing. On each side of the patient, the lowermost lateral port is placed two fingerbreadths anterior and superior to the iliac spine. The more superior lateral port is placed four fingerbreadths superior to the lower port (Fig. 52.1).

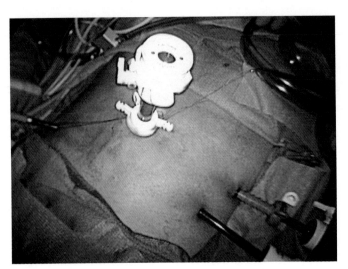

Figure 52.1 Port placement.

Technique

The operation begins by lifting the rectum toward the abdominal wall and retracting the proximal rectum superiorly and to the left. This motion creates tension on the redundant rectal mesentery. Positioning the patient in steep Trendelenburg will help remove the small bowel from the pelvis. Tilting the operating table to the left at this time will expose the right side of the rectum. The right lateral peritoneum overlying the mesorectum is then scored with electrocautery or scissors beginning at the sacral promontory. The retrorectal space is developed from proximal to distal and from right to left beneath the rectum. When only the peritoneum remains on the left, it is opened after retracting the rectum to the right. Rotating the table to the right at this time is helpful.

Division of the lateral stalks is undertaken according to individual surgeon's preference. Division of the stalks has been shown in several studies to promote constipation yet perhaps to decrease recurrence (2). If the surgeon elects to divide the lateral stalks, they may be divided with any one of the multiple new energy source devices.

Attachment of the fascia propria of the mesorectum to the sacral fascia is generally accomplished with interrupted sutures although the use of laparoscopic tacks to fasten the rectum into position has been reported to be associated with good results (3). The anterior rectum should be mobilized from the posterior vagina all the way to the anal canal, especially if the patient has a rectocele in conjunction with rectal prolapse.

POSTOPERATIVE MANAGEMENT

Clear liquids are instituted in the immediate postoperative period and continued until the passage of flatus after which a regular diet is offered. When a regular diet is tolerated the patient is discharged. Parenteral and enteral opiates are utilized in the postoperative period. Opiate intake is minimized, however, with liberal use of non-steroidal anti-inflammatory agents.

COMPLICATIONS

The overall major and minor complication rates with laparoscopic rectopexy are low. Complications identified in the literature include bleeding, infection, and a worsening of constipation.

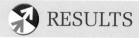

RESULTS

Studies comparing laparoscopic and open rectopexy have generally been small. Meta-analysis has been useful in determining morbidity and recurrence rates, as well as comparisons of length of hospitalization. Purkayastha et al. identified six studies, including a total of 195 patients (98 open and 97 laparoscopic) and found that there were no significant differences in recurrence or morbidity between laparoscopic abdominal rectopexy and open abdominal rectopexy (4). However, the length of stay was significantly reduced in the laparoscopic group by 3.5 days (95% confidence interval, 3.1–4; $P < 0.01$), whereas the operative time was significantly longer in this group, by approximately 60 minutes (60.38 minutes; 95% confidence interval, 49–71.8). Morbidity was the same for laparoscopic rectopexy and the open technique. Recurrence rates generally range from 0–10% in studies with 8–30 months follow-up.

CONCLUSIONS

Laparoscopic rectopexy is a reliable means to treat rectal prolapse. The laparoscopic technique results in a shorter hospital stay than does the equivalent open resection. Recurrence and complication rates are low and the absence of the need for an incision for specimen extraction as well as the absence of an anastomosis is theoretically appealing attributes of this approach. The technique of laparoscopic rectopexy requires knowledge of pelvic anatomy and the ability to laparoscopically mobilize the rectum and subsequently laparoscopically fix it to the presacral fascia.

Recommended References and Readings

1. Madib TE, Baig MK, Wexner SD. Surgical management of rectal prolapse. *Arch Surg* 2005;140:63–73.
2. Brazzelli M, Bachoo P, Grant A. Surgery for complete rectal prolapse in adults. *Cochrane Database Syst Rev* 2000;2:CD001758.
3. Nunoo-Mensah JW, Efron JE, Young-Fadok TM. Laparoscopic rectopexy. *Surg Endosc* 2007;21:325–26.
4. Purkayastha S, Tekkis P, Athanasiou T, et al. A Comparison of Open *vs.* Laparoscopic abdominal rectopexy for full-thickness tectal prolapse: a meta-analysis. *Dis Colon Rectum* 2005;48:1930–40.

Part XIV: Abdominal Operations for Rectal Prolapse

53 Abdominal Rectopexy: Hand-Assisted

Edward Borrazzo and Neil Hyman

 ## INDICATIONS/CONTRAINDICATIONS

Rectal prolapse may cause considerable life-altering disability including bleeding, pain, and fecal incontinence. Numerous remedial operations have been described with very few high quality studies available to facilitate evidence-based recommendations (1).

Generally speaking, abdominal approaches are recommended for fit patients and perineal procedures for the elderly and infirmed. Rectopexy allows for fixation of the rectum to the sacrum, thereby preventing the rectum from prolapsing out the anal canal. The role/need for concomitant resection remains uncertain and controversial (2,3).

Rectopexy can be performed utilizing open, laparoscopic, or hybrid techniques, such as the hand-assisted laparoscopic approach. It is our custom to perform rectopexies (with or without resection) using a purely laparoscopic approach. However, patients with recurrent prolapse after a previous abdominal approach (either open or laparoscopic) are often best-served by hand-assisted laparoscopic technique. Similarly, a hand-assisted laparoscopic rectopexy can be used to obviate the need for conversion to full open surgery when technical problems are encountered during laparoscopic rectopexy.

Extensive adhesions or previous pelvic sepsis can be considered a relative contraindication to hand-assisted laparoscopic rectopexy; however it is often difficult to predict a hostile pelvis based on history alone. Laparoscopic visualization with a forthright, considered assessment of the local conditions is often an appropriate first step.

As in all operative procedures, the surgeon must candidly assess their skill set and decide what is safest for the patient *in their hands*. Hand-assisted laparoscopic rectopexy may be the best and safest approach for many surgeons. The patient is primarily owed a safe and effective procedure to correct their prolapse and minimize the risk or recurrence. Whether the procedure is performed open, laparoscopically, or with hand assistance is truly a secondary consideration.

PREOPERATIVE PLANNING

Planning is similar to any other abdominal colorectal procedure. Patients should be suitable for laparotomy/laparoscopy or a perineal procedure should be chosen. It is important to consider why the patient has developed the prolapse and whether there are other manifestations of pelvic floor relaxation.

A careful history may elicit causative factors for the prolapse such as bulimia or a connective tissue disorder. Patients who strain excessively and/or have a defecation disorder such as a non-relaxing puborectalis can be appropriately counseled or referred for biofeedback to minimize the risk of recurrence after corrective surgery. Those individuals suspected to have slow-transit constipation may be scheduled for colonic transit studies and considered for colectomy at the time of rectopexy on a highly selective basis. Women with concomitant uterine prolapse or cystocele, for example, can be treated in a multidisciplinary manner with a joint surgical approach.

Flexible endoscopy (or suitable radiologic studies) should usually be performed, especially in age-appropriate patients, to make sure that the rectal prolapse is not caused by a neoplasm that is acting as the lead point for the prolapse.

If the patient has recurrent prolapse and/or has undergone previous pelvic surgery, review of the previous operative report(s) can be invaluable. Quite often, "recurrent" prolapse actually is persistent prolapse and represents a failure to adequately mobilize the rectum by an inexperienced pelvic surgeon.

 SURGERY

Hand-assisted laparoscopic techniques are helpful for dissection of the mid and lower rectum, especially in reoperative cases. An intracorporeal hand can facilitate identification of the ureters if stents are used, and also provides countertraction for dissection of the lower third of the rectum down to the pelvic floor. Tactile sensation affords better assessment of the true tension on the rectum and the appropriate degree of superior traction when fixing the rectum to the sacral promontory.

We position the hand-assisted device at the level of the umbilicus (Fig. 53.1). This keeps the hand from obscuring the field of view as compared to more inferior placement and provides acceptable cosmesis with the subsequent incision hidden in the umbilical fold. Ports are placed in the mid-abdomen on each side. An additional working port is placed in the right lower quadrant. The camera alternates between the two lateral ports to get a view on each side of the rectum as the dissection is performed in the pelvis.

In reoperative cases, anatomic planes are often difficult to identify visually at first. Use of the hand can help define the proper plane of dissection. It is often easiest to get

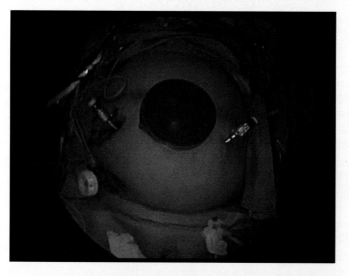

Figure 53.1 Port position. Operating surgeon stands on the patient's right side. The handport is positioned at the umbilicus. The two mid abdominal ports, here 5 mm, are used for the laparoscope and assistant retractor, alternating sides as needed. Right hand working port is in the right lower quadrant.

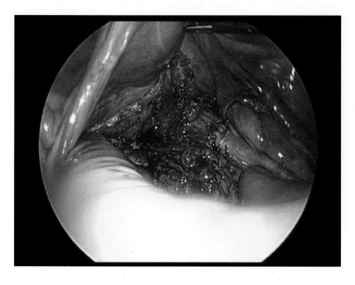

Figure 53.2 Dissection along left side of rectum in pelvis. The surgeon's left hand is seen in the foreground at the bottom of the picture. Fingers are used to splay tissues for dissection. The uterus is suspended anteriorly with a transabdominal suture that is released at the completion of the procedure. The rectum and mesorectum are retracted superiorly.

started along the White line of Toldt at the level of the descending colon, since this area has usually been untouched at the first operation even if a resection has been performed. The left ureter can then be traced inferiorly, while mobilizing the intact mesocolon and mesorectum off the retroperitoneum, pelvic brim, and lateral sidewall (Fig. 53.2).

In a similar fashion, the right ureter may be identified. Dissection is undertaken inferiorly along the lateral aspect of the rectum. (Fig. 53.3) The lateral stalks are usually divided in reoperative cases to facilitate mobilization of the distal third of the rectum and improve access to the pelvic floor. This may increase the risk of constipation, but appears likely to decrease the risk of another recurrence in these cases (4,5).

The most difficult part of the dissection is often the mobilization of the mesocolon and/or mesorectum off the sacrum in the previously dissected presacral plane, when some form of fixation has previously been attempted to the sacrum or sacral promontory. Care should be taken to identify and avoid the hypogastric nerves. Here, an energy source such as ultrasonic shears is particularly helpful in keeping the field relatively bloodless for optimal visualization. This posterior dissection is commonly the first to be completed down to the level of the pelvic floor (Fig. 53.4).

Often the most distal dissection is easiest in cases of recurrences, since the previous mobilization may not have extended to the lower rectum. After posterior dissection is completed to the level of the anal canal beyond Waldeyer's pelvic fascial reflection, the lateral stalks are divided or mobilized. Finally, the anterior dissection is performed behind the vagina in the rectovaginal septum as far as possible. The non-dominant hand is used to create traction-countertraction between the rectum and the vagina as well as the lateral

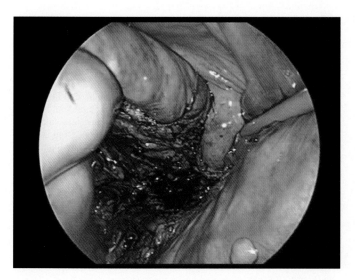

Figure 53.3 Dissection along right side of rectum in pelvis. Some of the posterior dissection has already been completed.

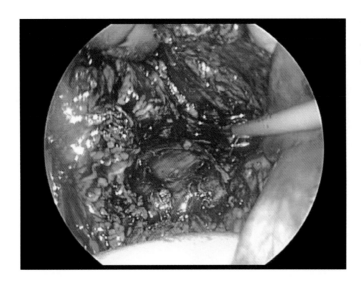

Figure 53.4 Dissection of distal posterior rectum is accomplished. The mesorectum is pushed anteriorly, countertraction is obtained posteriorly, all done with the left hand. The levator ani musculature is identified.

pelvic wall. The hand may also be useful in circumferential traction on the rectum to help in distal access to the very low rectum and surrounding soft tissue (Fig. 53.5).

Hand access can also facilitate fixation of the rectum to the sacrum. Tension is more easily assessed with tactile feedback (Fig. 53.6), and suturing is easy using the hand to create and secure knots (Fig. 53.7). The sacral promontory is palpated and tissue is splayed to allow precise fixation, by sutures and/or tacks. We do not use any form of mesh fixation as this does not appear to reduce recurrence rates (6–8). Figure 53.8 shows the completed rectopexy, sutured and tacked on each side to the sacrum.

POSTOPERATIVE MANAGEMENT

Patients undergoing hand-assisted rectopexy are started on clear liquids after surgery and advanced rapidly to regular diet as tolerated. No postoperative antibiotics are prescribed. Unless specifically indicated, no special diet or bowel supplement really needs to be provided. Hospital stay in uncomplicated cases is usually 1–2 days.

COMPLICATIONS

Complications after hand-assisted laparoscopic rectopexy are really no different than after other abdominal colorectal procedures. Wound infections, pelvic abscess, and

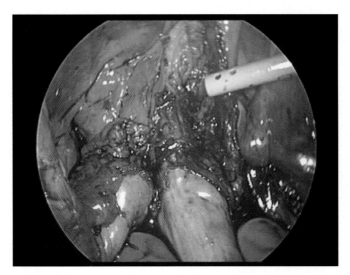

Figure 53.5 Anterior rectal dissection is performed. The left hand acts as an excellent retractor, and also helps create a plane between the vagina and rectum. If a cervical speculum or assistant's finger is used, the vagina can be palpated for identification and dissection of Denonvilliers' fascia. This area may be scarred if a previous resection has been performed, with the anastomosis adherent to the posterior cervix or vaginal wall. The hand may help identify and dissect the area of the previous anastomosis.

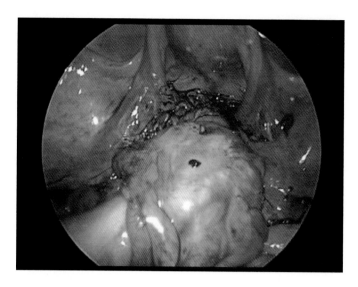

Figure 53.6 Tension assessed using tactile sensation with gentle superior traction. Fingers are seen in the left lower aspect of the photograph hooking the rectum.

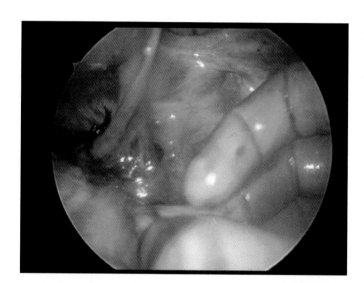

Figure 53.7 The hand port can facilitate fixation. With either hand, sutures can easily be tied, and adequacy of the tissue as well as tension on the rectum can be monitored continuously.

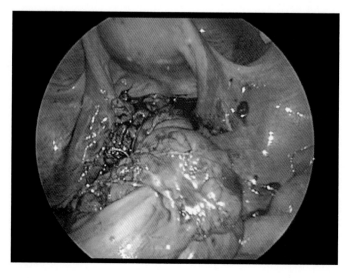

Figure 53.8 Completed rectopexy. The rectum is fixed to sacral promontory.

Part XIV: Abdominal Operations for Rectal Prolapse

inadvertent bowel injury are usually the major concerns. Long-term sequela, such as bowel obstruction or incisional hernias, appear to be lower in laparoscopic approaches than with open surgery (9,10).

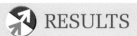 RESULTS

The reported recurrence rate after rectopexy is usually in the 10% range or lower. However, it must be acknowledged that the results reported in the literature are usually the best outcomes owing to publication bias and the recurrence rates in actual practice are likely much higher. Further, the incidence of recurrent prolapse clearly increases over time. As such, length of follow-up is a critical factor in interpreting the case series that are available in the literature.

CONCLUSIONS

Hand-assisted rectopexy is a valuable technique in the management of rectal prolapse. We find it particularly useful in cases of recurrent prolapse or to avoid conversion to open in cases where a purely laparoscopic approach has proven difficult or otherwise problematic. Long-term results should be similar to those that are achieved with open surgery, but there is little evidence to support this assertion. As with all laparoscopic techniques, proper training and individualized patient selection is critical.

References

1. Tou S, Brown SR, Malik AI, Nelson RL. Surgery for complete rectal prolapse in adults. *Cochrane Database Syst Rev* 2008;4:CD001758.
2. Lukkonen P, Mikkonen U, Jarvinen H. Abdominal rectopexy with sigmoidectomy versus rectopexy alone for rectal prolapse: a prospective, randomized study. *Int J Colorectal Dis* 1992;7(4): 219–22.
3. McKee RF, Lauder JC, Poon FW, Aitchison MA, Finlay IG. A prospective randomized study of abdominal rectopexy with and without sigmoidectomy in rectal prolapse. *Surg Gynecol Obstet* 1992;174(2):145–48.
4. Speakman CT, Madden MV, Nicholls RJ, Kamm MA. Lateral ligament division during rectopexy causes constipation but prevents recurrence: results of a prospective randomized study. *Br J Surg* 1991;78(12):1431–33.
5. Mollen RM, Kuijpers JH, van Hoeck F. Effect of rectal mobilization and lateral sphincter division on colonic and anorectal function. *Dis Colon Rectum* 2000;43:1283–87.
6. Novell JR, Osborne MJ, Winslet MC, Lewis AA. Prospective randomized trial of Ivalon sponge versus sutured rectopexy for full-thickness rectal prolapse. *Br J Surg* 1994;81(6): 904–906.
7. Winde G, Reers B, Nottberg H, Berns T, Meyer J, Bünte H. Clinical and functional results of abdominal rectopexy with absorbable mesh-graft for treatment of complete rectal prolapse. *Eur J Surg* 1993;59(5):301–305.
8. Galili Y, Rabau M. Comparison of polyglycolic acid and polypropylene mesh for rectopexy in the treatment of rectal prolapse. *Eur J Surg* 1997;163(6):445–48.
9. Boccasanta P, Rosari R, Venturi M, et al. Comparison of laparoscopic rectopexy with open technique in the treatment of complete rectal prolapse: clinical and functional results. *Surg Laparosc Endosc* 1998;8(6):460–65.
10. Solomon MJ, Young CJ, Eyers AA, Roberts RA. Randomized clinical trial of laparoscopic versus open abdominal rectopexy for rectal prolapse. *Br J Surg* 2002;89(1):35–39.

54 Nonresectional and Resectional Rectopexy

Scott R. Steele and Robert D. Madoff

INDICATIONS/CONTRAINDICATIONS

Full-thickness external rectal prolapse can be a distressing condition for both the patient and the surgeon alike. In addition to its unsightly and at times alarming appearance, rectal prolapse may cause progressive symptoms that affect both a patient's overall medical health and the quality of life (1). Full external prolapse occurs when the rectum descends beyond the anal verge, manifesting as concentric rings of rectal mucosa to the examiner. Severity varies, as the prolapse may progress from initial reduction with standing or cessation of straining, to full-thickness prolapse with even minimal activity, and finally, in certain cases, to continual prolapse. As time passes, chronic prolapse through the sphincter complex, along with the presence of concomitant pelvic floor dysfunction, can lead to problems with both continence and symptoms of constipation from outlet obstruction. When considering indications for intervention, it is important to distinguish overt from internal rectal prolapse (also known as hidden or occult intussusception) in which the prolapse contains the full thickness of the rectal wall but the intussusception does not extend beyond the anal verge.

Factors to consider in selecting the ideal therapeutic approach include the age and health of the patient, overall functional status, and the potential benefits and risks of a given surgical technique (2). In general, transabdominal procedures are recommended for fit patients, as they are associated with the lowest recurrence rates (3,4). Transperineal procedures are generally reserved for older patients and those with comorbid conditions who would gain the most benefit from a limited operation that is associated with lesser morbidity, a shorter length of hospital stay, and a faster recovery. Unfortunately, perineal repairs are not as durable as the transabdominal procedures, with reported recurrence rates of 16-40% depending on the particular procedure and follow-up time 5,6). Other factors may also play a role in procedure selection, such as the risk of sexual dysfunction from autonomic nerve damage during the pelvic dissection with an abdominal procedure.

The goal of abdominal rectopexy is to restore the rectum to its normal position in the pelvis by fixing it to the presacral fascia. This approach restores the normal posterior curve of the rectum in the hollow of the sacrum, though the physiologic benefits of this restoration are uncertain. Open abdominal rectopexy can be easily performed with or without resection of the redundant sigmoid colon.

While the main indication for prolapse repair is to address specific symptoms (mass, mucus discharge, incontinence, impaired defecation), the mere presence of rectal prolapse is reason enough to recommend repair because of the likely eventual progression of symptoms, particularly incontinence due to sphincter dysfunction, as well as a small risk of incarceration. Rectopexy is much less likely to alleviate symptoms associated with internal intussusception and is not indicated unless the patient has solitary rectal ulcer syndrome. For those patients with a large redundant sigmoid colon, history of symptomatic diverticular disease, and/or constipation-predominant symptoms, sigmoid resection can be considered as an adjunct to rectopexy.

 # PREOPERATIVE PLANNING

As this is an open transabdominal approach, patients undergoing consideration for this type of elective repair should be medically fit and able to tolerate a laparotomy. A detailed medical history is vital when evaluating patients with rectal prolapse, including a thorough review of bowel habits, as more than half of patients have coexisting incontinence and slightly fewer patients have constipation. Patients not only frequently report their rectal protrusion but also give a history of problematic bowel habits, abdominal discomfort, and mucus discharge. Many patients strain to initiate or complete defecation, experience incomplete evacuation, or require digital maneuvers to aid with defecation. This may be secondary to the rectal prolapse itself or pelvic floor dysfunction associated with either anatomical defects (rectocele, cystocele, enterocele) or functional abnormalities such as paradoxical or nonrelaxing puborectalis.

In addition to a general physical examination, digital rectal examination can detect the presence of attenuated sphincter tone and masses, as well as assess for concomitant pelvic floor pathology. The patient should be asked to both tighten her anal sphincter and "bear down" as a simulation of defecation to assess proper contraction and relaxation of the pelvic floor muscles. The perineum is assessed for associated increased perineal descent or bulge indicative of pelvic floor laxity that is often seen with increasing age, multiparity, or prior pelvic floor surgery. Examination of the vagina can also be helpful in identifying concomitant pelvic floor abnormalities such as rectocele, cystocele or uterine prolapse that may also need to be addressed.

Preoperative evaluation can include specific physiologic tests and imaging studies on a selective basis. Colonoscopy should be up-to-date for all patients aged 50 years or older and should be performed on a selective basis for younger patients or those with new symptoms since their last examination. Patients who complain of severe constipation with infrequent bowel movements should undergo a colonic transit study. Rectal prolapse patients have a high rate (approximately 15–30%) of concomitant pelvic floor disorders such as abnormal rectal emptying, nonrelaxing pelvic floor, enterocele and rectocele (7). When suggested by history or on physical examination, the dynamics of rectal evacuation and search for these concomitant findings may be studied with multicontrast defecography or dynamic magnetic resonance imaging. Anal manometry can serve as a useful baseline assessment for incontinent patients, though the findings rarely change the operative approach. Anal ultrasound can be considered to assess sphincter integrity in patients with associated fecal incontinence.

NONRESECTIONAL RECTOPEXY

Surgery

Prior to the procedure, in many cases, initial preparations for a nonresectional rectopexy consist of a mechanical bowel preparation, which may be often limited to enemas on the morning of surgery according to per physician preference. Preoperative intravenous antibiotics are routinely given and timed for adequate concentration during the initial skin incision. In addition, deep venous thrombosis prophylaxis including sequential compression devices and chemical prophylaxis such as heparin or low-molecular-weight heparin may be considered. In general, the most common types of nonresectional cases include rectal mobilization alone, mobilization with suture rectopexy, and mobilization with rectopexy involving mesh. As each of these have different risk and outcome profiles, preoperative counseling and discussion of the proposed procedure is important.

Positioning

In the operating room, the patients are positioned in the modified lithotomy position to provide access to the anus and the rectum, as well as to provide ideal positioning for retraction of the bladder, prostate, or vagina. Both the surgeon and the assistant should wear headlights to facilitate visualization during the pelvic dissection. Ureteral catheters may be especially helpful in patients who have had prior radiation, pelvic surgery, or adhesive disease, but their routine use is not necessary. All bony prominences are well padded and consideration should be given for a pad under the sacrum. Per physician preference, both arms may be tucked at the patient's side or extended for monitoring access.

Open Technique

The basic tenets of the abdominal approach include mobilization of the rectum to the pelvic floor with sacral suspension to hold it in place until it scars into position. The operation commences with a midline incision from the umbilicus to the pubis or a lower transverse (Pfannenstiel) incision; each of these incisions provides adequate exposure for most patients. After placement of self-retaining retractors, the small bowel is displaced superiorly and packed into the upper abdomen. Posterior mobilization is carried down to the level of the coccyx in the anatomic mesorectal plane. Proper identification of the avascular presacral plane is aided by application of forward traction on the rectum. Care is taken to preserve the hypogastric nerves at the level of the sacral promontory. Unintentional division of the hypogastric nerves, typically at the level of the inferior mesenteric artery takeoff or at the level of the sacral promontory, can cause sexual and urinary dysfunctions.

The proper amount of lateral and anterior dissection is subject to debate. Surgeons frequently discuss dividing the "lateral ligaments" or fixing them to the sacrum, but these ligaments do not exist as true anatomic structures. Thus, while failure to divide the lateral ligaments was shown to increase the recurrence rate in one small, randomized trial, exactly what structure was being divided is uncertain. Furthermore, the functional outcome of lateral ligament division is subject to debate: some authors have shown a worsening of constipation, but others have found no change in postoperative bowel function (8).

Anterior mobilization of the rectum allows it to be further displaced out of the pelvis, but its efficacy in preventing relapse or improving functional outcome is unknown. The anterior mobilization of the rectum begins with division of the peritoneal reflection. Dissection between the anterior aspect of the rectum and the posterior aspect of the anterior pelvic structures is facilitated by anterior retraction of the uterus or the bladder with a St. Mark's or a Wylie retractor, whereas posterior countertraction on the rectum is maintained by the surgeon's left hand. We generally carry our anterior dissection to the level of the mid to upper third of the vagina; more distal dissection, especially in men, increases the risk of parasympathetic nerve injury.

Rectal Mobilization Alone

In this procedure, mobilization of the rectum to the pelvic floor alone is performed as above, however there is no dedicated maneuver for sacral suspension. Rather, proponents feel the healing process that follows mobilization alone provides adequate ability for scar tissue to form and hold the rectum in place to avoid recurrence.

Suture Rectopexy

During the initial mobilization, emphasis is again placed on carrying the posterior dissection down to the level of the coccyx in the anatomic avascular mesorectal plane, preserving the hypogastric nerves, and opening the plane anterior to the rectum to varying extents based upon surgeon preference.

The rectopexy is then performed by first choosing a point approximately 4–5 cm below the sacral promontory for the inferior-most aspect of fixation. The rectum is then pulled posterior and superiorly toward the sacrum and the site for rectal fixation is chosen. The goal is to suspend the rectum without redundancy below the rectopexy sutures; excessive tension on the distal rectum should be avoided. While some authors advocate placement of fixation sutures on either side of the rectum, we prefer to place all the sutures on one side, because this approach avoids kinking of the rectum at the site of the rectopexy. We use two 2-0 Prolene mattress sutures, passed anterior to posterior through the mesorectum adjacent to the bowel wall, then through the presacral fascia, and finally back through the mesorectum (posterior to anterior) 1.5–2 cm from the initial bite. (Fig. 54.1A and B) Care must be taken to avoid both impalement of mesenteric vessels and injury to the presacral venous plexus. It is worth noting that the sutures' role is to provide temporary fixation until fibrosis from the scarring process fixes the rectum into place. The peritoneum is left open, and we do not routinely drain the pelvis. The abdominal wall is closed in layers once meticulous hemostasis has been ensured.

Mesh Rectopexy

Similar to the other nonresectional techniques, the rectal mobilization is as described above. However, in this case the mesh is placed to provide additional point of fixation and scarring to the sacral promontory. Various types of meshes have been described from polypropylene and PTFE to biologics. Similarly the mesh has been used in both posterior and anterior locations, as well as varying degrees of circumferential or partial wrapping of the rectum itself.

For a posteriorly based wrap, once the rectum has been fully mobilized, a rectangular-shaped piece of mesh is secured to the presacral fascia (Figs. 54.2 and 54.3). Three 2-0 Prolene interrupted sutures are placed in the middle of the mesh and secured to the presacral fascia. The mesh is wrapped from posterior to anterior and secured to the rectum using 2–3 rows of sutures, as the rectum is pulled posteriorly towards the sacrum and superiorly to reduce redundancy. (Fig. 54.4) Some surgeons prefer to place additional proximal and distal sutures along the margins of the mesh to prevent migration of the rectum underneath the mesh. The peritoneum is then closed and an extraperitoneal drain may be placed in the presacral space.

Anteriorly based wraps begin with the mesh placed over the anterior aspect of the rectum approximately 4–5 cm below the sacral promontory. The placement of sutures is divided into left and right sides and performed in sequential order, with three 2-0 Prolene interrupted sutures placed on one side of the mesh and secured to the ipsilateral presacral fascia. The same technique is repeated on the contralateral side. The rectum is then again pulled posterior towards the sacrum and superiorly to reduce redundancy. Prior to tying down the sutures, the tension on the rectum is inspected by having an assistant retract on the sutures while the surgeon places three to four fingers between the rectum and the sacrum. Finally, additional sutures are placed as necessary to secure the mesh and avoid slippage.

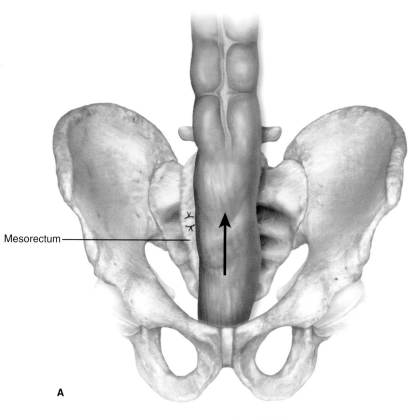

Mesorectum

A

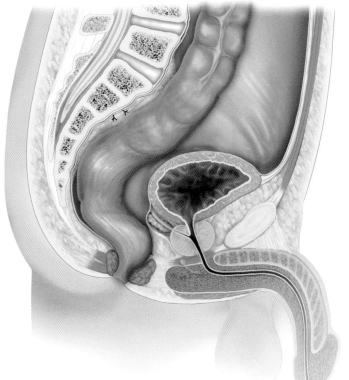

B

Part XIV: Abdominal Operations for Rectal Prolapse

Figure 54.2 Suturing the mesh to the sacrum.

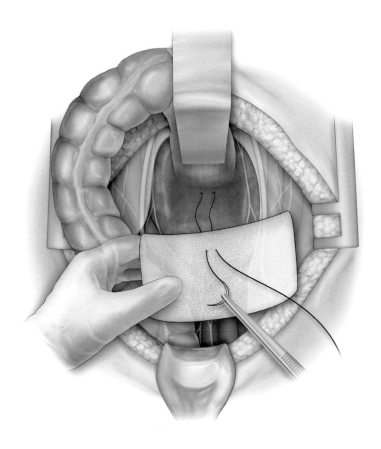

Figure 54.3 Posteriorly based mesh attached to the sacrum.

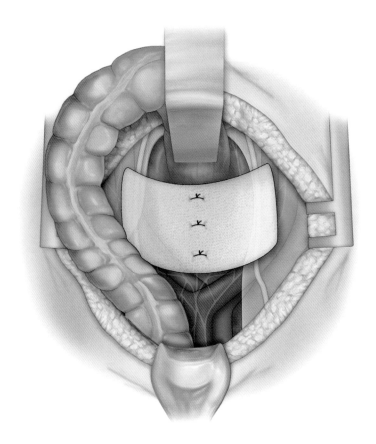

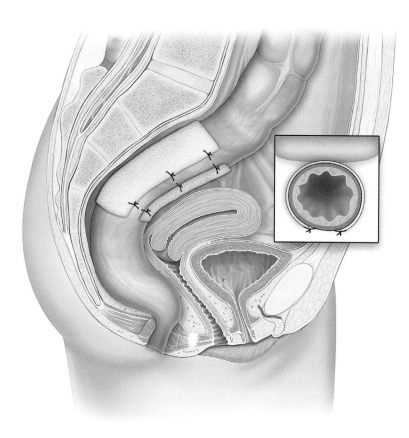

Figure 54.4 Completed mesh rectopexy with lateral view demonstrating the point of fixation.

 PEARLS AND PITFALLS

1. Since a resection is avoided, surgeons should place emphasis on the preoperative history to ensure a significant history of constipation is present that may warrant the addition of a resection.
2. Proper positioning of the mesh is imperative to ensure no loss of traction on the rectum.
3. Consideration may be made for tacking devices to fixate the mesh to the presacral fascia.
4. To reduce the chances of mesh infection, avoidance of any intraoperative spillage or inadvertent enterotomy is critically important.
5. Aggressive or tight wrapping should be avoided, as this may lead to constriction of the rectal vault with subsequent luminal narrowing.

 POSTOPERATIVE MANAGEMENT

Standard postoperative management includes early ambulation and initiation of enteral feeding as tolerated. Nasogastric tubes are not routinely used. The bladder catheter is usually removed on the first postoperative day. Patients are normally discharged in 3–6 days with clinical follow-up 7–10 days later.

COMPLICATIONS

Nonresectional repairs have a low rate in both morbidity (15–35%) and mortality (0.6–2%), while recurrent rectal prolapse has been reported in ~7–29%, (4,9,10) Potential complications from this repair include more generalized conditions such as small or large bowel obstruction, ureteral injury or fibrosis, damage to autonomic nerves, rectovaginal fistula, and fecal impaction. Other potential long-term complications from the addition of mesh include intractable constipation, fecal incontinence, and recurrence. Additionally, mesh erosion through the rectum has been reported up to six years following the sentinel procedure. Although rare, mesh migration may be corrected without further surgical intervention (11).

RESULTS

Rectal mobilization alone and simple suture rectopexy have been shown to improve continence in 15–82% of patients, with most studies demonstrating over 50% success rates (4). With the addition of mesh, most studies have demonstrated a wide range (3–92%) of patients to have restoration of continence, with the variability, in part, secondary to the type and location of mesh placement. Mean rates for most studies, however, demonstrate improvement most often between 20–60%. In looking at individual types of repair, the Ripstein procedure has demonstrated continence improvement 15–80%.

Mobilization with rectopexy alone has demonstrated a low rate of new-onset constipation. In general, most prospective studies have also demonstrated improvement in constipation ranging from 14 to 83% (12). Unfortunately, there continues to be small (11–31%) numbers of patients that will develop worsening of symptoms. Rectopexy with the use of mesh is similarly associated with a wide range of functional results in constipated patients (15–71%). Somewhat more commonly, mesh use has slightly higher rates of worsening constipation (14–50%) when compared with suture rectopexy.

RESECTION RECTOPEXY

Surgery

Initial preparations for a resection rectopexy is similar to that stated above for cases not involving sigmoid resection. In addition to issues concerning mechanical bowel preparation, preoperative intravenous antibiotic use, and thromboembolic prophylaxis, discussion of the addition of a sigmoid resection and its inherent risks is required.

Positioning

Positioning typically does not differ from that described for nonresectional cases. As a bowel resection is being performed, the modified lithotomy position allows access to the rectum from below as well as ideal positioning for retraction of the pelvic organs.

Open Technique

The addition of a sigmoid resection in appropriately selected patients can improve postoperative bowel habits. Indications for bowel resection with rectopexy include significant associated diverticular disease, substantial constipation and, less commonly, an excessively redundant sigmoid colon that appears to be at risk for volvulus following mobilization. Unfortunately, the effects of resection on constipation are both variable and poorly documented, and sigmoid resection alone is unlikely to mitigate severe slow transit constipation. Our preference is to preserve the superior rectal artery and to divide the sigmoid branches; care should be taken to properly identify the left ureter prior to mesenteric division. The point of distal transection of the bowel should be past the transition to the intraperitoneal rectum where the taeniae coli have splayed. (Fig. 54.5) Proximally, the transection point of the descending/sigmoid colon may be chosen by pulling the colon up toward the abdominal wall to identify the redundant element.

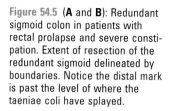

Figure 54.5 (**A** and **B**): Redundant sigmoid colon in patients with rectal prolapse and severe constipation. Extent of resection of the redundant sigmoid delineated by boundaries. Notice the distal mark is past the level of where the taeniae coli have splayed.

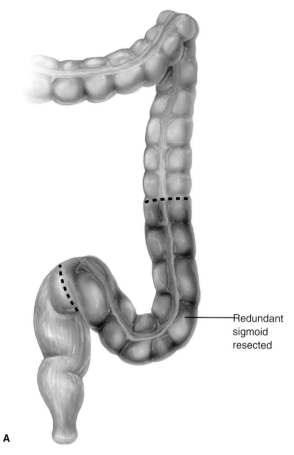

Redundant sigmoid resected

A

Part XIV: Abdominal Operations for Rectal Prolapse

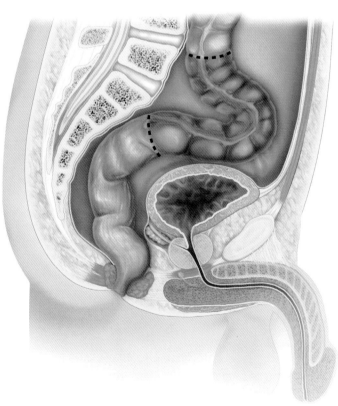

B

The proximal bowel should be soft and free of muscle hypertrophy associated with diverticular disease. Full mobilization of the splenic flexure may occasionally be required to ensure a tension-free anastomosis if an extensive sigmoid resection is required. A standard sutured or stapled end-to-end anastomosis is performed. Once the anastomosis has been fashioned, the anastomosis is checked for adequacy by insufflation of air via a rigid proctoscope placed transanally with the anastomosis submerged under saline. Additional information may be gathered by direct inspection via the proctoscope and ensuring that there are two complete "donuts" (rings) of tissue when using a stapled technique.

The rectopexy is then performed as detailed in the nonresectional section with 2 rows of 2-O Prolene mattress sutures placed though one side of the mesorectum and the presacral fascia. (Fig. 54.6A and B)

 # PEARLS AND PITFALLS

Surgeons should look for significant associated pelvic floor abnormalities that may need to be addressed at the time of prolapse surgery. Concomitant pelvic floor disorders such as enterocele, uterine or vaginal vault prolapse, cystocele, or rectocele can be present in up to 50% of patients with rectal prolapse. These anatomic abnormalities should be repaired only if they are symptomatic and have been adequately evaluated preoperatively. Correction of complex combined pelvic floor disorders is best performed with a multidisciplinary team that may involve a urologist, gynecologist or urogynecologist in addition to the colorectal surgeon.

 # POSTOPERATIVE MANAGEMENT

Standard postoperative management as in the nonresectional rectopexy patients remains the same with early ambulation, removal of the urinary catheter, antibiotics limited to the perioperative period, and early enteral feeding. Additionally, a bowel regimen that includes stool softeners and laxatives is initiated based on individual surgeon preference.

COMPLICATIONS

Similar to those cases that do not involve a sigmoidectomy, a resection rectopexy can be performed with minimal mortality (0–2.3%) and low morbidity (~15–35%) (13–16). The majority of early complications include urinary tract, wound, or respiratory infections with rates consistently in the 10–20% range. More significant problems requiring intervention such as presacral hemorrhage, fecal impaction, anastomotic leak, or deep space infections are less common (<5%). Of delayed complications, small bowel obstruction and severe constipation requiring hospitalization are also relatively infrequent. Other potential complications from this repair include ureteral injury or fibrosis, rectovaginal fistula, and worsening or new fecal incontinence.

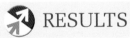 # RESULTS

Preoperative fecal incontinence is the major problem associated with long-standing rectal prolapse. Whether it is secondary to underlying sphincter tears, chronic stretch, or associated neuropathy, the majority of series have demonstrated some degree of fecal incontinence to be present in up to 75% of patients. In addition, 15–65% of patients with rectal prolapse also suffer from constipation or evacuation disorders (5).

The literature shows a wide range of improved continence (11–100%) following resection rectopexy, with mean rates approximating 50% (4,5). Yet, many patients,

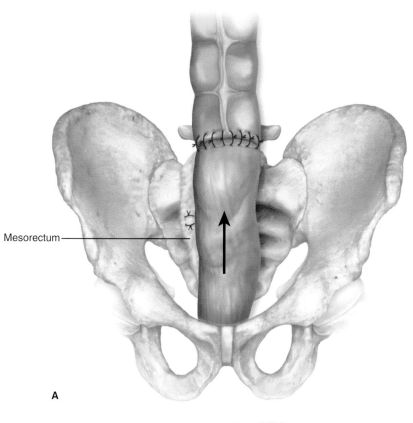

Mesorectum

A

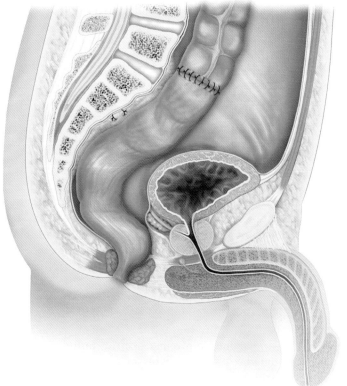

B

though improved, continue to have some degree of ongoing incontinence due to irreversible sphincter or pelvic nerve damage. As a practical matter, incontinent prolapse patients should have their prolapse corrected first and then undergo reevaluation and additional therapy if they have persisting problems.

For patients with preoperative constipation, results are variable. While many patients improve, a small number of patients develop new-onset or worsening of constipation following repair. Even in those patients who continue to have postoperative constipation, individual-related symptoms such as the feeling of incomplete evacuation, excessive time spent on the commode, need for enemas, and painful evacuation all tend to decrease after surgery. Although reported results and outcome measures vary, most series document decreased rates of constipation following rectopexy with sigmoid resection (18–80% improvement) (4,5). While there have been only two randomized prospective trials comparing rectopexy alone with rectopexy with sigmoid resection, both studies demonstrated lower rates of postoperative constipation with the addition of a sigmoidectomy.

Persisting constipation after rectopexy with sigmoid resection can be due to a number of causes. Some patients may have kinking at the level of the rectopexy, particularly when an anterior sling is utilized. Others have persisting slow transit constipation or a whole gut motility disorder. A third group may suffer from denervation of the rectal stump due to overly aggressive dissection. Finally, some patients have persisting or acquired pelvic floor dysfunction. Patients with persisting significant symptoms require repeat pelvic floor evaluation to determine the cause of the problem and a rational plan of therapy.

RECURRENT RECTAL PROLAPSE

It is generally accepted that recurrence rates following an abdominal prolapse repair (0–10%) are less than those after a perineal approach. Regardless of initial procedure performed, most recurrences are detected 1–3 years postoperatively, with up to one-third developing within the first 7 months. Although the cause of recurrence is not always clear, potential factors include technical errors associated with rectopexy and a failure to address concomitant pelvic floor defects. Additional reported risk factors for recurrence include concomitant psychiatric disease, male gender, older age, and higher body mass index.

A key factor affecting recurrence rates is length of time from surgery. In a large multicenter review of abdominal procedures, at a median follow-up of 43 months, recurrence occurred in 6.1% (9). In this series, 46 patients had only rectal mobilization, 130 patients had resection with rectopexy, and 467 had only rectopexy . The 1-, 5-, and 10-year recurrence rates were 1.06%, 6.61%, and 28.92%, respectively. Neither surgical technique, method of rectopexy (mesh *vs.* suture), nor means of access (open *vs.* laparoscopic) had any impact on the rate of recurrence—only length of follow-up. Therefore surgeons should be aware of not only to evaluate for recurrence even at extended follow-up intervals but also to counsel patients accordingly to ensure accurate expectations.

There are several important principles for managing patients with recurrent rectal prolapse. First, when possible, an abdominal repair of recurrent prolapse should be performed when the patient's risk profile permits. In the largest series specifically evaluating recurrent prolapse, despite the number of prior failures, abdominal approaches were consistently associated with lower rates of rerecurrence when compared with perineal repairs (6). Second, patients should be counseled that while successful repair of recurrent prolapse may alleviate the rectal protrusion, symptoms of constipation or fecal incontinence are likely to remain. Lastly, surgeons should make every effort to remove any prior anastomosis when performing resectional operations. Failure to do so may result in an interval ischemic segment, causing in mucosal sloughing, anastomotic leak, or stricture.

TABLE 54.1	Recurrence Rates with Open Resection Rectopexy			
Author	**Year**	**Patients**	**Recurrence (%)**	**Follow-up (months)**
Frykman	1968	80	0	–
Goldberg	1984	134	1.9	48
Watts	1985	102	1.9	6–360
Husa	1988	48	9	52
Luukkonen	1990	15	0	–
Madoff	1992	47	6.3	65
McKee	1992	9	0	3
Deen	1994	10	0	17
Huber	1995	39	0	54
Yakut	1998	19	0	38
Kim	1999	161	5	64
Kairaluoma	2003	30	0	12
Brown	2004	37	5	36
Raftopolous	2005	130	24	43
Johnson	2007	5	0	17
Byrne	2008	21	4.7	48
Hoel	2009	12	8.3	27
Pescatori	2009	6	12	61

Part XIV: Abdominal Operations for Rectal Prolapse

✦ CONCLUSIONS

Both resection rectopexy and nonresectional rectopexy are safe and effective operations indicated for rectal prolapse patients. The addition of a sigmoid resection is primarily reserved to those who suffer from constipation. Various nonresectional techniques exist that have unique benefits and risk profiles. Long-term data have demonstrated the reliability of these repairs with low recurrence rates, acceptable complication profile, and consistent improvement in both fecal incontinence and constipation (Table 54.1).

Recommended References and Readings

1. Karulf RE, Madoff RD, Goldberg SM. Rectal prolapse. *Curr Probl Surg* 2001;38:771–832.
2. Azimuddin K, Khubchandani IT, Rosen L, Stasik JJ, Riether RD, Reed JF 3rd. Rectal prolapse: a search for the "best" operation. *Am Surg* 2001;67:622–627.
3. Kim DS, Tsang CB, Wong WD, Lowry AC, Goldberg SM, Madoff RD. Complete rectal prolapse: evolution of management and results. *Dis Colon Rectum* 1999;42:460–466.
4. Madiba TE, Baig MK, Wexner SD. Surgical management of rectal prolapse. *Arch Surg* 2005;140:63–73.
5. Bachoo P, Brazzelli M, Grant A. Surgery for complete rectal prolapse in adults. *Cochrane Database Syst Rev* 2000;(2):CD001758.
6. Steele SR, Goetz LH, Minami S, Madoff RD, Mellgren A, Parker SC. Management of recurrent rectal prolapse: surgical approach influences outcome. *Dis Colon Rectum* 2006;49(4):440–5.
7. Mellgren A, Johansson C, Dolk A, et al. Enterocele demonstrated by defaecography is associated with other pelvic floor disorders. *Int J Colorectal Dis* 1994;9:121–124.
8. Speakman CT, Madden MV, Nicholls RJ, Kamm MA. Lateral ligament division during rectopexy causes constipation but prevents recurrence: results of a prospective randomized study. *Br J Surg* 1991;78:1431–1433.
9. Raftopoulos Y, Senagore AJ, Di Giuro G, Bergamaschi R, Rectal Prolapse Recurrence Study Group. Recurrence rates alter abdominal surgery for complete rectal prolapse: a multicenter pooled analysis of 642 individual patient data. *Dis Colon Rectum* 2005;48:1200–1206.
10. Tjandra JJ, Fazio VW, Church JM, Milsom JW, Oakley JR, Lavery IC. Ripstein procedure is an effective treatment for rectal prolapse without constipation. *Dis Colon Rectum* 1993;36:501–507.
11. Karagulle E, Yildirim E, Turk E, Akkaya D, Moray G. Mesh invasion of the rectum: an unusual late complication of rectal prolapse repair. *Int J Colorectal Dis* 2006;21:724–727.
12. Khanna AK, Misra MK, Kumar K. Simplified sutured sacral rectopexy for complete rectal prolapse in adults. *Eur J Surg* 1996; 162:143–146.
13. McKee RF, Lauder JC, Poon FW, Aitchison MA, Finlay IG. A prospective randomized study of abdominal rectopexy with and without sigmoidectomy in rectal prolapse. *Surg Gynecol Obstet* 1992;174:145–148.
14. Huber FT, Stein H, Siewert JR. Functional results after treatment of rectal prolapse with rectopexy and sigmoid resection. *World J Surg* 1995;19:138–43.
15. Luukkonnen P, Mikkonen U, Jarvinen H. Abdominal rectopexy with sigmoidectomy vs. rectopexy alone for rectal prolapse: a prospective, randomized study. *Int J Colorectal Dis* 1992;7: 219–22.
16. Madoff RD, Mellgren A. One hundred years of rectal prolapse surgery. *Dis Colon Rectum* 1999;42:441–50.

55 Laparoscopic Resection Rectopexy

Martin Luchtefeld and Dirk Weimann

 ## INDICATIONS/CONTRAINDICATIONS

There are many surgical options to choose from when treating a patient for rectal prolapse. The sheer number and diversity of choices suggests that there is no perfect answer for all circumstances. The choices can be broadly categorized into four: (a) sigmoid resection/rectopexy, (b) rectopexy with or without mesh, (c) perineal proctosigmoidectomy (Altemeier's procedure), and (d) Delorme procedure. The first two options, both abdominal procedures, can be done either open or laparoscopically. The first consideration while selecting the appropriate operation is whether or not the patient is medically fit to undergo a major abdominal operation. Abdominal approaches are felt to have a lower recurrence rate but are associated with a greater risk of complication. The perineal approaches are associated with a higher recurrence rate but are tolerated better with fewer complications.

If a patient is medically fit for an abdominal surgery, both sigmoid resection/rectopexy and rectopexy alone have good outcomes with low recurrence rates. However, rectopexy alone has a higher risk of postoperative constipation, even in patients with normal bowel habits prior to the procedure. Sigmoid resection/rectopexy is a better choice for the constipated patient but carries the small but real risk of anastomotic leak that is not an issue for the patient undergoing rectopexy alone. Sigmoid resection/rectopexy then is ideally suited for the medically fit patient who already suffers from constipation.

Sigmoid resection/rectopexy can be done as an open or laparoscopic procedure. Early in the history of laparoscopic colon and rectal surgery, rectal prolapse surgery was thought to be an ideal disease process for the laparoscopic approach: it is a benign illness, it is noninflammatory, and the mesentery tends to be redundant and relatively easy to address. Multiple studies of laparoscopic-aided sigmoid colectomy/rectopexy have now been published and when compared to the open version, the recurrence rates appear to be similar while short-term outcomes such as length of stay are superior.

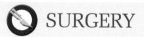 PREOPERATIVE PLANNING

Prior to surgery, the diagnosis of rectal prolapse must be verified during physical examination. Visualizing and identifying rectal prolapse is not always straightforward. Evaluating the patient on an examining table may not be sufficient to confirm rectal prolapse. If the diagnosis has not been made during the usual examination, the patient can be placed on the commode and then reexamined after several minutes of straining. Once the prolapse has been reproduced, the diagnosis is usually quite obvious. However, occasionally, it can be difficult to distinguish full-thickness rectal prolapse from mucosal prolapse or significant prolapsing hemorrhoidal disease. If uncertainty remains, identification of the circular folds of the full-thickness rectal prolapse will confirm the diagnosis.

Before making a final decision for a resection/rectopexy, it is important to evaluate the colon with colonoscopy (or some other form of full evaluation) to be certain that there is no other significant pathology present that might alter the surgical plan.

Anal physiologic studies also need to be considered preoperatively. For the patient with fecal incontinence, anal manometry, intra-anal ultrasound, and pudendal nerve terminal motor latency testing can provide documentation of the preoperative physiologic status. Conversely, for the patient with no impairment, these studies would add little value.

Many of these patients will suffer from constipation as well. In addition to the colonoscopy mentioned previously, colonic transit studies and defecography can be done.

SURGERY

Technique

Preoperative Preparation

The need for a mechanical bowel preparation is controversial. Many surgeons continue to use mechanical bowel preparations despite the fact that a multiple of prospective randomized trials have now been done and suggest that its use does not decrease surgical site infections. At a minimum, the rectosigmoid needs to be cleared of fecal matter with enemas to facilitate bowel handling and most importantly to allow the passage of an intraluminal stapling instrument.

The use of oral antibiotics as part of the bowel preparation has been abandoned by many surgeons. Meta-analysis of multiple trials has suggested that the addition of oral antibiotics will lead to a lower incidence of surgical site infections.

The administration of intravenous antibiotics within 1 hour of incision time is well documented to decrease surgical site infections and should be given routinely.

Positioning

Following general endotracheal anesthesia, the patient should be placed in the dorsal lithotomy position (Fig. 55.1). The legs should be in stirrups that can be easily positioned and changed if need be. An indwelling Foley catheter is also placed as well as a gastric tube (oro or nasogastric). It is important to have the patient secured to the operating room table in some fashion to ensure that the patient does not move excessively when being placed in steep Trendelenburg during the procedure. Although some surgeons will use a bean bag apparatus for this purpose, any effective method such as taping or use of straps is acceptable. Having the ability to safely place the patient in steep Trendelenburg is essential to allow the small bowel move out of the operative field.

Trocar Placement

The placement of trocars is an important part of the success of this operation and is essentially the same as for sigmoid or left colectomies (Fig. 55.2). A periumbilical port

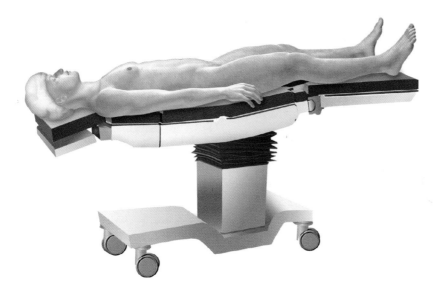

Figure 55.1 The patient is placed in dorsal lithotomy position with the legs in adjustable stirrups. The patient should be fixed in place with a beanbag mattress or some other combination of straps or fixation devices.

is used for the camera. Although usually the camera port is placed in an infraumbilical position, in a short patient with very little room between the pubis and the umbilicus, moving the port site to just above the umbilicus affords a better view with the laparoscope. Additional ports are placed as illustrated. The port in the right lower quadrant needs to be a 12-mm port to allow passage of an endoscopic linear stapler. The best rule for placement of this port is to place it 2 cm medial to and 2 cm superior to the anterior superior iliac spine. The other port on the right side can usually be a 5-mm port as this port is mostly used for passage of a grasper/dissector. An additional 5-mm port on the left side allows the assistant to provide retraction and countertraction for the primary surgeon.

Figure 55.2 The placement of the trocars is illustrated as well as possible extraction sites.

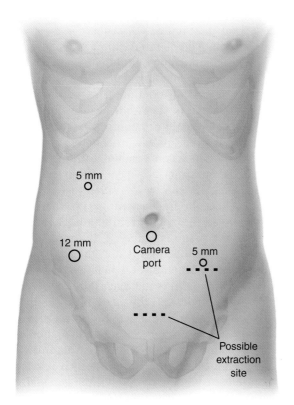

5 mm

12 mm

Camera port

5 mm

Possible extraction site

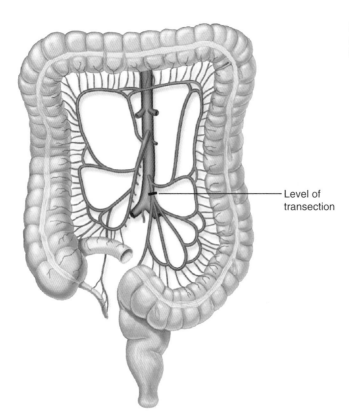

Figure 55.3 The vascular division occurs at the level of the superior hemorrhoidal vessels.

Level of transection

Vascular Division

Once all the trocars are in place, the patient is placed in steep Trendelenburg position to facilitate moving the small bowel out of the pelvis and thus optimizing the continued retraction of the small bowel. This simple maneuver will optimize visualization of the pelvic structures. The vascular division is done at the level of the superior hemorrhoidal vessels (Fig. 55.3) at the level of the sacral promontory. Dissection is most commonly undertaken in a medial to lateral fashion. The sigmoid colon is usually very redundant and the first step is to elevate the redundant colon out of the pelvis. By doing so, the superior hemorrhoidal vessels can be identified coursing over the sacral promontory. The mesentery can then be grasped and placed on traction. The simple step of placing the mesentery on tension makes the vasculature stand out even in the patient with a thick or very fatty mesentery (Fig. 55.4). The sacral promontory serves as a very useful and reliable landmark. The haptic feedback from touching this bony prominence helps identify anatomy even in the obese patient. Once comfortable with the anatomy, the peritoneum is then opened along the medial and inferior aspect of the vasculature so that the areolar tissue just behind the mesorectum can be identified just below the sacral promontory. Care should be taken to reflect the hypogastric nerves that course over the sacral promontory as injury here can lead to sexual dysfunction. Getting into the proper plane is very important. If the proper plane is obtained, the remainder of the dissection usually can proceed with very little difficulty. If not, the dissection is tedious, identification of anatomical landmarks is difficult, and it is easier to make technical errors and cause organ injury. If, at any time, it is not clear that one is in the right plane, it is well worth the time and effort to review all the anatomical landmarks until the correct plane is identified. Once the correct plane is entered, dissection can then be undertaken in a medial to lateral fashion (Fig. 55.5). This window should be made as large as possible to facilitate identification of retroperitoneal structures. This step can be accomplished by extending the peritoneal incision both inferiorly and superiorly. The dissection continues until important structures (the ureter, the gonadal vessels, and the iliac vessels) are identified and preserved. If the proper plane of dissection

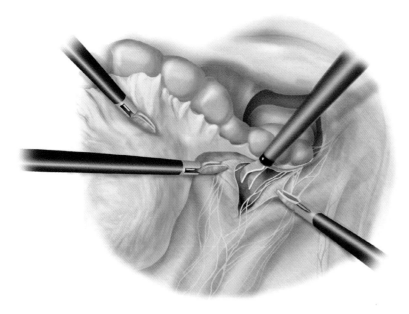

Figure 55.4 With the patient in steep Trendelenburg, the mesentery to the rectosigmoid is grasped and put on tension to put the superior hemorrhoidal vessels in relief. A peritoneal incision is then made over the vessels and down over the sacral promontory.

is difficult to identify or the ureter cannot be found after a reasonable amount of time and effort, the dissection can be initiated from the lateral aspect by incising the lateral peritoneal attachments and then reflecting the colon and mesentery medially.

Once the ureter and iliac vessels have been identified and reflected away from the mesentery, the vascular pedicle can be isolated with a combination of sharp and dull dissection. The vessels can then be ligated and divided by whatever means (stapler, clips, or energy device) the surgeon prefers (Fig. 55.6). Alternatively, since the procedure is for benign disease, some surgeons will opt to save the main trunk of the superior hemorrhoidal vessels and perform the dissection of the colon and division of the mesentery close to colon wall.

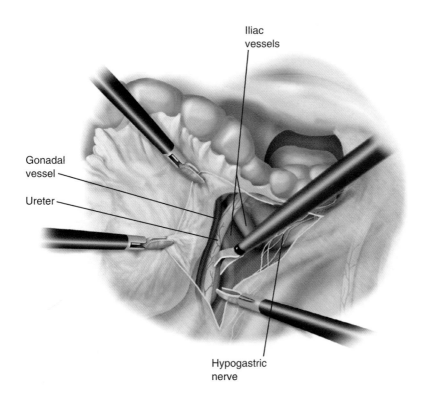

Iliac
vessels

Gonadal
vessel

Ureter

Hypogastric
nerve

Figure 55.5 The areolar plane behind the rectosigmoid mesentery is entered at the level of the sacral promontory and dissection is carried out in a medial to lateral fashion. The hypogastric nerves, left ureter, and iliac vessels should all be identified.

Part XIV: Abdominal Operations for Rectal Prolapse

Figure 55.6 The superior hemorrhoidal vessels are isolated, ligated, and divided (shown here with laparoscopic linear stapler).

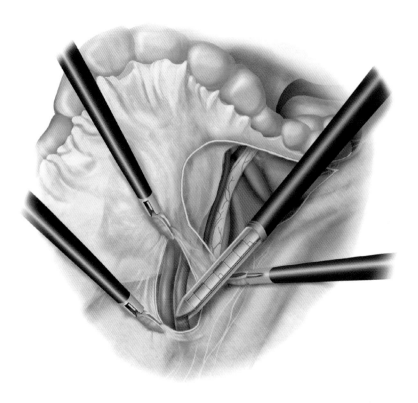

Rectal Mobilization

Once hemostasis is ensured at the level of the division of the vascular pedicle, attention is directed to mobilizing the rectum. The areolar tissue in the presacral space previously identified serves as an ideal entry point to start the dissection. With the assistant surgeon providing retraction of the rectosigmoid junction out of the pelvis and off the sacrum, the operating surgeon has an exceptional view to dissect in this plane posteriorly to the rectum and all the way to the pelvic floor (Fig. 55.7). In the course of this dissection, Waldeyer's fascia will be encountered and divided. If needed, the completeness of the dissection can be confirmed by having one surgeon go between the legs and do a digital

Figure 55.7 The dissection starts at the level of the sacral promontory and proceeds in the areolar plane just behind the mesorectum all the way down to the pelvic floor.

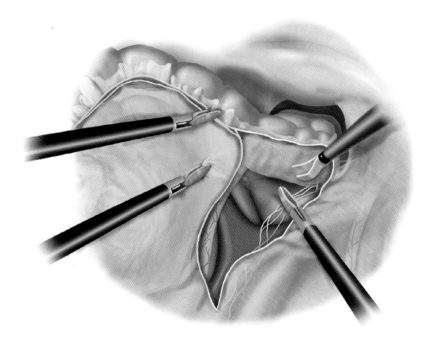

rectal examination. The examining finger can easily be seen with the laparoscopic view of the pelvis and the assistant can also feel the instruments doing the dissection through the rectal wall. Once sufficient posterior dissection has been carried out posteriorly, the lateral attachments can be readily identified and divided. There is controversy regarding the handling of the lateral stalks. Part of the controversy stems from the lack of consensus on the exact anatomy and even the existence of well-defined lateral stalks. Given this controversy it is not surprising that the literature is confusing regarding both the necessity of and the subsequent results of division of the lateral stalks. In our practice, it has been our habit to do a complete dissection posteriorly all the way to the pelvic floor but to leave the most distal of the lateral attachments untouched.

Division of Bowel with Extraction of Specimen

Once the dissection has been completed the next order of events is to decide at which level to perform the distal transection of the rectosigmoid. The division of bowel is planned to allow an anastomosis to be created at or slightly above the level of the sacral promontory. When identifying this level it is important that the mobilized rectum be pulled up out of the pelvis and be put on gentle but firm traction. This action will avoid marking a spot for transection that is too high. It is ideal to divide the bowel before dealing with the accompanying mesentery. To initiate the division, the peritoneal attachments at the proposed level of division are opened up both to mark the level and to help initiate dissection. The plane between the rectosigmoid and its mesentery is carefully identified and dissection carried out bluntly medially to laterally. A meticulous dissection is important here to minimize the risk of inadvertently entering the bowel. Once a plane has been developed all the way across, an endoscopic linear stapler can be used to divide the bowel at the previously identified level (Fig. 55.8). Oftentimes, it requires more than one firing of the stapler to completely transect the rectum. It is important to be meticulous in the placement of the stapler directly in the crotch of the previous staple line so that the subsequent stapler firing does not create an irregularity or dog ear on the rectal stump. After this portion is accomplished the only remaining tissue will be the mesorectum. At this level there are still significant large vessels that require division by whatever means the surgeon chooses. The distal end of the bowel to be resected will then be completely freed up and usually is quite mobile. Any remaining lateral attachments that need to be divided can now be identified and dealt with.

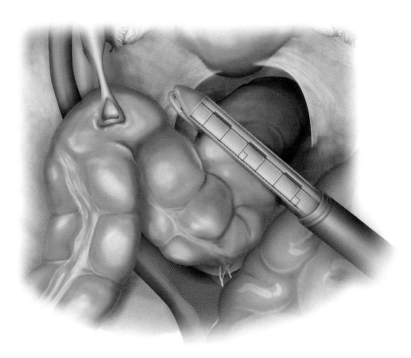

Figure 55.8 Once a plane has been developed between the rectosigmoid junction and its mesentery, the upper rectum can be divided with an endoscopic linear stapler.

Part XIV: Abdominal Operations for Rectal Prolapse

Exteriorization of the Bowel

The proximal point of resection now needs to be identified and marked in some fashion. Endoscopic clips, cautery, or simply using a locking grasper can serve this purpose. The level of proximal transection should allow for an anastomosis at the level of the sacral promontory. The bowel can then be exteriorized. There are several options for the site of exteriorization. A short transverse incision 2 cm above the pubis functions well. There are advantages of the suprapubic incision. Firstly, it serves as a second check on the level of the proximal resection margin. If the transected bowel can be bought to the skin level, it will also comfortably reach the sacral promontory for a tension-free anastomosis. Secondly, for the surgeon uncomfortable with certain parts of this procedure laparoscopically, this site can serve as an access site for transection of the rectosigmoid, placement of the rectopexy stitches, and performing an anastomosis.

Using a previous low midline or Pfannenstiel incision is a convenient option. If there are no existing incisions to use, the port site in the left lower quadrant can be extended and used as the extraction site.

Anastomosis

Once exteriorized, the bowel is transected at the site previously identified. The remaining mesentery is taken down under direct vision at the extraction site and then a purse-string suture placed into the cut end of the proximal bowel. An anvil from an appropriate-sized end-to-end stapling device is placed and the purse-string is pulled tight (Fig. 55.9). The proximal end is then placed back into the abdominal cavity, the extraction site closed to at least at the level of the fascia, and pneumoperitoneum reestablished. One surgeon then goes to the perineal position and places the end-to-end stapling device into the rectum. Under direct view with the aid of the laparoscope, the stapler is advanced up to the end of the rectal stump. The spike can then be advanced out through the rectal stump

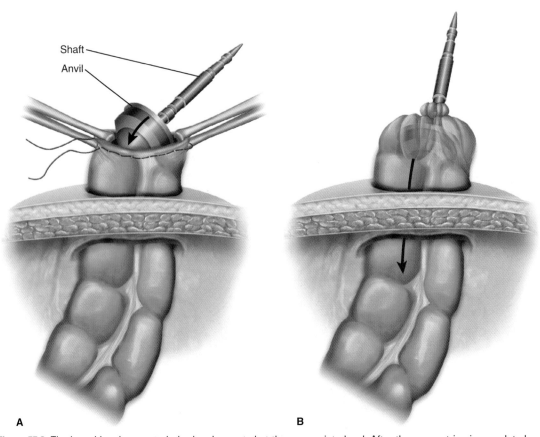

A   B

Figure 55.9 The bowel has been exteriorized and resected at the appropriate level. After the purse-string is completed the anvil of the stapling device is put in place and the purse-string tied down.

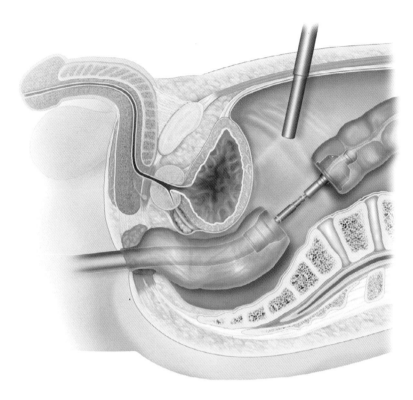

Part XIV: Abdominal Operations for Rectal Prolapse

Figure 55.10 Once pneumoperitoneum is reestablished, the circular stapler is passed up through the rectal stump and the spike advanced out through the end.

(Fig. 55.10). The other surgeon then needs to identify the proximal bowel with the anvil and then mate the two ends together (Fig. 55.11). The anastomosis is then carried out in the usual fashion. Once completed, the anastomotic rings are checked for completeness and the anastomosis itself is air-tested under water to check for leaks.

Rectopexy

Once the integrity of the anastomosis has been confirmed, attention can be directed to doing the rectopexy. The intent of the rectopexy is to fix the mobilized rectal stump to

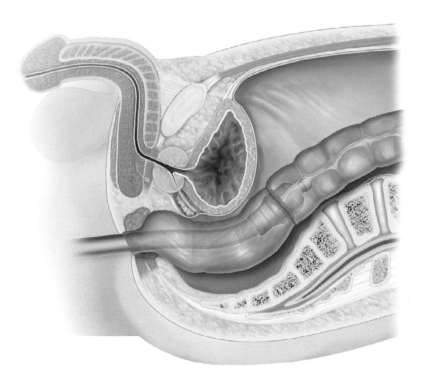

Figure 55.11 The two ends of the circular stapler are mated and the stapler fired to complete the anastomosis.

Figure 55.12 A permanent suture is passed through the lateral stalk and subsequently tacked to the sacral promontory to accomplish the rectopexy.

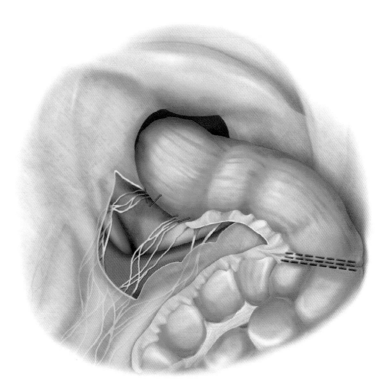

Figure 55.12 A permanent suture is passed through the lateral stalk and subsequently tacked to the sacral promontory to accomplish the rectopexy.

the sacral promontory so that the risk of recurrent prolapse is minimized. A permanent suture (0 or 2-0) is used to fix the lateral stalks of the rectum to the top of the sacral promontory (Fig. 55.12). The stitch into the sacral promontory needs to include the periosteum but at the same time be careful to avoid the sympathetic nerves and any vascular structures. At least two stitches should be taken to complete the rectopexy. Some surgeons have also used various other fixation devices such as a laparoscopic tack applier for this same purpose. Alternatively, the rectopexy sutures can be placed through the lateral stalks prior to rectosigmoid junction division or anastomosis creation. This latter method may limit excessive manipulation of the new anastomosis. Specifically, the sutures are placed through the lateral stalks and the sacral periosteum but left intact until after the anastomosis has been created.

An adjunctive approach is to close the entire length of the peritoneum to the rectum with absorbable suture. In closing the peritoneum, the lateral aspect of the bites of the peritoneum is more craniad. When the suture is tightened this closure serves to pull the rectum up and secure it in place higher in the pelvis.

POSTOPERATIVE MANAGEMENT

Postoperative management following a sigmoid resection/rectopexy is no different than after any other laparoscopic-aided colectomy. In our institution, like many others, an enhanced recovery program is instituted immediately postoperatively. While some of the details may vary from place to place, many of the elements are common: early feeding and early ambulation on the same day of surgery, and early removal of the Foley catheter (the morning following surgery). Of great importance is the effort to minimize narcotic analgesia by using gabapentin, acetaminophen, and nonsteroidal anti-inflammatory agents in various combinations. Prior to discharge, the patient needs to be tolerating solid food for at least two meals and taking enough fluids orally to avoid dehydration. The patient does not need to have a bowel movement prior to discharge but should at least be passing flatus. Successful implementation of this enhanced recovery program will require extensive staff education regarding the rationale, benefit, and safety of such an approach.

After recovery to normal work/life (usually 4 weeks) pelvic floor training by a specially trained physiotherapist for anal incontinence is often necessary. In cases of prolonged fecal incontinence of >6 months, it is likely that there are neuropathic pudendal nerves due to the preexisting descending perineum. In such cases, sacral nerve stimulation has been used with good results.

 COMPLICATIONS

Many of the complications that occur after this procedure are the same as can be expected after any segmental colectomy. Anastomotic leaks are feared but are fortunately uncommon. Because of the area of dissection, there can be injuries to the ureter and hypogastric nerves (with resultant sexual dysfunction). Even with the laparoscopic approach, ileus can occur and lead to a prolonged hospital stay. However, ileus is unusual enough in this setting that its occurrence should always make one search for an underlying cause of the ileus.

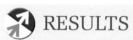 RESULTS

Both the short-term and the long-term results of laparoscopic-aided sigmoid resection/rectopexy are very good. Conversion to an open procedure is necessary in only a small percentage (5% or less) of the cases. While operative times are longer for the laparoscopic approach, the recovery of bowel function is quicker and length of stay is shorter than the open procedure. With long-term follow-up, the risk of recurrence is low (6–7% at 5 years in pooled studies).

Most patients see an improvement in their function. For those patients with incontinence, at least 50% will get better. For the patients with constipation, undergoing this procedure does not always resolve the constipation, but if the lateral stalks are not divided at least the condition does not typically worsen.

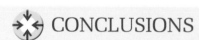 CONCLUSIONS

Laparoscopic-aided resection rectopexy is an excellent choice of a procedure for the medically fit patient with rectal prolapse accompanied by constipation.

Suggested Readings

Brazzelli M, Bachoo P, Grant. Surgery for complete rectal prolapse in adults. *Cochrane Database Syst Rev* 1999;4:CD001758. DOI: 10.1002/14651858.

Canfrere VG, des Barannos SB, Mayon J, et al. Adding sigmoidectomy to rectopexy to treat rectal prolapse: a valid option? *Br J Surg* 1994;581:2–4.

Luukkonen P, Mikkonen U, Jarvinen H. Abdominal rectopexy with sigmoidectomy vs rectopexy alone for rectal prolapse: a randomized prospective study. *Int J Colorectal Dis* 1992;7:219–22.

McKee RF, Lauder JC, Poon FW, et al. A prospective randomized study of abdominal rectopexy with and without sigmoidectomy in rectal prolapse. *Surg Gynecol Obstet* 1992;174:145–48.

Purkayastha S, Tekkis P, Aziz O, et al. A comparison of open vs. laparoscopic abdominal rectopexy for full-thickness rectal prolapse: a meta-analysis. *Dis Colon Rectum* 2005;48:1930–40.

Raftopoulos Y, Senagore AJ, Di Giuro G, et al. Recurrence rates after abdominal surgery for complete rectal prolapse: a multicenter pooled analysis of 643 individual patient data. *Dis Colon Rectum* 2005;48:1200–06.

Sayfan J, Pinbo M, Alexander-Williams J, et al. Sutured posterior abdominal rectopexy with sigmoidectomy compared with Marlex rectopexy for rectal prolapse. *Br J Surg* 1990;77:143–45.

56 Hand-Assisted Resection Rectopexy

William Timmerman

 ## INDICATIONS/CONTRAINDICATIONS

Rectal prolapse continues to be an interesting and challenging problem for both patients and surgeons alike. A myriad of procedures utilizing abdominal and perineal approaches have been developed, which serves as a testimony to the fact that no one procedure fits all patients, and therefore fitting the right patient to the right operation is important to obtain good results (1).

As a general rule, abdominal approaches are preferred for more healthy and fit patients, while perineal approaches are more often utilized in elderly and/or infirm patients (2).

A sigmoid resection and rectopexy offers the dual advantages of refixing the prolapsing rectum to the sacrum, *and* removing the usually redundant sigmoid, which not only helps prevent postoperative constipation (1,3–5), but also helps with prevention of recurrence by leaving the patient with a straightened left colon supported by the phrenicocolic ligament and left lateral peritoneal attachments (2,6). This anchoring in turn acts as a second point of fixation to help prevent rectal sliding and descent, and subsequent prolapse recurrence.

Sigmoid resection and rectopexy can be performed in open, pure laparoscopic, or hand-assisted laparoscopic fashion. Compared with open laparotomy, a laparoscopic approach offers the advantages of less pain, shorter hospitalization, and a faster recovery and return to work (2,3,7,8). It is our practice to perform resection/rectopexy in either pure laparoscopic or hand-assisted fashion, with the hand-assisted technique being especially useful in the more difficult patients with extensive adhesions from previous surgeries or pelvic conditions, in those patients with recurrences of prolapse following previous abdominal approaches, and when trying to avoid conversion to full open surgery when technical problems are encountered at operation. We also find it a very useful technique for those striving to obtain and improve their laparoscopic comfort, skills, and competency early in their laparoscopic careers (9,10).

Contraindications include all the usual contraindications to laparoscopic surgery, including labile cardiac disease, severe COPD, and conditions causing a general inability to tolerate position changes during surgery. The inability to safely dissect and operate at surgery, as caused by extensive adhesions or other technical factors is the most common contraindication to laparoscopic approaches. Therefore, as a first step at surgery, placing a single camera port with an honest assessment of the intra-abdominal "lay of the land", coupled with an honest assessment of one's technical skills, is crucial to a good, safe outcome for both patient and surgeon.

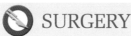 PREOPERATIVE PLANNING

As a first requirement, the patient must first be a suitable candidate for laparoscopic surgery. Significant cardiac and pulmonary problems must be accurately assessed and addressed, and the patient's previous surgical history thoroughly reviewed, especially previous pelvic or pelvic brim surgery. If the patient has had extensive previous pelvic surgery or inflammatory conditions, consider the placement of temporary ureteral catheters at the time of surgery, especially if early in one's laparoscopic career.

Preoperative workup goes to the reasons why the patient developed prolapse in the first place (11). Patients with significant constipation merit colonic transit studies, and may be candidates for concomitant total colectomy if severe colonic inertia is discovered.

Colonoscopy should be undertaken to exclude leading points for prolapse such as tumor, as well as to discover other covert or unrelated significant colonic problems that could be appropriately addressed at the same operation (e.g., a large right-sided villous neoplasm).

Concomitant pelvic floor abnormalities should be preoperatively identified, as they may affect surgical outcomes, and may on occasion be concomitantly treated at surgery. For example, uterine prolapse and cystoceles may be simultaneously treated in a multi-disciplinary fashion at the time of prolapse repair (12). Paradoxical puborectalis contractions may be a contributor to preoperative constipation, straining, and the formation of the prolapse, as well as a contributing factor to postoperative recurrence if unaddressed or unrecognized. Therefore, anal manometry and defecating proctography can play an important part of the workup.

⟩ SURGERY

Operative Technique

A hand-assisted technique can offer some significant advantages. For the less experienced laparoscopic surgeon, it offers the security of retained tactile feedback, improved eye-hand coordination, and help with learning depth perception while operating through a screen monitor (9,10). For surgeons at all skill levels it can offer improved exposure by traction and countertraction, and can be especially helpful with the ability to palpate and safely identify and delineate vital structures such as ureters, ureteral catheters, adhesed loops of bowel, and other significant structures, all of which may be partially obscured by adhesions and other operative conditions. It can aide in the control of bleeding vessels, and can help develop appropriate tissue planes during dissection. The tactile feedback with hand-assistance can help to more accurately assess tension across the colorectal anastomosis, and at the point of rectal fixation to the sacrum. In addition, it can also assist with intracorporeal suturing.

Patients are placed in supine lithotomy position, with both arms tucked, and orogastric and bladder catheters in place (Fig. 56.1); the operator stands at the patient's right side.

Placement of the hand-assisted device varies between "midline" locations (Fig. 56.2) and "off-midline" locations (Fig. 56.3), according to the preferences of the surgeon. We prefer placement in the left lower quadrant by an oblique transrectus muscle-splitting incision, as it helps us use the hand maximally as a retractor and dissecting aide, while keeping the hand away from the camera, and interfering less with the field of view. We place a supraumbilical port for the operating camera, and one to two right lower quadrant working ports for use of the laparoscopic instruments (or camera, if needed) (Fig. 56.4).

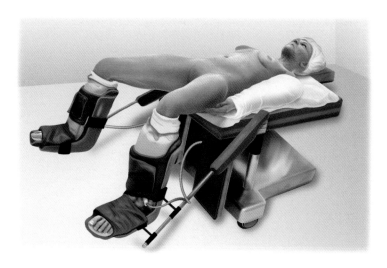

Figure 56.1 General positioning for laparoscopic resection rectopexy. Note supine lithotomy position, with both arms tucked at the sides, and orogastric tube and foley in place.

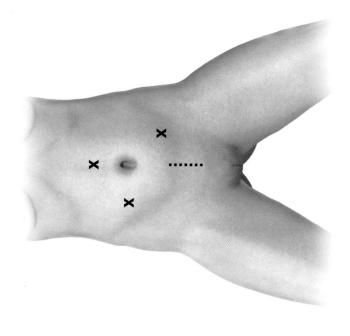

Figure 56.2 Midline placement of hand-assisted device, with typical port placements.

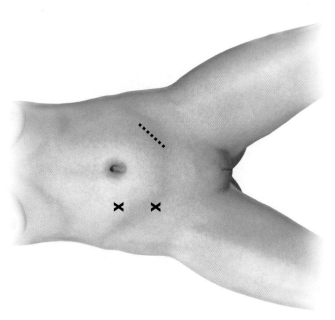

Figure 56.3 Off-midline placement of hand-assisted device in the left lower quadrant using an oblique transrectus muscle-splitting incision. Incision size is 1–2 cm smaller than the surgeon's numerical glove size.

Part XIV: Abdominal Operations for Rectal Prolapse

Figure 56.4 Our preferred port setup for hand-assisted resection/rectopexy.

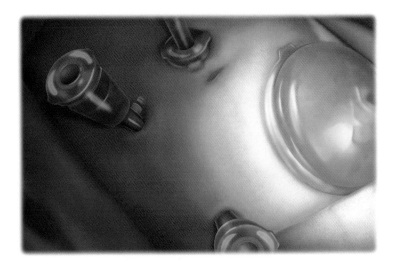

Incision size for the hand-assisted device is at most the same in centimeters as the surgeon's glove size. We prefer to incise 1–2 cm smaller than glove size, as the abdominal wall is plastic and will stretch during surgery. Hence, a size 7 glove would translate to a 5 cm incision size. We also always make the hand-port incision *after* the creation of the pneumoperitoneum, as incisions made before the creation of pneumoperitoneum will stretch, and may contribute to peri-device leakage of the pneumoperitoneum during the case.

We first mobilize the sigmoid, and identify the left ureter in all cases. Dissection may be in a medial-to-lateral (Fig. 56.5) or lateral-to-medial (Fig. 56.6) fashion, again depending on the surgeon's preference and local operative conditions. Unless the descending colon is loosely adherent to the lateral and posterior attachments, we do not routinely widely mobilize the descending colon, preferring to leave the majority of the descending colon's lateral and posterior attachments intact to act as a second point of "fixation" for the sigmoidectomy and rectopexy. The inferior mesenteric artery is elevated up away from the retroperitoneum, leaving the marginal branch intact and dropping the hypogastric nerves posteriorly (Fig. 56.7), taking the dissection over the sacral promontory and into the upper part of the retrorectal space.

While the peritoneum overlying the lateral stalks and lateral mesorectal tissue is divided to help elevate the rectum up out of the pelvis, we prefer to leave the lateral stalks themselves intact, not only for subsequent suturing to the presacral fascia, but to avoid denervating the rectum and potentially causing constipation postoperatively (2,5,7,11,13). The posterior presacral dissection is undertaken to the puborectalis sling at the pelvic floor (Fig. 56.8). Palpating the coccyx is a good anatomic landmark to ensure that the posterior

Figure 56.5 Initial sigmoid mobilization proceeding in a medial-to-lateral fashion, mobilizing the inferior mesenteric trunk cephalad.

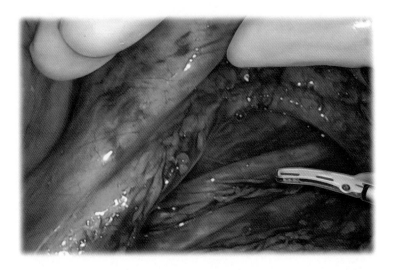

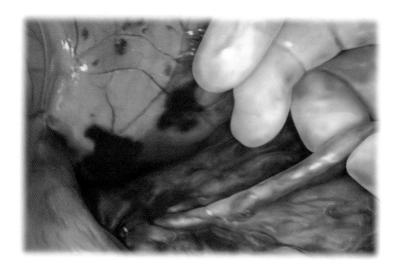

Figure 56.6 Initial sigmoid mobilization proceeding in a lateral-to-medial fashion, taking care to identify the left ureter, and not mobilizing more than the distal descending colon.

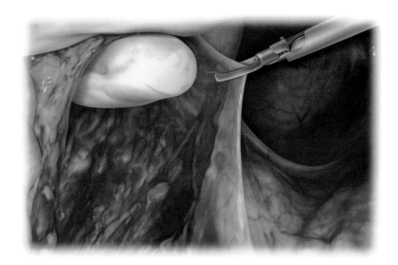

Figure 56.7 Dissection coming over the pelvic brim, elevating the inferior mesenteric system, while dropping the hypogastric nerves posteriorly, and entering the upper part of the retrorectal space.

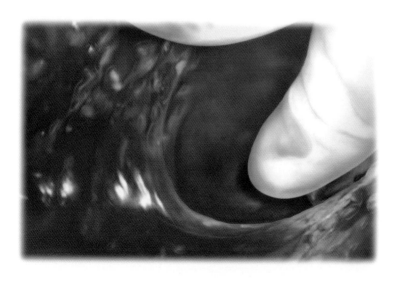

Figure 56.8 Posterior dissection is carried out caudally down to the puborectalis sling. The coccyx ought to be palpable with a fingertip, as a good check to confirm that the posterior dissection has gone far enough inferiorly. Anterior dissection is carried out 4–5 cm distal to the anterior peritoneal reflection.

Part XIV: Abdominal Operations for Rectal Prolapse

Figure 56.9 Rectal and sigmoid division away from the mesosigmoid and mesorectum. We like to leave the superior rectal branch to the rectum intact to increase vascular supply, and help avoid any damage to the hypogastric nerves.

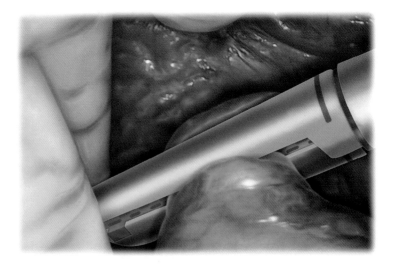

dissection has proceeded sufficiently inferiorly. Anteriorly, the peritoneal reflection at the cul-de-sac is divided and anterior rectal dissection taken 4–5 cm distally, to help elevate the rectum out of the pelvis for full rectal mobilization and subsequent fixation. The hand can be quite useful here for traction/countertraction, and exposure.

At this point, the uppermost rectum and sigmoid is dissected and divided away from the upper mesorectum and mesosigmoid, dividing segmental sigmoid branches, but again leaving the main inferior mesenteric system and inferiorly tracking superior rectal branch intact (Fig. 56.9). The uppermost rectum is then intracorporeally divided with a laparoscopic GIA stapler, and the redundant sigmoid is exteriorized by the hand-port and resected. A 29 or 33 mm anvil is placed in the distal colon, and the bowel is returned to the abdomen and pneumoperitoneum is reestablished. The rectul is tested with air insufflation for leakage both before and after the anastomosis is created with transanal stapling, to check for leaks at both the GIA and circular staple lines. The fixation of the rectum by its lateral stalks to the presacral tissues can now be accomplished, with the hand aiding in both the adjusting of the upward tension on the rectum, and with the placement of sutures or tacks (Fig. 56.10). The pelvic peritoneum is left open, and no drains are used.

 ## POSTOPERATIVE MANAGEMENT

We immediately start clear liquids, and rapidly increase to regular low residue diet as tolerated. Patients are ambulated by postoperative day one, and are discharged home when independently ambulating, tolerating regular diet, voiding, and passing stool or

Figure 56.10 We fix the rectum to the presacral tissues *after* the anastomosis has been created. The hand can help lift the rectum up to the proper location with the proper tension, and help with suture fixation.

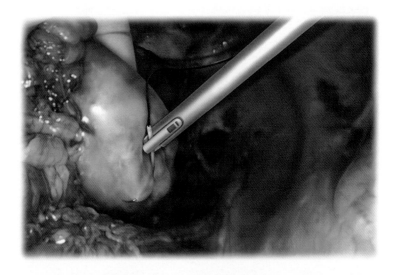

Part XIV: Abdominal Operations for Rectal Prolapse

flatus, with pain control by oral analgesia. Hospital stay is usually 2–4 days in uncomplicated cases.

 ## COMPLICATIONS

Complications following hand-assisted laparoscopic sigmoidectomy and rectopexy for rectal prolapse should be similar to those for elective sigmoid resections for diverticular and neoplastic disease. The most common are wound infections, pelvic infections, presacral bleeding, ileus, pneumonia, and anastomotic leak in the immediate postoperative period. The sigmoidectomy does not increase the morbidity of the procedure in terms of anastomotic leakage (rates reported as low as 0–1%) (1–4, 13). Potential long-term complications include hernias and bowel obstruction.

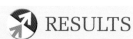 ## RESULTS

Prolapse recurrence rates with open or laparoscopic resection and rectopexy are generally better than those of rectopexy alone, with recurrence rates generally in the 0–10% range, depending on length of follow-up (3,13–15). However, as for all prolapse operations, recurrence increases over time, and the data is largely unavailable over 10 years out from surgery.

Constipation and incontinence are usually improved with resection/rectopexy compared to other techniques (2–4,11,13).

Preservation of the lateral ligaments appears to be important in reducing postoperative constipation, and improving continence (2,5,7,11,13).

Data on hand-assisted resection/rectopexy is sparse, but should be comparable to pure laparoscopic techniques.

 ## CONCLUSIONS

Hand-assisted laparoscopic sigmoidectomy and rectopexy is a useful technique for dealing with rectal prolapse, especially for those cases complicated by adhesions from previous surgery, cases of recurrent prolapse, and those in which operative conditions may otherwise mandate a conversion to open surgery. In addition, it may be a useful "bridge" for those surgeons who are still early in their laparoscopic experience, and who desire to improve their laparoscopic skill sets on surgically straight-forward patients.

References

1. Schiedeck TH, Schwandner O, Scheele J, Farke S, Bruch HP. Rectal prolapse: which surgical option is appropriate? *Langenbecks Arch Surg* 2005;390(1):8–14.
2. Madiba TE, Baig MK, Wexner SD. Surgical management of rectal prolapse. *Arch Surg* 2005;140:63–73.
3. Stevenson AR, Stitz RW, Lumley JW. Laparoscopic-assisted resection-rectopexy for rectal prolapse: early and medium follow-up. *Dis Colon Rectum* 1998;41:46–54.
4. Luukkonen P, Mikkonen U, Jarvinen H. Abdominal rectopexy with sigmoidectomy vs. rectopexy alone for rectal prolapse: a prospective, randomized study. *Int J Colorectal Dis* 1992;7:219–22.
5. Kessler H, Jerby BL, Milsom JW. Successful treatment of rectal prolapse by laparoscopic suture rectopexy. *Surg Endosc* 1999;13:858–61.
6. Fryckman HM, Goldberg SM. The surgical treatment of rectal pocidentia. *Surg Gynecol Obstet* 1969;129:125–30.
7. Kellokumpu IH, Kairaluoma M. Laparoscopic repair of rectal prolapse: surgical technique. *Ann Chir Gynaecol* 2001;90:66–69.
8. Senagore AJ, Duepree HJ, Delaney CP, Brady KM, Fazio VW. Results of a standardized technique and postoperative care plan for laparoscopic sigmoid colectomy: a 30-month experience. *Dis Colon Rectum* 2003;46(4):503–509.
9. Southern Surgeons' Club Study Group. Handoscopic surgery: a prospective multicenter trial of a minimally invasive technique for complex abdominal surgery. *Arch Surg* 1999;134:477–86.
10. Cobb WS, Lokey JS, Schwab DP, Crockett JA, Rex JC, Robbins JA. Hand-assisted laparoscopic colectomy: a single-institution experience. *Am Surg* 2003;69(7):578–80.
11. Madbouly KM, Senagore AJ, Delaney CP, Duepree HJ, Brady KM, Fazio VW. Clinically based management of rectal prolapse: comparison of the laparoscopic Wells procedure and laparoscopic resection with rectopexy. *Surg Endosc* 2003;17:99–103.
12. Ayav A, Bresler L, Brunaud L, Zarnegar R, Boissel P. Surgical management of combined rectal and genital prolapse in young patients: transabdominal approach. *Int J Colorectal Dis* 2005;20(2):173–79.
13. Bruch HP, Herold A, Schiedick T, Schwandner O. Laparoscopic surgery for rectal prolapse and outlet obstruction. *Dis Colon Rectum* 1999;42:1189–95.
14. Madoff RD, Williams JG, Wong WD, Rothenberger DA, Goldberg SM. Long-term functional results of colon resection and rectopexy for overt rectal prolapse. *Am J Gastroenterol* 1992;87(1):101–104.
15. Duthie GS, Bartolo DC. Abdominal rectopexy for rectal prolapse: a comparison of techniques. *Br J Surg* 1992;79:107–13.

57 Ripstein Procedure

Jason F. Hall, Helen M. MacRae, and Patricia L. Roberts

Introduction

Rectal prolapse is a full thickness protrusion of the rectum outside of the anal canal. It is an uncommon condition affecting an estimated 2.5 per 100,000 population (1). The condition predominantly affects women in the seventh and eighth decades.

Risk factors for the development of rectal prolapse include weak pelvic floor musculature, a deep pouch of Douglas, a redundant rectosigmoid, and lack of fixation of the rectum to the sacrum; nulliparity in women is also associated with prolapse. Other disease and conditions linked to rectal prolapse include connective tissue disorders, especially scleroderma, neurologic diseases, such as spina bifida, multiple sclerosis, spinal cord injury, and senility, prior surgery for congenital anomalies, especially imperforate anus, mental illness, and eating disorders, such as bulimia. A history of disordered defecation is often elicited.

Men affected by rectal prolapse tend to be younger than affected women. Rectal prolapse is also recognized in children under the age of 3 years and occurs in equivalent numbers of boys and girls. In young children, it is most often a self-limited condition associated with a diarrheal illness. The prolapse is often mucosal only and resolves with development of the sacral attachments to the rectum. The condition is also associated with cystic fibrosis, especially in Western countries.

The Ripstein procedure and its variations involve a rectopexy with the use of mesh. The Ripstein procedure previously was a common procedure for treatment of rectal prolapse because of its low recurrence rate, and the avoidance of a bowel anastomosis. However, the procedure has largely been supplanted by sigmoid resection and rectopexy or laparoscopic sutured rectopexy. Thus, although the Ripstein procedure and its variations are currently not a common operation for rectal prolapse, it still has specific indications, and should be in the armamentarium of any surgeon who treats rectal prolapse.

●●● INDICATIONS

The ideal operation for rectal prolapse should have low morbidity and should resolve the anatomic and physiologic abnormalities. Pursuit of this goal has resulted in over 100 procedures described for the correction or amelioration of rectal prolapse (2). These procedures have generally been grouped into two general categories; transabdominal and transperineal approaches. Traditionally, transabdominal approaches have been used for younger, healthy individuals to minimize recurrence, and transperineal procedures to elderly, frail populations, minimizing morbidity. It is difficult to make firm recommendations regarding the appropriateness of each technique for differing patient populations due to the lack of quality data on outcomes (3).

In the past, the Ripstein procedure was the abdominal procedure of choice for rectal prolapse. Currently, it is primarily used for patients in whom an abdominal procedure is indicated, but resection is either not indicated (those patients with no constipation), or where an anastomosis may be at high risk. The Ripstein procedure may also be undertaken in patients with recurrent rectal prolapse after other repairs. Patients who have failed previous perineal approaches, especially the Altemeier approach, may also be good candidates for a Ripstein type repair. In these patients, concern with the vascular supply may preclude an abdominal resection. Suture rectopexy is another option in these patient groups, with little evidence demonstrating superiority of one procedure over the other, but more long term data for the Ripstein procedure.

Ripstein first described an anterior sling rectopexy in 1952 (4). The procedure is typically performed through a transabdominal incision but can also be completed laparoscopically (5). Contraindications to the Ripstein procedure include the presence of medical comorbidities that would preclude a successful abdominal operation. Sepsis or fecal spillage at the time of surgery are also contraindications. A relative contraindication would be patients with preoperative constipation as the Ripstein procedure has increased the reported postoperative rates of constipation (6).

⟫ PREOPERATIVE PLANNING

The initial assessment begins with the demonstration of rectal prolapse in the surgeon's office. If the prolapse cannot be demonstrated on the exam table, the patient should be asked to strain on the toilet. The main differential diagnosis is prolapsing hemorrhoidal disease. Patients with rectal prolapse will generally have tissue with concentric prolapsing folds (Fig. 57.1), while patients with hemorrhoidal disease will have radial folds between the columns of Morgagni (Fig. 57.2). In full thickness rectal prolapse, two distinct walls of the rectum are palpable.

If a full thickness rectal prolapse cannot be demonstrated, defecography can be performed to assess for prolapse. Internal intussusception is a common finding on defecography, and not generally an indication for surgery.

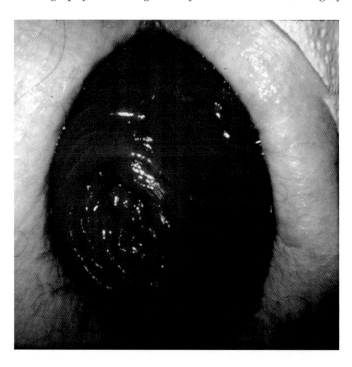

Figure 57.1 Concentric prolapsing folds characteristic of full thickness rectal prolapse.

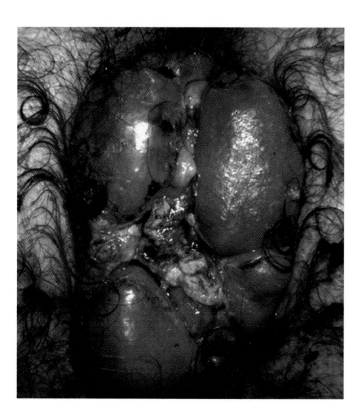

Figure 57.2 Radial prolapsing folds consistent with Grade III/IV hemorrhoids.

Digital rectal examination is performed to assess resting and squeeze pressures. Patients with rectal prolapse often have a patulous anus and weak anal sphincters. Women should be assessed for rectocele, enterocele, or other pelvic prolapse. Combined repair of other pelvic floor disorders, such as uterine and vaginal prolapse or cystocele are carried out with a multidisciplinary team. Approximately 5% of patients have an associated solitary rectal ulceration. This condition is believed to result from repeated mucosal trauma and resultant ischemia and generally occurs in the anterior rectum. It may be confused with rectal cancer and biopsy can easily confirm the diagnosis.

Up to 50% of patients with rectal prolapse suffer from fecal incontinence. This is thought to be secondary abnormalities in rectal compliance and distention (4). In these patients, anal manometry, endoanal ultrasonography, and electromyography are sometimes helpful in guiding the choice of operation, but not uniformly necessary prior to proceeding with repair.

About 15–65% of patients with rectal prolapse may suffer from constipation (7). The Ripstein procedure should be avoided in patients who report a history of constipation (6).

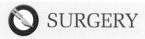 SURGERY

Positioning

After general anesthesia is induced, the patient is positioned either supine (if a split leg table is available), or in the lithotomy position, with padding of all potential pressure points; a urinary catheter is used in all cases.

Technique

For the open approach, a lower midline incision can be used. In patients without previous surgery, especially in slim females, all relevant structures can be accessed through a modest Pfannenstiel incision. A wound protector and appropriate retractor are placed.

Figure 57.3 Sutures are affixed to the sacrum to the right of midline.

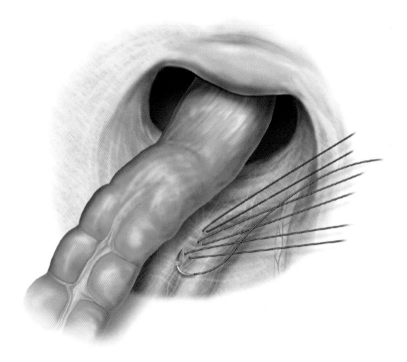

The patient is positioned in the Trendelenburg position, and the small bowel is packed into the upper abdomen. The sigmoid colon is mobilized along the white line of Toldt. The left ureter is identified and protected. The lateral peritoneal attachments of the mesosigmoid and mesorectum are incised beginning at the sacral promontory, and this incision is carried distally toward the pelvis, on both sides of the rectum (5). The rectum is lifted, allowing the mesorectum to be gently mobilized from the rectosacral fascia. The retrorectal areolar plane is entered posterior to the superior hemorrhoidal artery, dropping the sympathetic nerves posteriorly. The dissection is carried down sharply to the level of the coccyx and pelvic floor. Care must be taken to avoid the prescral venous plexus to avoid intraoperative hemorrhage (6).

The left colon and rectum receive innervation from nerve fibers coursing through the lateral ligaments. Some authors have suggested that division of the lateral ligaments leads to postoperative constipation (8). Others have pointed to decreased rates of recurrence in those who undergo lateral ligament division (9). Dividing the lateral ligaments can be individualized, based on the length of the prolapse, and ability to achieve secure placement of the sling.

To place the mesh anteriorly, a 5 cm strip of mesh is sutured to the sacrum to the right of midline. It is then passed over the anterior portion of the rectum, and affixed to the sacrum to the left of the midline. (Fig. 57.3) The mesh should be placed approximately 5 cm below the sacral promontory. The mesh is secured to the sacrum with nonabsorbable sutures (Fig. 57.4). The sutures are affixed approximately 1 cm from the midline on each side. Care is taken to avoid the presacral venous plexus. If bleeding does occur, tying the suture in place, rather than removing it, may be helpful. Packing or placement of further sutures may also help control bleeding. There should be sufficient width of mesh such that one can admit one finger between the sacrum and mesorectum. Once the mesh is sutured to the sacrum, the rectum should be proximally retracted until it is taut and the prolapse is well reduced. The mesh is then fastened to the rectum using fine 0 or 2–0 nonabsorbable sutures (Fig. 57.5). The sutures should be placed between the mesh and a muscular layer of the rectum. The lumen of the rectum should not be entered. The mesorectum should also be attached to the mesh, however, the mesorectum should not be completely encircled by the mesh. The mesh is then pulled to the left side and fastened to the rectum and sacrum using absorbable sutures (Fig. 57.6).

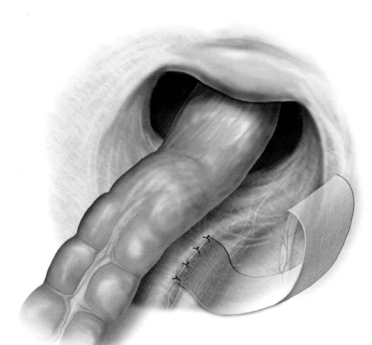

Figure 57.4 Mesh is affixed to the sacrum to the right of midline.

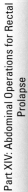

Because of a significant incidence of stricture and obstruction secondary to mesh constriction, Ripstein modified his procedure. Using this technique, the 5 cm long by approximately 10 cm wide Marlex or Gore-Tex mesh sling is placed posterior to the rectum, leaving the anterior rectal wall free to distend. The mesh is sutured to the sacrum first. Once again this is accomplished either by directly suturing the mesh to the sacrum, using interrupted nonabsorbable suture (such as 2-0 prolene), or alternatively,

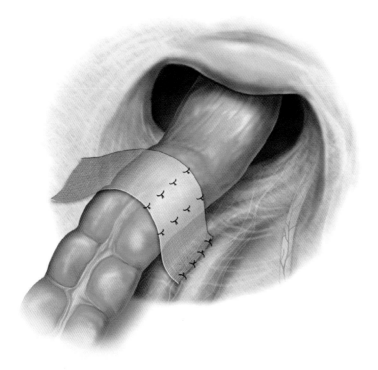

Figure 57.5 Mesh is affixed to the right side of the rectum using nonabsorbable sutures.

Part XIV: Abdominal Operations for Rectal Prolapse

Figure 57.6 Mesh is affixed to the left rectum and sacrum using non-absorbable sutures.

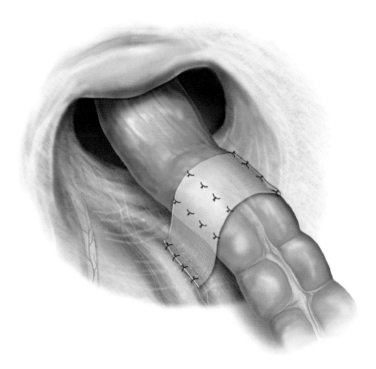

a hernia tacker may be used. The mesh is secured to the midline of the sacrum, facilitating avoidance of the venous plexus (Fig. 57.7). It is then sutured two-thirds to three-quarters of the way around the circumference of the rectum on either side, again taking care to avoid entering the rectal lumen. This leaves a gap in the mesh anteriorly which is designed to avoid narrowing of the rectum (Fig. 57.7).

Figure 57.7 A modification of the Ripstein procedure leaves a gap in the mesh anteriorly. This is designed to avoid strictures.

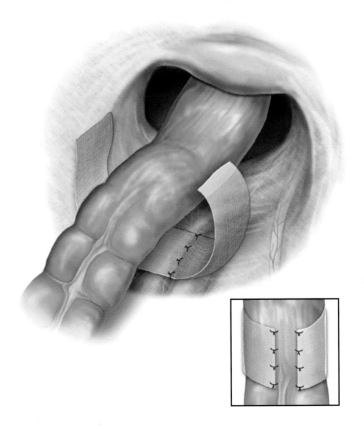

Kuminsky et al. (5) described the laparoscopic Ripstein repair in 1996. The essential elements of the operation are similar to an open procedure. Access is obtained using a supraumbilical 5 or 10 mm port for the camera. Two left lower quadrant ports are used. A 12 mm port medial and inferior to the anterior superior iliac spine, and a 5 mm port just lateral to the rectus, midway between the anterior superior iliac spine and the umbilicus. A 5 mm port at the level and medial to the left anterior superior iliac spine is also used. Steep Trendelenburg is used. The sigmoid colon is delivered from the pelvis. The rectosigmoid is held cephalad and anterior, and the inferior mesenteric artery (IMA) is visualized. The peritoneum is incised on the right side, posterior to the IMA, using laparoscopic scissors or the hook. The peritoneum is incised along this line, working inferiorly to the pelvic floor, and superiorly to the origin of the IMA. The presacral nerves are identified, and dropped posteriorly.

A grasper is placed posterior to the IMA, lifting it anteriorly. The plane posterior to the IMA is opened, using a combination of gentle blunt dissection and sharp dissection, in the avascular retrorectal areolar tissue.

This plane is developed over toward the left side. The left ureter is identified laterally as one comes under the IMA. The peritoneum to the left of the rectum is then incised, also to the pelvic floor. The pre-cut mesh is rolled and inserted through the right lower quadrant port. The mesh is affixed to the sacrum using a laparoscopic stapling device, or with intracorporeal sutures, and then secured to the rectum. Although this operation is technically feasible, there are no studies reporting long-term results following this technique.

 POSTOPERATIVE MANAGEMENT

Patients are started on a clear liquid diet postoperatively and advanced to a regular diet as they are able to tolerate it, usually within a few days. The urinary catheter is removed on postoperative day two.

 COMPLICATIONS & RESULTS

Although there is a significant body of literature regarding outcomes following the Ripstein procedure, there is a lack of randomized or prospective data. Mortality following this procedure tends to be low ranging from 0–2.8% and reported recurrence rates range from 0–13% (8). Roberts et al. reported the 22-year Lahey Clinic experience with the Ripstein procedure (135 patients). The most common complication associated with the procedure was hemorrhage from the presacral veins. Although the Ripstein procedure has been widely criticized because of concerns about stricture at the site of the sling, this complication was only reported in 2.2% of patients (10). Tjandra et al. (6) reported their experience with 169 patients undergoing surgical procedures for rectal prolapse, 142 of who underwent anterior mesh rectopexy. This group found that the persistence of constipation was higher after the Ripstein procedure than after resection rectopexy (57% vs. 17%). For this reason, they concluded that the Ripstein procedure should be avoided in patients with initial complaints of constipation. Although a laparoscopic Ripstein procedure has been described, no long term outcomes have been reported.

 CONCLUSIONS

The Ripstein procedure is an effective technique for the management of patients with full-thickness rectal prolapse. Because there are a number of options for the management of patients with rectal prolapse, the individual characteristics of each patient should be taken into account when choosing to apply this technique. Although this technique is associated with improved continence, it should be avoided in patients who present with constipation.

Recommended References and Readings

1. Kairaluoma MV, Kellokumpu IH. Epidemiologic aspects of complete rectal prolapse. *Scand J Surg* 2005;94(3):207–10.
2. Wexner SD, Cera SM. Surgery for rectal prolapse. In: Souba WW, Fink MP, Jurkovich GJ, et al., eds. *ACS Surgery: Principles and Practice* (6th ed). New York: Web MD Professional Publishing, 2007;949–962.
3. Tou S, Brown SR, Malik AI, Nelson RL. Surgery for complete rectal prolapse in adults. *Cochrane Database Syst Rev* 2008; (4):CD001758.
4. Ripstein CB. Treatment of massive rectal prolapse. *Am J Surg* 1952;83:68–71.
5. Kusminsky RE, Tiley EH, Boland JP. Laparoscopic Ripstein procedure. *Surg Laparosc Endosc* 1992;2(4):346–47.
6. Tjandra JJ, Fazio VW, Church JM, Milsom JW, Oakley JR, Lavery IC. Ripstein procedure is an effective treatment for rectal prolapse without constipation. *Dis Colon Rectum* 1993;36(5):501–507.
7. Schoetz DJ, Veidenheimer MC. Rectal prolapse. Pathogenensis and clinical features. In: Henry MM, Swash M, eds. *Coloproctology in the Pelvic Floor*. London: Butterworths, 1985.
8. Madiba TE, Baig MK, Wexner SD. Surgical management of rectal prolapse. *Arch Surg* 2005;140:63–73.
9. Siproudhis L, Bellisant E, Juguet F, et al. Rectal adaptation to distension in patients with overt rectal prolapse. *Br J Surg* 1998; 85:1527–32.
10. Womack NR, Williams NS, Holmfield JH, Morrison JF. Pressure and prolapse–the cause of solitary rectal ulceration. *Gut* 1987;28(10):1228–33.

Suggested Readings

McMahan JD, Ripstein CB. Rectal prolapse: an update on the rectal sling procedure. *Am Surg* 1987;53:37–40.

Mollen RM, Kuijpers HC, van Hoek F. Effects of rectal mobilization and lateral ligaments division on colonic and anorectal function. *Dis Colon Rectum* 2000;43:1283–87.

Roberts PL, Schoetz DJ, Coller JA, Veidenheimer MC. Ripstein procedure: lahey clinic experience 1963–1965. *Arch Surg* 1988;123: 554–57.

Speakman CT, Madden MV, Nichols RJ, Kamm MA. Lateral ligament division during rectopexy causes constipation but prevents recurrence: results of a prospective randomized study. *Br J Surg* 1991;78:1431–33.

Veidenheimer MC. Rectal prolapse. *Surg Clin North Am* 1980;60: 451–455.

Wang QY, Shi WJ, Zhao YR, Zhou WQ, He ZR. New concepts in severe presacral hemorrhage during pr. *Arch Surg* 1985; 120(9):1013–20.

58 Ventral Hernia

David B. Earle

 ## INDICATIONS/CONTRAINDICATIONS

The indications for treating a ventral hernia are no different when considered alone or in conjunction with a colorectal problem requiring an abdominal approach. Broadly, these indications are: (a) correcting of an existing problem, and (b) preventing problems from the hernia in the future.

Problems created from ventral hernia include:

- Pain
- Bowel obstruction (acute, recurrent)
- Abdominal wall deformity (poorly fitting clothes or ostomy appliance, cumbersome support garments)
- Skin ulceration
- Limitations in activities of daily living

Whether the patient is asymptomatic or has a problem, many untreated ventral hernias will progress in size over a period of months to years, have a progressively worsening symptom complex, and gradually become more difficult to repair. The rate of progression is unpredictable, and different among patients. As the difficulty level increases, the number of surgeons available with the necessary training and experience decreases.

Although it is acceptable to repair a ventral hernia that is asymptomatic, it is not mandatory to repair every ventral hernia, even when performing a concomitant abdominal procedure. When considering repair of a ventral hernia, it is important to explicitly establish the goals and objectives of the hernia repair separately, and align these goals and objectives with the patient and surgeon. In addition, there should be a separate discussion regarding the risks, benefits, and expected postoperative course regarding the hernia repair itself.

 ## PREOPERATIVE PLANNING

Once a ventral hernia has been diagnosed and the goals and objectives have been explicitly defined and aligned, planning may begin for either concomitant or deferred repair.

One must assess the existing problems and make a determination regarding the urgency of both the hernia repair in the colorectal procedure. An estimate of the complexity of the hernia repair will be required to make an appropriate determination. In general, large, incisional hernias (particularly recurrent with previous prosthetic repair) are the most difficult to fix. While there are no well-defined size parameters, ventral hernias larger than 5 cm in width are more difficult to repair, and hernias greater than 10 cm in width generally require a surgeon with hernia specific training and expertise.

Deferred repair should be considered if the patient is a poor surgical candidate, or the existing colorectal problem does not allow enough time to coordinate the operation with a surgeon that specializes in complex ventral hernia repair and:

- The hernia is minimal or asymptomatic.
- The hernia is recurrent.
- There has been previous synthetic mesh placed.
- The hernia is large.
- The hernia is from a previous large incision.

Under these circumstances, the primary goal of the operation would be a successful colorectal procedure. The addition of a separate, complex abdominal operation may be too risky, and put both procedures at risk for failure. Leaving the hernia alone for repair in the future will, however, require some planning regarding the incision. It would generally be safe to open the skin over the hernia sac and simply close the sac, subcutaneous tissues and skin at the end of the procedure, leaving the abdominal wall defect alone. This strategy should have a high success rate as long as the integrity of the skin is good.

Concomitant repair should be considered if: (a) the patient is a reasonable surgical candidate, and the hernia associated with an existing problem requires attention in a similar timeframe that colorectal problem does, or (b) the hernia is asymptomatic and there will be a multidisciplinary approach with a surgeon(s) specializing in abdominal wall reconstruction.

Selecting the proper technique for hernia repair will depend on the clinical scenario as a whole, in addition to the specific goals and objectives for the operation. The size of the hernia, however, will be one of the primary factors that will limit the available techniques. If there is an incisional hernia of any size, we know that recurrence rates will be much lower if a prosthetic is used compared to primary closure with "standard" suturing techniques which typically utilize at least 1 cm bites of tissue and advance at least 1 cm between sutures. Thus, the presence of an incisional hernia will either require a different suturing technique and/or prosthetic placement to maximize the successful closure of the abdominal wall.

If the prosthetic is going to be used, the choice of the specific prosthetic and placement location should be planned before the operation commences. This type of preoperative planning will help avoid intraoperative delays due to missing supplies and/or instrumentation. For example, if a retromuscular, extraperitoneal placement of a polypropylene prosthetic is planned, but intraoperative circumstances favor and intraperitoneal placement, but the operating room does not have a prosthetic designed for intraperitoneal use, the surgeon will be faced with the choice of significantly altering the technique, or utilizing a prosthetic in a manner in which it was not intended.

Ventral hernias with defects greater than 5 cm in width may also require a component separation prior to closure and prosthetic placement. Component separation requires the separation of the internal and external oblique muscles, division of the insertion of the external oblique, and sometimes mobilization of the posterior rectus sheath. This allows the rectus muscles to be advanced to the midline in the vast majority of cases, and may be used in combination with a prosthetic. Component separation techniques that preserve the blood supply to the skin significantly reduce the risk of wound complications. To accurately measure the size and shape of the defect, as well as to investigate for defects in other areas of the anterior abdominal wall, a CT scan without oral or IV contrast can be quite helpful. It may also sometimes be helpful to perform the scan with and without Valsalva maneuvers to look at the abdominal wall in a more dynamic fashion. If there is going to be a CT scan performed for other reasons, such as searching for metastatic disease, the proper CT protocol for that reason should be followed, and the abdominal wall may still be assessed. If a component separation is planned, a multidisciplinary approach is typically employed and will require substantial preoperative planning to align the operative plan and schedules.

In summary, the issues to be dealt with during the preoperative planning process include:

- Detailed assessment of hernia including symptoms and anatomic details (includes history, physical examination, and radiological studies)
- Establishment of goals and objectives related to hernia repair
- Determine appropriate technique to achieve the goals based on anatomic details (includes technique, prosthetic type, and placement location)
- Decision to perform hernia repair concomitant or subsequent to colorectal procedure

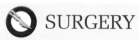 SURGERY

Technique

Before mentioning specific scenarios for prosthetic repair of ventral hernia, the appropriate suturing technique for midline laparotomy closure deserves mention. It has been shown that using smaller bites at smaller intervals increases the initial wound strength, reduces risk of wound infection, and dramatically reduces incisional hernia rate at 2 years. The appropriate depth of tissue and distance between sutures is 5–8 mm, significantly less than the 1–2-cm distances commonly utilized. It is also important to note the avoidance of muscle fibers and fat when placing each suture. This will slightly increase the time it takes to close the incision, but the long-term benefits that the patient will realize are worth the effort. It will be more difficult to precisely place the sutures in the aponeurosis during reoperative surgery than it will be with primary closure of a small defect. This so-called short suture technique should be used for closure of the vast majority (if not all) of laparotomy incisions.

Because there are an infinite number of clinical details, the discussion will be limited to specific techniques related to common clinical scenarios based on the size and type of ventral hernia. In addition, the term "extraction site" will be used to describe the specimen extraction site during laparoscopic procedures. Regarding the choice of prosthetic, there is no conclusive data supporting the use of one prosthetic over another. Clinical experience and existing data, however, suggests that microporous PTFE-based prosthetics have a relatively increased risk of infection, and bridging gaps with costly, non-cross-linked biologic prosthetics have a relatively increased risk of hernia recurrence. Synthetic prosthetics with an absorbable barrier on one side are designed for intraperitoneal use with a barrier side being placed towards the viscera to minimize adhesions. These types of prosthetics will be referred to as absorbable barrier prosthetics, and currently available products have a permanent structure made from polypropylene or polyethylene terephthalate (PET; polyester).

Small (<5 cm), Primary, Midline Ventral Hernia Such as Umbilical

If the laparotomy or extraction site incision is directly over the hernia defect, the defect may simply be closed utilizing the short suture technique described above. If a laparoscopic port is placed in the hernia, it should be placed under direct visualization, and the defect may again be closed utilizing a short suture technique if possible. As the size of the defect approaches 1 cm, the ability to utilize the "short suture" technique is lost, and there are a variety of techniques available for port site closure.

Small (< 5 cm), Midline Incisional Ventral Hernia

Proper repair of any incisional hernia requires a prosthetic in order to significantly lower the risk of recurrent hernia. In general, macroporous prosthetics made a polypropylene or polyester may be placed in the retromuscular, extraperitoneal ("sublay") position, and the overlying anterior rectus sheath either completely or partially closed utilizing the "short suture" technique. This technique may be used with concomitant colorectal procedure is with little risk for prosthetic infection or hernia recurrence. This technique requires complete closure of the posterior rectus sheath after it has been mobilized to expose the retromuscular space. If complete closure cannot be obtained, omentum would be necessary to suture to the edges of the closure to prevent herniation of bowel, and keep the prosthetic from being directly exposed to the viscera. Alternatively, absorbable barrier prosthetic may be used if the posterior rectus sheath cannot be fully closed, and/or if there is not enough omentum for visceral protection.

In addition, intraperitoneal placement of the prosthetic is a possibility, but may be at higher risk for fixation-related problems to the edges of the prosthetic, and tolerance of infection if one develops.

Placement of a prosthetic anterior to the abdominal wall musculature ("onlay") is another possibility, but essentially requires complete closure of the anterior rectus sheath and the development of some skin flaps which may increase the risk of wound-related complications and infection.

Medium-Sized (5–10 cm) Midline Incisional Hernia

Mobilization of the posterior rectus sheath with a "sublay" prosthetic and closure of the anterior rectus sheath over the prosthetic using the short suture technique would be considered the best approach for these types of hernias when considering repair with a concomitant colorectal procedure. The "onlay" technique may be technically easier, but does pose potential risks as mentioned above, particularly if the anterior rectus sheath cannot be closed.

Large (>10 cm) Midline Incisional Hernia

While there is no consensus, there is increasing opinion that proper repair of these types of incisional hernias requires a "component separation." This is accomplished by detaching the medial portion of the external oblique muscle bilaterally from the costal margin to the pubic symphysis, separating the oblique muscles, and mobilizing the posterior rectus sheath. This will allow medial release of the anterior rectus sheath that should bring the rectus muscles to the midline which should be closed using the short suture technique. Techniques that preserve the blood supply to the skin, such as an endoscopic component separation, has the advantage of avoiding large skin flaps, and reducing complications related to the midline wound. Nonendoscopic techniques that preserve the blood supply include limited skin flaps and laterally based incisions with the use of lighted retractors to improve visualization. There is no consensus as to whether a prosthetic should be placed in the "sublay" or "onlay" position. Placing a prosthetic in the "sublay" position has the theoretic advantage of better integration into host tissue and less risk of infection, particularly if there are complications related to the skin and subcutaneous tissues of the midline wound. These large hernias generally need to be repaired in an open fashion, particularly if a concomitant colorectal procedure being performed. A biologic prosthetic is also a possibility for use, but should usually not be used unless the midline can be closed completely.

For all of the above techniques, the patient may be in the supine position with or without lithotomy position. If a component separation is going to be performed endoscopically, it is usually best to tuck the arms at the patient's side. In addition, if the colorectal procedure is being done first, the patient can be re-positioned for the hernia repair to avoid lithotomy position for a prolonged time. It is important to make sure that all patient positioning equipment be fitted to the patient, and not vice versa. All appropriate precautions need to be taken to minimize the risk of positioning injury.

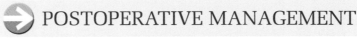 POSTOPERATIVE MANAGEMENT

Postoperative management of the hernia repair will depend on the technique used. For small- and medium-sized hernias that have been repaired with easy closure of the midline and either "sublay" or "onlay" prosthetic placement, the patient may advance their diet as tolerated, or dictated by the colorectal procedure. Activity may also advance as tolerated, without formal restriction. Large hernias that have been repaired with a component separation and prosthetic, generally, require activity restriction for 6–8 weeks, when the wound strength would be expected to be at approximately 90% of its maximum. Because this activity restriction is empiric, there is no consensus on exactly how to apply it. In general, it is important to educate the patient to avoid straining of their abdominal wall. This will include smoking cessation preoperatively, confirmed with preoperative nicotine testing. This may not only reduce coughing postoperatively, but should also improve wound healing. Because coughing and sneezing are involuntary, the patient should be instructed to attempt to cough and sneeze lightly possible. Nausea, also involuntary, should be treated anti-emetics, and liberal use of nasogastric decompression tubes. Constipation also creates scenarios requiring excess abdominal wall straining, and should be treated with laxatives. With large hernias, there are occasions when significant tension on the midline closure is unavoidable. Depending on the degree of tension, the following maneuvers are available to minimize the chance of a wound dehiscence:

- Keep the patient's torso slightly flexed at all times (even during transfers, bathing and ambulation) during the first postoperative week
- Placement of a properly fitting abdominal binder.
- Liberal use of medication for nausea, cough, and constipation.
- Only advance diet if not distended, and liberal use of NGT if distention develops.
- Maintain heavy sedation with endotracheal intubation for 2–4 days postoperatively (rare).
- Minimize activities which cause excessive abdominal wall straining for 6–8 weeks.

There should be liberal use of drains in the subcutaneous space, particularly if any flaps have been raised or there is excess skin and subcutaneous tissue that have created a potential space under the midline closure. The drain should be left in until it is draining less than 20–30 ml/24-hour period. While this usually occurs within the first 2 weeks, excessive drainage may persist for 6–8 weeks.

 COMPLICATIONS

Complications regarding prosthetic use for hernia repair may arise in the early (first 30 days) or late postoperative period, and include:

- Infection
- Inflammation
- Pain
- Seroma
- Hernia recurrence

Dealing with infectious complications is no different than with any operation, even in the presence of a prosthetic. Antibiotic use should be limited to tissue infection not amenable to drainage, such as cellulitis. If the infection or its treatment leaves the prosthetic exposed, negative pressure wound therapy and/or standard wound care may be employed without removing the prosthetic. This is generally true only for macroporous and biologic prosthetics, not macroporous prosthetics. Regardless of raw material, macroporous prosthetics appear to the naked eye like a screen, and microporous prosthetics appear like a solid sheet. Only portions of the prosthetic that do not incorporate with the surrounding tissue will eventually need to be excised. Systemic signs and symptoms of infection may indicate that the entire prosthetic is infected, and should prompt further investigation to make this determination, as removal of the entire prosthetic would then be necessary.

Occasionally, the skin of the anterior abdominal wall involving all or a portion of the area where the prosthetic was placed may develop an inflammatory reaction of unknown etiology, usually manifest with erythema and warmth of the skin that may be difficult to distinguish from infection. The erythema may become more intense when the patient is in an upright position compared to the supine position. Without systemic signs of inflammation such as fever, rigors, or leukocytosis, it is safe to treat this with observation and/or anti-inflammatory medications. Imaging studies may or may not reveal a fluid collection around the prosthetic, and may help serve as a baseline for future comparison.

As with any intra-abdominal procedure, uncontrolled enterotomy due to lysis of adhesions, anastomotic failure, fixation of the hernia prosthetic, or early postoperative obstruction is a possibility, and a potentially life-threatening complication. A high index of suspicion and low threshold to return to the operating room for a diagnostic laparotomy/laparoscopy are necessary to reduce morbidity and mortality from this complication. Return to the operating room should be considered if the patient is not following the typical postoperative course, and no other plausible explanation exists.

A seroma may be represented by a fluid collection around the prosthetic or in the subcutaneous space, and is a normal physiologic response to an operation with prosthetic implantation. Early in the postoperative course, this is not considered a complication, but the surgeon should be aware of its existence so it can be properly observed to determine if it resolves without treatment, causes any symptoms, or becomes infected in the future. Seromas that are thought to be causing significant symptoms or are infected should be drained. A seroma that persists beyond 12 months should be considered for a drainage procedure, even if it is asymptomatic, to avoid the possibility of infection from a distant site such as cellulitis or a dental infection. It is important to note, however, that percutaneous drainage of any seroma must entirely drain all of the material within the cavity. If there is solid material that is not drained, and a drain is left in place, it has a high risk of becoming infected. In the scenario where all of the material cannot be drained, it is best either to not leave a drain, or to return to the operating room for complete drainage.

Recurrence in the early postoperative period should not be ignored as a possibility. Diagnosis of hernia recurrence is no different in the early or late postoperative period, and include:

- Presence of the same symptoms related to the hernia compared to the preoperative state
- Presence of a reducible mass
- Excessive pain at the site of a presumed seroma
- Bowel obstruction

These findings from the history and physical examination may be complimented with radiologic studies, with CT scanning probably being the best study currently available.

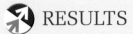 RESULTS

Results will vary depending on the technique. Most data looking at hernia repair lack adequate follow-up by physical examination. There are, however, a series of data that can be analyzed in a logical fashion related to abdominal wall closure. Incisional hernia formation after primary laparotomy closure using the "standard" suturing technique has a 15–20% incidence. This incidence is reduced to approximately 5% using the "short suture" technique. Primary repair of incisional hernia using the "standard" suturing technique has a recurrence rate of approximately 60%, and there is no data about primary repair of incisional hernia with the short suture technique, although presumably it would be lower. Recurrence rates from primary repair utilizing the "standard" suturing technique with a component separation (separation of internal and external oblique muscles, detachment medial border of external oblique, mobilization of posterior rectus sheath) are 20–30%.

Compared to "primary repair," a variety of techniques utilizing a prosthetic may reduce recurrence rates to 5–30%. Utilization of a component separation technique lowers recurrence rates with primary repair using the "standard" suturing technique, and presumably would have an even lower rate with the use of the "short suture" technique

TABLE 58.1

Technique	Advantages	Disadvantages	Expected recurrence rate	Comments
Primary repair ("standard" suture technique)	• Familiarity • Uncomplicated unless there is a large defect	• High failure rate • Increased wound infection rate	60%	Technique should be abandoned
Primary repair ("short suture" technique)	• Increased wound strength • Lower wound infection rate • Lower recurrence rate?	• Unfamiliar technique • Increased operative time	Unknown, but probably <60%	Should be used for closure of all laparotomy wounds
Prosthetic repair ("inlay" technique; edge of mesh sutured near edge of the defect)	• Technically simple	• High failure rate • Prosthetic becomes exposed of wound opened	60%	Technique should be abandoned
Prosthetic repair ("sublay" or intraperitoneal technique)	• Lower recurrence rate • Prosthetic not exposed if wound opened • Better tolerance of infection even if prosthetic involved (sublay only) • Does not require complete closure of midline	• Technically more difficult	5–10%	Sublay technique may require prosthetic designed for intraperitoneal use if posterior layer cannot be closed
Prosthetic repair ("onlay" technique)	• Technically easier than retromuscular techniques	• Requires complete closure of midline • Requires skin flaps • Prosthetic becomes exposed of wound opened	Unknown, probably around 15%	In general, prosthetics design for intraperitoneal use are not required
Component separation technique	• Able to close midline defects up to 20 cm in width • May be used with the prosthetic technique (retro muscular or onlay)	• Requires some training • Increases operative time	• 20–30% if midline closed using "standard" suturing technique • Probably 10–20% if "short suture" technique utilized • Probably 10% if utilized with "short suture" technique and a prosthetic	Standard open component separation associated with 20 to 30% major wound complication rate; endoscopic or may need—open techniques lower wound complication rates by avoiding large skin flaps to disrupt blood supply.

and/or a prosthetic. There is a paucity of data comparing the sublay versus onlay technique of prosthetic placement when used with or without a component separation, and the relative advantages and disadvantages have been described above. While accurate data are lacking, best available estimates of recurrence, along with the advantages and disadvantages of each technique are listed in Table 58.1.

CONCLUSIONS

In summary, many patients requiring an abdominal approach to a colorectal procedure will have a high risk for incisional hernia or an existing ventral hernia (primary or incisional). It is of vital importance to determine the patient's goals regarding hernia repair, and align these goals with the surgeon's objectives preoperatively. From a technical standpoint, proper technique of abdominal wall closure utilizing the "short suture" technique should be utilized in the vast majority, if not all cases. For small- and medium-sized midline incisional hernias, the best technique for prosthetic repair of hernia is probably the "sublay" technique utilizing a macroporous, permanent or biologic prosthetic. For large-sized incisional hernias, utilization of the component separation technique along with a "sublay" macroporous, permanent or biologic prosthetic, is probably the best technique. More data regarding the value of the prosthetic as it relates to cost and outcomes are necessary to make adequate recommendations regarding the use of specific prosthetics. Leaving the hernia alone during a colorectal procedure is also acceptable, and requires adequate closure of the skin and subcutaneous tissues. This decision will depend on the overall circumstances.

It is also important to realize that there is no definitive proof regarding the best technique of hernia repair in general, let alone in combination with a colorectal procedure. If the surgeon is going to incorporate incisional hernia repair in his or her practice, it is imperative to continually stay updated with hernia repair techniques. It is also useful for the colorectal surgeon to utilize a multidisciplinary approach regarding concomitant ventral hernia repair, particularly for large hernias, if there is local expertise regarding hernia repair available.

Suggested Readings

Burger JW, Luijendijk RW, Hop WC, et al. Long-term follow-up of randomized controlled trial of suture versus mesh repair of incisional hernia. *Ann Surg.* 2004;240(4):578–83; discussion 583–5.

den Hartog D, Dur AH, Tuinebreijer WE, Kreis RW. Open surgical procedures for incisional hernias. *Cochrane Database Syst Rev.* 2008;(3):CD006438.

Halm JA, de Wall LL, Steyerberg EW, et al. Intraperitoneal polypropylene mesh hernia repair complicates subsequent abdominal surgery. *World J Surg.* 2007;31(2):423–9; discussion 430.

Jänes A, Cengiz Y, Isrealsson LA. Preventing parastomal hernia with a prosthetic mesh: a five-year follow-up of a randomized study. *World J Surg.* 2009;33(1):118–21; discussion 122–3.

Millbourn D, Cengiz Y, Israelsson L. Effect of stitch length on wound complications after closure of midline incisions: a randomized controlled trial. *Arch Surg.* 2009;144(11):1056–1059.

Strzelczyk JM, Szymański D, Nowicki ME, et al. Randomized clinical trial of postoperative hernia prophylaxis in open bariatric surgery. *Br J Surg.* 2006;93(11):1347–50.

59 Finney and Jaboulay Techniques

Hasan T. Kirat and Feza H. Remzi

 INDICATIONS/CONTRAINDICATIONS

Crohn's disease (CD) is an inflammatory condition without known cure. CD may manifest in one of the three principal patterns: obstructive, inflammatory, and perforating. Surgery is needed for at least half of patients with CD during their lifetime (1). While extensive surgical resection does not reduce recurrence of the disease, it may place the patients at risk for the development of short-bowel syndrome (2). Strictureplasty, which was adapted from pyloroplasty for the treatment of tuberculous stricture, has become a valuable choice in patients affected by diffuse obstructive CD, since it conserves the bowel (3). Some studies found no difference in the recurrence rate following strictureplasty and resection (4,5). Others showed significantly shorter reoperation-free survival for patients undergoing strictureplasty alone or strictureplasty with resection than those who underwent resection alone (6). While the most preferred strictureplasty is the Heineke-Mikulicz (H-M) for the strictures <10 cm in length (7), Finney or Jaboulay strictureplasties are most applicable to patients with longer strictures (8,9). Some studies found higher rate of recurrence following Finney or Jaboulay techniques compared to H-M strictureplasty (8,10). However, a meta-analysis of 1,825 strictureplasties showed that the proportion of patients requiring additional surgery was decreased when a Finney strictureplasty was used (7). Strictureplasty has also become the preferred technique for obstructive duodenal CD, when complications develop. This chapter describes techniques and outcomes of Finney and Jaboulay strictureplasties for small-bowel and duodenal CD.

Duodenal Strictureplasty

Although CD rarely involves the duodenum, when complications such as bleeding, perforation, or obstruction develop, surgery is needed. Bypass surgery has been abandoned after strictureplasty has become the preferred technique for obstructive duodenal CD. H-M or Finney procedures are used depending upon the length and position of the stricture. For strictureplasty, a full Kocher maneuver is used to completely mobilize the duodenum. During strictureplasty, simultaneous strictures should be assessed by passage of a deflated urinary catheter, especially at the junction of the third and fourth parts of the duodenum. Gastrostomy and vagotomy, when pyloroplasty was performed, are no longer used (11).

Worsey et al. (11) reported 13 CD patients with duodenal stricture. Two patients had post-operative complications. At a median follow-up of 3.6 years, one patient underwent reoperation for recurrence. They concluded that strictureplasty is a safe and effective operation for duodenal CD. Use of Finney-type anastomosis also has been reported for duodenal stricture in CD with good results (12). However, a study including 13 patients with strictureplasty showed that strictureplasty for duodenal CD is associated with a high incidence of postoperative complications and restructure, since nine patients required further surgery with a follow-up of 9 years (13). The difference in the duration of follow-up may explain these different results. Further studies investigating recurrence after duodenal strictureplasties with longer follow-up and greater number of patients are needed.

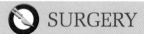 SURGERY

Technique for Finney Strictureplasty

Finney strictureplasty is performed for strictures between 10 and 20 cm long. It can be performed with either the stapler or hand-sewn technique. In the hand-sewn technique, first, a stay suture is placed on the mid portion of the stricture. This area is folded over onto itself, and a U-shaped enterotomy is made through the stricture using scalpel or cautery (Fig. 59.1). Another suture is placed on the normal side of the bowel to hold the U-shape in place. After the posterior edges are sutured in a continuous fashion (Fig. 59.2), anterior edges are sutured together in an interrupted fashion using long-term absorbable sutures in one layer (Fig. 59.3).

Technique for Jaboulay Strictureplasty

Jaboulay Strictureplasty is similar to the Finney procedure. It is a side-to-side enteroenterostomy and used for medium-length strictures in which the strictured area is folded over onto itself. The posterior layer of strictureplasty is done using an interrupted row of Lembert sutures. Two incisions are made into small-bowel loops using electrocautery (Fig. 59.4). The inner layer of the posterior row of the strictureplasty is sutured using a continuous absorbable suture material (Fig. 59.5). The anterior row is then closed with a series of interrupted full-thickness nonabsorbable suture (Fig. 59.6). Jaboulay strictureplasty can also be performed with the stapler technique.

Figure 59.1 A U-shaped enterotomy is made through the stricture.

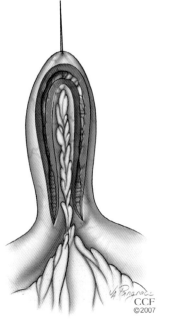

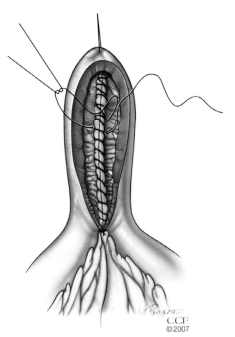

Figure 59.2 The posterior edges are sutured in a continuous fashion.

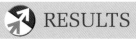# RESULTS

Small-Bowel Strictureplasty

After a successful report of strictureplasty for multiple strictures involving the small intestine due to tuberculosis by Katariya et al. (14), strictureplasty has been the preferred technique by many surgeons for the strictures of the small bowel. The H-M and Finney have been the two most commonly used strictureplasties. Fazio et al. (15) reported 42 CD patients with 225 strictureplasties. Long strictures were treated with Finney and short strictures with H-M. Sixty percent of the patients also had bowel resection due to acute inflammation with phlegmon or fistulae. Sixteen percent of the patients developed complications. They concluded that strictureplasty minimizes the necessity for bowel

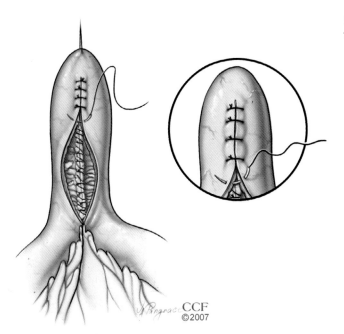

Figure 59.3 Anterior edges are sutured together in an interrupted fashion.

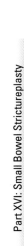

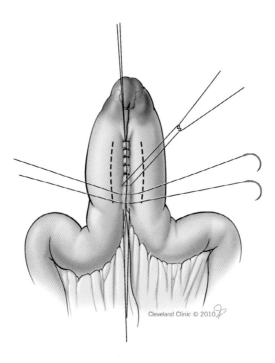

Figure 59.4 The posterior layer of strictureplasty is sutured and two incisions are made into small-bowel loops.

resection in patients with short strictures resulting in recurrent small-bowel obstruction. After long-term follow-up, Fazio et al. (16) reported 24% of symptomatic recurrence and 17% need for reoperation in 116 obstructive CD patients with 452 strictureplasties including 405 H-M and 47 Finney procedures. Tonelli et al. (17) reported 44 patients with strictures treated by H-M, Finney, and Jaboulay techniques. Of these, 8.8% patients required reoperation. They concluded that strictureplasty is a valuable adjunct to resection. In another study with a median follow-up of 99 months, 57% of patients undergoing strictureplasty after resection for CD (ileocolonic strictureplasty) had a symptomatic recurrence and 50% of them required surgery. The authors stated that strictureplasty is a safe and efficacious procedure for ileocolonic anastomotic recurrence in patients with CD (18). In a study of 44 patients with 174 strictureplasty, H-M was used in strictures 1–8 cm

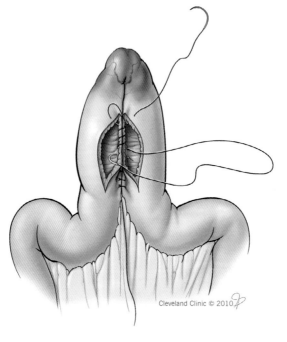

Figure 59.5 The inner layer of the posterior row of the strictureplasty is sutured using a continuous absorbable suture material.

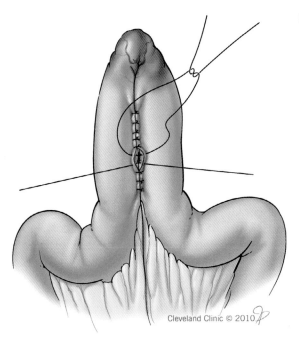

Figure 59.6 The anterior row is closed.

long, Finney strictures 10–30 cm long, and Jaboulay strictures 10–18 cm long. The authors concluded that given the low rate of postoperative complications and of symptomatic recurrences, strictureplasty is an effective mean of preserving the small bowel (9).

No difference was reported in the recurrence rate following strictureplasty and resection (4,5). Also, no statistically significant difference was observed in the reoperation rate among patients treated only by strictureplasty or with an associated resection (17). In contrast, significantly shorter reoperation-free survival was shown for patients undergoing strictureplasty alone or strictureplasty with resection than those who underwent resection alone (6). In a review, which included seven studies comprising 688 CD patients, Reese at al. (19) reported that patients undergoing resection had a greater risk for development of complications following surgery than those with strictureplasty alone. However, surgical recurrence after strictureplasty was more likely than following resection.

In terms of comparison of the techniques for strictureplasty, Futami et al. (8) reviewed 103 patients with obstructive CD who underwent 293 strictureplasty including 235 H-M, 22 Finney, 35 Jaboulay, and 1 side-to-side isoperistaltic strictureplasty. Sixty-two patients underwent synchronous other surgical procedures. A total of 265 strictures were located in small bowel. At a mean length of follow-up of 80.3 months, the 5- and 10-year reoperation rates were 45% and 62%, respectively. Forty-three percent had further operation due to recurrence. Perforating disease for recurrence was more common at the site treated by the Jaboulay or Finney technique compared to H-M procedure, 6 (50%) of 12 versus 2 (14.3%) of 14 patients. In another study, Ayrizono et al. (10) reported 28 patients with 116 strictureplasties (81% H-M, 13% Finney, and 6% side-to-side ileocolic strictureplasty). They found clinical and surgical recurrence rates of 63% and 41%, respectively. Recurrence occurred at strictureplasty site in 3.5%—the Finney procedure being the most frequent one. Meanwhile, a meta-analysis of 15 studies (7) included 506 patients who underwent 1,825 strictureplasties (85% H-M and 13% Finney). Of 15 studies included, 11 reported both procedures. Two studies reported only H-M while two others only the Finney technique. A total of 14 patients with H-M developed recurrence and 13 patients needed reexploration in the studies that broke down the outcomes based on the technique of strictureplasty. There was an increased rate of recurrence and reoperation in patients with H-M. The patients who underwent Finney strictureplasty were found to have a decreased rate of additional surgery. Also, this meta-analysis showed that studies including only patients with H-M technique reported higher rate of recurrence (32%) and reoperation (23%) compared to studies consisted of only patients with Finney procedure, which reported 0% recurrence and 0% reoperation rate. Dietz et al. (20) reported 1,124 strictureplasties, 88% H-M (for strictures less than 10–12 cm) and 11% Finney procedures (for longer strictures), for obstructing small-bowel CD. There was no perioperative mortality. Postoperative complications included septic complications (5%), prolonged ileus (4%), mechanical small-bowel obstruction (1%), and luminal bleeding requiring transfusion (7%). Four patients underwent reoperation in the early postoperative period. Recurrence that required surgery was occurred in 116 patients (37%). The factors might have an influence on morbidity or recurrence was examined. It was found that the type of strictureplasties performed did not influence morbidity and recurrence. Also, another study with 123 CD jejunoileitis patients (21) reported 615 H-M (88%) and 86 Finney (12%) procedures. Seventy percent of the patients underwent concomitant bowel resection. The overall morbidity rate was 20%. Thirty-five patients (28%) had recurrence that required reoperation with a median follow-up of 6.7 years. Various factors were studied to determine their impact on morbidity or recurrence. It was shown that type of strictureplasty was not the predictive of morbidity or recurrence. Meanwhile, one concern with respect to the Finney technique compared to other techniques is the development of bacterial overgrowth in the resultant diverticulum. To overcome this concern, a procedure that involves features of both Finney and H-M strictureplasties was reported (22).

✧ CONCLUSIONS

Finally, the length of stricture and the multiplicity of stricture in a long segment dictate the type of strictureplasty that needs to be done. Finney procedure is a good option with favorable outcomes for long strictures in small bowel. Jaboulay technique can be performed for medium-length strictures although it is rarely preferred by surgeons. Further studies report that recurrence after duodenal strictureplasties with longer follow-up is needed.

References

1. Farmer RG, Whelan G, Fazio VW. Long-term follow-up of patients with Crohn's disease. Relationship between the clinical pattern and prognosis. *Gastroenterology* 1985;88:1818–25.
2. Yamamoto T. Factors affecting recurrence after surgery for Crohn's disease. *World J Gastroenterol* 2005;11:3971–79.
3. Ozuner G, Fazio VW, Lavery IC, Church JM, Hull TL. How safe is strictureplasty in the management of Crohn's disease? *Am J Surg* 1996;171:57–60; discussion 60–61.
4. Sampietro GM, Cristaldi M, Porretta T, et al. Early perioperative results and surgical recurrence after strictureplasty and miniresection for complicated Crohn's disease. *Dig Surg* 2000;17:261–67.
5. Broering DC, Eisenberger CF, Koch A, et al. Quality of life after surgical therapy of small bowel stenosis in Crohn's disease. *Dig Surg* 2001;18:124–30.
6. Borley NR, Mortensen NJ, Chaudry MA, et al. Recurrence after abdominal surgery for Crohn's disease: relationship to disease site and surgical procedure. *Dis Colon Rectum* 2002;45:377–83.
7. Tichansky D, Cagir B, Yoo E, et al. Strictureplasty for Crohn's disease: meta-analysis. *Dis Colon Rectum* 2000;43:911–19.
8. Futami K, Arima S. Role of strictureplasty in surgical treatment of Crohn's disease. *J Gastroenterol* 2005;40(Suppl 16):35–39.
9. Tonelli F, Ficari F. Strictureplasty in Crohn's disease: surgical option. *Dis Colon Rectum* 2000;43:920–26.
10. Ayrizono Mde L, Leal RF, et al. Crohn's disease small bowel strictureplasties: early and late results. *Arq Gastroenterol* 2007;44:215–20
11. Worsey MJ, Hull T, Ryland L, Fazio V. Strictureplasty is an effective option in the operative management of duodenal Crohn's disease. *Dis Colon Rectum* 1999;42:596–600.
12. Takesue Y, Yokoyama T, Kodama T, et al. Surgical treatment for duodenal involvement in Crohn's disease: report of a case. *Surg Today* 1997;27:858–62.
13. Yamamoto T, Bain IM, Connolly AB, et al. Outcome of strictureplasty for duodenal Crohn's disease. *Br J Surg* 1999;86:259–62.
14. Katariya RN, Sood S, Rao PG, Rao PL. Strictureplasty for tubercular strictures of the gastro-intestinal tract. *Br J Surg* 1977;64:496–98.
15. Fazio VW, Galandiuk S, Jagelman DG, Lavery IC. Strictureplasty in Crohn's disease. *Ann Surg* 1989;210:621–25.
16. Fazio VW, Tjandra JJ, Lavery IC, et al. Long-term follow-up of strictureplasty in Crohn's disease. *Dis Colon Rectum* 1993;36:355–61.
17. Tonelli F, Ficari F, Bagnoli S. Repair of stricture in Crohn's disease: treatment of choice? *Chir Ital* 1995;47:15–23.
18. Yamamoto T, Keighley MR. Long-term results of strictureplasty for ileocolonic anastomotic recurrence in Crohn's disease. *J Gastrointest Surg* 1999;3:555–60.
19. Reese GE, Purkayastha S, Tilney HS, et al. Strictureplasty vs resection in small bowel Crohn's disease: an evaluation of short-term outcomes and recurrence. *Colorectal Dis* 2007;9:686–94.
20. Dietz DW, Laureti S, Strong SA, et al. Safety and longterm efficacy of strictureplasty in 314 patients with obstructing small bowel Crohn's disease. *J Am Coll Surg* 2001;192:330–37; discussion 337–38.
21. Dietz DW, Fazio VW, Laureti S, et al. Strictureplasty in diffuse Crohn's jejunoileitis: safe and durable. *Dis Colon Rectum* 2002;45:764–70.
22. Fazio VW, Tjandra JJ. Strictureplasty for Crohn's disease with multiple long strictures. *Dis Colon Rectum* 1993;36:71–72.

60 Heineke-Mikulicz, Finney, and Michelassi Strictureplasty

Alessandro Fichera, Fabrizio Michelassi, and Sharon L. Stein

 ## INDICATIONS/CONTRAINDICATIONS

Surgical treatment of Crohn's disease is complicated by the recurrent nature of the disease. Many patients require multiple operations throughout their lives for failure of medical management, treatment of symptoms or complications of the disease including sepsis, stricture, bleeding, and cancer. Repeated intestinal resections may leave patients with inadequate intestinal mucosal surface leading to malabsorption of nutrients, vitamins, and fluids, resulting in malnutrition and chronic dehydration, a condition known as short gut syndrome.

Strictureplasty preserves intestinal absorptive surface area. Although the length of intestine may be reduced by modification of the shape of the bowel, total surface area remains the same in the preserved segment of bowel. Currently, it is not known whether the previously diseased segment regains absorptive function after strictureplasty, but studies demonstrate normalization of endoscopic and radiographic appearance in follow-up examinations after strictureplasty (1,2).

The concept of strictureplasty was first introduced by Katariya et al. to treat ileal strictures secondary to intestinal tuberculosis. In the 1980s, Emmanuel Lee began using this technique to treat fibrostenotic Crohn's disease strictures in patients with extensive intestinal disease. Since that time the use and indications for strictureplasty have continued to expand.

Strictureplasty techniques were initially used only for quiescent small bowel disease; recently their use has been extended to duodenal disease as well as recurrent disease on small bowel anastomoses or ileocolic anastomoses. Strictureplasty can be coupled with bowel resections and several strictureplasty techniques can be used simultaneously to maximize bowel preservation.

Contraindications to strictureplasty include patients with generalized sepsis, cancer, or dysplasia. Severely diseased segments with luminal obliteration or unyielding intestinal wall, and intestinal segments with inflammatory phlegmonous masses or significantly thickened mesentery are probably best resected. Although the presence of fistulous disease or localized sepsis was initially thought to be contraindications, several studies have demonstrated that strictureplasty is safe when the degree of acute inflammation associated with fistulae or sepsis is limited. An unstable patient should not undergo strictureplasty secondary to the length and complexity of the operation. At this time there is limited data regarding the use of strictureplasty in primary colonic disease.

PREOPERATIVE PLANNING

Appropriate preoperative evaluation for patients with Crohn's disease includes thorough assessment of extent of disease. Although patients may present with a single symptomatic area of disease, preoperative knowledge of extent of disease aids in operative planning and in patient preparation.

A computed tomography (CT) scan is often the initial imaging study performed to evaluate symptomatic Crohn's disease. CT scan is useful in that it evaluates both intraluminal and extraluminal findings including obstruction, edema, abscess, and fistula. CT enterography provides greater detail on intraluminal findings and presence of mucosal disease. Small bowel follow through, when performed and interpreted by experienced personnel, provides even greater accuracy for extent of disease. Endoscopic evaluation, including colonoscopy with ileal intubation, esophagogastroduodenoscopy, and capsule endoscopy can help in assessing the disease. In patients with narrow strictures, a capsule endoscopy is contraindicated as the capsule could be retained in an area of stenosis requiring surgical retrieval.

Despite the increased accuracy of modern preoperative radiographic and endoscopic imaging, appropriate selection of operative procedures (strictureplasty, resection, by-pass or intestinal diversion) can only be performed after accurate visualization at the time of the operative intervention. Therefore preoperative discussions and informed consent should include all of the above options.

SURGICAL PROCEDURE

Preparation

The use of preoperative bowel preparation varies depending on the location of the disease. Mechanical bowel preparation is necessary for colonic disease, but may be avoided for small bowel and ileocolonic disease. In the presence of chronic obstructive small bowel disease, a preoperative period of clear liquids may be useful to reduce the amount of intraluminal-retained fluid.

Patients are given appropriate antibiotic coverage for clean-contaminated or contaminated surgical procedures prior to incision. Sequential compression devices are used perioperatively for deep venous thrombosis prophylaxis along with administration of subcutaneous low-molecular-weight heparin.

Positioning

The patient is usually placed in the supine position on the operative table. If access to the perineum is anticipated, the patient can be placed supine on the operating table and moved to the lithotomy position at the appropriate time. In this case, the patient's hips and buttocks are placed protruding over the break of the operating table to ensure easy access to the perineum once moved to the lithotomy position. Alternatively the patient can be positioned in the modified lithotomy position for the entire procedure.

Technique—General Principles

Upon entering the abdomen, a thorough exploration of the abdominal cavity and a careful examination of the entire small and large intestine are mandatory. The total length of intestine should be noted. Any diseased areas should be examined and the length and extent of disease should be recorded. If many areas of disease are found, it can be helpful to mark each one with sutures to facilitate subsequent planning. With a complete "road map" created, an operative strategy is then formulated.

Short isolated segments of stricture are appropriate for Heineke-Mikulicz (less than 7 cm) or Finney (up to 15 cm) strictureplasties. Longer segments or chain of lake formation may be considered for a Michelassi strictureplasty. Several different strictureplasty techniques with or without simultaneous bowel resections may be used in the same patient to maximize intestinal preservation.

Several maneuvers are universally used during strictureplasty to help minimize contamination of the operative field by enteric contents. Use of a wound protector may help to prevent subcutaneous contamination. While operative towels or laparotomy pads are placed under the isolated bowel loop to prevent soilage into the abdominal cavity. An atraumatic intestinal clamp is placed several centimeters proximal to the operative segment, where it will not hinder the surgeon, but prevents continued leakage of enteric contents into the operative field. An assistant should be assigned to handle suction following enterotomy.

After opening the disease segment in preparation for a strictureplasty, the mucosa must be inspected. If findings suspicious of cancer or dysplasia are found, a biopsy should be sent immediately to pathology for frozen section: if confirmed, the segment should be resected and strictureplasty aborted.

Meticulous hemostasis of the intestinal wall and overlying mucosa must be achieved. Diseased segments are often quite friable and bleed easily. Suturing of the intestinal wall during the performance of the strictureplasty may help with hemostasis, but any on-going bleeding should be treated with precise application of electrocautery prior to starting fashioning the strictureplasty.

At the end of the procedure, small metal clips are used to mark the strictureplasty site extraluminally for future identification in case of recurrent obstructive symptoms. Metals clips can be visualized radiographically on subsequent investigations or intraoperatively at successive operations.

Areas distal to the segment of diseased bowel should be intraoperatively examined. When patients have symptomatic proximal disease, strictures distally may be asymptomatic and may not cause bowel dilation. If areas of stenosis are suspected but not evident on inspection, a bladder catheter with a balloon inflated to a 2-cm diameter inserted through the enterotomy to be used for the strictureplasty can be used to assess the size of the internal lumen of the suspected sites.

Inspection of the bowel, identification of diseased segments, and mobilization of the intestinal loops may be laparoscopically performed. However, the authors suggest that performance of the actual strictureplasty be done through a limited abdominal incision through which the diseased loop of intestine has been exteriorized. The severely thickened mesentery, the strictured and fibrotic intestinal wall, and the disparity between wall thickness of normal and diseased intestine are all challenges which are best confronted through an open approach during which tactile feedback and control of the intestines are crucial to minimizing postoperative complications including hemorrhage, sepsis, and anastomotic dehiscence.

Operative Technique

Heineke-Mikulicz Strictureplasty (In-Situ Strictureplasty)

The most commonly performed strictureplasty is the Heineke-Mikulicz strictureplasty (2). This type of strictureplasty is most appropriate for isolated short segments, no longer than 5–7 cm in length. After isolation of the diseased segment, two stay sutures are placed on either side of the strictured area at the midpoint. A longitudinal incision is made along the antimesenteric border of the stricture (Fig. 60.1a) and is extended for 1–2 cm into the normal pliable bowel on either side of the stricture. The longitudinal enterotomy is then closed in a transverse fashion (Fig. 60.1b) with either a single or double suture layer (Fig. 60.1c).

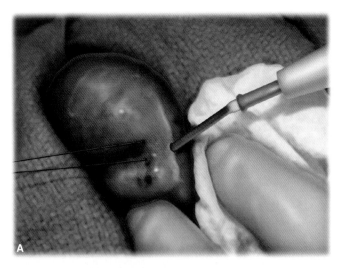

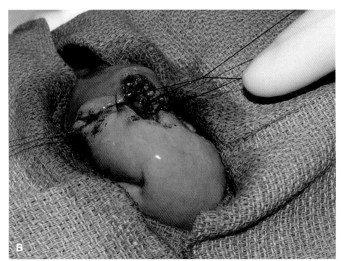

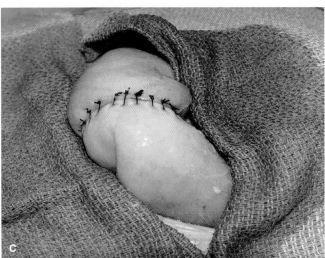

Figure 60.1 A. Heineke-Mikulicz strictureplasty. A longitudinal incision is made along the strictured segment of bowel. **B.** After extending the strictureplasty for 1–2 cm into normal pliable bowel, the longitudinal enterotomy is then closed in a transverse fashion. **C.** Completed Heineke-Mikulicz strictureplasty.

Finney Strictureplasty (Side-to-Side Strictureplasty)

The Finney strictureplasty is appropriate for strictures up to 15 cm in length (3). A stay suture is placed on the midportion of the strictured site. The strictured segment is then folded onto itself into a U-shape (4). A row of interrupted seromuscular sutures is placed between the two arms of the U (Fig. 60.2a) and a longitudinal U-shaped enterotomy is made paralleling the row of sutures. Full thickness sutures are then placed in a continuous running fashion beginning at the apex of the posterior wall of the strictureplasty and continued to approximate the proximal and distal ends of the enterotomy (Fig. 60.2b). This full-thickness suture line is continued anteriorly to close the strictureplasty (Fig. 60.2c). A row of seromuscular Lembert sutures is then placed anteriorly. One drawback of this procedure is that a very long Finney strictureplasty may result in a functional bypass with a large lateral diverticulum, which can be at risk for stasis and bacterial overgrowth, occasionally the cause for a subsequent resection of the strictureplasty.

Michelassi Strictureplasty (Side-to-Side Isoperistaltic Strictureplasty)

The side-to-side isoperistaltic strictureplasty (SSIS) was first described in 1996 by Michelassi to treat long segments of diseased bowel, and has been performed on segments from 20 to 75 cm in length. SSIS eliminates the need for multiple short strictureplasties

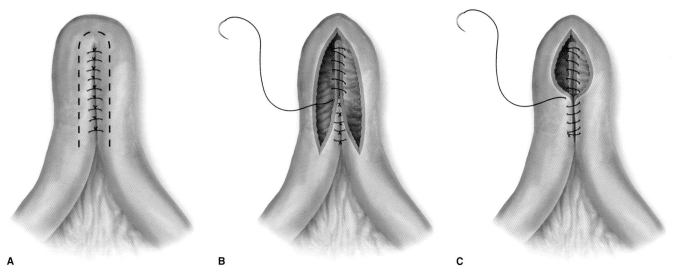

A   **B**   **C**

Figure 60.2 **A–C.** Finney strictureplasty. After a row of interrupted sutures is placed between the two loops of bowel, a longitudinal enterotomy is created along the antimesenteric border of the strictured segment. The enterotomy is then closed using a running suture from the posterior wall of the strictureplasty; then on the anterior wall of the strictureplasty.

in close proximity that may create a bulky, awkward repair. The SSIS has the benefit of a more uniform repair without intestinal or mesenteric bulking.

The mesentery of the small bowel loop to undergo a SSIS is divided at its midpoint. The mesentery is often thick with inflammation and lymphadenopathy and may require suture ligation between Kelly clamps for hemostasis. The midpoint of the small bowel is severed between atraumatic intestinal clamps.

The distal loop of small intestine is overlaid on the proximal loop in a side-to-side isoperistaltic fashion (Fig. 60.3a). The stenotic segments of one loop are aligned with dilated areas of the other loop to balance intestinal diameter and allow for adequate intestinal flow through the strictureplasty (Fig. 60.3b). The back wall of the two loops are approximated using a layer nonabsorbable 3-0 sutures in interrupted seromuscular Lembert sutures and extends approximately 1 cm into healthy tissue of the proximal and distal ends.

An enterotomy is performed on both loops, into healthy tissue on proximal and distal ends (Fig. 60.3c,d). The mucosa of the two loops is inspected to evaluate for possible malignancy and meticulous hemostasis is obtained. The ends of each loop of intestines are gently tapered to avoid blind stumps at the proximal and distal margins of the strictureplasty (Fig. 60.3e).

Two full thickness running 3-0 absorbable suture lines are started on the posterior wall of the strictureplasty. This inner layer is run from the midpoint toward each end and continued on the anterior wall (Fig. 60.3f). Following closure of the entire anterior wall, an outer layer of nonabsorbable Lembert sutures is placed to complete the two-layer side-to-side isoperistaltic enteroenterostomy (Fig. 60.3g).

POSTOPERATIVE MANAGEMENT

Postoperatively, patient management is similar to patients undergoing bowel anastomosis. Antibiotics are terminated within 24 hours of operation. Patients on steroids preoperatively should receive appropriate stress dose steroids to prevent adrenal insufficiency after surgery. Early ambulating, pulmonary toilet, and incentive spirometry are encouraged. Diet may be advanced based on clinical signs. Because of extent of disease and intestinal manipulation, patients may develop ileus postoperatively and should be monitored for abdominal distension. Consultation with a gastroenterologist familiar with Crohn's disease should be obtained for consideration of maintenance therapy.

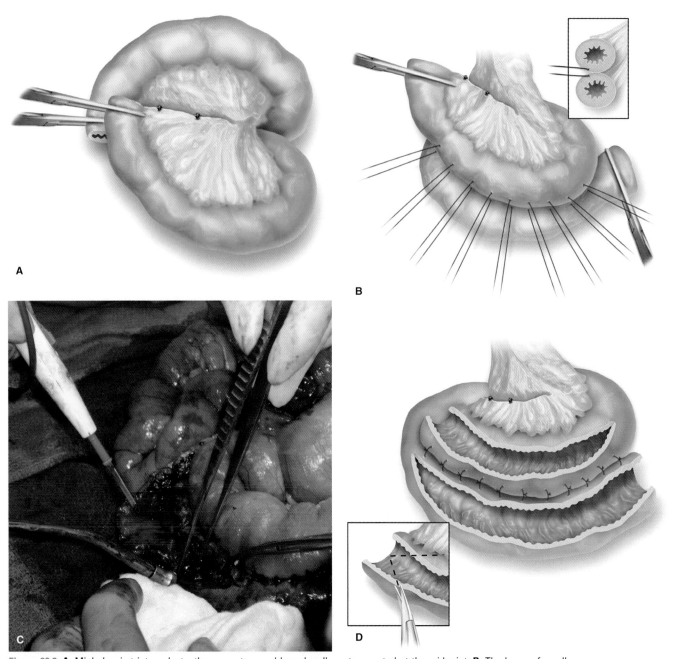

Figure 60.3 A. Michelassi strictureplasty: the mesentery and bowel wall are transected at the midpoint. **B.** The loops of small intestine are overlaid, with dilated segments of the proximal loop aligned with stenotic segments of the distal segment. **C.** After a row of interrupted Lembert sutures is placed along the back row of the segment, a longitudinal enterotomy is made on the antimesenteric border. **D** and **E.** The ends of the strictureplasty are tapered to prevent creation of diverticula with stasis as the corners of the strictureplasty. (*continued*)

COMPLICATIONS

The safety of strictureplasty techniques in Crohn's patients was initially questioned. Unlike resection with primary anastomosis where the diseased tissue is removed to grossly normal margins and sutures are placed in healthy bowel, strictureplasties are fashioned in affected bowel and suture lines are placed within scarred and diseased tissue. In addition, many patients with Crohn's disease are on immunosuppressants, parental nutrition or preoperatively malnourished. These factors raised concerns for

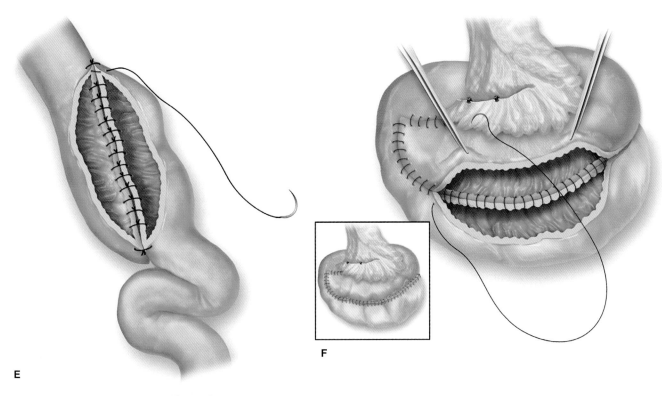

E

F

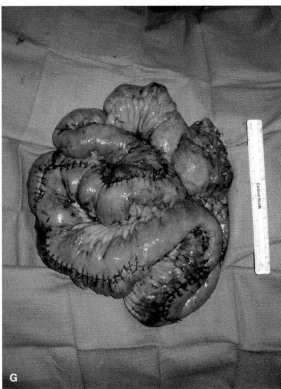

G

Figure 60.3 (*Continued*) **F.** The inner layer is completed on the back wall and run medially from the end of the strictureplasty.
G. The completed side-to-side isoperistaltic strictureplasty.

increased rates of perioperative complications. However, strictureplasty has been demonstrated to be safe in appropriately selected patients.

Complications for patients after strictureplasty are similar to patients who undergo intestinal resection and include anastomotic dehiscence, suture line hemorrhage, and wound infections. The incidence of anastomotic dehiscence has been measured at 2–4% in large series and the rate of postoperative bleeding in need of blood transfusions occurs in 2–3% of cases. A meta-analysis by Yamamoto et al. demonstrated overall complication rate of 13%. Risk factors for complications included older age, emergency surgery, abscess with intraabdominal contamination, anemia, and preoperative weight loss (5).

Results from our own series demonstrate an overall complication rate of 12%, with a dehiscence rate of 1.7% (6). A multicenter trial of SSIS demonstrated complication rates of 5–21% with the incidence of gastrointestinal hemorrhage (2.1%), suture line dehiscence (3.9%), and bowel obstruction (1%) within the range of intestinal resections (7).

Although considerable concern has been expressed over the risk of adenocarcinoma developing at strictureplasty sites, this remains a rare complication. Adenocarcinoma of the small bowel occurs in less than 2% of gastrointestinal malignancies, and although the risk in Crohn's disease appears to be higher, accurate numbers are difficult to discern. Only four cases of adenocarcinoma at the site of a prior strictureplasty have been described to date in the literature and typically present 2–8 years after the initial operation (8). For this reason, the authors recommend biopsies in any suspicious segments of intestine during strictureplasty.

RESULTS

Despite the magnitude of some of these procedures, the mean length of stay varies from 6 to 17 days in multiple series. Most importantly, studies have demonstrated that strictureplasties result in prompt resolution of symptoms and weight gain when compared to traditional intestinal resections.

The realization that gross Crohn's disease is deliberately left unresected during a strictureplasty has raised concerns of early recurrence. Yet longitudinal studies have demonstrated that this is not the case. Yamamoto listed a 3% site-specific recurrence rate in their meta-analysis, and the SSIS multicenter trial had a 7.6% rate of recurrence within the strictureplasty. Interestingly, several studies have reported that on postoperative endoscopic, radiographic, and operative observations there is evidence of normal appearing mucosa, quiescent disease, loss of fat wrapping, and recovery of submucosal vascular patterns in the majority of patients (1,9–11). Further data are needed to evaluate the possibility of restitution of absorptive function in previously diseased segments of bowel.

CONCLUSIONS

Strictureplasties alleviate obstructive complications of Crohn's disease and preserve intestinal mucosal surface, thus minimizing the risk of short gut syndrome secondary to repeated resections. Strictureplasty techniques may be used in duodenal disease, short or long segment small bowel disease, and recurrent disease at previous enteroenteric or ileocolonic anastomoses. Relative contraindications to strictureplasty include extremely fibrotic intestinal wall and intestinal fistula. Absolute contraindications are limited to free perforation, unstable patients, and cancer. Strictureplasty can be performed in appropriately selected patients with minimal morbidity when compared to resection. Site-specific recurrence rates appear to be lower in patients who undergo strictureplasty than traditional bowel resection.

Recommended References and Readings

1. Poggioli G, Stocchi L, Laureti S, et al. Conservative surgical management of terminal ileitis: side-to-side enterocolic anastomosis. *Dis Colon Rectum* 1997;40:234–39.
2. Roy P, Kumar D. Strictureplasty. *Br J Surg* 2004;91(11):1428–37.
3. Milsom JW. Strictureplasty and mechanical dilation in strictured Crohn's disease. In: Michelassi F, Milson JW, eds. Operative Strategies in Inflammatory Bowel Disease. New York: Springer-Verlag, 1999:259–67.
4. Sharif H, Alexander-Williams J. The role of strictureplasty in Crohn's disease. *Int Surg* 1992;77:15–18.
5. Yamamoto T, Fazio VW, Tekkis PP. Safety and efficacy of strictureplasty in Crohn's disease: a systematic review and meta-analysis. *Dis Colon Rectum* 2007;50:1968–86.
6. Hurst RD, Michelassi F. Strictureplasty for Crohn's disease: techniques and long-term results. *World J Surg* 1998;22(4):359–63.
7. Michelassi F, Taschieri A, Tonelli F, et al. An international, multicenter, prospective, observational study of the side-to-side isoperistaltic strictureplasty in Crohn's disease. *Dis Colon Rectum* 2007;3(50):277–84.
8. Menon AM, Mirza AH, Moolla S, et al. Adenocarcinoma of the small bowel arising forma previous strictureplasty for Crohn's disease: report of a case. *Dis Colon Rectum* 2007;50:257–9.
9. Tjandra JJ, Fazio VW. Strictureplasty for ileocolonic anastomotic strictures in Crohn's disease. *Dis Colon Rectum* 1993;36:1099–1104.
10. Stebbing JF, Jewell DP, Kettlewell MG, et al. Recurrence and reoperation after strictureplasty for obstructive Crohn's disease: long-term results. *Br J Surg* 1995;82:1471–4.
11. Michelassi F, Hurst RD, Melis M, et al. Side-to-side isoperistaltic strictureplasty in extensive Crohn's disease. *Ann Surg* 2000;232:401–8.

Suggested Readings

Fazio VW, Tjandra JJ. Strictureplasty for Crohn's disease with multiple long strictures. *Dis Colon Rectum* 1993;36:71–2.

Lee EC, Papaioannou N. Minimal surgery for chronic obstruction in patients with extensive or universal Crohn's disease. *Ann R Coll Surg Engl* 1982;64(4):229–33.

Michelassi F. Side-to-side isoperistaltic strictureplasty for multiple Crohn's strictures. *Dis Colon Rectum* 1996;39(3):345–9.

Recommended References and Readings

1. Poggioli G, Stocchi L, Laureti S, et al. Conservative surgical management of terminal ileitis: side-to-side enterocolic anastomosis. *Dis Colon Rectum* 1997;40:234–39.
2. Roy P, Kumar D. Strictureplasty. *Br J Surg* 2004;91(11):1428–37.
3. Milsom JW. Strictureplasty and mechanical dilation in strictured Crohn's disease. In: Michelassi F, Milson JW, eds. Operative Strategies in Inflammatory Bowel Disease. New York: Springer-Verlag, 1999:259–67.
4. Sharif H, Alexander-Williams J. The role of strictureplasty in Crohn's disease. *Int Surg* 1992;77:15–18.
5. Yamamoto T, Fazio VW, Tekkis PP. Safety and efficacy of strictureplasty in Crohn's disease: a systematic review and meta-analysis. *Dis Colon Rectum* 2007;50:1968–86.
6. Hurst RD, Michelassi F. Strictureplasty for Crohn's disease: techniques and long-term results. *World J Surg* 1998;22(4):359–63.
7. Michelassi F, Taschieri A, Tonelli F, et al. An international, multicenter, prospective, observational study of the side-to-side isoperistaltic strictureplasty in Crohn's disease. *Dis Colon Rectum* 2007;3(50):277–84.
8. Menon AM, Mirza AH, Moolla S, et al. Adenocarcinoma of the small bowel arising forma previous strictureplasty for Crohn's disease: report of a case. *Dis Colon Rectum* 2007;50:257–9.
9. Tjandra JJ, Fazio VW. Strictureplasty for ileocolonic anastomotic strictures in Crohn's disease. *Dis Colon Rectum* 1993;36:1099–1104.
10. Stebbing JF, Jewell DP, Kettlewell MG, et al. Recurrence and reoperation after strictureplasty for obstructive Crohn's disease: long-term results. *Br J Surg* 1995;82:1471–4.
11. Michelassi F, Hurst RD, Melis M, et al. Side-to-side isoperistaltic strictureplasty in extensive Crohn's disease. *Ann Surg* 2000;232:401–8.

Suggested Readings

Fazio VW, Tjandra JJ. Strictureplasty for Crohn's disease with multiple long strictures. *Dis Colon Rectum* 1993;36:71–2.
Lee EC, Papaioannou N. Minimal surgery for chronic obstruction in patients with extensive or universal Crohn's disease. *Ann R Coll Surg Engl* 1982;64(4):229–33.

Michelassi F. Side-to-side isoperistaltic strictureplasty for multiple Crohn's strictures. *Dis Colon Rectum* 1996;39(3):345–9.

Part XVIII: Small Bowel Strictureplasty

Note: Page numbers followed by "*f*" denote figures; those followed by "*t*" denote tables.